Innovative Teaching Strategies in Nursing and Related Health Professions

Fifth Edition

Edited by

Martha J. Bradshaw, PhD, RN
Professor
Louise Herrington School of Nursing
Baylor University
Dallas, Texas

Arlene J. Lowenstein, PhD, RN
Professor and Director
Health Professions Education Doctorate Program
Simmons College
Boston, Massachusetts

Professor Emeritus
MGH Institute of Health Professions
Boston, Massachusetts

JONES AND BARTLETT PUBLISHERS
Sudbury, Massachusetts
BOSTON TORONTO LONDON SINGAPORE

World Headquarters
Jones and Bartlett Publishers
40 Tall Pine Drive
Sudbury, MA 01776
978-443-5000
info@jbpub.com
www.jbpub.com

Jones and Bartlett Publishers
Canada
6339 Ormindale Way
Mississauga, Ontario L5V 1J2
Canada

Jones and Bartlett Publishers
International
Barb House, Barb Mews
London W6 7PA
United Kingdom

Jones and Bartlett's books and products are available through most bookstores and online booksellers. To contact Jones and Bartlett Publishers directly, call 800-832-0034, fax 978-443-8000, or visit our website, www.jbpub.com.

Substantial discounts on bulk quantities of Jones and Bartlett's publications are available to corporations, professional associations, and other qualified organizations. For details and specific discount information, contact the special sales department at Jones and Bartlett via the above contact information or send an email to specialsales@jbpub.com.

The authors, editor, and publisher have made every effort to provide accurate information. However, they are not responsible for errors, omissions, or for any outcomes related to the use of the contents of this book and take no responsibility for the use of the products and procedures described. Treatments and side effects described in this book may not be applicable to all people; likewise, some people may require a dose or experience a side effect that is not described herein. Drugs and medical devices are discussed that may have limited availability controlled by the Food and Drug Administration (FDA) for use only in a research study or clinical trial. Research, clinical practice, and government regulations often change the accepted standard in this field. When consideration is being given to use of any drug in the clinical setting, the health care provider or reader is responsible for determining FDA status of the drug, reading the package insert, and reviewing prescribing information for the most up-to-date recommendations on dose, precautions, and contraindications, and determining the appropriate usage for the product. This is especially important in the case of drugs that are new or seldom used.

Production Credits
Publisher: Kevin Sullivan
Acquisitions Editor: Amy Sibley
Associate Editor: Patricia Donnelly
Editorial Assistant: Rachel Shuster
Production Editor: Amanda Clerkin
Marketing Manager: Rebecca Wasley
V.P., Manufacturing and Inventory Control: Therese Connell
Composition: DSCS/Absolute Service, Inc.
Cover Design: Scott Moden
Cover Image: © Photodisc
Printing and Binding: Malloy, Inc.
Cover Printing: Malloy, Inc.

Library of Congress Cataloging-in-Publication Data
Innovative teaching strategies in nursing and related health professions /
[edited by] Martha J. Bradshaw and Arlene J. Lowenstein.—5th ed.
p. ; cm.
Includes bibliographical references and index.
ISBN-13: 978-0-7637-6344-2 (alk. paper)
ISBN-10: 0-7637-6344-6 (alk. paper)
1. Nursing—Study and teaching. I. Bradshaw, Martha J.
II. Lowenstein, Arlene J.
[DNLM: 1. Education, Nursing—methods. 2. Teaching—methods. WY 18
I589 2011]
RT71.F84 2011
610.73071—dc22

2009038851

6048

Printed in the United States of America
14 13 12 11 10   10 9 8 7 6 5 4 3 2 1

Dedication

To teachers—past, present, future.
May you always inspire, uplift, and transform.

Contents

Preface

This edition of *Innovative Teaching Strategies in Nursing and Related Health Professions* continues the theme of interdisciplinary collaboration in health professions education. The need to capitalize on the contributions of numerous healthcare professionals is increasingly more important in light of the current, complex healthcare system. Education has a knowledge base that crosses over disciplinary lines and is one we need to understand in order to be effective in our work.

This book incorporates educational principles and techniques suitable for students in all higher education settings, at the graduate or undergraduate levels. More attention has been given to use of various forms of technology, although it is never possible to present all methods and versions that are available. What needs to be remembered by educators is that technology is the means, not the ends, to teaching effectiveness. It is the individual teacher who makes decisions based upon best educational principles, about what strategy or form of technology to use in order to meet goals in the learners. The diversity of learners has increased on all levels of higher education. A new chapter in this book covers generational diversity in both learners and faculty, and provides approaches for greater accord in the teaching–learning process among age groups.

It is our intent that this book will be a useful resource for educational programs in all health professions.

Martha J. Bradshaw
Arlene J. Lowenstein

Contributors

Stephanie S. Allen, RN, MSN
Louise Herrington School of Nursing
Baylor University
Dallas, Texas

Catherine Bailey, PhD, RN
College of Nursing
Texas Woman's University
Dallas, Texas

Kathy P. Bradley, EdD, OTR/L, FAOTA
Medical College of Georgia
Professor and Chairperson
Department of Occupational Therapy
Augusta, Georgia

Martha J. Bradshaw, PhD, RN
Louise Herrington School of Nursing
Baylor University
Dallas, Texas

Deborah Casida, MSN, RN
West Texas A & M University
Canyon, Texas

Patricia R. Cook, PhD, RN
University of South Carolina–Aiken
School of Nursing
Aiken, South Carolina

Sharon M. Cosper, MHS, OTR/L
Medical College of Georgia
SAHS, Department of Occupational Therapy
Augusta, Georgia

Mariana D'Amico, EdD, OTR/L
Medical College of Georgia
SAHS, Department of Occupational Therapy
Augusta, Georgia

Lisa A. Davis, PhD, RN
West Texas A & M University
Canyon, Texas

Brian M. French, RN, MS, BC
The Institute for Patient Care
Massachusetts General Hospital
Boston, Massachusetts

Clive Grainger
Harvard-Smithsonian Center for Astrophysics
Cambridge, Massachusetts

Miriam Greenspan, RN, MS
Brigham and Women's Hospital
Boston, Massachusetts

Alex Griswold, AB
Harvard-Smithsonian Center for Astrophysics
Cambridge, Massachusetts

Jill M. Hayes, PhD, RN
Professor Emeritus
School of Nursing
North Georgia College and State University
Dahlonega, Georgia

Carol Holtz, PhD, RN
Kennesaw State University
Kennesaw, Georgia

Lynn Jaffe, ScD, OTR/L
Medical College of Georgia
SAHS, Department of Occupational Therapy
Augusta, Georgia

Judy Johnson-Russell, EdD, RN
Clinical Educator, Medical Education Technologies, Inc.
Professor Emerita, Texas Woman's University, Dallas
Sarasota, Florida

Charlotte J. Koehler, RN, MSN
Mary Black School of Nursing
University Center Greenville
University of South Carolina, Upstate
Spartanburg, South Carolina

Ellen M. Landis, PhD, ADTR
Adjunct Faculty Lesley University
Division of Expressive Therapies
Clinical Director, Sharevision Inc.
Family Counseling and Consulting Group
Amherst, Massachusetts

Kimberly Leighton
Bryan LGH College of Health Sciences
Lincoln, Nebraska

Arlene J. Lowenstein, PhD, RN
Professor and Director, Health Professions Education Doctoral Program
Simmons College
Professor Emeritus
MGH Institute of Health Professions
Boston, Massachusetts

Jennifer E. Mackey, MA, CCC-SLP
MGH Institute of Health Professions
Department of Communication Sciences and Disorders
Boston, Massachusetts

Hendrika Maltby, PhD, RN, FRCNA
College of Nursing and Health Sciences
University of Vermont
Burlington, Vermont

Gail Matthews-DeNatale, PhD
Associate Dean, Graduate and Professional Programs
Emmanuel College
Formerly Interim Director
Academic Technology
Simmons College
Boston, Massachusetts

Lesley Maxwell
MGH Institute of Health Professions
Department of Communication Sciences and Disorders
Boston, Massachusetts

Marjorie Nicholas, PhD
MGH Institute of Health Professions
Department of Communication Sciences and Disorders
School of Health and Rehabilitation Sciences
Boston, Massachusetts

Eric Oestmann, PhD, PT
OEI Consulting
Bradenton, Florida

Dr. Joanna Oestmann, LMHC, LPC, LPCS
OEI Consulting
Bradenton, Florida

Shawna Patrick, RN, MS
Nurses for Nursing
Snowmass, Colorado

Lynda M. Pesta, RN, MSN
Louise Herrington School of Nursing
Baylor University
Dallas, Texas

Llewellyn S. Prater, RN, MSN
Louise Herrington School of Nursing
Baylor University
Dallas, Texas

Jeannie Salfi, PhD, RN
McMaster University
School of Nursing
Faculty of Health Sciences
Hamilton, Ontario, Canada

Judith Schurr Salzer, PhD, MBA, RN, CPNP
Medical College of Georgia
School of Nursing
Augusta, Georgia

Patricia Solomon, PhD, PT
McMaster University
Faculty of Health Sciences
School of Rehabilitation Science
Hamilton, Ontario, Canada

Richard L. Sowell, PhD, RN, FAAN
Kennesaw State University
WellStar College of Health and Human Services
Kennesaw, Georgia

Suzanne Sutton, RN, MSN
Mary Black School of Nursing
University Center Greenville
University of South Carolina, Upstate
Spartanburg, South Carolina

Deborah Tapler, PhD, RN, CNE
College of Nursing
Texas Woman's University
Dallas, Texas

Traci D. Taylor, RN, MSN
West Texas A & M University
Canyon, Texas

Karen H. Teeley, MS, RN, AHC-BC, CNE
Simmons College
Boston, Massachusetts

Barbara C. Woodring, EdD, RN
Georgia State University
Byrdine F. Lewis School of Nursing
Atlanta, Georgia

Richard C. Woodring, BA, MDiv, DMin
Medical College of Georgia
Division of Continuing Education
Augusta, Georgia

SECTION I

FOUNDATIONAL APPROACHES TO TEACHING AND LEARNING

Creating an effective learning environment is not an easy task in today's world, and it is even more complex in education programs for the health professions. Students entering the field of health care are extremely diverse. Traditional undergraduates, entering college directly from high school, interact with a vast variety of nontraditional students returning to school after experiences in the workplace and/or having completed previous college degrees. There is a wide range of ages and experiences within the student body. Educators are challenged to recognize different learning needs and respect and utilize the knowledge and experiences that students bring to the learning settings. The teaching strategies and examples throughout this book may be adapted for use in a variety of situations, at undergraduate and graduate levels, taking into account the diversity of learning needs.

The chapters in Section I provide a foundation for understanding, selecting, and adapting specific teaching strategies to the educator's setting and student body. The contributors provide a theory base for learning and critical thinking and bring in various dimensions of effective learning that include creativity, humor, and exploration of diverse viewpoints and ways of processing information.

CHAPTER 1

Effective Learning: What Teachers Need to Know

Martha J. Bradshaw

Knowing is a process, not a product.
—*Jerome Bruner (1966)*

What brings about effective learning in nursing students? Is it insight on the part of the student? A powerful clinical experience? Perhaps it is the dynamic, creative manner in which the nurse educator presents information or structures the learning experience. Effective learning likely is the culmination of all of these factors, in addition to others. In this chapter, dimensions of effective learning will be explored as a foundation for use of the innovative teaching strategies presented in subsequent chapters. The monumental growth in the use of technology has definitely changed the teaching–learning environment. Learners also have changed in the ways they access and use information and their expectations regarding feedback. The field of health professions education is experiencing a growth in the variety of students, yet how individuals learn is essentially unchanged.

THEORIES OF LEARNING

We approach learning individually, based largely on cognitive style (awareness of and taking in of relevant information) and preferred approaches to learning, or learning style. Some students are aware of their style and preference, some gain insight into these patterns as they become more sophisticated learners, and some students have never been guided to determine how they learn best.

Theoretical underpinnings classify learning as behavioristic or cognitive. Behavioristic learning was the earliest pattern identified through research. Psychologists, such as Skinner and Thorndike, described learning as a change in behavior and used stimulus response actions as an example. Subsequent theorists have described more complex forms of behaviorist learning. Bandura's (1977) theory of social learning describes human learning as coming from others through observation, imitation, and reinforcement. We learn from society, and we learn to be social. This type of learning is evident when we describe the need to "socialize" students to the profession of nursing.

Robert Gagne (1968) formulated suggestions for the sequencing of instruction, conditions by which learning takes place, and outcomes of learning, or categories in which human learning occurs. These learning categories are based on a hierarchical arrangement of learning theories, moving from simple to complex learning, and include intellectual and motor skills, verbal information, cognitive strategies, and attitudes. For example, within the category of intellectual skills are the following stages:

- Discrimination learning: distinguishing differences in order to respond appropriately
- Concept learning: detecting similarities in order to understand common characteristics
- Rule learning: combination of two or more concepts, as a basis for action in new situations

Gagne's ideas seem to combine behaviorism and cognitive theories. Use of behaviorism in nursing education was especially popular in the 1970s and early 1980s through the use of concrete, measurable, specific behavioral objectives. Even though nursing education has moved away from the concrete methods of learning and evaluation, use of the hierarchical arrangement is seen in curriculum development and learning outcomes.

Cognitive theories address the perceptual aspect of learning. Cognitive learning results in the development of perceptions and insight, also called gestalt, that brings about a change in thought patterns (causing one to think, "Aha") and related actions. Jerome Bruner (1966) described cognitive learning as processes of conceptualization and categorization. He contended that intellectual development includes awareness of one's own thinking, the ability to recognize and deal with several alternatives and sequences, and the ability to prioritize. Bruner also saw the benefit of discovery learning to bring about insights. Ausubel's (1968) assimilation theory focuses on meaningful learning, in which the individual develops a more complex cognitive structure by associating new meanings with old ones that already exist within the learner's frame of reference. Ausubel's theory relies heavily on the acquisition of previous knowledge. These principles are useful for introducing the new student to the healthcare environment by relating information to what the student knows about health and illness. The same principles are fundamental to curriculum development based on transition from simple to complex situations.

Gardner's theory of multiple intelligences recognizes cognition as more than knowledge acquisition. Based on his definition of intelligence as "the ability to solve problems or fashion products that are valued in more than one setting" (Gardner & Hatch, 1990, p. 5), Gardner has described seven forms of intelligence:

1. Linguistic: related to written and spoken words and language, and use and meaning of language(s)
2. Musical/rhythmic: based on sensitivity to rhythm and beat, recognition of tonal patterns and pitch, and appreciation of musical expression
3. Logical/mathematical: related to inductive and deductive reasoning, abstractions, and discernment of numerical patterns
4. Visual/spatial: ability to visualize an object or to create internal (mental) images, thus able to transform or re-create
5. Bodily kinesthetic: the taking in and processing of knowledge through use of bodily sensations; learning is accomplished through physical movement or use of body language
6. Interpersonal: emphasizes communication and interpersonal relationships, recognition of mood, temperament, and other behaviors
7. Intrapersonal: related to inner thought processes, such as reflection and metacognition; includes spiritual awareness and self-knowledge (Gardner & Hatch, 1990)

Cognitive theories that address learning stages appropriate for college students include Perry's (1970) model of intellectual and ethical development. This model recognizes four nonstatic stages in which students progress: (1) dualism (black vs white), (2) multiplicity (diversity and tolerance), (3) relativism (decision made by reasoned support), and (4) commitment to relativism (recognition of value set for decision making). Perry's ideas can serve to explain how critical thinking is developed over time.

APPROACHES TO LEARNING

Emerging from learning theories are descriptions of preferred styles or approaches to learning. Categorized as cognitive styles and learning styles, these approaches to learning are the ways that individuals acquire knowledge, which are concerned more with form or process than content (Miller & Babcock, 1996). Cognitive style deals with information process, the natural, unconscious internal process concerned with thinking and memory. It is the consistent way in which individuals organize and handle information (DeYoung, 2009). The most common example of cognitive style is Witkin and colleagues' field dependent–field independent style (Witkin, Moore, Goodenough, & Cox, 1977). The field dependent–field independent style describes one's field of perception, or how one takes in information or data. Whereas one style generally predominates, people possess the capacity for both styles. Field-dependent individuals are more global, are open to external sources of information, are influenced by their surroundings, and therefore see the situation as a whole, rather than identifying and focusing on the separate aspects of it. Field-dependent people tend to be social, people oriented, and sensitive to social cues. Learners in which the field-dependent style predominates may be externally motivated and therefore take a more spectator or passive role in the learning process, preferring to be taught rather than to actively participate. Field-independent individuals are less sensitive to the social environment and thus take on a more analytical approach to information. By identifying aspects of the situation separately, they are able to restructure information and develop their own system of classification. Field-independent learners enjoy concepts, challenges, and hypotheses, and are task oriented (Miller & Babcock, 1996).

An aspect of learning style related to student behavior is response style. Kagan (1965) pioneered work, with school-age children, on the concepts of reflection and impulsiveness. These dimensions of cognitive response style describe personal tendencies regarding possibilities to solutions and choice selection. Individuals who have the impulsivity tendency prefer the quick, obvious answer, especially in highly uncertain problems, thus selecting the nearly correct answer as first choice. Reflective individuals identify and carefully consider alternatives before making a decision or choice. The implications for nursing education are apparent and will be discussed further. One problem that emerges with individuals who have a strong tendency in one of these dimensions is that the impulsive individual acts too quickly, based on an instant decision. On the other hand, the reflective individual may be immobilized in decision making, which has outcomes implications.

Reflection, as associated with learning, was described as early as 1916 by John Dewey as being a process of inquiry (Miller & Babcock, 1996). To reflect on a situation, experience, or collection of information is to absorb, consider, weigh, speculate, contemplate, and deliberate. Such reflection serves either as a basis for reasoned action or to gain understanding or attach meaning to an experience. The most notable descriptions of reflection, especially as related to nursing, have been presented by Schön (1983). In his work, Schön related reflection to problem solving. He pointed out that traditional means of teaching and learning result in structured problem solving where the ends are clear and fixed. In the reality of health care, such ends are not always so concrete.

Schön also believes that professionals in practice demonstrate a unique proficiency of thinking, and he has described three aspects of this thinking: (1) knowing-in-action (use of a personally constructed knowledge base), (2) reflection-in-action (conscious thinking about what one is doing, awareness of use of knowledge), and (3) reflection-on-action (a retrospective look at thoughts and actions, to conduct self-evaluation and make decisions for future events). Reflection results in synthesis. This outcome is evident when the individual carries over thoughts, feelings, and conclusions to other situations. Teaching includes reflection-in-action, in which the teacher spontaneously adapts to learner reactions. Thus, reflection is the foundation for growth through experience. Reflection, as a form of thinking and learning, can be cultivated. Educators improve their teaching when they reflect on episodes of teaching that were successful, as well as those that were failures (Pinsky, Monson, & Irby, 1998).

One of the best known descriptions of learning styles is Kolb's, which emerged from Dewey's seminal theory on experiential learning (Kolb, 1984). Dewey pioneered educational thinking regarding the relationship between learning and experience. The relationship between the learning environment and personal factors such as motivation and goals can lead the learner through a stream of experiences that, once connected, bring about meaningful learning (Kelly & Young, 1996). Using these ideas, Kolb went on to describe learning as occurring in stages: concrete experiences, observation and reflection on the experience, conceptualization and generalization, then theoretical testing in new and more complex situations. Learning is cyclical, with new learning coming from new experiences. Consequently, learning occurs in a comprehensive means, beginning with performance (concrete experience) and ending with educational growth. Kolb further explained that individuals go about this learning along two basic dimensions: grasping experiences (prehension) with abstract-concrete poles and transforming, with action-reflection poles (Kelly & Young, 1996). Applying his experiential learning theory to his dimensions, Kolb identified four basic learning styles:

1. Convergers prefer abstract conceptualization and active experimentation. These individuals are more detached and work better with objects than people. They are problem solvers and apply ideas in a practical manner.
2. Divergers prefer concrete experience and reflective observation. Individuals with this tendency are good at generating ideas and displaying emotionalism and interest in others. Divergers are imaginative and can see the big picture.
3. Assimilators prefer abstract conceptualization and reflective observation. Assimilators easily bring together diverse items into an integrated entity, sometimes overlooking practical aspects or input from others. Theoreticians likely are assimilators.
4. Accommodators prefer concrete experience and active experimentation. These individuals, while intuitive, are risk takers and engage in trial-and-error problem solving. Accommodators are willing to carry out plans, and they like and adapt to new circumstances (Miller & Babcock, 1996).

Gregorc's (1979) categorization of learning styles is similar to Kolb's, except that Gregorc believes that an individual's style is static, even in light of the changing educational setting. Thus, even through maturity and further learning, an individual still approaches learning in the same way. Gregorc uses the learning style categories of concrete sequential, concrete random, abstract sequential, and abstract random. In his research, Gregorc determined that individuals have preferences in one or two categories. In studying both first-year and fourth-year baccalaureate nursing students, Wells and Higgs (1990) discovered that these students have preferences in the concrete sequential and abstract random categories (total 81% of first-year students, 74% of fourth-year students).

USE OF LEARNING STYLES AND PREFERENCES: APPLICATION OF RESEARCH

Theoretical foundations regarding learning and descriptive studies of cognitive and learning styles provide insight and understanding of self. It would be difficult to address research on all modes of learning in this one chapter. A summary application of information from the vast field of knowledge about learning theory and cognitive and learning styles has been developed by Svinicki (1994) as six operating principles:

1. If information is to be learned, it must first be recognized.
2. During learning, learners act on information in ways that make it more meaningful.
3. Learners store information in long-term memory in an organized fashion related to their existing understanding of the world.
4. Learners continually check understanding, which results in refinement and revision of what is retained.
5. Transfer to new contexts is not automatic but results from exposure to multiple applications.
6. Learning is facilitated when learners are aware of their learning strategies and monitor their use (Svinicki, 1994, p. 275).

To understand one's own learning styles helps understand one's own thinking, to be aware of a fit between style and strategies for learning, and thus to select the most effective and efficient means to go about learning. Some students are aware of how they learn best and gravitate toward that strategy. Instructors see this process in students who choose to sit in the front row of the class, take many notes, and feel involved with the topic, or students who prefer online learning, choose to not come to class but instead read course material, watch

Internet clips or videos, and acquire information as it pertains to a clinical assignment. Some students adhere to tradition-bound forms of learning, such as lecture and reading, yet do not maximize their learning. This result explains why these students benefit more from direct clinical experiences. Many students find learning to be more powerful when they experience something new or significant in a clinical environment, then explore information and reflect on the experience. Learning experiences can be adapted to the environment and are influenced by the environment in which they occur. Awareness and comprehension of one's style of learning enables one to tailor the learning environment for optimal outcomes. A simple test that will guide the student in discovering his or her learning style(s) is presented in the teaching example at the end of this chapter.

Feedback from an observer, such as the instructor, can heighten awareness of personal styles. The knowledgeable educator also can guide the student in enhancing predominant styles or in cultivating additional dimensions of thinking and responding. For example, a student who is predominantly impulsive in decision making should be guided to explore outcomes of decisions and encouraged to increase reflection time, as appropriate. Conversely, the student who is highly reflective may need to explore reasons that bring about hesitancy or prolonged deliberation and the outcomes of such behaviors.

EFFECTIVE TEACHING FOR EFFECTIVE LEARNING

A knowledgeable and insightful educator is the key to effective learning in many situations. Consequently, the educator should have a knowledge base in learning and teaching as well as an extensive repertoire of useful strategies to reach learning goals. Faculty in health professions education are challenged to be directive in their teaching, addressing measurable learning outcomes that are directly linked to professional standards. This is juxtaposed with the importance of freeing the student from linear thinking and encouraging broader approaches to learning that are accomplished through dialogue, expression, and attribution of meaning. Instructors must determine best use of time, both for themselves and for students. So, difficult decisions must be made regarding what to leave in and what to omit from teaching episodes. In the health professions, faculty have to choose between teaching for practical judgment or for disciplinary knowledge. Specialized knowledge from within the discipline can clarify issues involved in practical situations, but it cannot determine judgment or a course of action (Sullivan & Rosin, 2008). This is where the role of the instructor, as a seasoned practitioner, is indispensible.

In their research to discover attributes of successful teachers at the rank of full professor, Rossetti and Fox (2009) developed four categories this teaching success:

Presence of the teacher: "being there" or available for the students, becoming acquainted with students, and cultivating mutual respect and trust

Promotion of learning: interested in students' learning and finding meaning in their education

Teachers as learners: staying current in the discipline and teaching strategies, and continually updating and refreshing courses

Enthusiasm: conveying an interest in the subject and passion for the work

Regardless of setting—traditional classroom, clinical care, synchronous or asynchronous electronic instruction—these principles of teaching success are applicable.

As students advance in their education, their established, comfortable ways of knowing, thinking, and reflecting are challenged. This is especially true in the health professions, where students explore value systems that differ from their own and identify ethical dilemmas in practice, circumstances in which there is more than one right answer or no clear choice. In situations in which the research evidence diverges from existing paradigms that are known to students, and thus cause conflict in thinking, the instructor should be prepared to adapt and modify teaching to address this conflict (Fryer, 2008). Therefore, the instructor needs to be patently aware of their own teaching styles and how to amend style for the circumstances.

Underlying assumptions regarding the nature of professional education are derived, in part, from principles on adult learning, as formulated by Knowles (1978). Key principles include assuming responsibility for one's own learning and recognizing the meaning or usefulness of information to be learned. Students in health professions are career oriented and need to see practical value in their educational endeavors. As consumers, adult students need to believe that they are receiving the maximum benefit from learning experiences. Furthermore, taking charge of one's own learning is empowering. Students who gain a sense of self-responsibility can feel empowered in other areas of their lives, such as professional practice. Faculty, in turn, have the responsibility to cultivate empowerment and to affect learning outcomes.

The teaching–learning experience, whether it is in a classroom environment or online, should be fresh and challenging each time the class convenes. Faculty should endeavor to provide variety in the manner in which they teach, rather than the same, predictable, albeit comfortable method of telling rather than teaching. As providers of information, instructors need to remember that learning is best brought about by a combination of motivation and stimulation. The effective instructor should be the facilitator of learning in the students. In professional education, motivation is gained when the relationship to the well-being of the client is pointed out. The value of faculty experience is evident when the nurse-teacher shares from his or her own professional experiences and uses these anecdotes as examples for client outcomes. Nursing students and faculty agree that nontraditional strategies such as collaborative or cooperative learning, active involvement, and participation in the learning experience are desirable for effective learning. Students in professional education programs do respond positively to opportunities to choose or structure some of their learning experiences (Melrose, 2004). This approach should be used frequently by the teacher to not only promote active learning but to instill in students a sense of empowerment, which is an important attribute for the clinical setting. Technology-based learning activities direct the student to engage in independent learning, research, and use visual cues, such as video, to enhance comprehension.

Students are more likely to remember information with which they can agree or relate, and if they can attach meaning to the item or information (DeYoung, 2009). Disagreement or disharmony should be explored in an objective fashion. Viewpoints can then be strengthened or altered. Questioning and discussion should be based on the diversity that exists among the students. An instructor who is able to establish a sense of trust and confidence with the students can promote the expression of different perspectives likely to be found in the group. Professional educators should support students who are at various levels of cognitive growth, looking upon students from a criterion framework rather than a normative one. Faculty should show that various viewpoints are welcome, legitimate, and worthy of discussion.

Effective educators guide students to see how their thought processes occur. They ask "what do you know about . . . ?" and "how did you arrive at that answer/conclusion?" Teachers cultivate further development in individual learners by demonstrating how to critique a theory, develop a rationale, or work through the steps of problem solving. These strategies will facilitate growth in students who are in an early cognitive stage such as dualism, or will challenge more advanced students to a commitment to realism (Perry, 1970).

Delivery of information should be based on instructional theory in addition to content expertise. Using Ausubel's (1968) principles of advanced organizer, the teacher can develop inductive discovery by which students can build on previously acquired, simplistic knowledge to develop new or broader concepts. This strategy operationalizes some of Svinicki and Dixon's (1987) cognitive principles.

Effective learning experiences that emerge from identified styles should be developed and used in both classroom and clinical settings. Information from Kolb's four dimensions serves as an excellent example. Students who are convergers readily become bored with straight lecture, especially with topics that are abstract in nature. These individuals work better by themselves, so they are less likely to participate well in group projects. Learners with the diverger style learn from case studies and will actively participate in discussion, but they may have difficulty detaching personal values from the issue. These students often are visionary group leaders. Individuals with the assimilator style manipulate ideas well, so they will participate well in discussion or write comprehensive papers; however, these students may be less practical and have difficulty with some of the realism of clinical practice. Accommodators usually enjoy case studies, new or unusual teaching strategies, skills lab, and tinkering with new equipment. These learners will be most responsive to a challenging, complex client. With the multitude of learning opportunities available through electronic resources and patient simulation, teachers can readily craft a learning experience that meets most learning styles and preferences.

Skiba, Connors, and Jeffries (2008) cite nursing education as the field considered by many to be the pioneer in the use of educational technology. Nursing, along with the other health professions, must face the challenges of incorporating core competencies, using emerging technologies, and practicing in informatics-intensive healthcare environments. However, one-way learning, such as Web-based instruction, will not fully replace competency-based instruction and verification that is needed in the applied disciplines of health care (Knapp, 2004).

In the clinical setting, the instructor may wish to provide introductory motivation through discovery learning. One way to accomplish this goal is to have each student observe or follow an individual in the clinical setting to gain exposure to the myriad tasks and responsibilities of a professional healthcare provider. Whereas students may have some rudimentary ideas of what healthcare providers do, they discover the depth and demands required in day-to-day work by observing actual practice. This strategy should broaden their perspectives and set the stage for meaningful learning, which includes increased retention of material and greater inquiry.

As students develop clinical written summaries about their clients, instructors should be flexible with the type of written work submitted. Traditionally, nursing students develop some form of a care plan based on the nursing process. The structured, linear method has taken criticism as the only way to look at clients. As a concrete, methodical strategy, the nursing process care plan is effective for students who are field independent and who can readily discern the data and related information needed for each step.

Additional methods of client summary or analysis should be introduced, and students should be encouraged to try each method. In doing so, students may broaden their ways of seeing clients and nursing problems, thus setting the stage for increased insight, analysis, and confidence. For example, use of the concept map is a way in which a student can envision the client or care situation in a holistic manner. Concept maps provide a fluidity that enhances the ability to determine relationships and make connections. Therefore, this strategy likely will be used positively by students who demonstrate Gardner's categories of visual/spatial or interpersonal intelligence. Learners who are field dependent also should do well with the concept map strategy because of their tendency to see the situation as a whole. Concept mapping should be effective for learners with all of Kolb's styles, but for different reasons and with different outcomes.

Guided reflection, especially reflection-on-action, helps the student bring closure to the clinical experience, as well as conduct self-evaluation and gain from the experience. Journal writing is one of the most effective means by which the student can capture thoughts and responses and preserve these ideas in writing for subsequent consideration. This strategy is particularly useful as a means by which students can identify and modify impulsive-reflective tendencies. Journal writing will have the best results with divergers and assimilators, and some students may benefit from open discussion about the experiences entered into their journals. Again, feedback from the faculty is crucial and should be as thoughtful as the entries provided by the student. Faculty reading journals should guide the student in growth of insight and patterns of reflection.

Effective teachers in the health professions are those who possess content expertise, create an active learning environment, and use carefully selected teaching strategies (Wolf, Bender, Beitz, Wieland, & Vito, 2004). One of the greatest challenges for faculty is in developing the blend of strategies to bring about effective learning in all students. Part of the challenge is the fit between the faculty's styles and learning preferences and that of each of the learners. Faculty especially should be on guard against favoritism to students who possess the same attributes as the instructor. Conversely, the congruency between styles of the teacher and of the student may enhance a relationship that is especially meaningful and may evolve into professional mentoring.

FUTURE CONSIDERATIONS

The majority of research on cognitive styles, learning style, and learning preferences was conducted in the 1970s and 1980s. This was before the widespread accepted use of electronic technology. The use of technology in teaching and learning may be influenced by learning preferences, such as in visual and kinesthetic learners. Have some students learned to modify their preferences in order to become more comfortable with technology? Online education is widely accepted, and the role of the instructor is changing. The extent to which learners continue to value the presence of the instructor for spontaneous teaching is worthy of investigation. Currently, there is a shift in education toward student-centered, active learning for the development of critical thinking, coupled with generations of students who are used to immediate feedback and a variety of stimulation. Educators must determine if selected strategies are useful for genuine learning or, if not used properly, merely providing entertainment.

CONCLUSION

Effective learning is more than merely the result of good teaching. It is enhanced by a learning environment that includes active interactions among faculty, students, and student peers. Effective learning is achieved through the use of creative strategies designed not to entertain but to inform and stimulate. The best ways faculty can bring about effective learning are by recognizing students as individuals, with unique, personal ways of knowing and learning, by creating learning situations that recognize diversity, and by providing empowering experiences in which students are challenged to think.

TEACHING EXAMPLE

How Do I Learn Best?

This instrument typically takes 4 to 6 minutes to complete and can be self-scored. The style categories are visual, aural, read/write, and kinesthetic, which correspond with categories found in Gardner's multiple forms of intelligence. Students are directed to answer the brief questions, then are shown the learning modalities that best fit predominant styles.

HOW DO I LEARN BEST?

This test is to find out something about your preferred learning method. Research on left brain/right brain differences and on learning and personality differences suggests that each person has preferred ways to receive and communicate information.

Choose the answer that best explains your preference and put the key letter in the box. If a single answer does not match your perception, please enter two or more choices in the box. Leave blank any question that does not apply. Once you have completed the test, find the totals for each of the letters (V, A, R, K) that correspond with a learning preference. Then look at the table of learning modalities (Table 1-1) to see what strategies best support your learning preference.

1. **You are about to give directions to a person. She is staying in a hotel in town and wants to visit your house. She has a rental car. Would you:**
   (V) draw a map on paper?
   (R) write down the directions (without a map)?
   (A) tell her the directions by phone?
   (K) collect her from the hotel in your car?

2. **You are staying in a hotel and have a rental car. You would like to visit a friend whose address/location you do not know. Would you like him to:**
   (V) draw you a map on paper?
   (R) write down the directions (without a map)?
   (A) tell you the directions by phone?
   (K) collect you from the hotel in his car?
3. **You have just received a copy of your itinerary for a world trip. This is of interest to a friend. Would you:**
   (A) call her immediately and tell her about it?
   (R) send her a copy of the printed itinerary?
   (V) show her the itinerary on a map of the world?
4. **You are going to cook a dessert as a special treat for your family. Do you:**
   (K) cook something familiar without need for instructions?
   (V) thumb through the cookbook looking for ideas from the pictures?
   (R) refer to a specific cookbook where there is a good recipe?
   (A) ask for advice from others?
5. **A group of tourists has been assigned to you to find out about national parks. Would you:**
   (K) drive them to a national park?
   (R) give them a book on national parks?
   (V) show them slides and photographs?
   (A) give them a talk on national parks?
6. **You are about to purchase a new stereo. Other than price, what would most influence your decision?**
   (A) A friend talking about it.
   (K) Listening to it.
   (R) Reading the details about it.
   (V) Its distinctive, upscale appearance.
7. **Recall a time in your life when you learned how to do something like playing a new board game. Try to avoid choosing a very physical skill (e.g., riding a bike). How did you learn best? By:**
   (V) visual clues—pictures, diagrams, charts?
   (A) listening to somebody explaining it?
   (R) written instructions?
   (K) doing it?
8. **Which of these games do you prefer?**
   (V) Pictionary
   (R) Scrabble
   (K) Charades
9. **You are about to learn to use a new program on a computer. Would you:**
   (K) ask a friend to show you?
   (R) read the manual that comes with the program?
   (A) telephone a friend and ask questions about it?
10. **You are not sure whether a word should be spelled *dependent* or *dependant*. Do you:**
    (R) look it up in the dictionary?
    (V) see the word in your mind and choose the best way it looks?
    (A) sound it out in your mind?
    (K) write both versions down?

11. Apart from price, what would most influence your decision to buy a particular textbook?
    (K) Using a friend's copy.
    (R) Skimming parts of it.
    (A) A friend talking about it.
    (V) It looks okay.
12. A new movie has arrived in town. What would most influence your decision to go or not go?
    (A) Friends talked about it.
    (R) You read a review about it.
    (V) You saw a preview of it.
13. Do you prefer a lecturer/teacher who likes to use:
    (R) handouts and/or a textbook?
    (V) flow diagrams, charts, slides?
    (K) field trips, labs, practical sessions?
    (A) discussion, guest speakers?

Source: Gardner, H., & Hatch, T. (1990). *Multiple intelligences go to school: Educational implications of the theory of multiple intelligences* (Technical Report No. 4). New York: Center for Technology in Education.

Table 1-1 Learning Modality

	In Class	When Studying	For Exams
Visual	Underline Use different colors Use symbols, charts, arrangements on a page	Recall visual aspects of presentation Reconstruct images in different ways Redraw pages from memory Replace words with symbols and initials	Recall the pictures on the pages Draw, use diagrams where appropriate Practice turning visuals back into words
Aural	Attend lectures and listen Discuss topics with students Use a tape recorder Discuss overheads, pictures, and other visual aids Leave space in notes for later recall	May take poor notes because of preference for voices Expand your notes by talking out ideas Explain new ideas to another student Read assignments out loud	Speak your answers/tutorials Practice writing answers to an old exam Read questions to self or have someone read them to you
Reading/ Writing	Use lists, headings Write out lists and definitions Use handouts and textbooks	Write out the words Reread notes silently Rewrite ideas in other words Use lecture notes/read	Practice with multiple-choice questions Write paragraphs, beginnings, endings Organize diagrams into statements
Kinesthetic: Use All Your Senses	May take notes poorly because topics do not seem relevant Go to lab, take field trips Use trial-and-error method Listen to real-life examples	Put examples in note summaries Talk about notes, especially with another kinesthetic person Use pictures and photos to illustrate	Write practice answers Role-play the exam situation in your head

REFERENCES

Ausubel, D. P. (1968). *Educational psychology: A cognitive view*. New York: Holt, Rinehart and Winston.

Bandura, A. (1977). *Social learning theory*. Morristown, NJ: General Learning Press.

Bruner, J. (1966). *Toward a theory of instruction*. New York: W. W. Norton & Co.

DeYoung, S. (2009). *Teaching strategies for nurse educators* (2nd ed.). Upper Saddle River, NJ: Prentice-Hall.

Fryer, G. (2008). Teaching critical thinking in osteopathy: Integrating craft knowledge and evidence-informed approaches. *International Journal of Osteopathic Medicine, 11*(2), 56–61.

Gagne, R. M. (1968). Learning hierarchies. *Educational Psychologist, 6*, 1–9.

Gardner, H., & Hatch, T. (1990). *Multiple intelligences go to school: Educational implications of the theory of multiple intelligences* (Technical Report No. 4). New York: Center for Technology in Education.

Gregorc, A. F. (1979). Learning/teaching styles: Their nature and effects. In *Student learning styles* (pp. 19–26). Reston, VA: National Association of Secondary Principals.

Kagan, J. (1965). Reflection-impulsivity and reading ability in primary grade children. *Child Development, 36*, 609–628.

Kelly, E., & Young, A. (1996). Models of nursing education for the 21st century. In K. Stevens (Eds.), *Review of research in nursing education* (pp. 1–39). New York: National League for Nursing.

Knapp, B. (2004). Competency: An essential component of caring in nursing. *Nursing Administration Quarterly, 28*, 285–287.

Knowles, M. A. (1978). *The adult learner: A neglected species* (2nd ed.). Houston, TX: Gulf Publishing.

Kolb, D. A. (1984). *Experiential learning theory*. Englewood Cliffs, NJ: Prentice-Hall.

Melrose, S. (2004). What works? A personal account of clinical teaching strategies in nursing. *Education for Health, 17*, 236–239.

Miller, M. A., & Babcock, D. E. (1996). *Critical thinking applied to nursing*. St. Louis, MO: Mosby.

Perry, W. G. (1970). *Forms of intellectual and ethical development in the college years: A scheme*. New York: Holt, Rinehart and Winston.

Pinsky, L. E., Monson, D., & Irby, D. M. (1998). How excellent teachers are made: Reflecting on success to improve teaching. *Advances in Health Sciences Education, 3*, 207–215.

Rossetti, J., & Fox, P.G. (2009). Factors related to successful teaching by outstanding professors: An interpretive study. *Journal of Nursing Education, 48*(1) 11–16.

Schon, D. A. (1983). *The reflective practitioner: How professionals think in action*. New York: Basic Books.

Skiba, D. J., Connors, H. R., & Jeffries, P. R. (2008). Information technologies and the transformation of nursing education. *Nursing Outlook, 56*(5), 225–230.

Sullivan, W. M., & Rosin, M. S. (2008). A life on the mind for practice: Bridging liberal and professional education. *Change, 40*(2), 44–47.

Svinicki, M. D. (1994). Practical implications of cognitive theories. In K. A. Feldman, & M. B. Paulsen (Eds.), *Teaching and learning in the college classroom* (pp. 274–281). Needham Heights, MA: Ginn Press.

Svinicki, M. D., & Dixon, D. M. (1987). The Kolb model modified for classroom activities. *College Teaching, 35*, 141–146.

Wells, D., & Higgs, Z. R. (1990). Learning and learning preferences of first and fourth semester baccalaureate degree nursing students. *Journal of Nursing Education, 29*, 385–390.

Witkin, H. A., Moore, C. A., Goodenough, D. R., & Cox, P. W. (1977). Field-dependent and field-independent cognitive styles and their implications. *Review of Educational Research, 47*, 1–64.

Wolf, Z. R., Bender, P. J., Beitz, J. M., Wieland, D. M., & Vito, K. O. (2004). Strengths and weaknesses of faculty teaching performance reported by undergraduate and graduate nursing students: A descriptive study. *Journal of Professional Nursing, 20*, 118–128.

CHAPTER 2

Diversity in the Classroom

Arlene J. Lowenstein

Today's classrooms are very different from those in the past. Immigration, both forced and voluntary, has shaped the face of this country. Each new wave of immigrants adds to the mosaic that is the United States. A mosaic is made up of many pieces, each different in size and shape, some may be brightly colored, others pale, transparent, or no color added. Each piece does not mean much by itself but, when put together, they change, forming new designs and an overall effect very different from its component pieces. The strength of that mosaic is the ability to capitalize on new and different ideas. Its weakness is the clash between cultures that feeds prejudice and discriminatory behaviors. Health professions educators and leaders have recognized this change, and cultural competence of practitioners is now being stressed in both education and service. By using the strengths and originality of diverse students, the final classroom product can be much stronger than the product of an assimilated, cookie-cutter one.

A new emphasis on civil rights, feminism, sexuality, and morality issues in the late 1960s and 1970s brought about drastic change in what had been considered accepted societal behavior. Those changes shaped the move toward increased diversity of both patients and student body in our world today, and provided new and different opportunities and challenges from those of the past. Change continues as we speak, and classrooms in the future may look very different. Educators need to be flexible, aware of trends and patterns, and able to respond to continuing challenges. This chapter presents a brief glimpse at some of the diversity issues in the past and present day, and discusses some of the issues and strategies involved in working with a diverse classroom population.

THE PAST

In the 1950s, healthcare professional education was almost nonexistent for African Americans (Blacks), other minorities, and persons with disabilities. Men went into medicine, while women became nurses. Other health professions may have had some of each gender, but women were often in the majority (Moffat, 2003). Educational facilities were often segregated culturally and religiously, not only in the South, which had a history of legal segregation at that time, but in the North as well (Carnegie, 1991, 2005). Catholic and Jewish hospitals often had their own schools of nursing, and there were religious and ethnic student quotas in many colleges and universities. This meant that most classes were homogenized, with a large majority of Caucasian (White) and Protestant students in all but the religious-sponsored or minority-established programs, and those were few and far between. Very few Hispanic, Asian, Islamic, or Muslim students were admitted to the schools. For minorities that were admitted, retention rates were often low (Carnegie, 1991).

Nursing education was founded in hospital diploma programs using the apprentice system of education. From the early days in the late 1800s through the 1950s there were very few graduate nurses in hospitals. Most graduate nurses moved into private duty after graduation, with some going into public health and a few staying on primarily in managerial or teaching positions. Student nurses were the major providers of care for hospital patients. Very ill patients on the hospital wards were most often assigned a private duty nurse to care for them, usually paid for by the patients and their families, although hospitals absorbed the cost in some instances.

In 1946, shortly after World War II, the Hill-Burton Act was passed by Congress and signed into law. It provided funds to hospitals for renovation, expansion, capital projects, and new hospital buildings. As hospitals expanded, more nurses and other healthcare professionals were needed. Another trend of the time was the development of intensive care units in the mid-1950s, and skilled nurses were needed for those areas as well. The nursing students and nurses in the labor pool during those years were still primarily Caucasian and Protestant with few minorities.

During that time, although it seems hard to believe in today's world, very few nursing schools admitted married students. Female students were dismissed from the program if they chose to get married, especially if the "secret marriages" that occurred were found out by school authorities, and even if they were almost ready to graduate. In the few schools where married students were permitted, pregnant women were excluded and pregnancy out of wedlock was an unforgivable sin for health professions education.

Nursing was viewed as a women's profession and few men were permitted in, and those that were had severe restrictions in clinical experiences, such as in obstetrics and gynecology, but could be welcomed in psychiatric facilities because it was thought that they were stronger and could work better with distraught and violent patients. It was generally considered that students with disabilities would not be able to participate in providing all aspects of care and, therefore, were not admitted to programs. There were no allowances made.

In Augusta, Georgia, from the early 1900s through the early 1960s, University Hospital had two schools of nursing, the Lamar School for Blacks and the Barrett School for Whites (Lowenstein, 1990, 1994). The two schools joined together in 1965, after the passage of civil rights legislation. The Barrett School accepted more nursing students and had a higher graduation rate than the Lamar School. One year, three Asian students applied and were admitted to the Barrett School, but only one graduated. In Augusta, as in most of the South and often in the North (although no one talked about that), Black students were assigned to the units with Black patients, and White students with White patients. Supervisors, administrators, and teachers were almost always White.

The late 1960s and early 1970s brought a revolutionary change, which has continued expanding since that time. The Civil Rights Movement sparked a feminist movement, and those movements opened previously closed doors in education. Women had more opportunities to be admitted to healthcare professions that were previously male dominated. A few men were admitted into programs that had only women students, although the numbers were still small and discrimination prevalent, especially the belief that male nurses were homosexual. The sexual revolution of those years also brought a change in thinking about sexual orientation, although many attitudes of the past still exist today and discrimination still occurs. In nursing, the rules against marriage were dropped and women could attend school while pregnant. Although the changes have been gradual, the face of the classroom is continuing its transformation.

During this period of time, the community college movement began, which provided more access to minorities, to those who could not afford private college tuition, and to students who needed educational facilities closer to their homes. This was a boon to older women, including minority women, and those with families who could now attend less expensive schools that were closer to home. Part-time attendance was possible in some programs, and nursing students no longer needed to live at the hospitals. Graduates of associate degree programs in nursing were eligible for licensure as registered nurses and took less time to graduate than the typical 3-year diploma program students. Many hospital diploma schools began to close, although that was a prolonged fight. During those years, nursing leaders recognized the discrimination against women in college and university admissions. They were pleased that nursing education had moved out of the hospital program, but were not satisfied. In an effort to raise the status of women in the profession, they began a move toward baccalaureate collegiate education for all nurses by 1984, which also helped the demise of hospital programs. However, for many reasons, the baccalaureate goal was not achieved.

The physical therapy profession and its professional organization, the American Physical Therapy Association (APTA), were begun by women, but men were recognized in the profession by the 1920s. However, even with the feminist movements of the 1960s and 1970s, it took until the early 1990s for the APTA to feel it important enough to address women's issues and the inequities in the profession as it pertained to the disparities in the professional and economic status of women. The board of directors appointed the first Committee on Women in Physical Therapy and, in 1994, an Office of Women's Issues was created at APTA headquarters in Alexandria. The Office of Minority Affairs also became an integral part of the APTA headquarters at this time, as the profession tried to recruit more minorities (Moffat, 2003).

Those years also saw the beginning of affirmative action and an increased number of minorities began to be admitted to colleges, although the numbers were still small. The end of the Vietnam War began an Asian migration to the United States, and we have seen other migrations since that time creating increased Latino/Hispanic, Muslim, Indian, and Russian-Jewish populations, among others. Those migrations have meant more diverse students accepted into health professions programs.

In 1991, the American Disability Act (ADA) was passed by Congress and signed into law. This Act required educators to think differently about what could be done to provide access and retention for disabled persons who would be able to work in some, if not all, aspects of their chosen health profession, and thereby provide a valuable service for the profession and its patients.

THE PRESENT

So where has this history led us in the classroom in today's world? The health professions classroom is more diverse than ever before. However, diversity no longer means ethnic background alone. The age range may be wide and gender ratios may have changed, although nursing still has a minority of male students. In medicine it worked the other way around, and more women have gone into that field than ever before. There is diversity in sexual orientation, which can expose students to discrimination.

There are diverse social and family issues in the classroom. Many divorced and single parents have gone back to school, but often have great responsibility in raising their children alone, and that may interfere with the amount of time that can be allotted to school work (Grosz, 2005; Ogunsiji & Wilkes, 2005). In some places, disadvantaged students have come into the health professions classrooms as new economic relief programs are put into place (Wessling, 2000). Students, especially older ones, may have caretaker responsibilities for their parents or other relatives, including children with disabilities. Those in the "sandwich generation" may have caretaker responsibilities for both their parents and their children.

We also have wealthy students, for whom textbook purchases and other expenses are not a problem, and need-based scholarship students and other students who may have real concerns about financial issues, which can impact their progress and completion of their program. Tuition increases and the spectre of repayment of student loans may create additional stress. Financially secure students do not always have it easy just because they have the financial means, but may have other family and social problems that affect them and their classroom abilities.

The numbers of disabled students, with both physical and/or learning disabilities, has increased. Due to technological advances and better awareness, educational institutions are now able to provide more accommodations for students with disabilities. This may include policy modifications, equipment, and physical changes to increase handicap access. Students with disabilities often have concerns about how they are being perceived by others, and worry that other students and faculty are expecting them to fail. Research has shown that creative problem solving and faculty support can be developed for students with disabilities, and health professions education programs can be enriched by their presence (Carroll, 2004).

Colleges and universities are being encouraged to promote diversity in both hiring faculty and in student recruitment and admissions, although success rates are still low (Barbee & Gibson, 2001; Silver, 2002). Even though affirmative action has been under fire, it is recognized that there is still a need to make higher education more accessible for both minorities and students with disabilities. Although diversity in admissions and hiring may be strongly encouraged, retaining diverse students and faculty is often difficult. However, Splenser and his colleagues (2003), in a study of physical therapy educational programs, found that when schools provided special retention efforts, they were effective in increasing the numbers of graduating minority students. They also found a positive correlation between increased minority applications and the presence of minority faculty in a program.

Other researchers have found that many minority students experience significant culture shock when entering the collegiate world, which may be very different from their previous life experiences. In schools or programs with low numbers of diverse students and faculty, the recruited minority students often had feelings of isolation, loneliness, and anxiety. These feelings could be compounded by impersonal, and sometimes hostile, treatment from faculty, who were still predominately White. Minority faculty also face these feelings, and, in turn, this often leads to students dropping out of school and faculty leaving educational positions (Evans, 2004; Kosowski, Grams, Taylor, & Wilson, 2001; Vasquez, 1990).

Kirkland (1998) found a difference in psychological stress between Black and White nursing students. Blacks often felt more stress and perceived their environment differently. Because of the history of discrimination and their previous experiences with discrimination, Blacks may perceive discrimination, even though White students, employers, or other employees in a healthcare setting do not feel that discrimination exists (Lowenstein & Glanville, 1995). Kosowski et al. (2001) noted that the failure rate for Black students can be higher than their White counterparts.

There are many causes for the lack of success. Because Blacks are frequently in the minority in such a classroom, feelings of isolation, alienation, and loneliness, as well as perceived racism, can cause academic difficulties. Inadequate academic preparation for the rigor of college, family conflicts, and lack of financial resources can contribute to that failure. In many cases, support services are offered by institutions, but may not be used (Kosowski et al., 2001). Bain (2004) reported that negative stereotypes are often internalized by minority students. That can apply to disabled persons as well. Think about the term *minority*. What does that label mean to students? The connotation is that they are out of the mainstream, not as good as the "majority" students, and are often expected to fail. Bain noted that even students who had a strong self-image could fall into the trap of feeling that they needed to prove themselves, leading to increased anxiety and stress and, eventually, failure. Teachers who have been successful with this population have set up situations where positive expectations are verbalized and integrated into the classroom. Letting minority students know that there is respect for their abilities has been shown to lead to improvement in pass rates (Bain, 2004).

These issues are not limited to Blacks, but often affect other minorities, as well as White students from poorer economic strata. Evans (2004) found Hispanic/Latino and Native American nursing students struggled with similar feelings. Those in the study described the impact of perceived lack of options for minorities. Even before they entered the program, it was difficult for them to imagine themselves successful in a healthcare profession. Language issues can be difficult to overcome. Lack of family support due to financial or cultural expectations and ignorance of academic demands was also identified as a barrier to success for some students, especially those who were the first in their families to attend college. Students who successfully confronted those barriers were helped by faculty who recognized these stressors, worked to respect students' intense obligation to family and community, and provided long-term, personal encouragement to continue in the program (Evans, 2004).

WORKING WITH A DIVERSE STUDENT BODY

Diversity can have a positive impact on teaching and learning. When encouraged by faculty, recognition and understanding of differences and an introduction to other cultures can broaden viewpoints and stimulate discussion and ideas (Villaruel, Canales, & Torres, 2001). However, it is important to point out that, although this chapter talks about some cultural traits, there is a wide range in cultural responses and traits within a single culture. Members of a racial or cultural group may or may not adhere to some of the traditions of their background culture and ethnic group, and may not even identify as a member of that group. Faculty members must remember that people are individuals who react differently and must be treated individually. Students who are members of a cultural group cannot be expected to be a spokesperson for their group. There are too many variations within the groups themselves, and what is appropriate for one sect within a group may not be acceptable to another sect in that group.

Discrimination is always a difficult issue and faculty, staff, administrators, and patients are not immune. We all have our likes, dislikes, and moral beliefs. Because of their previous experiences, many minorities will see discrimination where others do not. That needs to be respected and cannot be brushed off, but sometimes it also needs to be faced, corrected, or worked with. The major thrust here needs to be concentration on providing appropriate learning opportunities and meeting learning objectives. Seeking ways to help students learn about each other can be a positive force in changing discriminatory attitudes. Many myths of prejudice and discrimination can be dismantled and dismissed when students who have led sheltered backgrounds begin to know those who are different from them and understand that, although there are cultural differences, there are also many similarities.

However, conflict between cultural groups does occur in the classroom. There can be other sources for conflict that have nothing to do with ethnicity, as well as conflicts that are ethnicity and values led. In some instances, mediation may be helpful to define limits and focus the groups back on the learning tasks at hand. Separation may work for other groups, but that is usually a temporary situation until the strong feelings calm down. Encouraging groups to learn about each other is a strategy that can be used to defuse potential conflict, but this strategy needs to be carefully managed and the instructor needs to observe group dynamics and be on the alert for peer influenced negative ideas and peer pressure to adopt those ideas.

Baumgartner and Johnson-Bailey (2008) note that traditionally we, as teachers, work to avoid emotions in working with diversity and that negative emotions were to be avoided and emotions to be kept under control. They stress that, while it is important to not get mired in emotions when discussing challenging issues, there is also an opportunity for a good teaching moment to explore.

> Positive emotions can enhance the learning process. Moreover, emotions are always to be acknowledged, not judged. We contend that emotions that are on display are a sign that students care and are engaged. When a student expresses a strong emotion, it is a good time to take an intellectual breather, not a break or a recess, and

> say, "Do you mind if we explore that?" "I missed that side of it," or "How about we step back from this emotional terrain and deconstruct this premise." Take advantage of the energy that learners bring to your classroom even when it means departing from the syllabus. These rare challenging teachable moments should be embraced as opportunities to knock down walls (Baumgartner & Johnson-Bailey, 2008, p. 52).

Developing a welcoming and supportive environment is essential, not only for ethnic minority students, but also for the other groups mentioned as part of the diverse classroom, including single parents, disabled students, and age and gender disparities. Faculty availability and interest are critical elements in developing a positive environment. Instructors need to be aware of potential issues, know their students, and demonstrate interest in them and their success in the program. The importance of cultural and linguistic role models (e.g., community health professionals of varied ethnicity and/or those from minority-based professional organizations, including those who speak a similar language) cannot be overemphasized because it has a universal effect on overcoming obstacles and achieving academic success for ethnically diverse students and students for whom English is a second language (ESL) (Heller & Lichtenberg, 2003; Yoder, 1996). Mentoring has shown success, whether it comes from outside the school or from an advanced student of one's own ethnic group or cultural origin, especially when there are no faculty members of color. Those same principles apply to gender-based minorities in programs who may also feel isolated or unwelcome in the profession.

When learning difficulties appear in any group of students, it is important to look for behavioral patterns that may be impacting their success or other stresses or anxieties that seem present. Some students may need to be encouraged to be tested for learning disabilities. A diagnosis of a learning disorder, confirmed by testing, allows the student access to the resources required under ADA regulations. Faculty need to learn about student support services in their college. They need to know to whom and how to make referrals for students in areas such as financial aid, study skills, test taking skills and tutorial assistance, mental and physical health services, and social services. It is extremely important that students are supported and encouraged to take advantage of those services.

Age Range

Older students will have a sense of history during their lifetime that is very different from 18-year-old students, and they have learned how to deal with many situations that 18 year olds have not yet faced, which can be valuable when there are opportunities for sharing. However, depending on their success or frustration levels in working with those situations, older students can also hold a cynical or ingrained view that comes through and needs to be worked with and mediated at times. Older students may not value the young lifestyle and may find younger students immature. Building on some of the strengths of the younger group having grown up in the technology age can be helpful to older students who are not comfortable with the technology.

Young students can be bored by the older students' experiences, tired of listening to them, not relate those experiences to their own, or they can be interested and learn from them. Younger students may relate to older students as parental figures (which can be good or bad), view them as caring, or view them as the other extreme of dictatorial or authoritarian, which is often based on their experiences with other older adults. The most important task is getting students in different age groups to respect and learn from each other. Small group work can create diverse working groups. Monitoring group work is important to identify conflict areas. However, when students in different age levels get to know each other better and have success in working together toward a common goal of meeting learning objectives, negative perceptions can change and they can be a positive support for each other.

Communication

Communication can be problematic between cultural and ethnic groups and the majority group. The learning goals and objectives need to be clearly understood by both students and teacher in a diverse classroom. Communication is often an issue and, at the same time, is the key to understanding and accepting those goals. Diverse students may have their own individual goals and objectives based on their interest and learning experiences, and may or may not be willing to share them with the instructor. An instructor needs to be open to listening to and encouraging ideas that can be different than the ones he/she planned for the class and allow for appropriate analytic, creative, and practical knowledge to be utilized. It may be easier for ESL students to read English than it is to understand spoken English, so written instructions or handouts may be helpful and allow students more time to clarify concepts. Instructors need to speak slowly and clearly in classroom presentations, and conversational pauses may need to be longer so that students can be encouraged to speak up, and to also allow them to catch up with what is being said and with note taking.

Some minority students come from cultures where eye contact and/or active participation are not normal experiences and may be uncomfortable for them (Suinn, 2006). This can include minimal participation in class discussion and they may sit back and not offer comments in class—even when they have a good understanding of the material and would have information that would be helpful to the class, or need clarification and additional help with a concept. Many of these students may do better in small discussion groups. Some cultures feel strongly about and use collaboration as a norm and participants may not want to stand out from the group, while the American culture tends to be more individualistic and often competitive, with class discussion more acceptable because it is familiar and offers an opportunity to show off their knowledge base. Of course students raised in the American culture can also be shy or nonparticipating, especially in large classes, and small group discussions can be helpful for them as well.

Students and faculty may have a difference in perception, especially if English is not the primary language. Ideas may not translate well. I had the experience of presenting a lecture in Taiwan, and worked with a Taiwanese nurse who spoke English well and was responsible for translating my comments to the audience in their native language. We met together and went over my lecture notes while she wrote her translations, and I thought things seemed to be going very well, until she asked me, "what is custodial care?" I immediately realized that I had assumed she understood everything I was talking about, but that was not necessarily the case. We went over the speech again, until I was comfortable that she understood the concepts and would be able to translate them appropriately.

American ideals and values may be different from what some students are used to. One of the most important aspects in working with all students, but especially with minorities and ESL students, is what I call "know your PVCs." This is not the cardiac term most of us are familiar with, but instead stands for *Perception, Validation,* and *Clarification*. Each person perceives an event differently. An inquiry to see if there are any questions or areas they do not understand needs to be more in-depth than just asking if the students understand and expecting and getting an affirmative answer. Students need to be encouraged to articulate what they think was said, and that is where the differences show up. Formal classroom assessment techniques can also be helpful in identifying problem areas (Angelo & Cross, 1994).

When an instructor feels a student lacks understanding of the materials, it is important to question that *perception* with the student, *validate* that what was meant to be communicated is in reality what the student understood to be communicated, and, when there is a difference, *clarification* is in order. Students who are not proficient in English may smile and seem to understand but often do not, and they may not want to ask in front of the whole class for clarification or statements to be repeated. It is important for faculty to be aware of this possibility, and follow through outside of the classroom environment may be necessary.

Accommodation

The passage of the American Disabilities Act, in 1991, has made a major difference in today's classrooms. Instructors need to adjust to accommodations that may be necessary. Think about the following: If a health professional is injured or comes down with a debilitating illness or is wheelchair-bound, can accommodations be made so they can continue working? In most cases employees can and will be accommodated in various jobs within the profession, even those employees that become deaf or legally blind. These jobs may not be the usual clinical care, but are still jobs that need a health professional to perform and are essential for quality care. Think about jobs that a disabled person could perform in your specialty—those that may be possible, despite the fact that some jobs will be limited or unable to be performed. Assistive devices can often be used to allow the employee to perform safely and appropriately in limited activities, if they have the appropriate clinical knowledge required for the specific position. If that is true, why does the door to the profession need to be closed and applicants with disabilities be turned away? Think about ways in which a disabled student could be prepared to work in those jobs within the profession, and the types of clinical experiences that a disabled student can carry out that will provide appropriate experiences for a future job. The technology field is rapidly expanding and assistive devices are improving and becoming more cost effective and more available.

Faculty must become well aware of the disability regulations and student support services that colleges have set up because of those regulations. Faculties need to develop awareness of the barriers and regulations that are present for disabled students and need to be addressed, and where resources can be found to help both faculty members and students. One problem that needs to be worked with in a positive manner is "are these accommodations fair to the students that are not disabled?" What does "fair" mean? A disability may not be visible to others, in particular learning disabilities or certain physical disabilities such as back problems. Rules of privacy may not allow a faculty member to discuss a disabled student's condition, but they can encourage the student to discuss this with others and provide support as necessary.

For many, many years teachers were authoritarians in the classrooms, with rigid standards and rules and regulations. Things are different today. Student demonstrations in the late 1960s and early 1970s began a student right's movement that altered college cultures. But some questions need to be asked. How much can be compromised, and how do we work within regulated issues? A very positive part of student's rights has been that faculties have had to look at what they were doing and assess whether they were working by ritual or providing real learning opportunities. Those faculties have learned to work successfully with students who, in the past, would not have had the opportunities available to them today.

Making accommodations is also an important concept to those with heavy personal responsibilities. Older students may be faced with family issues, such as caring for children and/or elderly parents. They and single parents may have responsibilities that interfere with their ability to meet deadlines or come to class. Rigid attendance policies are often more ritualistic than real. The focus needs to be on what is necessary for the learning experience. Sitting in a class does not guarantee that a student is attentive and learning. Teachers are well aware that students daydream, have conversations with their classmates, and even fall asleep, and that they will forget a good portion of what was presented, even though we as teachers believe that every word we give them is valuable. It may be more important for a student to attend a small seminar type class because the learning is dependent on participation in discussion than it is for sitting in a large lecture session. The important determining issue is what are the goals and objectives for the course, and are there other ways to meet them without perfect attendance? That may sound heretical, but there are other ways for conscientious and motivated students to meet learning objectives and set priorities. The use of the Internet, library services, and out-of-class assignments can afford some flexibility if needed. Attendance in clinical experiences may be more problematic because of the need for scheduling and faculty availability, but there are ways to design a program with a student that may afford some flexibility for specific instances. Again, it is important to keep the learning goal of the experience or class in mind and consider creative and flexible ways to work with students to plan for what they feel they can accomplish.

Financially challenged students may not be able to participate in some activities because they may need to work, along with their school responsibilities. They may have difficulty in buying books and special or technological equipment or participating in outside learning opportunities, such as conferences or lectures that have a fee attached. These students may not be able to spend hours in the library because of their work and family schedules, and finding study time may be difficult. Anxiety and worry over finances can impact their learning experience.

There is no easy answer to these issues but, again, student services can often be an ally. Student lives outside the classroom need to be respected, but the responsibility for learning is theirs, not yours. Student and faculty can work together to assess what is needed to achieve the objectives of the learning experiences and to facilitate their learning. Are there alternative ways of achieving those objectives that do not meet up with the "is it fair to others?" question. It is important for instructors to meet with student services to find out just what they do, and how they do it. Student services can help students set up workable schedules, tutorial services, and study and testing guidance. They can also counsel students on student life issues and refer students to outside resources when needed. Faculty should also be familiar with financial aid issues and regulations, which can be quite complicated because of differences in government and private sources, and with outside services for referrals when appropriate.

Academic Issues

Students with academic problems need to be identified early and encouraged to discuss the issue with faculty without the spectre of punishment or embarrassment. It is important to discover patterns of negative behavior, discuss them directly with the student involved, and develop a plan on which the student and faculty agree and believe can be implemented and carried out. Unfortunately, not all students can be helped and some will drop out or fail out, but others will be successful and benefit from the encouragement.

Students with learning disabilities and ESL students may have problems with timed tests. ESL students may need more time to read and digest test questions, because they may be translating the questions back into their language, and some words and phrases do not translate well. The learning disability students are supported in the need for additional time by the ADA regulations, but that is not true for ESL students. In order to evaluate and accurately grade the level of knowledge, faculty can provide opportunities for various types of testing other than timed tests—take home tests being one example. There may be a limit to this, however, when students need to improve in timed testing because they will be subjected to that in the licensure testing. Again, students with learning disabilities can have additional time because the regulations support them, but ESL can be a cause for failure in timed tests and those students may need practice and/or tutorial assistance to become more proficient in testing in order to pass a licensing exam and enter the profession.

Although working with diverse students can be challenging, it can also be stimulating and exciting. As healthcare professionals, we and our students are in a clinical environment, and learning about new cultures and disabilities can hopefully be translated into increased cultural competence when working with patients. In summary, remember that the responsibility for learning lies with the learner, but feelings of anxiety and isolation can cause stress that impacts the learning process and may affect graduation rates and successful entrance into the profession. Family responsibilities can also interfere with a student's ability to carry out the required work. Faculty members need to learn to develop sensitivity and awareness of issues that impact the learning process and work with students to meet the learning goals. They need to develop their knowledge of services and resources that can be utilized by students. Flexibility, patience, and creativity are needed to develop a supportive environment that enhances learning. A major role of faculty is offering support, guidance, and referrals, as appropriate, and developing a community of students that view diversity as a strength that provides an opportunity to learn from each other as well as from their teachers. It is painful but necessary to understand that this will not work for all students, but it will be appreciated by and benefit many students. Our reward for efforts expended is that we can rightly celebrate and be proud of the successful students that we have helped enter the profession and who are now providing a valuable service to their patients, communities, and profession.

REFERENCES

Angelo, T. A., & Cross, K. P. (1994). *Classroom assessment techniques: A handbook for college teachers* (2nd ed.). San Francisco, CA: Jossey-Bass.

Bain, K. (2004). *What the best college teachers do*. Cambridge, MA: Harvard University Press.

Barbee, E., & Gibson, S. (2001). Our dismal progress: The recruitment of non-whites into nursing. *Journal of Nursing Education, 40*, 243–244.

Baumgartner, L. M., & Johnson-Bailey, J. (2008). Fostering awareness of diversity and multiculturalism in adult and higher education. *New Directions for Adult & Continuing Education, 120*, 45–53.

Carnegie, M. E. (2005). Educational preparation of Black nurses: A historical perspective. *The ABNF Journal, 16*(1), 6–7.

Carnegie, M. E. (1991). *The path we tread: Blacks in nursing 1834–1990*. New York: National League for Nursing.

Carroll, S. M. (2004). Inclusion of people with physical disabilities in nursing education. *Journal of Nursing Education, 43*(5), 207–212.

Evans, B. C. (2004). Application of the caring curriculum to education of Hispanic/Latino and American Indian nursing students. *Journal of Nursing Education, 43*(5), 219–228.

Grosz, R. (2005). The forgotten (?) minority. *The Internet Journal of Allied Health Sciences and Practice, 3*(3). Retrieved November 8, 2009, from http://ijahsp.nova.edu/articles/vol3num3/grosz_commentary.htm

Heller, B. R., & Lichtenberg, L. P. (2003). Addressing the shortage: strategies for building the nursing workforce *Nursing Leadership Forum, 8*(1), 34–39.

Kirkland, M. L. S. (1998). Stressors and coping strategies among successful female African American baccalaureate nursing students. *Journal of Nursing Education, 37*(1), 5–13.

Kosowski, M. M., Grams, K. M., Taylor, G. J. & Wilson, C. B. (2001). They took the time. . . they started to care: Stories of African-American Nursing students in intercultural caring groups. *Advances in Nursing Science, 23*(3), 11–27.

Lowenstein, A. (1994, September). *Racial segregation and nursing education in Georgia: The Lamar experience*. Paper presented at the annual convention of the Transcultural Nursing Society, Atlanta, Georgia.

Lowenstein, A. (1990, March 28–April 1). Racial segregation and nursing education in Georgia: The Lamar experience. *Proceedings of the National Association for Equal Opportunity in Higher Education's (NAFEO's) 15th National Conference on Blacks in Higher Education*, Washington, DC.

Lowenstein, A. J., & Glanville, C. (1995). Cultural diversity and conflict in the health care workplace. *Nursing Economics, 13*(4), 203–209, 247.

Moffat, M. (2003). The history of physical therapy practice in the United States. *Journal of Physical Therapy Education, 17*(3), 15–25.

Ogunsiji, O., & Wilkes, L. (2005). Managing family life while studying: Single mothers' lived experience of being students in a nursing program. *Contemporary Nurse, 18*(1–2), 108–123.

Silver, J. H., Sr. (2002). Diversity issues. In R. Diamond (Ed.), *Field guide to academic leadership* (pp. 357–372). San Francisco: Jossey-Bass.

Splenser, P. E., Canlas, H. L., Sanders, B., & Melzer, B. (2003). Monirity recruitment and retention strategies in physical therapist education programs. *Journal of Physical Therapy Education, 17*(1), 18–26.

Suinn, R. M. (2006). Teaching culturally diverse students. In W. J. McKeachie, & M. Svinicki (Eds.), McKeachie's teaching tips (12th ed., pp. 152–171). Boston: Houghton Mifflin.

Vasquez, J. (1990). Instructional responsibilities of college faculty to minority students. *Journal of Negro Education*, *59*, 599–610.

Villaruel, A. M., Canales, M., & Torres, S. (2001). Educational mobility of Hispanic nurses. *Journal of Nursing Education, 40*(6), 245–251.

Wessling, S. (2000, Fall). Coming home: two unique programs are giving homeless and disadvantaged persons an opportunity to start again as nursing professionals. *Minority Nurse*, 32–35.

Yoder, M. (1996). Instructional responses to ethnically diverse nursing students. *Journal of Nursing Education*, *35*, 315–321.

SUGGESTED READING

Byrne, M. (2001). Uncovering racial bias in nursing fundamentals textbooks. *Nursing and Health Care Perspectives*, *22*, 299–303.

Dickerson, S., & Neary, M. (1999). Faculty experiences teaching Native Americans in a university setting. *Journal of Transcultural Nursing, 10*(1), 56–64.

Edward, J. (2000). Teaching strategies for foreign nurses. *Journal for Nurses in Staff Development, 16*(4), 171–173.

Griffiths, M., & Tagliareni, E. (1999). Challenging traditional assumptions about minority students in nursing education. *Nursing & Health Care Perspectives*, *20*, 290–295.

Maruyama, G., Moreno, J. F., Gudeman, R. H., & Marin, P. (2000). *Does diversity make a difference? Three research studies on diversity in college classrooms*. Washington, DC; American Association of University Professors.

Maville, J., & Huerta, C. (1997). Stress and social support among Hispanic student nurses: Implications for academic achievement. *Journal of Cultural Diversity*, *4*(1), 18–25.

Miller, J. E., & Hollenshead, C. (2005). Gender, family, and flexibility—why they're important in the academic workplace. *Change, 37*(6), 58–62.

Taylor, V., & Rust, G. (1999). The needs of students from diverse cultures. *Academic Medicine, 74*, 302–304.

Weaver, H. (2001). Indigenous nurses and professional education: Friends or foe? *Journal of Nursing Education*, *40*, 252–258.

Yurkovich, E. (2001). Working with American Indians toward educational success. *Journal of Nursing Education*, *40*, 259–269.

ELECTRONIC RESOURCES

Center for Teaching and Learning. (1997). *Teaching for Inclusion: Diversity in the college classroom*. Chapel Hill, NC: University of North Carolina at Chapel Hill. Retrieved November 8, 2009, from http://cfe.unc.edu/pdfs/TeachforInclusion.pdf

Gurin, P., Dey, E. L., Hurtado, S., & Gurin, G. (2002). Diversity and higher education: Theory and impact on educational outcomes. *Harvard Educational Review, 72*(3). Retrieved November 8, 2009, from http://gseweb.harvard.edu/~hepg/gurin.html

U. S. Department of Justice. (2009). *ADA regulations and technical assistance materials*. Retrieved November 8, 2009, from http://www.usdoj.gov/crt/ada/publicat.htm

CHAPTER 3

Strategies for Innovation

Arlene J. Lowenstein

The scope of change in health care has been enormous, and the rate at which change occurs continues to accelerate. Today's technology and therapeutics were inconceivable even a few decades ago. Over time, the growth of the health professions has been influenced by those new technologies and therapeutics, but there are many other influencing factors and forces, including, but not limited to:

- The appearance of new diseases, such as H1N1 flu, HIV/AIDS, and Lyme disease.
- War and its consequences, which brought new techniques to care for burns and radiation, growth in the use of penicillin and other antibiotics, treatment for posttraumatic stress disorder, growth of nursing and rehabilitation services in the military, and veterans' systems.
- Sociocultural issues—including the Civil Rights Movement, the feminist movement, the consumer revolution of the late 1960s and 1970s, and changing immigration and demographic patterns—that brought dramatic changes in maternity care from shortened length of stay to sibling visitation and increased focus on care of the elderly and end-of-life care. Diversity has increased in healthcare education and practice, and more emphasis has been placed on culturally competent care.
- Religious issues brought in ethical components of care and the development of parish nursing.
- Changing economics, as evidenced in the recession of 2008/2009, and political/legal issues brought us Medicare, Medicaid, managed care, legalized abortion, and the debate over healthcare reform.
- Changes in education brought nursing into academic settings and gave rise to nursing science and nursing research, thereby changing practice and creating new roles, such as advanced practice nursing and the newest, the

Doctor of Nursing Practice (DNP). Physical therapy embraced the Doctor of Physical Therapy (DPT) as an entry-level degree and other health professions have developed and evolved as well.

These forces are not isolated but are part of the total environment in which we live and work. They are ever-changing and interacting, challenging health professions educators to keep on top of the trends, technologies, and resources, while enabling self-directed student learning. Graduates who are self-directed learners understand and are responsive to healthcare system changes when they are in practice and out of the school setting, where there are no faculty members with whom to consult.

Healthcare educators straddle the fields of healthcare practice and education. They need to be knowledgeable about changes in practice and technology in both fields. What healthcare practitioners learn, as well as how they are taught, must keep pace with the changing milieu. The field of education has also changed over the years because of many of the same forces that affected health care. Technology and therapeutics in health care can be compared to a new understanding of learning theories and teaching methods in education. The student entering a healthcare profession from high school today is most likely much more comfortable with the use of computers than the registered nurse (RN) returning to school or an older student who has chosen a health profession as a second career. Online courses are now in the mainstream.

Health professions classrooms are also more culturally diverse than ever before. More men are entering the nursing profession and more women are going to medical schools. Younger students may have had very different cultural experiences in the secondary schools than did older students. Older students may be dealing with the added stress of parenthood and job responsibilities. Different cultures and experiences may produce different expectations of teaching and learning. Respecting learning-need differences and establishing an innovative climate in the classroom can help to prepare students for the changes they will face in practice. An educational climate that values different viewpoints and experiences among students encourages those students to create their own innovations. Those innovations will serve them in good stead by enhancing positive interactions with the wide variety of persons for whom they will be caring and with whom they will be working.

Sources of information have multiplied. The Internet has introduced the possibility of learning over long distances. The barrier of geography has been breached. Even nurses in rural communities have access to continued learning by highly qualified nurse educators. Innovative computer-based materials can provide technical training within the classroom—audio and video combining to offer a breadth of exposure previously only available through many hours at the bedside.

Instant messaging is available, and we can listen to lectures over podcasts and locate reference material instantly through our very own personal digital assistants (PDAs). We can have two-way access between health settings and homes with the use of SKYPE—a software application that provides the ability to make voice calls, complete with pictures, over the Internet—and telemedicine, so a person many miles away can join you in your living room or in a health facility. The use of simulators has increased. This capability is becoming much more important as productivity pressures make clinical sites for student experience harder and harder to find.

How do we teach more and more information to our students without overwhelming them? And how do we maintain the underlying paradigm of care and compassion? How do we maintain the threads of patient-centered, holistic, and compassionate care within the complex scientific information our students must master? In this textbook, we hope to provide health professions educators with ideas and examples that will allow students to master the facts and theory as well as the perspective of a caring professional. Implementing and adapting these methods will lead to further discovery of successful teaching strategies to keep pace with changes in the profession.

EXAMPLES OF INNOVATION

Innovative teaching strategies can range from simple to complex. Innovations can be developed for an exercise within a course or for the method by which the entire course is taught. Teaching innovations can be developed for whole programs, or even whole schools. They can be developed by one faculty member or by groups of faculty members. The prime objective is that the teaching strategies selected must address what needs to be learned in relation to the learning needs of students.

Think back to a favorite teacher or any strongly remembered event. Why does it stand out? What makes it unique among similar events? A major factor can be the realization that one object was completely different or out of its usually defined place, whereas the surrounding objects appeared normal. The teachers we remember often stood apart from our perception of others by only one or two details, but these details were out of the normal range. We remember the different much more than the normal, yet we can grasp only a small amount of different and a large amount of the usual. The occasional nondigestible, completely different piece in the sea of the expected forces us to analyze not just the different piece, but also the other 99% rote material normally not given much attention and easily forgotten. Kirp, a professor of public policy, asked a former student, who was now a college professor, what she remembered about his teaching. He was astonished to hear that she remembered his baseball stories. She elaborated that the baseball anecdotes prodded her into thinking of him as more approachable and more human. Once she felt that way, she began to pay attention (Kirp, 1997).

Exhibit 3-1 is an example of using something different in a lesson: an analogy of pain management to the sinking of the Titanic. The objective is to allow students to apply what they already know to other situations. Students will remember more if they can make their own discovery.

Art, literature, storytelling, humor, and technology-assisted learning can all be used in innovative ways. Whitman and Rose (2003) had students choose a media to express their nursing philosophy. This technique required students to think

EXHIBIT 3-1

Analogy: Pain Management and the Sinking of the Titanic

The aftermath of bone surgery, such as ankle fusion, is a very painful procedure for patients. An analogy was used to create a more dynamic understanding of a patient's experience with pain and the need for appropriate pain relief measures. The choice of the Titanic disaster as an analogy actually came from a patient's description of the pain he felt in the postoperative period and his feeling that the nursing staff needed to pay more attention to pain relief. He felt there were times when he was totally immersed with the pain, and relief could have been started sooner and on a more even keel.

The Titanic was constructed with six watertight compartments that were expected to withstand a breach and keep the ship afloat. The compartments had very high walls but, unfortunately, no top. The design was appropriate for most possibilities, except the accident that actually happened. Students were told to think of the walls as the job of the pain medication and water as the pain. The wall of the pain medication isolates the water from the ship and the passengers' realization that they are surrounded by water. The pain is hidden. The danger lies in what happens if the water in the first compartment overflows its limit and then starts filling the second compartment. If up to three of these compartments fill with water (pain), it may not interfere with the ship's normal function; however, as the effect cascades into more of the compartments, the ship sinks by the bow until "all hands lost."

Patients initially do not understand that a sea of pain surrounds them. As the pain relief diminishes and they suddenly (perhaps by waking from sleep) find themselves immersed, a fear of this unexpected and uncomfortable situation is formed. This fear becomes a constant presence even after pain relief is restored, leading to anxiety and apprehension over the possibility of a repeat experience. In very painful procedures, this fear can result in "clock watching" over the medication schedule as well as a compulsion to do anything to stay ahead of the pain curve. Appropriate pain relief measures, timing of administration, and other nursing measures can be discussed—all the while continuing use of the analogy (e.g., use of lifeboats in the pain relief cycle). Students can also be taught to develop and share their own analogies to improve learning retention.

differently about what they were doing and what they believed. One student used a guitar and song to express his philosophy of healing. Another painted a brain within a heart, which symbolized her need to incorporate compassion as well as intellect into patient care. A third wrote a poem to express her feelings and beliefs. This technique used sight, touch, and movement in addition to listening, which encouraged retention post class for both the creator of the piece and the viewer.

DEVELOPING INNOVATIVE STRATEGIES

Innovation can occur at all levels of an educational organization. Support for innovation in education may begin at the top of the organization or be developed and implemented at program or individual class levels. Success is enhanced when administrators and faculty members work side by side to plan strategically and implement changes to improve the educational milieu (Woods, 1998).

Innovation at the school level was demonstrated by a group of business school educators. These schools chose to focus more on entrepreneurship and to move away from the traditional management that prepared students to work in large organizations. This strategic innovation recognized the realities of the marketplace in a changing world. These schools set the pace for others to follow ("They create winners," 1994). In working with social workers, Michael Chovanec (2008) recognized an educational need that was not being met. While group process may be in the curriculum for social workers, they often need to work with involuntary groups, such as court-ordered programs in domestic abuse and chemical dependency. There is a very different process needed to work with people who do not want to be there, but are forced to attend. Chovanec developed three innovative frameworks to teach social work students about this type of work. His article describes those frameworks as *reactance theory* for working with the reactions of those who do not want to be in the group, a *stages of change* model, and *motivational interviewing*, which encourages working with clients to improve their self-motivation. His model provides guidelines and exercises for students to mock up unpleasant experiences that they may be exposed to in their practice.

Nursing education has grown through innovation. Mildred Montag's introduction of the associate degree program in nursing, developed through research to meet an assessed need, changed the landscape of nursing education. The introduction of nurse practitioner programs also created a revolution in the profession. The physical therapy profession has endorsed the Doctor of Physical Therapy (DPT) as the entry-level degree and strongly encouraged schools to provide transition programs for physical therapists currently in practice. The introduction of distance learning in all of the health professions is the latest revolution and growing rapidly, offering students different choices that are unfettered by the barrier of geography.

EXHIBIT 3-2

The Process of Innovation

Assessment

What is the content to be learned? What are the student learning needs? How are those needs being met? What is working and what is not?

Define Options

How else can I look at this? Does the literature provide suggestions that would address the identified needs? Do students or other faculty members have suggestions that I could utilize?

Plan

1. Does this change require working with curriculum committees, collaborating with other faculty members, or individual instructor planning? How should this change be approached?
2. Will there be a need to work with technical specialists in the use of computer technology? Do I need additional technological knowledge to carry out this change?
3. How can I best use change theory in this planning? Who are the stakeholders that need to be considered? How and where will I meet resistance? How will I develop support?
4. How will I plan to evaluate the effectiveness of this innovation?

Gain Support for Innovation

What resources will be needed? How will they be acquired and funded? What is the level of administrative support required and available? What strategies will I use to gain additional support if needed?

Prepare Students for the Innovation

Do I need written student instructions? If so, are they clear? Have I provided a mechanism for troubleshooting problems, and do students know how to address problems?

Prepare Faculty Members for the Innovation

If other faculty members are involved, do they need additional education? How will that be carried out? Is everyone in agreement as to how the strategy will be run? Is rehearsal time needed?

Implement the Innovation

How much flexibility is available if the intervention is not going well? Will follow up be needed?

Evaluate the Outcome

How will I measure the learning outcome? How have students reacted to the strategy, and can they provide input for change or improvement? If other faculty members are involved, can a consensus be reached about the direction for needed change and/or support for continuation?

Successful innovation does not come easily and requires creativity, planning, and evaluation. Exhibit 3-2 describes a process educators can use to develop innovative teaching strategies. Just as health professions call for patient assessments, the educational process calls for learning and program assessments. ***Assessment*** of a course requires a look at both strengths and problems. How can the strengths be enhanced? What needs to be changed? Educators must focus on the expected learning outcomes and be aware of learning theory and student learning styles and needs. Specific content requirements change often in health care, as new techniques, technologies, and research bring new knowledge needs. With the overwhelming amount of information available in today's healthcare world, it will not be possible to include everything students need. They will need to have appropriate resources to supplement classroom or clinical learning. The instructor must decide what and how much content will be needed, a decision that is often difficult. While addressing the content to be learned, it is also important to consider student learning needs. An understanding of the diversity in learning needs provides a foundation for the development of effective strategies.

To ***define options*** the literature should be searched for research, suggestions, or techniques that could address the identified needs. Asking students or other faculty members for suggestions can also be helpful. This is the place where creativity reigns. It is important to look at the many different ways to address the learning objective, before selecting one. Asking the question "is there another way to look at this?" can be fun and lead to additional options.

Once a strategy has been selected, ***planning*** is all-important. Understanding who the stakeholders are and their investment in the status quo or in change can be helpful in planning strategies to bring them on board. Many stakeholders, including students, do not like change and will resist new approaches. Using change theory can assist in demonstrating need and provide information that can make resisters more amenable to change. Some strategies will require curricular change, which is a complicated process and one that needs to be started early to avoid implementation delays. It is important to take time to develop support for the strategy. If this is a simple change within a course, then the instructor will need students to participate effectively and not sabotage the effort. In more complex strategies, it may be important to bring in other faculty members or administrators.

Some strategies will need help from technical specialists who may be able to offer support and/or instruction for using the required equipment. Time must be allotted for adequate instruction to enable faculty members and students to reach a comfort level. Most importantly, the technical staff must be available to help solve problems, which are bound to occur. Planning strategies for troubleshooting and providing access for problem solving for both faculty members and students need to be thought out in advance of implementation.

Another phase of the planning process is planning for the evaluation of the strategy. This is the time to decide what needs to be evaluated and how it should be done. This phase can range from how the strategy will be used in student grading to evaluating learning outcomes for the class as a whole; it needs to be developed to allow student and faculty input for future development. This can also be the time to develop an educational research project, if appropriate. Educational research and publication of results are needed and can assist all of us in understanding and applying an effective educational process.

Gaining support for the innovation is the next step. Some strategies require little or no resources to implement, whereas others require significant physical and/or financial resources. If resources are needed, then gaining support for acquisition of those resources is essential. Looking at alternative sources of funding is helpful. Grants can provide a good funding source but require time and effort to secure and may be available for a limited time. Administrative support may be required, but administrators may also be an excellent resource to tap for potential funding or acquisition of physical resources. Once the project has been developed, it is important to validate the support of stakeholders.

Class preparation is a given in education. ***Preparing students for the innovation*** is an important step. Student instructions need to be clear and specific. This is the time for motivating students to want to try this process and for gaining their support. Students need to know how to address problems, especially when technology is involved. There may be a learning curve required with some strategies. Students need to feel comfortable that they will not be punished for mistakes, but rather will benefit from those mistakes as part of the learning process. Evaluation methods or grading must be made clear.

Faculty members may also need preparation for the innovation. For some strategies, rehearsal time may be needed, or additional education may be required. Planning sufficient time for those activities will increase everyone's comfort level with the process. This is the time to be sure that everyone agrees about how the strategy will be run. Use of *perception*, *validation*, and *clarification* (I use the mnemonic *PVCs* when I teach students about this) can be valuable here. Health professionals are familiar with cardiac premature ventricular contractions as PVCs, but using this term in a different context can help students relate to the term and remember it better. Too often, people interpret statements differently. Checking that everyone has the same perceptions (validating) and clarifying any differences can provide unity in the approach to students and reduce the problem of students playing one instructor against another. "Remember your PVCs" reminds us to think about this issue.

The best part of the process is ***implementing the innovation***. It is hoped that things will go well, but flexibility may be required if problems arise. Sometimes, unintended consequences, such as surfacing of emotional issues, can occur. Instructors should be alert to the need for follow-up or referral if problems arise.

Evaluating the outcome is the final step in the process. Remember that learning can continue to occur long after implementation of the strategy. It may be possible to measure short-term attainment of learning outcomes, but it may or may not be possible to explore long-term effects. For certain strategies that were developed to provide a foundation for other learning experiences, it may be possible to remeasure students at the end of their program. Students and faculty members should be able to provide input for future development and use of the strategy. A strong evaluation process provides an opportunity to participate in educational research. Even if a strategy is not suitable for research, it still may be appropriate for publication. Sharing teaching strategies presents the opportunity to improve the educational process. A catchword in health care today is "evidence-based practice." We also need evidence-based practice in education.

Teaching Example

Interdisciplinary Case Study Analysis

An example of an innovative strategy at the school level was the introduction of interdisciplinary case studies to health profession students. Healthcare providers interact daily with members of other disciplines. The mission statement of the health professions school, with programs in nursing, physical therapy, and communications sciences disorders, included the following:

> While health professionals must be prepared to provide expert care within their respective disciplines, they contribute to evaluating and improving health care delivery by working in close cooperation with professionals from other disciplines. Students educated in an interdisciplinary setting, one that integrates academic and clinical pursuits, will be well-equipped to function as members of the health care team. The involvement of active practitioners from different fields in program planning, student supervision, and teaching supports such an integrated program (MGH Institute of Health Professions, 2000, p. 13).

Faculty members and administrators felt the need to strengthen the manner in which students interacted with other disciplines. Although students were exposed to a few multidisciplinary courses, such as research and ethics, there was overall agreement that they needed more useful exposure to other disciplines within a clinical context. An interdisciplinary faculty task force was developed to explore possibilities. The academic dean staffed the task force and provided administrative support. After much discussion, the task force settled on a series of four required interdisciplinary clinical seminars as the preferred method.

The mechanics of developing and implementing the program were daunting, but the group was committed to the project. They enlisted other members of their departments to develop four case studies—one for each seminar. The subject of the case study would require care from each of the three disciplines: nursing, physical therapy, and speech pathology. Thought was given to the need for students to be involved with different age groups and various clinical settings. Teams of faculty members with expertise in each area developed the following cases:

- **Seminar Case 1:** Pediatric patient with cerebral palsy who is starting school.
- **Seminar Case 2:** Elderly patient with cerebral vascular accident and dysphagia in an acute care setting.
- **Seminar Case 3:** Middle-aged adult in the community with HIV (end stages of illness) and family issues.
- **Seminar Case 4:** Young teen with traumatic brain injury in a rehabilitation center.

The intensive involvement of many faculty members in the development of the cases had some very beneficial effects. Interdisciplinary cooperation was necessary as the cases were developed. Faculty members were able to learn from each other and appreciate the roles of the other disciplines. The faculty members who developed the cases were invested in the project and were able to support and commend it to other faculty members and to students in their classes, which reduced some resistance.

Each program was responsible for determining which students would be required to attend the seminars. The nursing program selected students who were in the spring semester of the second year of an entry-level master's program and were enrolled in the Primary Care I course. Nursing students in this program held a baccalaureate in any field prior to entry into the program. They had completed the first year and second fall semester in the generalist level of the nursing program. They were in the process of taking the RN licensing exam during this semester (they all passed). They were now in advanced-level course work that would lead to a Master's of Science in Nursing degree and eligibility to sit for certification as a nurse practitioner. Interdisciplinary seminar attendance was mandatory and counted as part of the clinical component in the Primary Care I course, so that students would not be required to add hours to the course. Compromise and negotiation were needed on the part of the course faculty to recognize and accept that the interdisciplinary seminar was a legitimate learning experience appropriate to the course.

Scheduling the seminars was a major problem. Coordinating three programs with students in different classes and in clinical sites was very difficult. The seminars were held in the late afternoon, and students in clinical placements were asked to leave their clinical site early enough to return to the school. There is no easy answer to this problem. Each student was sent a letter outlining the purpose of the seminars and given the dates and times. The letter explained that attendance was mandatory and that the seminar would count as class hours.

Approximately 60 students were expected to attend the seminars. Four faculty members from each department were recruited to facilitate each seminar. In smaller departments, this meant that department faculty members participated in more than one seminar. The case discussions were designed so that students had an opportunity to participate in multidisciplinary groups, meet with their own specialty, and meet as a total group. The sessions were planned to last for 2 hours each.

The role of the faculty members was to facilitate but not to lead the discussion among students. Faculty members were available to correct wrong information, but the focus was to have students take responsibility for explaining their discipline's role in working with the patient. Faculty members were not expected to be experts in the area under discussion or to introduce new material. The faculty role was explained to the students at the beginning of the session.

Previously prepared case materials presented assessment tools used by each discipline and questions to be addressed. The goals of the seminar were presented and clarified to all of the students before breaking students into groups. Students presented their assessments and plans for working with the patients, defining priorities of care. Faculty facilitators encouraged participation by all. Each small group took notes to be presented to the entire group for general discussion.

Evaluations of the seminars from both faculty members and students were excellent. The time selected for the seminars was problematic for many participants and seemed to be the major concern of students. Some students had various excuses for not being able to attend. Snow forced the cancellation of one session. All students attended a minimum of one seminar, but most attended the sessions as scheduled. Students remarked that the discussions were excellent and that they had learned new knowledge from each other as the different disciplinary approaches were presented. Faculty members also benefited from the discussions, and interdepartmental communications were enhanced. Some faculty members were uncomfortable at first with the expectation of their role and were concerned that they did not know enough about specific cases; however, most soon realized that the objectives of the session were valid for the level of their expertise and the expectation of facilitation, not instruction. Overall, the project was deemed a strong success and was presented again, with minor changes.

The program has now evolved, but the commitment to interdisciplinary education remains and has expanded. For this year, students will have at least one interdisciplinary learning experience in each year. Each department is responsible for developing the experience for their students and school-wide presentations will be carried out each semester. A full evaluation will be completed at the end of the spring semester.

REFERENCE

MGH Institute of Health Professions. (2000). Mission statement. *MGH Institute of Health Professions Self-Study*, 13.

CONCLUSION

Innovative teaching strategies must be based on both learning objectives and student learning needs. The wide diversity of student learning needs means that educators must recognize that, although most students will benefit from the new approaches, some will not. This perspective can be disappointing, but it is realistic, and educators must take pride in what they have accomplished. Problems will occur that no amount of planning could foresee. These problems, although disturbing at the time, are often humorous memories in the future and can be addressed to improve future offerings. Developing effective teaching strategies is challenging and requires effort and persistence but can also be exceedingly rewarding and fun. Sharing those strategies with others will benefit students and faculty alike. We hope you will take advantage of the strategies presented in this book and go on to develop, implement, and share your own innovative strategies.

REFERENCES

Chovanec, M. (2008). Innovations applied to the classroom for involuntary groups: Implications for social work education. *Journal of Teaching in Social Work, 28*(1/2), 209–225.

Kirp, D. L. (1997). Those who can't: 27 ways of looking at a classroom. *Change 29*(3), 10–19.

They create winners. (1994). *Success, 41*(7), 43–46.

Whitman, B. L., & Rose, W. J. (2003). Using art to express a personal philosophy of nursing. *Nurse Educator, 28*(4), 166–169.

Woods, D. R. (1998). Getting support for your new approaches. *Journal of College Science Teaching, 27*(4), 285–286.

ADDITIONAL RESOURCES

Butell S. S., O'Donovan, P., & Taylor. J. D. (2004). Educational innovations. Instilling the value of reading literature through student-led book discussion groups. *Journal of Nursing Education, 43*(1), 40–44.

Jesse, D. E., & Blue, C. (2004). Mary Breckinridge meets Healthy People 2010: a teaching strategy for visioning and building healthy communities. *Journal of Midwifery & Women's Health, 49*(2), 126–131.

Nof, L., & Hill, C. (2005). On the cutting edge - A successful distance PhD degree program: A case study. *The Internet Journal of Allied Health Sciences and Practice*, 3(2). Retrieved November 8, 2009, from http://ijahsp.nova.edu/articles/vol3num2/nof.htm

Travis, L., & Brennan, P. F. (1998). Information science for the future: An innovative nursing infomatics curriculum. *Journal of Nursing Education,* 37(4), 162–168.

CHAPTER 4

Critical Thinking in the Health Professions

Patricia R. Cook

INTRODUCTION

Let us set the stage: The patient is a 62-year-old woman admitted with anemia. Twenty-four hours prior to admission the patient fainted in the grocery store. Because of the patient's history of uterine cancer 6 years ago and the possibility of metastasis, she is admitted for a comprehensive evaluation. As a registered nurse (RN), you admit the patient to the unit and conduct your initial interview. The patient informs you that her stools have been very dark and that she has been taking an anti-inflammatory drug for her swollen knee. Is this information related to her admitting diagnosis? What components of the patient's history should the nurse consider as relative to the current situation?

Every day healthcare providers are faced with situations such as this example. Nurses are required to think critically in order to deliver safe and competent nursing care. The challenge facing healthcare education today is to develop a curriculum that contains effective teaching/learning strategies for students to develop skills in critical thinking. Utilization of critical thinking gives a care provider the advantage of looking at things from a point of view that is grounded in purposeful and methodical thinking. This challenge seems at face value to be fairly simple, but this task is difficult and complex for those responsible for educating tomorrow's healthcare professionals.

DEFINITION OF CRITICAL THINKING

Scholars from various disciplines have examined the concept of critical thinking to gain a better understanding of this process. Dewey (1933) used the phrase reflective thinking to describe this process. Following Dewey's contributions to understanding critical thinking, Watson and Glaser (1980) looked at critical thinking and identified three elements that make up this thinking process, namely, attitude, knowledge, and skill. First, the critical thinker must have the attitude or desire to approach the problem and to accept that the problem needs to be solved. Next, the critical thinker must have knowledge of the problem's subject matter. The critical thinker then must have the necessary skills to use and manipulate this knowledge in the problem-solving process.

Ennis (1985) studied critical thinking and defined it as "reflective and reasonable thinking that is focused on deciding what to believe or do" (p. 45). He added that critical thinking is a practical activity that requires creativity in identifying hypotheses, questions, options, and ways of experimentation. Based on a philosophy background and an in depth study of critical thinking, Paul (1993) identified critical thinking as thought that is "disciplined, comprehensive, based on intellectual standards, and as a result, well-reasoned" (p. 20). Paul related seven characteristics of the critical thinker.

1. It is thinking which is responsive to and guided by intellectual standards such as relevance, accuracy, precision, clarity, depth, and breadth.
2. It is thinking that deliberately supports the development of intellectual traits in the thinker, such as intellectual humility, intellectual integrity, intellectual perseverance, intellectual empathy, and intellectual self-discipline, among others.
3. It is thinking in which the thinker can identify the elements of thought that are present in all thinking about any problem, such that the thinker makes the logical connection between the elements and the problem at hand.
4. It is thinking that is routinely self-assessing, self-examining, and self-improving.
5. It is thinking in which there is integrity to the whole system.
6. It is thinking that yields a predictable, well-reasoned answer because of the comprehensive and demanding process that the thinker pursues.
7. It is thinking that is responsive to the social and moral imperative to not only enthusiastically argue from alternate and opposing points of view, but also to seek and identify weaknesses and limitations in one's own position (pp. 20–23).

Probably the most substantial definition of critical thinking was developed in the late 1980s by a group of theoreticians and published by the American Philosophical Association (APA) in 1990. This group identified the critical thinker as one who is:

> Habitually inquisitive, well-informed, trustful of reason, open-minded, flexible, fair-minded in evaluation, honest in facing personal biases, prudent in making judgments, willing to reconsider, clear about issues, orderly in complex matters,

diligent in seeking relevant information, reasonable in the selection of criteria, focused in inquiry, and persistent in seeking results which are as precise as the subject and the circumstances of inquiry permit (p. 3).

Nursing has used these critical thinking definitions from education and philosophy to formulate its own view of this important concept. Facione and Facione (1996) described critical thinking as purposeful, self-regulatory judgment that gives reasoned consideration to evidence, content, conceptualization, methods, and criteria. Using the APA's definition of critical thinking, Facione and Facione identified the role of one's disposition in this thinking process. Within one's disposition there are seven elements: truth seeking, open mindedness, analyticity, systematicity, self-confidence, inquisitiveness, and maturity. Using these seven elements, Facione and Facione (1994) developed *The California Critical Thinking Disposition Inventory (CCTDI) Test Administration Manual*. This inventory was specifically put together to assess "one's opinions, beliefs, and attitudes" (p. 3).

Bandman and Bandman (1995) discussed the issue of critical thinking and the role of reasoning in this thinking process. If individuals are critically thinking, then they will "examine assumptions, beliefs, propositions, and the meaning and uses of words, statements, and arguments" (p. 4). They continued by identifying four types of reasoning that constitute critical thinking, namely deductive, inductive, informal, and practical reasoning.

Alfaro-LeFevre (2004) discussed critical thinking and noted that critical thinking is a synonym for "reasoning . . . that involves distinct ideas, emotions, and perceptions . . ." (p. 4). She delineated a description of critical thinking and noted that critical thinking in nursing:

1. Entails purposeful, outcome-directed (results-oriented) thinking that requires careful identification of key problems, issues, and risks involved.
2. Is driven by patient, family, and community needs.
3. Is based on principles of nursing process and scientific method (e.g., making judgments based on evidence rather than guesswork).
4. Uses both logic and intuition, based on knowledge, skills, and experience.
5. Is guided by professional standards and ethics codes.
6. Requires strategies that make the most of human potential (e.g., using individual strengths) and compensate for problems created by human nature (e.g., overcoming the powerful influence of personal views).
7. Is constantly reevaluating, self-correcting, and striving to improve (p. 5).

Scheffer and Rubenfeld (2000) used a four-round Delphi technique to reach a consensus among nursing faculty regarding a definition of critical thinking. This approach resulted in cluster labels for critical thinking called "habits of the mind" and "skills" (p. 358). Specifically, critical thinking in nursing was defined as:

Habits of the mind			
Confidence Contextual perspective Creativity	Flexibility Inquisitiveness Intellectual integrity	Intuition Open mindedness Perseverance	Reflection
Skills			
Analyzing Discriminating Logical reasoning	Applying standards Information seeking Predicting	Transforming knowledge	

IMPORTANCE IN THE HEALTH PROFESSIONS

Enter any healthcare setting today and the need for critical thinking is clearly evident. Situations in typical healthcare settings present a level of complexity that requires all care providers to make rational and responsible decisions. Specific reasons critical thinking is needed in health care today include:

1. Situations require the care provider to process and utilize a great deal of information.
2. Information related to health care continues to expand on a daily basis.
3. Trends in health care have forced sick patients home prematurely, requiring extensive and complex home health care.
4. Changing staffing patterns in acute care facilities challenge nurses and other providers to care for high acuity patients.
5. Changes in health care—many of which we cannot begin to imagine—will continue to occur.
6. Trends in technology show continued advances in diagnostics and treatment modalities.
7. Society continues to grow in complexity, with many diverse cultures represented in American society.

Health professionals of today and of the future must have the ability to use valuable time to think in an effective, organized, goal-directed, and open-minded manner. Clinicians must solve problems using a variety of mental processes, such as reasoning, reflection, judgment, and creativity. Health professions education has the responsibility to produce graduates who possess and utilize critical thinking. In addition to critical thinking and clinical reasoning, students need to develop skills in personal assessment, peer assessment, and to recognize the value of lifelong learning (Candela, Dalley, & Bensel-Lindley, 2006). Furthermore, the future of the graduate depends on educational programs that continuously evaluate their programs and implement needed changes to ensure graduates' success on licensure exams and success as a member of the healthcare workforce. Therefore, teaching/learning strategies that promote the development of critical thinking need to be identified.

THE ROLE OF HEALTH PROFESSIONS EDUCATION

In education for the health professions, the challenge of producing students who think critically needs to be met by first examining all components of the teaching/learning process: curriculum, teaching/learning strategies, and evaluation measures. Critical thinking is a process that is developed over time in the individual; thus, teaching strategies and learning experiences must be learner-centered. For learner-centered education to take place, the student must be motivated, self-directed, and able to make decision that result in appropriate actions—that is, take responsibility for their own learning outcomes. Seasoned educators recognize that learners vary in motivation, influential personal experiences, and learning styles (Candela et al., 2006).

If the education program implements an effective and comprehensive curriculum, identifies useful teaching/learning strategies to teach critical thinking, and applies appropriate evaluation measures, then students will be assured that they are exiting their programs with skills in critical thinking. Teaching/learning strategies can be identified based on key elements of critical thinking identified by Watson and Glaser (1980), namely, attitude, knowledge, and skill.

Attitude

Given any situation in health care, students must first recognize that a problem exists and is worthy of solving. Faculty must utilize teaching/learning strategies that instill an attitude of curiosity and caring. From the first day of class until graduation, faculty should present common healthcare problems and relate them to needed interventions. Clinical experiences provide students with opportunities to apply the concepts of patient care in real life situations. This introduction to real life situations promotes the interest of students and develops awareness of the many problems to be solved. Instructors play an important part in developing an attitude of inquiry by guiding students to ask questions, examine or challenge current practices, look for answers, and evaluate various factors in the delivery of care.

Knowledge

The issue of what to include in a curriculum continues to frustrate faculty. Today's knowledge of disease and illness has never been greater. Therefore, faculty must evaluate the content of their curricula and include concepts that focus on developing a knowledge base that is applicable to multiple situations. Curriculum forms the structure for presenting concepts that provide for the development of critical thinking skills.

With a sound curriculum in place, nursing education is faced with identifying teaching/learning strategies that promote learning and the development of critical thinking. Unfortunately, there is no simple answer to developing the skill called "critical thinking." In her discussion of teaching methods, Klaassens (1988) identified four principles for teaching critical thinking. First, the teaching method should move systematically through the stages of readiness, introduction, reinforcement, and extension. Second, it should be focused, moving from introduction of task and explanation of steps to presentation, supervised practice, and return demonstration by the student. Third, this method should blend with the typical topics and, fourth, it should guide students through the steps of knowledge acquisition—ending in formal thinking.

The traditional strategy for imparting knowledge in a nursing classroom has been lecture. Although students often prefer this teaching strategy, it does little to stimulate critical thinking.

In 1979, Steinaker and Bell identified an experiential taxonomy for use in planning and evaluating educational programs. Using a taxonomy reinforces that teaching/learning strategies should be evaluated and implemented based on the strategy's ability to reinforce learning where the student is at the time of the expected learning. The taxonomy developed by Steinaker and Bell (1979) has five categories, with varying levels within each category. These categories are exposure, participation, identification, internalization, and dissemination. The categories of exposure, participation, and identification are used to discuss the framework for appropriate teaching/learning strategies. The categories of internalization and dissemination are not being used because they require more experience within the practice of nursing following graduation from nursing programs.

Exposure

The category of exposure is used at the introduction level, at which the student is aware of the experience, begins to form mental reactions to the stimuli, and becomes prepared for more experience. At this level, the instructor is setting the stage for learning—in other words, presenting basic concepts. The goal is to develop skill in applying knowledge in the delivery of nursing care, but students must acquire knowledge prior to application. At this stage in learning, lecture is an effective strategy for the introduction of the content; however, students need additional teaching/learning strategies that offer them the opportunity to manipulate and process basic content.

The following strategies are effective tools in applying basic concepts:

1. Study guides: In this strategy, students seek out basic information related to the subject topic. The guide directs students to answer questions about the subject. Instructors can be creative in developing study guides and can use patient scenarios to promote beginning application thinking. Use of study guides encourages students to independently seek out information, which was supported by Rubenfeld and Scheffer (2006) in their comment that educators must "move toward learning partnerships focused on students discovering things for themselves" (p. 85). For many students, this beginning level of empowerment encourages them to be more responsible for their learning—a basic need for the critical thinker. As students study new material, ample opportunity that encourages students to ask why or how must be provided because this increases the value of one's learning new information (Nugent & Vitale, 2004).
2. Case studies: Using case studies to apply concepts is nothing new to nursing education. Using examples of how concepts are applied in a clinical setting encourages students to think about how concepts relate to real life situations. Case studies can be developed with varying levels of difficulty—ranging from the simple application of principles of hot and cold to the application of multiple concepts in the care of the burn patient. When using case studies at the exposure level, simple situations, focusing on specific focus concepts, should be included. Although case studies are often used as independent work for the student, they also are useful in the classroom. Case studies can be used as a class activity to teach students to think on their feet and to reinforce the need to understand concepts in real life situations. In other words, case studies take facts and use them in practical ways. This type of application shows students how selected interventions focus on outcomes for the patient (Youngblood & Beitz, 2001).
3. Group discussions: While participating in classroom discussions, students learn from other students while developing their personal thinking skills. In this setting, students challenge each other's ideas and opinions, which is an important component to critical thinking (Linderman & McAthie, 1999). When using an in-class activity such as group discussions, faculty need to continuously monitor the use of thinking and thoughtfulness and intervene as appropriate to redirect the group.

4. Writing: Students at all levels of a nursing curriculum can benefit from writing. At the basic level, students use concepts and build them into current knowledge as well as previous experiences. Development of papers requires the application of various tools of critical thinking, such as blending of concepts, determining priorities, and formulating conclusions (Nugent & Vitale, 2004). Using writing assignments provides the faculty with an opportunity to assess what students are learning and how well they process the new concepts.

Participation

At the second level of the taxonomy, students have purposeful interaction with the experience. Many of the exposure strategies also are suitable for the participation level, namely, writing, case studies, and computer-based interactive programs. Teaching/learning strategies at the participation level require recurrent thinking, because previously learned foundational concepts need to be used as students build on and learn beyond the basics. Writing, for example, requires students to move beyond the basic concepts and to use or apply them to a situation. Writing at the participation level promotes student recognition that patient situations are not textbook and that they require the selection of interventions appropriate to that specific patient. In her discussion of a writing project conducted in California, Olson (1992) identified four levels or domains of writing—sensory/descriptive, imaginative/narrative, practical/informative, and analytical/expository. The domain of sensory/descriptive is writing built on concrete concepts or points. The goal at this level is to center and focus on basic information. At the next level, students construct a story by means of identifying, sequencing, and capturing significant details. At the practical/informative level, students "learn accuracy, clarity, attention to facts, appropriateness to tone, and conventional forms" (p. 23). At the last level of the domain, students are expected to use the tasks of analysis, interpretation, and persuasion. Olson noted that these domains are not completely separate, and interdependency does exist among the levels.

Case studies used at the participation level should involve more creativity and reasoning than those used at the exposure level. With more knowledge, students can be challenged to bring together concepts that have an increasing number of variables. For example, at the exposure level, students learn to identify the role of vital signs in the assessment of their patients. At the participation level, students should begin identifying the alterations in vital signs that occur when diseases affect the body and should identify needed interventions.

Other teaching/learning strategies appropriate for the participation level include:

1. Problem-solving team: Using groups to work as a team provides an opportunity for the students to share ideas and knowledge while working on a common goal or outcome. For this strategy to be effective, the instructor must provide clear objectives with specific instructions. Brookfield (1987) identified themes characterizing critical thinking. One of those themes related to critical thinkers is the use of imagination and exploration of alternatives. Teamwork provides ample opportunity to spark imagination and creativity for the situation presented. Typically, group discussion leads to the identification of many alternatives; the group then evaluates and selects the needed interventions. This type of teaching/learning strategy promotes a second theme identified by Brookfield: the importance of context in critical thinking. No nursing or patient care situation is identical to another. Students must be able to assess each situation and to implement the required interventions. According to Linderman and McAthie (1999), when knowledge guides practice, it takes into consideration all other information gained through complementary means.
2. Reflective journals: Students' use of journals is an important tool to encourage reflection on an experience and to evaluate one's performance and/or responses to the experience. Reflection provides an opportunity to weigh, consider, and choose (Adams & Hamm, 1994). Use of a reflective journal encourages students to think about their experiences and to examine the components as well as the overall experience. To be effective, instructors need to give specific guidelines on what information to include in the journal. For example, the student first describes the patient care situation. Next, students provide an analysis of significant events in the delivery of patient care and an exploration of feelings, reactions, and responses. Critical thinking is developed further when students are asked to identify decisions made or priorities set during the clinical experience. In the last phase of journal writing, students "examine the outcomes of the reflective process" (Bratt, 1998, p. 1). After this examination, students often identify changes to be made in future experiences.
3. Problem-based learning: This teaching/learning strategy focuses primarily on process. A small student group works on a case study with the assistance of a faculty facilitator. This strategy links theory with clinical situations and encourages reasoning in a realistic situation using collaboration and negotiation within the group. See Chapter 9 for more information on this strategy.

4. Mind (concept) mapping: This simple but effective teaching/learning strategy requires students to develop word pictures for a specific patient problem. There are a variety of ways these maps can be constructed, but they all focus on helping students to reason, prioritize, and link the various components to a patient problem with nursing actions. Students conclude this activity with a holistic view of the situation at hand (Schuster, 2002). See Chapter 27 or more information on this strategy.
5. Questioning: Using questioning to reinforce learning is an excellent tool in the development of critical thinking. The use of questioning as a teaching tool can be traced back to Socrates in ancient Greece. Socratic questioning examines basic concepts or points, explores deeper into these concepts, and attends to problem areas of one's thinking (Paul, 1993). One effective way to use questioning is in a game format. It is easy to adapt popular games to the content being discussed. Gaming can be very effective because it infuses fun into learning.

Identification

At the identification level, students become more active learning partners. Students identify with the experience at an emotional and personal level. As the experience becomes a part of the students, they desire to share the experience with others. As previously noted, teaching/learning strategies, such as writing or case studies, continue to be important learning tools in the category of identification. With each of these strategies, there needs to be increasing complexity with more variables.

Additional teaching/learning strategies at the identification level should focus on organizing and applying concepts. Instructors play an important role at this level because they must rely on teaching/learning strategies that engage students to think in complex situations with more variables. Other teaching/ learning strategies for the identification category include:

1. Defensive testing: Students at this level need to be challenged more on why they select one option over another. They need to recognize that nursing care is based on principles and know which principle matches a specific situation—in other words, matching knowledge to the appropriate context. This strategy also provides students the opportunity to reflect on their understanding of the material being tested. Additionally, they are providing rationalization to their answers.
2. Debates and critiques: Having students critique an article or other type of work provides a means of reinforcing the six critical thinking abilities

identified by Linderman and McAthie (1999). These abilities include identifying possibilities/innovations, formulating and analyzing arguments, constructing meaning, using knowledge as context, negotiating, and critically reflecting on one's thoughts and actions. Seeking information and analyzing its meaning moves students beyond basic concepts and challenges traditional uses of these concepts. The strategy of debating is effective to developing critical thinking because it prepares students "to doubt, to challenge what is held to be true" (Smith, 1990, p. 104). If a student is required to debate the issue of abortion, he or she will formulate in depth critical thinking about the purpose of abortion, its impact on a woman, and how society views access to this intervention. See Chapter 11 for information on the use of debate.

3. Problem-based learning: With this teaching/learning strategy, students actively participate in problem solving. Discussion focuses on the problems presented in the case study and the identification of knowledge from previous experience with the identified problem(s).

Skill

Once students have developed an attitude of inquiry and the knowledge base needed, they need an opportunity to develop and apply knowledge in real life (clinical) situations.

The learning lab provides a tremendous opportunity for simulated learning. Although the learning lab traditionally has been used for learning psychomotor skills, it offers students a safe, controlled environment to develop critical thinking (see Chapter 15). As students' nursing knowledge increases over the span of the curriculum, instructors can use a high-fidelity patient simulator to create situations in the learning lab that promote student exploration into the various options available for nursing care (without injury to the patient). In this nonthreatening environment, students are provided the opportunity to question, explore, and experiment using a simulated patient scenario. Students can apply reasoning skills without the constraints of limited time and reflect on decisions made during the course of the experience. See Chapters 14 and 16 for more discussion of the use of high-fidelity simulators to promote student learning.

The clinical setting is identified as any setting where students provide nursing care to real patients. Today, clinical settings range from in-hospital units to homeless clinics in the community. In these clinical settings, learning opportunities to develop critical thinking abound. The challenge of all clinical instructors is to construct clinical experiences that maximize student learning. The clinical setting requires students to be familiar with their patients' health problems, medications, procedures, and lab data. Using their knowledge of the textbook patient, students are challenged to develop skills in critical thinking in their efforts to implement appropriate care for an actual patient.

Care of patients in real life situations reinforces that critical thinking is contextual. Although the textbook lists specific interventions for patients with pneumonia, students must recognize the care needed for a specific patient at a specific time. Using a variety of mental processes, such as reasoning, prioritizing, judging, and inferring, students are able to select needed interventions. As knowledge and clinical skills develop, students' skills in critical thinking increase.

There is no best style for instruction in the clinical setting; however, several points should be considered to increase the effectiveness of the clinical experience.

1. Questioning by the instructor is an important part of the clinical experience. This process encourages students to think about the options available and to select an intervention appropriate to a specific patient. A good technique to use when questioning students is asking the student to talk aloud while answering the instructor's questions (Corcoran, Narayan, & Moreland, 1988). Using this technique assists instructors in evaluating students' processing skills. Did they use appropriate reasoning skills? Was there a logical correlation between data and problem identification? Was the nursing process used appropriately, with logical sequencing of data, problem, goals, strategies or interventions, evaluation, and follow up with changes? Was there effective prioritization for the patient?
2. Students should be encouraged to test their thinking. Many healthcare alternatives are available today, and students need to explore what is best for their patients. The clinical setting provides the instructor with the opportunity to teach students on a one-on-one basis. Instructors need to verbally praise the student when the student performs correctly. Although clinical training is stressful and challenging, students need and deserve positive reinforcement of effective problem solving using critical thinking.
3. Instructors need to empower students to think critically. Students who feel a sense of empowerment take responsibility for the process of problem solving.
4. Instructors must see the importance and impact of role modeling. Using the teaching/learning strategy of modeling includes "leading the student through thoughts and experiences to one's own conclusions" (Reilly & Oermann, 1992, p. 331).
5. Written work related to clinical experiences is an important component in developing critical thinking. Students have the opportunity to take textbook patients and to select suitable interventions for their patients. The exercise of

individualizing nursing care reinforces the conceptuality of critical thinking and the need to explore all available options for patient care.

Kurfiss (1988) discussed the elements of what she called cognitive apprenticeship, which include modeling or demonstration, coaching or assisting, guiding with gradual removal of the guidance, articulating or reasoning, reflecting or comparing, and exploring goals and options. All of these elements can be accomplished with clinical experiences. Clinical experiences expose students to the dynamic world of health care and practice with multiple concepts. Whether collecting data and relating their role to the patient's condition or developing an argument on why one intervention is better than another, students are developing skills in critical thinking. See Chapters 25, 26, and 28 for more discussion of clinical instruction.

EVALUATION OF CRITICAL THINKING

In 1991, the National League for Nursing revised its criteria for accreditation and incorporated the need for evaluation of critical thinking in undergraduate nursing programs. The National League for Nursing Accrediting Commission (2005) recently reiterated its support of the need for critical thinking as noted in its core competencies for nursing educational programs. The American Association of Colleges of Nursing (1988) also emphasized critical thinking. Because of this notable recognition of critical thinking and its role as a competency for nursing, educators have explored, pondered, and discussed how critical thinking should be evaluated. While there is agreement on the need for critical thinking for all nurses, a consensus is absent on how critical thinking is defined and how it can be measured (Ali, Bantz, & Siktberg, 2005); however, evaluation of critical thinking is an important component of nursing education. Work within nursing education over the last few years has seen the identification of alternative options to evaluating critical thinking skills, such as concept maps and context-dependent testing (Daley, Shaw, Balistrieri, Glasenapp, & Piacentine, 1999; Oermann, Truesdell, & Ziolkowski, 2000).

Teaching and evaluation clearly go hand in hand. Nursing education is challenged to identify and/or develop tools for evaluating critical thinking that reflect the individual program's definition and philosophy. With the use of multiple means of evaluation, nursing education gains a better understanding of teaching critical thinking and the impact of this instruction on student learning. Students should see evaluation as a learning tool; it is a positive means for determining the need for additional learning, further clarification, and/or added directions by instructors.

CONCLUSION

Professional education's challenge to produce a care provider who can think critically has never been greater. Changing health care, increased acuity of patients, and a dynamic culture offer a tremendous challenge for nurses. Nursing education must attune itself to the task of reexamining the concept of critical thinking. This reexamination includes evaluation of all components of the teaching/learning process—curriculum, teaching/learning strategies, and evaluation measures.

Critical thinking is best advanced through learner-centered teaching approaches, some of which are described in this book: service learning, learning through discussion, team-based teaching, and a structured research course. These methods aid in the development of engagement, critical thinking, clinical reasoning, and innovative practice. Outcomes from these teaching approaches are that students take more responsibility for their own learning and show more maturity as learners (Kramer et al., 2007). In selecting approaches to develop critical thinking skills, faculty can assure their students that, as the healthcare workers of tomorrow, they will possess the necessary skills needed to deliver safe and competent patient care.

REFERENCES

Adams, D. M., & Hamm, M. E. (1994). *Cooperative learning: Critical thinking and collaboration across the curriculum*. Springfield, IL: Charles C Thomas Publisher.

Alfaro-LeFevre, R. (2004). *Critical thinking and clinical judgment: A practical approach*. Philadelphia: W. B. Saunders.

Ali, N. S., Bantz, D., & Siktberg, L. (2005). Validation of critical thinking skills in online responses. *Journal of Nursing Education, 44*(2), 90–96.

American Association of Colleges of Nursing. (1998). *The essentials of baccalaureate education for professional nursing practice*. Washington, DC: Author.

American Philosophical Association. (1990). *Critical thinking: A statement of expert consensus for purposes of educational assessment and instruction*. The Delphi report: Committee on pre-college philosophy (ERIC Document Reproduction Service No. ED 315–423). Millbrae, CA: The California Academic Press.

Bandman, E. L., & Bandman, D. (1995). *Critical thinking in nursing*. Norwalk, CT: Appleton & Lange.

Bratt, M. M. (1998). Reflective journaling: Fostering learning in clinical experiences. *Dean's Notes, 20*(1), 1–3.

Brookfield, S. (1987). *Developing critical thinkers: Challenging adults to explore alternative ways of thinking and acting*. San Francisco: Jossey-Bass.

Candela, L., Dalley, K., & Bensel-Lindley, J. (2006). A case for learning-centered curricula. *Journal of Nursing Education, 45*(2), 59–66.

Corcoran, S., Narayan, S., & Moreland, H. (1988). Thinking aloud as a strategy to improve clinical decision making. *Heart & Lung, The Journal of Critical Care, 17*(5), 463–468.

Daley, B. J., Shaw, C. R., Balistrieri, T., Glasenapp, K., & Piacentine, L. (1999). Concept maps: A strategy to teach and evaluate critical thinking. *Journal of Nursing Education, 38*(1), 42–47.

Dewey, J. (1933). *How we think: A restatement of the relation of reflective thinking to the educative process*. Chicago: Regnery.

Ennis, R. N. (1985). A logical basis for measuring critical thinking skills. *Educational Leadership, 43*(2), 44–48.

Facione, N., & Facione, P. A. (1994). *The California Critical Thinking Disposition Inventory (CCTDI) test administration manual*. Millbrae, CA: The California Academic Press.

Facione, N., & Facione, P. A. (1996). Externalizing the critical thinking in knowledge development and clinical judgment. *Nursing Outlook, 44*(3), 129–136.

Klaassens, E. L. (1988). Improving teaching for thinking. *Nurse Educator, 13*(6), 15–19.

Kramer, P., Ideishi, R.I., Kearney, P.J., Cohen, M.E., Ames, J.O., Shea, G.B., et al. (2007). Achieving curricular themes though learner-center teaching. *Occupational Therapy in Health Care, 21*(1–2), 185–198.

Kurfiss, J. G. (1988). *Critical thinking: Theory, research, practice, and possibilities*. College Station, TX: Association for the Study of Higher Education.

Linderman, C., & McAthie, M. (1999). *Fundamentals of contemporary nursing practice*. Philadelphia: W. B. Saunders.

National League for Nursing. (1991). *Criteria and guidelines for evaluation of baccalaureate nursing programs*. New York: Author.

National League for Nursing Accrediting Commission. (2005). *Accreditation manual with interpretive guidelines*. New York: Author.

Nugent, P. M., & Vitale, B. A. (2004). *Test success: Test-taking techniques for beginning nursing students*. Philadelphia: F. A. Davis Company.

Oermann, M., Truesdell, S., & Ziolkowski, L. (2000). Strategy to assess, develop, and evaluate critical thinking. *The Journal of Continuing Education in Nursing, 31*(4), 155–160.

Olson, C. B. (1992). *Thinking/writing: Fostering critical thinking through writing*. New York: HarperCollins.

Paul, R. W. (1993). *Critical thinking: What every person needs to know to survive in a rapidly changing world*. Pohnert Park, CA: Center for Critical Thinking.

Reilly, D. E., & Oermann, M. H. (1992). *Clinical teaching in nursing education*. New York: National League for Nursing.

Rubenfeld, M. G., & Scheffer, B. K. (2006). *Critical thinking TACTICS for nurses: Tracking, assessing, and cultivating thinking to improve competency-based strategies*. Sudbury, MA: Jones and Bartlett Publishers.

Scheffer, B. K., & Rubenfeld, M. G. (2000). A consensus statement on critical thinking in nursing. *Journal of Nursing Education, 38*(8), 352–359.

Schuster, P. M. (2002). *Concept mapping: A critical-thinking approach to care planning*. Philadelphia: F. A. Davis Company.

Smith, R. (1990). *To think*. New York: Teachers College Press.

Steinaker, N. W., & Bell, M. R. (1979). *The experiential taxonomy: A new approach to teaching and learning*. New York: Academic Press.

Watson, F., & Glaser, E. M. (1980). *Watson-Glaser critical thinking appraisal*. Dallas: Psychological Corporation.

Youngblood, N., & Beitz, J. M. (2001). Developing critical thinking with active learning strategies. *Nurse Educator, 26*(1), 39–42.

CHAPTER 5

The Teaching–Learning Experience from a Generational Perspective

Lynda Pesta

I hear babies cry, I watch them grow,
They'll learn much more, Than I'll ever know,
And I think to myself, What a wonderful world.
—Sung by *Louis Armstrong*

INTRODUCTION

Much has been written in pedagogical and business literature about the learning differences among generations. Each generation is shaped in part by the cultural, technological, and political events that have transpired during formative years. Therefore, each generation carries its own unique imprint from specific generational influences. Most of the college classrooms are filled by Generation X and Y (Xers and Yers) students, with the minority group being Baby Boomers. However, Boomers have heavy influence on both of the younger generations as their parents and teachers.

Projection data from the US Bureau of Labor Statistics (BLS) indicate that job growth is expected in all areas of healthcare occupations and health care will generate more than 3 million new wage and salaried positions by the year 2016. It is estimated that more than 1 million new and replacement nurses and 200,200 physicians will be needed by 2016. Universities, colleges, and training centers that prepare people for health occupations may find several challenges in recruiting, admitting, and retaining a workforce prepared to meet the expected demand. Tension may arise between learners and educators of differing generations who may have conflicting expectations of each other.

GENERATIONAL PERSPECTIVES OF FACULTY AND STUDENTS

Several generations are bound together for the transference of essential knowledge, skills, and attitudes for the health professions. Faculty typically consist of three generations: the ***Veterans/Traditionalist/Silent Generation (Veterans)*** who were born in the years between 1922 and 1945, the ***Baby Boom Generation (Boomers)*** who were born between 1946 and 1964, and ***Generation X (Xers)*** who were born between 1965 and 1981, and the ***Generation Y (Yers)*** who were born between 1982 and 2002. There is some overlap of years for each generation, depending on the source. Many healthcare programs, especially nursing, attract a wide group of students: the traditional student who enters college after high school graduation, the slightly older student who has worked after high school or perhaps has a young family, and the seasoned individual who decides to pursue a career after raising a family or deciding to change professions. To help meet future predictions for health-care professions, recruitment efforts will remain focused on appealing to a younger demographic, fostering the idea throughout secondary educational settings that health care is an attractive career choice (Cohen et al., 2006). The majority of nursing students are either Yers or Xers. Only a minority of students today are Boomers.

The Veteran

Cultural Setting

Most Veterans experienced the effects of the Great Depression where an estimated 25 to 30% of the US population experienced unemployment or displacement. This ended when World War II broke out in 1941. The Social Security Act of 1935 was new. Medicare and Medicaid were still decades away. Credit cards had not arrived. Veterans are known for patriotism, loyalty, and duty. Many families were just beginning to afford a family car and the Interstate Highway System that linked remote areas of the nation had not been built. People listened to swing and the big band sounds of Tommy Dorsey and Glenn Miller on 78 rpm records. The whole family sat near the radio and listened to President Roosevelt's "Fireside Chat" or was spellbound by the "Shadow" series and other radio shows. Reel-to-reel tape recorders and televisions were new and extremely expensive. Any adult could correct a youngster and it was not considered extraordinary by a parent. The virtues of frugality, thriftiness, and self-restraint were necessary for survival.

Rapid advances in health care came about during and after World War II. However, polio and tuberculosis killed or crippled thousands of people during this era. Many died from infection or sepsis from simple traumas. The widespread availability of penicillin during the 1940s reduced infection death rates (Smith & Bradshaw, 2008).

Despite the United States being the "melting pot" of the world, cultural diversity was not the norm or routine part of life for Veterans, especially in smaller cities, towns, or isolated rural communities. Most Americans lived in homogenous neighborhoods that were segregated by cultural practice, religious belief, race, or ethnicity. Family farms were still a way of life and Veterans were often isolated from outside influences. Life for Veterans was simpler but they grew up in a more formal and ordered society where manners and decorum were prized. They were taught not to question those in authority. Information from the outside world came from movie newsreels, *Life Magazine*, newspapers, and postal delivery of handwritten letters. The digital age has made the world a smaller place, yet the Veterans may not be as accepting of cultural differences as are the younger generations.

Characteristics/Work Ethics/Learning Styles

Veterans are known to be disciplined, hard working, patriotic, and loyal. Veterans are known to be team players. There is an almost universal belief within this generation in the motto "All for one and one for all" to ensure that the group good surpasses individual desires. They believe that history has important lessons to follow and use them as bridges to the future. Veterans have reached retirement age but many work due to longer life expectancies and changes in retirement goals. Workplace stability and longevity in the work environment is prized by this cohort. This has supported the expectation of retirement security. Being raised in an environment that valued deference for established rules, Veterans will usually follow the status quo. Veterans appreciate the wisdom of experienced leaders and elders and they appreciate the mentor/mentee aspects in personal and professional relationships. Finally, Veterans prefer a hierarchical structure in the workplace where lines of authority and responsibility are well defined. Veterans spent most of their lives without the convenience (or headaches) associated with personal computers, laptops, personal digital assistants (PDA), instant messaging, email, or Facebook. In fact, they often view technology suspiciously or as an intrusion. They put a higher value on face-to-face interaction, well-written notes, and telephone conversations.

The educational system in place during a Veteran's upbringing placed a heavy emphasis on reading, writing, and arithmetic. Most learning acquisition occurred with an emphasis on process. Knowledge was obtained through sequential, step-by-step instruction and through memorization drills. Because of this, there may be a higher comfort level among Veterans in using these strategies in teaching. There are few Veteran faculty but their influences persist in traditional healthcare curricula, policies, and teaching strategies.

The Baby Boomer

Cultural Setting

Boomers are generally classified as being born between the years of 1946 and 1964. During this time, the middle class was growing along with the economy.

Growth meant more resources to purchase goods. Automobiles, time saving appliances, electronics, and store-bought clothing became the norm. This generation learned that credit cards could provide more purchasing power and adopted a "buy now pay later" mindset with respect to homes, cars, and big ticket items (Johnson & Romanello, 2005). Advances in medicine and health care meant the average life expectancy continued to rise. Health insurance was an expected benefit when you worked for a company or corporation.

Boomers were born prior to digital technology. Because Veterans and Boomers needed to learn these digital technologies, often as a result of employer mandates, they are sometimes called digital immigrants (Prensky, 2001). Boomers needed to adapt and catch up to the rapid changes brought about by the introduction of the public Internet in the early 1990s and the ubiquitous presence of personal computing, email, distance learning, cellular telephones, and rapid information access through powerful search engines. Boomers learned that some of their previous prized skills for penmanship and spelling were now antiquated. Predigital education had an emphasis on punctuation, writing, spelling, drills, rules, and memorization. Learners were taught in a highly structured, teacher-centered educational system that called for obedience to the rules. Computers were behemoths and, because of their large size, needed entire rooms to house them. The average person could neither afford nor use a personal computer. Simple arithmetic could not be done on calculators. Manual typewriters created important documents. Correction fluid was considered a major time saver when correcting typed mistakes. In recent decades, learners have the distinct advantage of the delete key and can cut and paste large volumes of information into documents. Early television was not created as an educational tool but as entertainment where viewers watched on small, 9-inch screens in black and white with metal antennae. In the educational setting, challenging a teacher or parent was not expected or tolerated. Corporal punishment was not considered child abuse and was often used for a disobedient child.

Boomers used telephones to communicate when face-to-face encounters were not possible. Like learning a new language, the Boomers had to adjust to new technologies, such as email and computer networks, as a necessity of work life and not a choice (Sherman, 2006). The Boomers are not like the younger generations who are fascinated with new technology and often view these inventions as time savers and vital connections to significant others (Oblinger, 2003). For the Boomer, Friday nights meant attending a chaperoned dance at school. London's Twiggy was the epitome of fashion. Boomers relied on eight-track tapes or AM/FM radios for music. Now digital MP3 players provide a wide variety of music in an instant to almost every Xer and Yer. Boomers were enthralled with a variety of musical styles, the most influential being rock. The energetic sounds from a multitude of rock and roll bands emerged. The Woodstock music festival was a celebration of youth and freedom but with a downside of a culture laced with the idealization of illicit drugs, anger sparked by the Vietnam War, and the promotion of casual sex.

There were other events of the day that influenced the Boomer generation. Following World War II, the tension between Russia and the United States escalated the threat of nuclear war. Other major events that shaped the attitudes of the Boomer were the mandatory draft, the Vietnam War, the Kent State massacre, the Civil Rights Movement, the assassination of Martin Luther King, the assassination of President Kennedy, the feminist movement, and President Nixon's Watergate scandal. Protests occurred in the street and on college campuses across the nation. Boomers are seen as idealists who want to right the wrongs of an unjust world (Gardner, Deloney, & Grando, 2007). The overall discontent of the era created an upheaval in the mores of society. Unlike their parents, many Boomers came to mistrust authority figures and loudly questioned the wisdom of the institutions of organized religion, government, military, and marriage.

Characteristics/Work Ethics/Learning Styles

It is interesting that, as working adults, the Boomers became known as the generation to put in long and hard hours—often at the expense of their families. Often referred to as the "me" generation, Boomers sought individual accomplishment over the group good (Benedict, 2008). They often equate work with self worth. In general, Boomers expect positive acknowledgment for work performed and thrive on praise for their efforts. They prefer a more casual style of dress and have an uneasy relationship with authority. The healthcare profession continues to have optimistic growth potential and many Baby Boomers dispossessed from another industry, job, or profession may find changing to health care both an attractive and challenging alternative. Boomers are known to be committed, lifelong learners and solve problems by action.

Generation X

Cultural Setting

There are differences among authors as to the exact years that define Xers. Some authors use the years between 1960 and 1977 while other ranges exist in the literature, such as 1965 to 1976 (PEW, 2009). The most agreed upon years are in the range of 1965 to 1981. Regardless of the difference in defining age ranges, Xers comprise a much smaller group when compared to the Boomers that preceded them and the Yers who came after them. Culturally, this group was shaped by the important events of the time including *Roe v. Wade* (1973), which legalized abortion.

Xers were mostly raised by Boomer parents. Demographic shifts meant many Generation X children were not raised near extended family or even by both parents. Many children were raised by single parents or parents who both worked. Xers grew up on the experiment of the Children's Workshop Network, known as *Sesame Street*. Some of these children participated in after-school programs manned by unrelated adults. The term "latchkey kid" was coined for the Xer child was left alone after school hours while a parent or both parents remained at work. Left home often without adult supervision, they entertained themselves with television shows, computer games, and videos.

Xer children were exposed to a higher level of violence in movies, music, and in video games. During this time, various musical styles emerged. Music Television (MTV) first aired in 1981. Musical influences such as grunge, heavy metal, and rap entered the mainstream American culture during the typical Xer's formative years. These musical styles and videos contained graphic violence and obscene material that needed close monitoring from busy parents. They grew up in unprecedented economic prosperity and severe downturns in the economy. Middle class children were exposed to more marketing commercialism for brand name clothes, toiletries, and shoes than any other generation before them. Drugs such as ecstasy, heroin, and cocaine became prolific across the country. Major cities had increasing violence with gang warfare and violent initiation rites. Nationally, unwed teen pregnancy and divorce rates trended upward while marriage rates dropped (Boonstra, 2002; Stockmayer, 2004). The problems of acquired immune deficiency syndrome (AIDS) and homelessness were part of public discussions. Influential events included the Los Angeles riots of 1991, the Challenger space shuttle explosion, and the environmental disaster at Valdez. Overseas, the Tian'anmen Square protests of 1989, the unraveling of apartheid in South Africa, the Chernobyl nuclear accident, and the fall of communism helped shape this generation. Communication was instantaneous and brought to life in living color within moments of occurring. The Internet was introduced during this time. Xers became acclimated to learning on personal computers at home, at school, and during after school hours.

Characteristics/Work Ethics/Learning Styles

There are many conflicting characteristics that are attributed to Xers. Generally they feel more comfortable working alone and are considered independent. Due to their upbringing and isolation, it has been said that Xer have learned they can only "rely on themselves." They readily identify friends as extended family. As a learning group, Xers have come to expect instant gratification because of the advances in technology and obtaining information at the click of a button. They tend to see themselves as consumers of education and tend to mistrust authority figures, which could include faculty. Xers become bored in meetings where there is much discussion prior to making decisions (Sherman, 2006).

Leisure and time off to enjoy other interests is particularly critical to Xers. Unlike their parents who worked long hours, only to watch them lose out on what they consider to be the fun of living, Xers jealously guard free time and view requests to work overtime as intrusions. Because of the higher value they place on personal time over the needs of their employers, they have been viewed as undependable. They highly value their individuality but, as a group, widely adopted bizarre hairstyles, tattoos, and body piercings as a sign of independence from the norm. This generation witnessed companies increasingly grow in international markets, thereby supplanting the local American worker for cheaper labor overseas. They realized that the years of loyalty their grandparents and parents had in return for job security and a guaranteed pension no longer existed and, as a result, view government programs with skepticism and do not believe that social programs like Social Security will be available for them when they retire. Xers are described as cynical, ironic, clever, pragmatic, and resourceful (Johnson & Romanello, 2005). If there is a collective mantra that sums up the attitude of work versus leisure among Xers, it is "Work to live, not live to work."

Generation Y

Cultural Setting

Depending on the writer, there are many names and descriptions for Generation Y. They are referred to as Nexters, Generation N, Millenials, and "Digital Natives." Collectively, Yers are usually placed as being born between 1981 and 2001. Despite variations in date, what is certain is that most Yers have never known a time before the age of digital technology. Culturally, Yers have been shaped by such events as the 1995 Oklahoma City bombing, the 1996 Summer Olympics bombing, the mass shootings at Columbine High School in 1999, and the terrorist attacks of September 11, 2001. The War on Terror, with efforts in Iraq and Afghanistan, continues to affect the paradigm of this generation. Generation Yers show a taste in diverse music from rap, alternative, and socially conscious groups such as Coldplay, Yellow Card, or Green Day. Music and videos from Yers' favorite bands can be instantly accessed on YouTube on wirelessly connected laptops, all while performing other tasks.

The US birthrate continued to decline in this era. Most children born in this generation were planned and "wanted." The parents of this generation are known to be very involved in their children and are often coined "helicopter" parents because they hover around their children. The hovering behavior is evidenced by high level of involvement with every aspect of their children's lives and imparting on them more material goods than previous generations. As a benefit of caring and involved parents, Yers are secure and value family relationships.

Characteristics/Work Ethics/Learning Styles

Yers, however, are thought to be more sociable than Xers. While Veterans and Boomers are referred to as "digital immigrants" because they were not exposed to the digital world until adulthood, Xers and Yers are comfortable with new technologies and are referred to as digital natives (Prensky, 2001). MP3 players, blogs, personal computers, Internet searches with Google or Yahoo, cell phones, instant messaging, text messaging, interactive gaming, video cameras, game technology such as Wii and PlayStation, Wikis, Twitter, Flickr, YouTube, and Facebook/My Space seem foreign to the "digital immigrant." Digital natives are those who were exposed to the benefits of computer and digital technology and cannot remember a time before them. Many attributes have been assigned to Yers, including a high comfort level with computers and an insistence on being connected to family and friends technologically. There is no doubt that our world is becoming increasingly interconnected with wireless technology. Since Yers have never known a life without the presence of computers, cable, satellite radio, wireless connections, or cell phones they are comfortable "surfing" the Web, use digital music sources to download to MP3 players, and are usually experts in uploading or downloading videos through YouTube or other sources. Using Twitter, texting, and Facebook are as essential as breathing air to the majority of Yers. Technological advances continue to grow at unprecedented rates, but Yers enjoy the latest advances. As the Xers rode the wave of MTV, the next wave brought YouTube to the Yers.

Parents of Yers have been known to involve their children in a multitude of activities: sports, music, private tutoring, and group activities. Therefore, Yers often have multiple and diverse talents. Generation Yers generally are considered more optimistic than Xers. They have lived structured, scheduled lives and generally are much closer to their parents and feel more comfortable in a structured environment than their earlier X counterparts. They are known to be enthusiastic learners but want to know that "what they are learning is connected to the bigger picture" (Sontag, 2009). Yers are known to be deeply committed to causes of justice, environmentalism, and volunteerism for the greater good. They are the most ethnically and racially diverse generation and readily accept persons who are different from themselves. Diversity is often celebrated and prized. Yers consider themselves to be global citizens (Johnson & Romanello, 2005).

Yers are comfortable in group settings and feel isolated when unable to have instant access to friends through communication devices. There are similarities and differences described in the literature between the two youngest generations, Xers and Yers. Both groups have usually been exposed to a high degree of computer and digital technology in their formative years. Because of the preponderance of technology for communication, Xers and Yers may not have the verbal communication skills of their predecessors (Prensky, 2001).

There are similarities and difference among each of the generations. Although each generation is made up of individuals with unique characteristics, it is helpful to list some common characteristics that have been attributed to each generational cohort as outlined here. Table 5-1 summarizes characteristics associated with each generation.

GENERATIONAL CONSIDERATIONS FOR EDUCATORS

Changes in behavior, and thus learning, take place more readily when the student is fully engaged and can actively participate in the learning process. Faculty should plan teaching experiences carefully in order to achieve successful outcomes. With generational considerations in mind, an educator might ask the following questions:

What factors influence each generation involved in educational settings?

What are the typical characteristics for each generation?

How do my generational preferences and characteristics merge or differ from the newer generations?

What are the best teaching strategies to engage each generation of learner?

How do generational differences affect communication?

Could generational differences simply be maturity issues?

How does technology affect the new learner?

Who are digital natives and who are digital immigrants?

Do digital natives think differently than other learners?

What strategies can engage the new generation of learners?

Table 5-1 Generational Characteristics

Attributes/Characteristics/Interpersonal Relationships/Communication Style			
Veterans, 1922–1945	**Boomers, 1946–1964**	**Xers, 1964–1981**	**Yers, 1982–2001**
• Unselfish; group oriented; loyal; patriotic; will delay gratification; responsible; accepts line authority • Prizes the group welfare over individual needs; honors tradition; formal and proper • Prefers personal or written communication; not as comfortable with electronic style; prefers to communicate along established lines of authority	• Self-seeking behaviors; "me" generation • Inconsistent love–hate relationship with authority • Ambitious; challenge status quo; informal; casual; likes fewer rules; idealistic • Early wave accused of sacrificing family for work obligations • Prefers face-to-face communication; Adapts to technology as a necessity	• Confident; direct; assertive; fearless; adaptable; diverse; impatient; fun; informal; independent; pragmatic; outcome oriented • Challenges authority • Body piercings and tattoos popular forms of expression; pessimistic tendencies • Sees friends as extensions of family • Hesitant to commit to marriage and long-term relationships • Prefers technology-driven over face-to-face communication	• Instant access to desires; technology integrated into life • Assertive; ethnically diverse; optimistic; self confident in most areas; embraces diversity; civic minded; consumer oriented; self reliant; enthusiastic; easily bored; idealistic; patriotic; expects respect; optimistic; friendly; cooperative; open minded; talented; less mature; interested in others; collegial. • More respectful of rules and authority than Xers and Boomers • Closer to parents than predecessors • Enjoys face-to-face; craves social connections via technology • Informal but schedule driven; being smart is cool; team players/ collaborative

Learning/Work Styles			
• Dependable; follows established rules; prefers hierarchy • Educated in teacher-centered settings • Values mentorship with established leader or experienced person • Less likely to embrace newer technology than successors; more process oriented; expects work security; very loyal to employer	• Prefers text over graphics; linear thinking; process oriented; step by step • Likes contact with faculty • Lifelong learning commitment; ties learning with life experiences; expects rewards for work done; enjoys titles and accolades for achievements; willing to work long hours to get job done • Seeks secure retirement; loyal to employer • Technology reluctant • Does not enjoy games or being put on the spot	• Education began in student-centered settings; processes quickly; multitaskers; enjoys fast pace; focused; expects clear instructions; parallel/mosaic thinking; nonlinear thinking; concrete thinkers • Prefers to work alone; needs safe environment to participate; experiential; embraces technology • Little tolerance for extraneous information; dislikes assignments—does not view them as learning enhancements; discounts contact with faculty as important • Desires work and school flexibility; expects instant results for efforts; self directed; entrepreneurial • Values free time over work hours; little loyalty to employer; wants success and ambition on their own terms; may overestimate contributions to an organization; expects rapid advancement	• Parallel/mosaic thinking; multitaskers; expresses doubts about academic abilities; processes quickly; prefers graphics over text; likes to work in groups; curious; experiential; thrives on discovery; shorter attention spans; higher incidences of ADD/ADHD diagnoses • Enjoys interactive learning and games with immediate response; expects 24/7 access to learning/faculty; learns best by trial and error; prefers more structure than Xers. • Likes creatively presented learning materials; enjoys entertainment aspect to learning; no tolerance for delays in class beginning and endings. • Has expressed concerns regarding academic abilities; enjoys mentoring relationships from experienced leaders; likes stories that are relevant to content; eager to learn new requirements for work/school for the expectation of reward • Prefers audio/visuals over reading; expresses higher reading comprehension than Xers

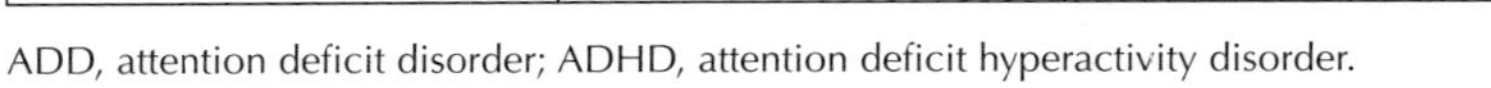
ADD, attention deficit disorder; ADHD, attention deficit hyperactivity disorder.

Educational Expectations of Teachers

Traditional teacher-centered learning has given way to a more student-centered approach (Brown, 2008). Within nursing programs, there are decades of separation from the authoritarian, quasi-military chain-of-command programs that dominated the training for most of the Veterans and Boomers, but little changes have resulted in nursing curricula (National League for Nursing [NLN], 2003). Faculty expects students to meet learning objectives in order to successfully meet program outcomes. The hospital-based apprenticeship model of nursing education has long since moved into colleges and universities wherein students are expected to read and interpret complex written material while giving less weight to actual clinically based education with live patients. The emphasis from administration to hospital staff is to shorten lengths of stay and to provide safe, skillful, and efficient care. Providing the appropriate intensity of service according to the severity of illness is stringently applied by insurance payers.

A well-trained professional must be prepared and equipped to manage the complexities of the system or become overwhelmed by role performance demands. Faculty, armed with the knowledge and experience of the profession's challenges, expect students to meet the expectations set out in program curricula. Faculty expect students to attend class, remain honest when preparing assignments, meet assignment deadlines, arrive on time to class, pass exams, demonstrate appropriate communication skills, and perform psychomotor skills satisfactorily. Students who arrive late or do not attend class, communicate poorly, or appear to be inattentive in class are viewed circumspectly. Students who text message, shop online, do not keep appointments, talk in class, or use a disrespectful tone of voice are seen as uncivil by most Boomer or Veteran faculty. To maintain a positive rapport between faculty and students of different generations, the faculty member must clearly define behaviors that are acceptable in the classroom and clinical areas (Suplee, Lachman, Siebert, & Anselmi, 2008).

Educational Expectations of Students

Parent and student expectations have undergone radical changes in primary, secondary, and postsecondary educational settings in the past decades. Advances in technology, the view that education is a commodity, developing maturity, tight schedules, previous life experiences, values, and cultural backgrounds will influence the expectations of learners. Education is no longer seen as a revered institution incapable of being criticized, as much as it is a product—the result of a consumer-oriented culture. Whereas Boomers appreciate a mentoring relationship with faculty, Xers believe they can teach themselves if given the right tools while Yers view experienced faculty with admiration but not awe. Generation Y students, sheltered by doting parents, are said to be more grade conscious than earlier counterparts. They are confident and not fearful of challenging faculty over a grade disagreement. They will quite readily voice dissent and demand their consumer rights. Younger students expect respect and to be listened to when their opinions are expressed. They prefer an egalitarian approach in the learning environment (Gardner et al., 2007).

Generation Xers and Yers do expect that faculty be experts and have recent relevant experience in the subjects they teach (Oblinger, 2003). They also expect rationales as to why material is to be learned. That expectation coincides with adult learning theory and is not a foreign concept to experienced educators. They like personal attention and expect immediate constructive criticism for their performance. Above all, students seek a connection with faculty (Gardner et al., 2007). Younger generations expect 24/7 access to their instructors (American Association of State Colleges and Universities [AASCU], 2004). One study indicated that 64% of college students indicated they would be interested in communicating with faculty outside of the class schedule in postings created in blogs (Junco & Cole-Avent, 2008). Today, schools, colleges, and universities are striving to keep pace by placing the required technological infrastructures in place to support online access for students and faculty. Communication networks supported by colleges and universities enable communication methods to support the desire for increased learning activities or faculty support outside of the classroom.

Generation Yers expect support and nurturing from faculty (Gardner et al., 2007). Both generations will adapt to a variety of teaching methods with Xers being more comfortable with computer, online, and distance learning and self-paced modules. Experiential learning is an expectation of both generations. Yers have a special penchant for hearing personal stories to illustrate points (e.g., analogies, humor, and wit) and expect an entertainment quality to teaching sessions. Despite their apparent addiction to new technologies, some studies indicate that nursing students actually prefer a well-designed and entertaining PowerPoint with elements of multimedia imbedded into the lecture material. They also expect that a complete set of notes and slides will be provided. Younger students prefer this over other teaching methods (Paschal, 2003; Walker et al., 2006). This is especially true for difficult content topics and this traditional method is often preferred by students over group work. Undergraduate baccalaureate students younger than 25 years preferred to *read* about the subject first, followed by an expert's *lecture*, despite self-reports of reading comprehension difficulties (Walker et al., 2007). When attempting to learn a psychomotor skill, students in these cohorts favored demonstration over a lecture covering the material. Experiential learning fits easily within all three cognitive domains of nursing and is a valued methodology among all generations. Experiential learning is described as learning through experiences (Kolb, 1984). Xers actually value *doing* over *knowing* according to one author. Younger generation learners have been reported to prefer to perform the skill first under the direction of the faculty and then independently rather than hear a lecture over the material (Walker et al., 2007).

Barriers to the Teaching–Learning Experience

Education in a health professions program is challenging, especially for the incoming student. The sheer amount of reading and material can intimidate even the most scholarly student, yet it is inherent that, to be successful in the program, one must be able to comprehend, analyze, and write well (Arhin & Cormier, 2007). The typical Yers will have difficulty reading and studying for long periods of time (Gardner et al., 2007). Multitasking is second nature to the Yers, but sitting and reading for long periods of time is difficult. It is estimated that by the time students reach college, they will have spent 5,000 hours reading compared to 10,000 hours playing video games and 20,000 hours watching television (Prensky, 2001). There is no doubt that Yers have had more sensory input since childhood than earlier generations. Scientific evidence does support that environmental influences alters brain structures (Draganski et al., 2004; Sontag, 2009). It has also been supposed that the newer generations do learn differently from their predecessors because of the excessive amounts of visual stimulation they received throughout childhood.

Parallel/Mosaic Thinking Patterns

Mosaic thinking was coined by media theorist Marshall McLuhan (1978) who hypothesized that the electronic age sparked a revolutionary, or mosaic, way of processing information. Western civilization was formerly characterized by the dominance of reading and writing, which is now giving way to electronic media. Linear reasoning relies on a phonetic/alphabetical structure and its use is foundational to logical and sequential thought processes. Mosaic thinking is a consequence of visual symbols and images that are found in media today. According to McLuhan and others, this change in communication has radically altered the way information is processed and society functions. Similarly, parallel thinking is the ability to process information from a variety of sources simultaneously. These thinking/learning patterns have been ascribed especially to the newer generational cohorts who are comfortable in a fast paced, technologically connected world.

Our newest cohorts connect with various digital technologies as they become available. Digital natives are said to gather information in parallel or a mosaic pattern. They process quickly and have the ability to take in information simultaneously from various sources. Therefore, they do not always learn in a step-by-step sequential manner. Younger students have been exposed to endless hours of digitally enhanced games (Prensky, 2001). In gaming, trial and error methods meet with failure or reward. Quick motor reflexes, for conquering spatial barriers, and problem solving are rewarded and positively reinforced. A consequence of this is students' reduced tolerance for quiet reading, reflection, and listening. There is evidence that, because of changes in brain activity, technologically dependent students have a shorter attention span and poorer reading abilities than digital immigrants. As a result, boredom is not conducive to active learning.

Another downside to the reliance on instant feedback is the accuracy of Internet sources. Easy distractibility due to the constant habit of multitasking is often observed in younger students. To engage today's learner, the experienced generations will need to understand their learners' preferred learning styles and adapt or enhance teaching strategies help them connect with the material. The new generation prefers learning strategies that encourage exploration, discovery, and trial and error. Unfortunately, trial and error problem solving takes time and resources. It is not ideal in patient scenarios where the ultimate goal is to protect the patient's safety and comfort within limited time constraints. Current nursing education may be outdated for digital natives as well as future generations of students. Curricula in health profession programs include a large demand for reading and sequencing. There is an emphasis on step-by-step processes to achieve learning outcomes. This method does not take into account new learner's propensity for a fast paced, parallel, and mosaic thinking patterns. Online access, virtual reality, simulation, and computer games could solve these needs. Because of this, many nursing leaders question whether current nursing curriculums are preparing a viable workforce. The American Association of College Nurses and the NLN have published position papers calling for major changes to incorporate the technology of this younger generation (NLN, 2008). More schools are going online to adjust to the ever increasing demand from students for increasing class schedule flexibility. It is estimated that online and distance nursing programs will continue to rise and remain a viable option for many. Despite the plethora of options for students today, recent studies indicate Boomers and Yers prefer face-to-face communication over distance learning–type arrangements.

Strategies for Teaching Across the Generations

To best serve our successors, it will be necessary for faculty to understand our personal biases, learning styles, and preferred methods of teaching (Pardue & Morgan, 2008). The methods used to teach students are going through a radical upheaval because of changes in societal expectations, technological advances, and increased access to information. Adult learning theory rests on the accepted principle that learners will retain and retrieve information when meaning is associated with it. Another important principle of adult learning theory is the idea that adults want to learn what is applicable to them at the moment (Knowles, 1973). Knowledge of the technological advances in a digital age and methods to employ them in the classroom, lab, or clinical site will become increasingly important over time. To say that it would be a necessity to engage the students would be an understatement. Foreknowledge of general attributes of the digitally engaged student is useful for nurse educators who have been a product of a different generation. For any generation, faculty creativity, an open honest dialogue, and availability will help create a positive environment for students to thrive. From a learning perspective, Xers jealously guard their time; they prefer the bullet point version of subjects. They want to know precisely what they need to know to pass to get good grades in the shortest way possible. They enjoy the presentation of specific information through email, blogs, and instant messaging (Gibson, 2009). Xers have little tolerance for inefficiency and do not want their time wasted. They prefer brief learning episodes followed by group interaction and, because of their independence, will research information easily online (Gibson, 2009). They enjoy online courses because it provides more flexibility in scheduling. Xers are determined to complete tasks but see it only as a means to an end, not as learning for the sake of learning.

Yers learn best in an environment where there are multiple choices for obtaining the information, especially when the subject matter is difficult; choices include detailed notes, recordings of lectures, PowerPoint lectures, and video tapes of lectures that can be reviewed later. Yers enjoy the joy of discovery more than their older counterparts. They are known to enjoy hearing experiences from teachers whom they consider mentors. This trait may be especially heartening to the educator who has a rich history and experiences to share. Yers may need to be more directed by their educators than Xers (Gardner et al., 2007). Yers appreciate being asked for their opinions and relish opportunities to be part of a discussion. They demand respect from those who are in leadership roles. The Yer is more likely to be engaged when teaching strategies involve creative solutions (Gibson, 2009). The Yer prefers immediate feedback and expects instructors to be available beyond the classroom schedule. The use of classroom clickers is a method to enhance classroom participation and may appeal to all generations within the classroom. They allow anonymous responses to classroom activities and provide immediate feedback to problems. (Skiba & Barten, 2006). The risk for exposure is minimal and would appeal to a Boomer student who chooses an incorrect response.

Technology and the increasing role it plays in our lives will continue to expand, which may be sometimes intimidating and frustrating for the older generations but not so for the younger generations. In the workplace, the trend for increasing reliance on electronic and digital equipment and electronic medical records underscores the fact that technology marches forward. It will be necessary to utilize the technology already in the workplace to prepare future health professionals. The Technology Informatics Guiding Education Reform (TIGER) initiative started in 2007 is a national plan to move nursing practice and education into the digital age. Members and experts from nursing education, informational technology, practice areas, and government agencies are collaborating to meet a 10-year strategic plan. The TIGER vision is twofold. First, to "allow informatics tools, principles, theories and practices to be used by nurses to make healthcare safer, effective, efficient, patient-centered, timely and equitable" and, second, to "interweave enabling technologies transparently into nursing practice and education, making information technology the stethoscope for the 21st century" (TIGER, 2007).

There are countless ways of involving and engaging students in experiential methods with or without technology enhancements. Virtual clinical experiences and lab practice are becoming more affordable, reliable, and evidence-based. They may be essential educator extensions as the shortage of qualified educators in the health professions continues. They blend well with the traditional methods to assist the learner in gaining psychomotor skills. The power of multisensory experiences imbedded in curricular teaching strategies cannot be overestimated because it increases the long-term memory retention and retrieval of the material for the learner. Increased networking with other faculty in distant universities through Internet listserves or blogs are viable ways for faculty to network and increase teaching method repertoires.

Computer-based video games have been part of entertainment and primary education for many years. Students are exposed to simulation experiences at increasingly younger ages. They become experts at manipulating objects in spatial environments repetitively throughout their childhoods. Applying trial and error methods in a safe environment allow the participant to practice necessary skills until perfection is achieved. Sources indicate that most of younger students, especially digital natives, expect and thrive on this type of learning. Older students may not embrace game playing as valuable, especially if they are not attuned to this particular modality. Fast-paced gaming may be threatening to an older student. There should be alternatives to this format if the class consists of multiple generations. Older students may need more time to practice or prefer a one-to-one self-paced computer experience that focuses on decision making to enhance clinical reasoning skills. Simulation games have long been used for training purposes in aviation and the military. The learner will play out scenarios repetitively and receive immediate feedback for correct or incorrect responses. The game HotZone© was developed by Noblis for first responders during a biohazard terrorist scenario (Noblis, 2007).

As the technology becomes more sophisticated and realistic, it is not hard to imagine the possibilities for all areas of the healthcare professions. Learning and creative expression can also be taken into the virtual world of Second Life (Junco & Cole-Avent, 2008; Linden Research, Inc., 2009). Second Life is a virtual reality world where "players" interact with each other locally or from across the world. Through the combination of enhanced video games, role play, simulation, and case studies comes a potential new learning methodology using this system. The educational goals might be collaborative skill development, communication, reasoning abilities, and practicing complex psychomotor skills. An exciting dimension to simulation learning has great potential in the healthcare professions. In 2005, Texas A&M University–Corpus Christi partnered with Breakaway Ltd., a gaming company, to launch a virtual reality simulation lab for training military and civilian emergency medical personnel in trauma care. This teaching modality immerses the learners in a high fidelity three-dimensional world that allows for multiple realistic patient scenarios to be played out in an emergency room setting. These experiential scenarios encourage critical thinking, psychomotor skill acquisition, and collaboration with other healthcare personnel—all in a low risk virtual environment ("Pulse!!," 2005). Educators should expect virtual simulations to become more widely used as they become increasingly available and reliable (Schmidt & Stewart, 2009). It should be noted that students are more receptive when experiential learning takes place in a low stress environment.

There are many teaching strategies that can be employed to engage the younger generations of learners. Narrative pedagogy is a way of interpreting information from different perspectives; using a deconstruction (analytical) approach may work in classes that welcome and expect student participation, analysis, and dialogue (Diekelmann, 2001). Concept maps use parallel/mosaic thinking to promote clinical reasoning (Vacek, 2009). Reflection and critical thinking can be powerful and generationally relevant for promoting clinical thinking by experienced faculty. Students are guided in "examining every angle" through organized brainstorming techniques (Kenny, 2003). Another strategy that encourages clinical reasoning is engaging in Edward de Bono's six hat game (de Bono, 1999; Kenny, 2003). This encourages parallel thinking processes by looking at a problem from six different perspectives and discussing them.

CONCLUSION

Conflicts of younger generations with their elders have been documented for millennia. It may be debated that root causes are student immaturity, undeveloped reasoning abilities, preferred learning styles, or alterations in brain structure.

On the other hand, faculty reluctance to change or generational unawareness will impact communication and learning. It will become increasingly requisite for healthcare curricula to change, modify, and adapt to strategies that coincide with technological advances and the societal expectations of the new generations (Li, 2006). Whatever the causes, these differences must be reckoned with. The timeless determinate for true educational success will most likely remain the connections from teacher to learner and from learner to teacher that transcend generational differences.

REFERENCES

American Association of State Colleges and Universities. (2004). *The key to competitiveness: Understanding the next generation learner—A guide for college and university leaders*. Washington, DC: Author.

Arhin, A. O., & Cormier, E. (2007). Using deconstruction to educate generation Y students. *Journal of Nursing Education, 46*(12), 562–567.

Benedict, S. I. (2008). How practitioners do and don't communicate: Part II. *Integrative Medicine, 7*(2), 54–59.

Boonstra, H. (2002). Teen pregnancy: Trends and lessons learned. *The Guttmacher Report on Public Policy*, 5(1). Retrieved from July 5, 2009, from http://www.guttmacher.org/pubs/tgr/05/1/gr050107.html

Brown, B.L. (1997). New learning strategies for generation x. *ERIC Digest*, (184). Retrieved July 3, 2009, from http://www.ericdigests.org/1998-1/x.htm

Cohen, R., Burns, K., Frank-Stromborg, M., Flanagan, J., Askins, D., & Ehrlich-Jones, L. (2006). Educational innovation. The kids into health careers (KIHC) Initiative: innovative approaches to help solve the nursing shortage. *Journal of Nursing Education, 45*(5), 186–189.

de Bono, E. (1999). *Six thinking hats*. Boston: Back Bay Books.

Diekelmann, N. (2001). Narrative pedagogy: Heideggerian hermeneutical analyses of lived experiences of students, teachers, and clinicians. *Advances in Nursing Science, 23*(3), 53–71.

Draganski, B., Gaser, C., Busch, V., Schuierer, G., Bogdahn, U., & May, A. (2004). Neuroplasticity: changes in grey matter induced by training. *Nature, 427*(6972), 311–312.

Gardner, E. A., Deloney, L. A, & Grando, V.T. (2007). Nursing student descriptions that suggest changes for the classroom and reveal improvements needed in study skills and self-care. *Journal of Professional Nursing, 23*(2), 98–104.

Gibson, S. E. (2009). Enhancing intergenerational communication in the classroom: Recommendations for successful teacher-student relationships. *Nursing Education Perspectives, 30*(1), 37–39.

Johnson, S. A., & Romanello, M.L. (2005). Generational diversity teaching and learning approaches. *Nurse Educator, 30*(5), 212–216.

Junco, R., & Cole-Avent, G. A. (2008). An introduction to technologies commonly used by college students. *New Directions for Student Services, 124*, 3–17.

Kenny, L. J. (2003). Using Edward de Bono's six hats game to aid critical thinking and reflection in palliative care. *International Journal of Palliative Nursing, 9*(3), 105–112.

Knowles, M. S. (1973). *The adult learner: A neglected species*. Houston, TX: Gulf Publishing Company.

Kolb, D. (1984). *Experiential learning: Experience as the source of learning and development*. Englewood Cliffs, NJ: Prentice-Hall.

Li, S., & Kenward, K. (2006). A national survey of nursing education and practice of newly licensed nurses. *JONA's Healthcare Law, Ethics & Regulation, 8*(4), 110–115.

Linden Research, Inc. (2009). What is second life? Retrieved November 9, 2009, from http://secondlife.com/whatis/?lang=en-US

McLuhan, M. (1978). The brain and the media: The Western Hemisphere. *Journal of Communication, 28*(4), 54–60.

National League for Nursing. (2003). *Innovation in nursing education: A call to reform*. New York: National League for Nursing.

National League for Nursing. (2008). *Preparing the next generation of nurses to practice in a technology-rich environment: An informatics agenda*. New York: National League for Nursing.

Noblis. (2007). HotZone—First responder game. Retrieved June 1, 2009, from http://www.noblis.org/MethodsTools/AreasofExpertise/Documents/HotZone.pdf

Oblinger, D. (2003). Boomers gen-xers millenials: Understanding the new students. *EDUCAUSE Review*, July/August, 37–47. Retrieved November 9, 2009, from http://net.educause.edu/ir/library/pdf/erm0342.pdf

Pardue, K. T., & Morgan, P. (2008). Millennials considered: A new generation, new approaches, and implications for nursing education. *Nursing Education Perspectives, 29*(2), 75–79.

Paschal, J. (2003). *Understanding generation Y—expectations of nursing education*. Unpublished thesis submitted to the graduate faculty of Baylor University (UMI#1414800).

PEW, 2009 Pew Internet and American Life Project. (2009, January). Jones, S. (2009, January) Generations online in 2009. Retrieved December 11, 2009, from http://pewresearch.org/pubs/1093/generations-online

Prensky, 2001 *Prensky, M. (2001, October). Digital natives, Digital immigrants, Part II. Do they really think differently? On the Horizon. Vol. 9, No. 5: NCB University Press.* Retrieved December 11, 2009, from*:* http://www.marcprensky.com/writing/

Pulse!! (2005). Retrieved August 10, 2009, from http://www.sp.tamucc.edu/pulse/info-multimedia.asp.

Schmidt, B., & Stewart, S. (2009). Implementing the virtual reality learning environment second life. *Nursing Educator, 34*(4), 152–155.

Sherman, R (2006). Leading a multigenerational nursing workforce: Issues, challenges, and strategies. *Online Journal of Issues in Nursing, 11*(2), 1–13.

Skiba, D., & Barton, A. (2006). Adapting your teaching to accommodate the net generation of learners. Online Journal of Issues in Nursing, 11 (2), Retrieved December 11, 2009, from CINAHL with full text database.

Smith, D., & Bradshaw, B.S. (2008). Reduced variation in death rates after introduction of antimicrobial agents. *Population Research and Policy Review, 27*(3), 343–351.

Sontag, M. (2009). A learning theory for 21st century students. *Journal of Online Education, 5*(4). Retrieved April 12, 2009, from http://www.uh.cu/static/documents/STA/A%20Learning%20Theory%20for%2021st-C%20Students.pdf

Stockmayer, G. (2004). Demographic rates and household change in the United States, 1900–2000. Presented at Population Association of America Annual Meeting, Boston, MA, April 3. Retrieved August 1, 2009 from http://paa2004.princeton.edu/download.asp?submissionId=41802

Suplee, P., Lachman, V., Siebert, B., & Anselmi, K. (2008). Managing nursing student incivility in the classroom, clinical setting, and on-line. *Journal of Nursing Law, 12*(2), 68–77.

Technology Informatics Guiding Education Reform. (2007). Evidence and informatics transforming nursing: 3-year action steps toward a 10-year vision. Retrieved June 3, 2009 from http://www.aacn.nche.edu/Education/pdf/TIGER.pdf

Vacek, J. (2009). Using a conceptual approach with concept mapping to promote critical thinking. *Journal of Nursing Education, 48*(1), 45–48.

Walker, J., Martin, T., Haynie, L., Norwood, A., White, J., & Grant, L. (2007). Preferences for teaching methods in a baccalaureate nursing program: how second-degree and traditional students differ. *Nursing Education Perspectives, 28*(5), 246–250.

CHAPTER 6

Esthetic Action: Creativity as a Collaborative Process

Ellen Landis

Encouraging healthcare practitioners to share insights of sensory-emotional values, or esthetics, can contribute to more creative collaboration in the field. In the classroom or on location, the call to be creative often inspires feelings of excitement or something to be guarded against, as if a no-win outcome would inevitably occur. These responses make way for important conversations on personal, cultural, and institutional judgments based on deeply felt sentiments and corresponding actions. While research, theory, and protocol are of immense importance to practitioners, inevitably, we are faced with the unexpected and a lack of apparent solutions. These junctures present the opportunity to develop new ideas, relationships, and practices.

Early in his career, the philosopher Gaston Bachelard (Thiboutot, Martinez, & Jager, 1999) adopted the prevalent attitude of the sciences at the onset of the 20th century: that creative imagination stood in the way of scientific objectivity. One needed to get beyond impulses to do scientific work. At that point, he thought imagination was important in intimate and informal settings but it was a hindrance in the workplace. He later replaced these essentialist views with the opinion that creative imagination joins together the opposites of self and other, mankind and nature, and what is and what is not. In doing so, he testified to the belief that creative imagination provides us with the capacity to unify our experience of living.

Approaches to collaborative creativity that help build reflexive practice and outcomes in health care can benefit the range of stakeholders. Why is it then that collaboration, and especially collaborative reflection, is considered a luxury by some and a burden by others? Generally speaking, we value the actions we perform over reflection on those actions. This focus on performance is linked to commerce and money making. "Time is money" and "time is not to be wasted" are familiar phrases exemplified in the healthcare workplace. Look at all the time a mental health clinician works in isolation seeing clients and doing billing-related paperwork. Then, compare that with the time spent reflecting with colleagues on those actions. Some smart businesses build in time for group reflection. Google, for example, encourages people to spend time together in activities such as ping pong and pool during work as ways to support stress relief, relationship building, and, of course, creativity. This is based on an understanding that performance is enhanced in a collaborative–reflective work environment.

Findings from cognitive science demonstrate that emotional support is at the heart of educational processes. When people feel safe, listened to, and understood, their performance is enhanced. Professor Julia Byers, art therapist and family therapist at Lesley University, begins graduate school classes not with the expectations laid out in a syllabus. Rather, she begins with introductions, a process that bridges the gap between academic hierarchical knowing and cognitive/kinesthetic recognition and empathy. This immediately breaks down alienation among students who will be learning how to perform in the classroom and workplace together.

All too often, as new ideas emerge, they are credited to either a small number of people or an individual. Ideas have veins whose sources are vital, like fresh water springing up from the earth, whose underground sources may be hard to trace. For instance, everyone has had an experience of going unrecognized for a contribution that he or she made in resolving a difficult situation. We may also remember sensations of hiding our involvement in the development of an idea because of concerns about reverberations that may come with recognition.

People often seek health care when there is an acute situation—a crisis or emergency. Evidence-based, theory-driven, reflective practice can offer healthcare practitioners a work environment that brings the best out in people, whether that is the patient or the professional. Collaborative creativity can bring forth unexpected resources from others. Despite our limited knowledge of what practitioners in health care will face in the coming years, we encourage students to explore the mystery of creativity as a collaborative process in school and at work.

THEORETICAL RATIONALE

The development of skills for creativity in the classroom includes personal agency, divergent thinking, and assessment of patterns. According to social philologist John Shotter (1993), to avoid becoming entrapped within the confines of narratives, metaphors, and theories about life, new practices for "multivoiced tradition(s) of argumentation" (Shotter, 1997, p.10) must be invented. The extent to which someone is enmeshed in, or estranged from, a system can influence their ability to be effective in that system (Pearce & Cronen, 1980). Catherine

Bateson (1994) believes that to emphasize a single activity, such as taking down an instructor's information, listening for diagnostic criteria from a client, or finding answers to specific questions, teaches us to devalue multisensory awareness. She emphasizes the learning potential of attending to relational as well as technical information. To this end, Barbara Vacarr (2001) approaches her role as an educator with a strategy that includes public expressions of vulnerability. By normalizing unexpected actions and self-revelations, she helps her students to become aware of transformational opportunities.

Any group that listens to each other's perspectives on a given situation brings attention to variables that would otherwise be missed. Nursing educator Carol Picard believes that recognizing one's own patterns, making meaning of them, and considering their ramifications is especially important in turbulent times. Therefore, she invites healthcare professionals into partnerships with their patients.

Practitioners may find compassion to be a great asset to their work. They may also find a cost of caring (Figley, 2002), burnout (Maslach, 1982), compassion fatigue (Joinson, 1992), or secondary traumatic stress (Stamm, 1999). These factors may include unwanted stressors, such as intrusive thoughts and nightmares about their patients, and distancing themselves from various sorts of intimacy. Maintaining high standards for client care while simultaneously attending to the costly impact of healthcare work on practitioners is a major concern for healthcare employers. Job-related stress and exhaustion are linked to extensive health challenges, including dysregulation of the hypothalamic-pituitary-adrenal axis and impaired immunity functions (Melamed, Shirom, Toker, Berliner, & Shapira, 2006; Toker, Shirom, Shapira, & Berliner, 2005). An evolving consensus suggests that rates of distress might be lowered by the use of collaborative–reflective practices (Landis, 2007b). Baldwin (2005) says:

> Collaborative creativity is one of the most powerful resources we have for transforming difficult situations into opportunities for growth. Yet, when we are overwhelmed by situations we feel we cannot resolve, we tend to lose this capacity, reacting, instead of responding reflectively, narrowing our range of behavior, often isolating ourselves from others. (p. 1)

Inherent to collaboration are clashing experiences with diversity, difference, and conflict. Circumstances that bring people to health practitioners can be thought of as social phenomena. Conditions arise in patterns of perception that demonstrate multiple social constructions, including economics, policy, tradition, law, environment, gender, ethnicity, race, religion, sexual orientation, and class. Anderson and Goolishian (1988, 1992) propose that practitioners facilitate problem-dissolving conversations, rather than problem-solving ones. Instead of approaching clients with the aim of fitting them into preestablished hypotheses, they recommend that practitioners take a stance of "not knowing."

Dance and health care have a shared history that offers an appealing example of this type of sensory-emotional healing. Pioneer dance therapist Marion Chace brought elements of her earlier dance career into working with psychiatric patients from the 1940s through the 1960s. She met with servicemen who had returned from war and were unable to speak, severely withdrawn individuals, and people who had schizophrenia. By observing their signature movements, she mirrored back to them in the gestures and emotions of their own expressions. These collaborative movement relationships Chace offered to her patients reflected her deep emotional acceptance and an ability to "meet each person where he/she is" and then move onward (Levy, 1988).

The invention of the reflecting team by Tom Andersen (1990) took the collaborative reflective process to a new level. Clients and practitioners would take turns listening to each other, highlight what was positive, and encourage each other. Katz and Shotter (1996) found that asking follow-up questions about arresting moments often suggests the social, as well as medical, explanations for which patients seek help. These practices are echoed in Hoffman's quote from Russian philologist Mikhail Bakhtin ". . . there is no knowledge of the subject but [the] dialogical" (2002, p. 161). Another proponent of this idea is the philosopher of reflectiveness, Donald Schon. Schon (1983) strongly states the case for becoming active learners through reflection-in-action. In order to engage in dialogue, we must be present with clients and use our senses to navigate the exchange. To all this Hoffman writes, "it occurred to me that this communal perspective rests on a change in the definition of what needs to change. . . . and since an environment is communally experienced, the antidote must be communal too" (2002, p. 271).

SHAREVISION: A PRACTICAL EXAMPLE OF COLLABORATIVE CREATIVITY

The Sharevision approach is an example of creativity generated through collaborative-reflection. It was developed among family therapy practitioners who were meeting families in their homes after the state had investigated charges of child neglect and abuse. This approach was facilitated by consultant Lynn Hoffman. Sharevision is currently being applied in graduate healthcare training and in healthcare facilities.

In 1987, family therapist and social worker Lynn Hoffman brought her critique of the helping professions' flawed "power-over idea versus power-with" approach to working with teams of professionals and their clients. In meetings at the family services agency People's Bridge Action in western Massachusetts, Hoffman was able to reduce ideological battles among staff by simply making time for each participant to speak and by honoring listening as much as speaking. Participants learned to value gestures and affect as much as words. The emphasis on hierarchy, reductionism, and convergent thinking was exchanged for personal experience, stories, and associative thinking. If the group was too large, participants were divided up into smaller groups. While there is a much larger conversation on the practice and theory of Sharevision (Baldwin, 1999, 2004a, 2004b, 2004c, 2006, 2008; Baldwin & Thompson, 1989; Fontes, 1995; Hoffman, 1993, 2002; Landis 2004, 2005, 2006, 2007a, 2007b, 2008; Landis, Baldwin, & Thompson, 2004), a premise is that, with more ideas on the table, better informed decisions would be made. It seems that the use of the model is linked to innovative programming, low staff turnover, and high morale.

RESEARCH ON COLLABORATIVE CREATIVITY

Research on Sharevision in hospitals and clinics was conducted with small groups of graduate interns and highly skilled clinicians who scored at extremely high risk for compassion fatigue on the Compassion Satisfaction/Fatigue Self Test for helpers and the Silencing Response Scale (Baranowsky, n.d.; Stamm,1999). Sharevision research includes the integration of movement and arts activities based on their positive impact with people in resilience programs when trauma had been involved (Berrol, 2006; Fisher & Ogden, 2009; Kisiel et al., 2006; Milliken, 2004; Murrant, Rykov, Amonite, & Loynd, 2000; Newman & Holzman, 1999; Ray, 2006; Rothschild, 2006; Shapiro, Brown, & Biegel, 2007; Stokrocki, Andrews, & Saemundsdottir, 2004; Van der Kolk, 2006).

Part of the research on this collaborative-reflection approach includes an arts-integrated group social action project. Social action to interrupt the cycle of violence on behalf of one's self and others is effective in trauma recovery and building resilience (Freire, 1970; Golub, 2005; Harvey, 2007; Junge, Alvarez, Kellogg, & Volker, 1993; Kaplan, 2007; Powell & Marcow-Speiser, 2005; Schutzman & Cohen-Cruz, 1994. Choosing an arts-integrated group project stimulates sensory-emotional dialogue on values and aspirations, helping participants bridge their isolation to a community. This practice of Sharevision appears to correlate with a decrease in compassion fatigue, a decrease in silencing the responses of clients, and an increase in compassion satisfaction.

The Sharevision group project is called *Esthetic Action* (Landis, 2008). The term esthetic action emerged in dialogue between Richard Baldwin, one of the originators of Sharevision and myself, the researcher, during a 2005 conversation about an early adaptation of Sharevision, which was focused on relieving compassion fatigue through arts and social action. *Esthetic action* is a process wherein the group examines existing patterns and builds ideas about new ones, then realizes these ideas through action in different contexts. Diverse communication media are used in this process to support nonlinear connections. The focus is to evolve a pattern that "feels right" or "fits" the group and the context. Once the esthetic action is accomplished, the group gathers and reflects on the results. In this way, an esthetic loop can be developed. These practices have roots in Gregory Bateson's ecological esthetics, ". . . esthetics is this glimpse that makes us aware of the unity of things which is not consciousness" (Bateson & Bateson, 1987, p. 300).

SHAREVISION: COLLABORATIVE-REFLECTION IN THE CLASSROOM

In classroom adaptations of Sharevision, students have a chance to hear from each other about dilemmas they present in small groups. Sharevision can take place for 15 to 20 minutes during 2½ hour classes. In large classes, students can miss opportunities to pose questions and hear from each other. Often, it is the more outspoken students that are the ones to regularly speak up. Sharing the time equitably provides each student with the opportunity to present her perspective. There is time for differing ideas and different ways of expressing oneself. Classroom practice in posing sensitive and concise questions and responses provides learning opportunities for develops listening and speaking skills that healthcare professionals need. Students also gain an awareness of the vulnerability patients have when they are asked to identify their thoughts and feelings in front of a group. The experience of receiving affirming responses from others in their small group can be crucial.

In smaller seminar classes, the teacher–student hierarchy is flattened in favor of timed periods of collaborative-reflection. Students report that they:

- Like having a structure where everyone's issues can be addressed
- Feel listened to
- Feel safe enough to bring any questions and concerns about internship
- Getting lots of creative ideas from others on how to approach challenges during internship
- Feel encouraged

CREATIVE ARTS LEARNING AND COLLABORATION IN THE CLASSROOM: PRACTICAL EXAMPLE

During a class on self-care for healthcare professionals, a collaborative arts-integrated experience enriches the dialogue on the topic. Here is an example of a classroom activity that encourages collaboration. A class begins with a lecture on burnout prevention, addressing the risk and frequency of secondary trauma for professionals, as well as thoughts and behaviors to watch out for in oneself and colleagues. An experience of self-care follows, addressing the elements of creating an environment that meets the needs of a multicultural workforce.

The class divides into small groups of four people. One box is full of inexpensive supplies such as balloons, ribbon, color markers, and paper and scissors are made available. The task is to create a safe place where students and professionals can decompress from the stress of their jobs. Their rich conversation about the range of possible priorities and ways to express their ideas using these simple supplies is limited by time. The goal is to create a performance piece that would include the development of this counterstress environment they have been asked to establish. Each group takes supplies, discusses their concerns, and comes up with a product that communicates their situation. This activity is followed by a group discussion. Themes that have emerged include bringing a spirit of fun to difficult work, feeling and emitting a sense of calm, being a good listener, offering new ideas to the discussion, as well as engaging conflict resolution skills.

Teaching Example

Developing Collaborative Creativity Skills

This activity by Ellen Landis was first used in a play therapy course for master's candidates in a variety of healthcare professions at Lesley University in Cambridge, Massachusetts. Most of these students had worked professionally in the healthcare field prior to returning to school or had experiences in the field through internships. The theme for the day was self-care for the professional. The class began with a lecture on burnout prevention, introduced the frequency and risk of secondary trauma for professionals as well as thoughts and behaviors to watch out for. An experience on self-care followed, addressing the sociocultural elements of creating an environment that meets the needs of a diverse workforce.

Landis brought out just one box full of inexpensive supplies such as balloons, ribbon, colored markers, paper, and scissors. The class divided into small groups of four people. They were all instructed to collaboratively create a safe place for them as students and professionals to decompress from the stress of their job. They needed to make decisions about their priorities and find a way to express their ideas using the simple supplies. They were asked to create a performance piece that could include the development of creating a safe place. Each group took supplies, discussed their concerns and came up with a performance piece. The activity was followed up with a group discussion. Themes that emerged include bringing a spirit of fun to difficult work, bringing a sense of calm to the job, being a good listener, bringing ideas to the table, as well as bringing conflict resolution skills to the job.

Since people often seek health care when there is an acute situation, a crisis, or an emergency, students recognize the inherent stress related to their work. This trilogy of evidence-based, theory-driven, reflective practice brought students together in affirmation of their goal to be part of a work environment that brings out the best in people, whether that is the patient or the professional.

REFERENCES

Andersen, T. (1990). *The reflecting team: Dialogues and dialogues about the dialogues*. Kent, UK: Borgman Publishing, Ltd.

Anderson, H., & Goolishian, H. (1988). Human systems as linguistic systems. *Family Process, 27*, 371–393.

Anderson, H., & Goolishian, H. (1992). The client is the expert. In S. McNamee & K. Gergen (Eds.), *Therapy as social construction*. Newbury Park, CA: Sage Publications.

Baldwin, R. (1999). *Sharevision: A clinical group supervision model*. Amherst, MA: Sharevision Inc.

Baldwin, R. (2004a). *Historical threads of Sharevision Inc*. Amherst, MA: Sharevision, Inc.

Baldwin, R. (2004b). *Reflective performance*. Amherst, MA: Sharevision, Inc.

Baldwin, R. (2004c). *Some ideas about the arts & clinical/educational practice*. Amherst, MA: Sharevision, Inc.

Baldwin, R. (2005). *Sharevision*. Hadley, MA: Sharevision.

Baldwin, R. (2006). *Sharevision: A story of its inception*. Hadley, MA: Sharevision.

Baldwin, R. (2008). *Sharevision: The process*. Hadley, MA: Sharevision.

Baldwin, R. & Thompson, L. (1989). Sharevision: An alternative to Supervision in Clinical Practice. Unpublished paper. Baranowsky, A. (2002). In C. Figley (Ed). *Treating compassion fatigue*. (pp. 155–170). New York: Brunner-Routledge.

Baranowsky, A. (n.d.) *Silencing response scale*. Retrieved September 5, 2006, from http://www.psychink.com/insite.htm

Bateson, M.C. (1994). *Peripheral visions: Learning along the way*. New York: Harper Collins.

Bateson, G., & Bateson M.C. (1987). *Angels fear*. New York: Dutton.

Berrol, C. (2006). Neuroscience meets dance movement therapy: Mirror neurons, the therapeutic process and empathy. *The arts in psychotherapy, 33*(4), 302–315.

Figley, C. (2002). *Treating compassion fatigue*. New York: Brunner-Routledge.

Fisher, J., & Ogden, P. (2009). Sensorimotor psychotherapy. In C. Courtois, & J. Ford (Eds.), *Treating complex traumatic stress disorders* (pp. 312–328). New York: The Guilford Press.

Fontes, L.A. (1995). Sharevision: Collaborative supervision and self-care strategies for working with trauma. *The Family Journal, 3*, 249–254.

Freire, P. (1970). *Pedagogy of the oppressed*. New York: Continuum.

Golub, D. (2005). Social action art therapy. *Art Therapy Journal of the American Art Therapy Association, 22*(1), 17–23.

Harvey, M. (2007). Towards an ecological understanding of resilience in trauma survivors: Implications for theory research and practice. *Journal of Aggression, Maltreatment and Trauma, 14*(1).

Hoffman, L. (1993). *Exchanging voices: A collaborative approach to family therapy*. London: Karnac Books.

Hoffman, L. (2002). *Family therapy: An intimate history*. New York: W.W. Norton.

Joinson, C. (1992). Coping with compassion fatigue. *Nursing, 22*(4), 116, 118–119, 120.

Junge, M., Alvarez., J., Kellogg, A., & Volker, C. (1993). The art therapist as social activist: Reflections and vision. *Art Therapy: Journal of Art Therapy Association, 10*(3), 148–155.

Kaplan, F. (2007). *Art therapy and social action*. Philadelphia: Jessica Kingsley.

Katz, A. M., & Shotter, J. (1996). Hearing the patient's 'voice': Towards a social poetics in diagnostic interviews. *Social Science and Medicine, 43*, 919–931.

Kisiel, C., Blaustein, M., Spinazzola, J., Schmidt, C., Zucker, M., & Van der Kolk, B. (2006). Evaluation of a theater-based youth violence prevention program for elementary school children. *Journal of School Violence, 5*(2), 19–36.

Landis, E. (2004). Sharevision: Looking through the lens of social construction theory.

Lesley University Expressive Therapies Field Training Supervisors, Cambridge, MA.

Landis, E. (2005). Moving into Family Therapy: A Collaborative Approach. Annual New England Chapter of the American Dance Therapy Association, Keene, NH.

Landis, E. (2006). *Building social action into group therapy with children.* Family Institute of Cambridge, Watertown, MA.

Landis, E. (2007a). *Concepts of wellness: Reflective performance builds resilience.* Northampton Veterans Affairs Medical Center, Northampton, MA.

Landis, E. (2007b). Effects of a collaborative reflective model to ameliorate secondary trauma. Unpublished paper. Cambridge, MA: Lesley University.

Landis, E. (2008). A collaborative approach to eliminating secondary trauma: Pilot study findings. Lesley University Doctoral Student Conference, Cambridge, MA.

Landis, E., Baldwin, R., & Thompson, L. (2004). Expressive arts therapy: A voice from the USA. *Context.* London: The Invicta Press.

Levy, F. (1988). *Dance movement therapy. A healing art.* Reston, VA: The American Alliance for Health, Physical Education, Recreation, and Dance.

Maslach, C. (1982). *Burnout the cost of caring.* New York: Prentice-Hall.Melamed, S., Shirom, A., Toker, S., Berliner, S., & Shapira, A. (2006). Burnout and risk of cardiovascular disease: Evidence, possible causal paths, and promising research directions. *Psychological Bulletin, 132*(3), 327–353.

Milliken, R. (2004). Dance movement therapy as a creative arts therapy approach in prison to the treatment of violence. *The Arts in Psychotherapy, 29*(4), 203–206.

Murrant, G., Rykov, M., Amonite, D., & Loynd, M. (2000). Creativity and self-care for caregivers. *Journal of Palliative Care, 16*(2), 44–49.

Newman, F., & Holzman, L. (1999). Beyond narrative to performed conversation ('In the beginning' comes much later). *Journal of Constructivist Psychology, 12,* 23–40.

Pearce, B., & Cronen, V. (1980). *Communication, action and meaning: The creation of social realities.* Westport, CT: Praeger.

Powell, M. C., & Marcow-Speiser, V. (2005). *The arts, education and social change: Little signs of hope.* New York: Peter Lang.

Ray, S. (2006). Embodiment and embodied engagement: Central concerns for the nursing care of contemporary peacekeepers suffering from psychological trauma. *Perspectives in Psychiatric Care, 42*(2), 106–113.

Rothschild, B. (2006). *The psychophysiology of compassion fatigue and vicarious trauma: Help for the helper: Self-care strategies for managing burnout and stress.* New York: W.W. Norton.

Schutzman, M., & Cohen-Cruz, J. (1994). *Playing boal.* New York: Routledge.

Schon, D. (1983). *The reflective practitioner: How professionals think in action.* London: Temple Smith.

Shapiro, S., Brown, K., & Biegel, G. (2007). Teaching self-care to caregivers: Effects of mindfulness-based stress reduction on the mental health of therapists in training. *Training and Education in Professional Psychology, 1*(2), 105–115.

Shotter, J. (1993). *Cultural politics of everyday life.* Buffalo, NY: University of Toronto Press.

Shotter, J. (1997). The social construction of our 'inner lives.' *Journal of Constructivist Psychology, 21*(1), 7–24.

Stamm, B. (1999). *Secondary traumatic stress; Self-care issues for clinicians, researchers, and educators* (2nd ed.). Baltimore: Sidran Press.

Stokrocki, M., Andrews, S., & Saemundsdottir, S. (2004). The role of art for homeless women and survivors of domestic violence. *Visual Arts Research, 29*, 73–82.

Thiboutot, C., Martinez, A., & Jager, D. (1999). Gaston Bachelard and phenomenology: outline of a theory of imagination. *Journal of Phenomenological Psychology, 30*(1), 1–17.

Toker, S., Shirom, A., Shapira, I., & Berliner, S. (2005). The association between burnout, depression, anxiety, and inflammation biomarkers: C-Reactive protein and fibrinogen in men and women. *Journal of Occupational Health Psychology, 10*(4), 344–362.

Vacarr, B. (2001). Voices inside schools: Moving beyond polite correctness: Practicing mindfulness in the diverse classroom. *Harvard Educational Review*, Summer 2001.

Van Der Kolk, B. (2006). Clinical implications of neuroscience research in PTSD. *Annals of the Academy of New York Sciences*, 1–17.

ADDITIONAL RESOURCES

Anderson, H., Gergen, K., McNamee, S., Cooperrider, D., Gergen, M., & Whitney, D. (2001). *The appreciative organization*. Chagrin Falls, OH: Taos Institute Publication.

Bradshaw, M. J., & Lowenstein A. J. (2007). *Innovative teaching strategies in nursing and related health professions* (4th ed.). Sudbury, MA: Jones and Bartlett.

Figley, C. (1997). *Burnout in families: The systemic costs of caring*. Boca Raton, FL: CRC Press.

Figley, C. (1995). *Compassion fatigue: Coping with secondary traumatic stress disorder in those who treat the traumatized*. New York: Brunner/Mazel.

Figley, C. (1995). Compassion fatigue. In B. H. Stamm (Ed.), *Secondary traumatic stress: Self-care issues for clinicians, researchers and educators* (pp. 3–28). Baltimore: Sidran Press.

Figley, C., & McCubbin, H. I. (1983). Looking to the future: Research, education, treatment, and policy. In C. R. Figley, & H. I. McCubbin (Eds.), *Stress and the family, Volume I: Coping with catastrophe* (pp. 185–196). New York: Brunner/Mazel.

Figley, C., & Stamm, B. H. (1996). Psychometric review of the Compassion Fatigue Self Test. In B. H. Stamm (Ed.), *Measurement of stress, trauma & adaptation*. Baltimore: Sidran Press.

Gergerson, M. (2007). Creativity enhances practitioners' resiliency and effectiveness after a hometown disaster. *Professional Psychology: Research and Practice, 38*(6), 596–602.

Kakkad, D. (2005). A new ethical praxis: Psychologists' emerging responsibilities in issues of social justice. *Ethics & Behavior, 15*(4), 293–308.

Keeney, B. (1983). *Aesthetic of change*. New York: The Guilford Press.

Picard, C., & Jones, D. (2005). *Giving voice to what we know: Margaret Newman's theory of health as expanding consciousness in nursing practice, research, and education*. Sudbury: MA: Jones and Bartlett.

Stamm, B. H., & Figley, C. (1996). Compassion satisfaction and fatigue test. Retrieved September 5, 2006, from http://www.psychink.com/insite.htm

White, M. (2004). *Narrative practice and exotic lives: Resurrecting diversity in everyday life*. Adelaide, South Australia: Dulwich Centre Publications.

CHAPTER 7

Lighten Up Your Classroom

Mariana D'Amico and Lynn Jaffe

Humor is also a way of saying something serious.
—*T. S. Eliot*

He who laughs most, learns best.
—*John Cleese (Priest, 2007)*

INTRODUCTION

Most educators take learning very seriously, especially those in health care. They overlook the fact that humor is a lifeline to sanity and reality. Humor is not a primary teaching strategy and it is quite difficult to measure the educational effect of humor in isolation from other teaching methods. The judicious use of humor can influence the cognitive and behavioral aspects of learning by engaging at least six of Gardner's seven forms of intelligence (as identified in Chapter 1). Research on humor has been a multidisciplinary endeavor, including a focus on use in classrooms and health care (Adamle, Chiang-Hanisko, Ludwick, Zeller, & Brown, 2007; Chauvet & Hofmeyer, 2007; Garner, 2006; Kher, 2003; Kher, Molstad, & Donahue, 1999; Wrench & McCroskey, 2001; Ziegler, 1998). Well-placed humor can make the classroom environment a safe, comfortable, and effective arena for cognitive and professional growth. Educators have used humor to alleviate classroom stress and facilitate knowledge acquisition and application for decades. Humor contributes to a positive affect and, to that end, humor has been used as a teaching tool for generations. Effectively using humor in the classroom requires knowledge, art, and skill, all of which may be learned (Garner, 2005, 2006; Hellman, 2007; Hillman, 2001; Kher, 2003; Ziegler, 1998). This chapter will highlight humor as an educator's tool and describe specific strategies for humor use in the classroom.

DEFINITION AND PURPOSE

Humor is a communication that induces amusement. Thus, it must be shared. It makes the learning environment a shared, pleasurable experience. In education, the most positive forms of humor are funny stories or comments, jokes, and professional humor. Sarcasm has been recorded as common in the classroom, but tends to be a negative form of humor. Wit is the cognitive process that elicits humor. Mirth is the emotional reaction to humor, joy, and pleasure. Laughter or smiling is a physical expression of humor. With all these elements, the formal study of humor in the classroom has been a challenge. A decade ago, the literature on the use of humor in healthcare education was predominantly opinion pieces or reviews as opposed to actual evidence, although at least a dozen studies of humor were conducted in educational settings (Ziegler, 1998). Whether the evidence is as sound as it should be remains equivocal, but lately the majority of authors praise its contributions to the educational experience (Chauvet & Hofmeyer, 2007; Dormann & Biddle, 2006; Garner, 2005, 2006; Hillman, 2001; James, 2004; Priest, 2007; Southam & Schwartz, 2004; Torok, McMorris, & Lin, 2004).

Humor has been studied and discussed from a variety of approaches—the physiologic, psychologic, emotional, and cognitive. Recent reviews have summarized these studies (Southam & Schwartz, 2004; Torok et al., 2004) and confirmed that humor can promote health as well as learning through the physical benefits of reduced stress, increased productivity, and enhanced creativity. Humor has been deemed a primary vehicle for enhancing the learning environment through enlivening potentially dreary topics, keeping lectures engaging and enjoyable, and humanizing faculty in students' perceptions. The cultivation of the abilities to laugh at oneself and with others bridges many gaps between people and broadens the pathway from student to professional as well as professional to client/patient (Adamle et al., 2007; Flowers, 2001; Priest, 2007).

The use of humor in the classroom can be productive, promoting comfortable, safe interactions between faculty and students. It has been shown to increase teacher credibility (Garner, 2006; Torok et al., 2004). The effective use of humor promotes creativity, learning, retention, and enculturation of professionals (Adamle et al., 2007; Chauvet & Hofmeyer, 2007; Boerman-Cornell, 2000; Dormann & Biddle, 2006; Flournoy, Turner, & Combs, 2001; Girdlefanny, 2004; Southam & Schwartz, 2004; Thorne, 1999). Counterproductive humor can cause fear and hostility, decrease self-esteem and motivation, and disrupt the community within the classroom and work settings (Boerman-Cornell, 2000; Ciesielka, Conway, Penrose, & Risco, 2005; Girdlefanny, 2004; Hurren, 2006; Meyer, 1997; Weber, 2000).

Both White (2001) and Torok et al. (2004) studied whether perceptions regarding the use of humor were correlated between professors and students, whether students thought more favorably of professors who used humor, and what types of humor were preferred. Their findings had strong correlations between perceptions in the use of funny stories, funny comments, jokes, and professional humor. Students were not supportive of humor in testing, nor the use of sarcasm.

Shibles' (1989) analysis of humor declares ridicule and sarcasm are used as a superiority differentiation or as a defense mechanism and therefore do not qualify as types of humor. Educators need to be cognizant of this because such a misuse of humor will be counterproductive in the classroom. Students often found humor facilitated attention, morale, and comprehension. Gender differences in student's perceptions of humor use, with female faculty's use of humor less likely to be recognized, has also been noted (White, 2001). White's study identified agreement between professors and students regarding humor as a tool to relieve stress, create a healthy learning environment, gain attention, and motivate students. An item of greatest variation between faculty and student perceptions was in the use of humor to handle unpleasant situations—students believed it could be used, but faculty did not.

THEORETICAL FOUNDATIONS

Humor is a complex phenomenon with a long and rich history. While no one has been able to establish when the first joke actually occurred, we know the Greek theatre used both comedy and drama to entertain and enlighten. Many authors, such as Dickens and Swift, used satire to comment on society. Theoretical foundations of humor are multiple (Shibles, 1989). They have been categorized by discipline (biological, cognitive, physiological, linguistic, etc.) and construct (incongruity, superiority, etc.) (Ziegler, 1998). Boyd (2004) purports that humor and laughter relate to play theory and, thus, create a sense of shared playfulness. He suggests that this sense of playfulness opens the participants to creative and critical thinking and action, while simultaneously alerting and disarming them in an environment of mutual trust and enjoyment. Effective use of humor may be a component of all learning theories. Humor and laughter contribute to all necessary principles of learning: enjoyment; creativity; interest; motivation; a relaxed, open, warm environment; a positive student–teacher relationship; and decreased tension and anxiety. To be authentic is one of the most important qualities of an educator. Having a sense of humor is an aspect of authenticity (Hellman, 2007; Lottes, 2008). Humor used constructively builds a positive self-image (Chauvet & Hofmeyer, 2007; Garner, 2005, 2006; Hellman, 2007; Priest, 2007).

Cognitive and affective theories appear the most important for education, as they account for linguistic, intellectual, and emotional aspects of learning. Some humor theories state that laughter or amusement occurs as an intellectual reaction to something unexpected, illogical, or inappropriate in some way (Boyd, 2004; Shibles, 1989). Cognitive theory focuses on an understanding of language, knowledge, situation, and reasoning that addresses recognition of mistakes, incongruity, and wordplays. Research indicates that the recognition of incongruity begins in infancy (Boyd, 2004; Wild, Rodden, Grodd, & Ruch, 2003). Puns, irony, and satire require analysis and synthesis of words, knowledge, and context (Boyd, 2004; Wild et al., 2003). Without such understanding, students do not perceive the humor and may take affront or feel put-down by the instructor. When students understand a concept well they can make jokes or funny remarks about it, indicating their synthesis of the material. Cognition is shaped by culture and humor has been defined as culturally appropriate incongruity (Boyd, 2004; Chauvet & Hofmeyer, 2007; Wrench & McCroskey, 2001).

According to Bloom, affect is an important domain of learning. Those theorists who subscribe to affective theory stress emotional components of humor. However, it seems inadequate to treat affect as separate from cognition, because emotion is largely constituted by thought (Shibles, 1989). There has been extensive discussion regarding the emotional and physiologic benefits of releasing psychic energy through laughter. Because of this, humor is an invaluable contribution to the educational process. Its use creates an affirmation of shared understanding and experience (Boyd, 2004). Research supports its use to reduce anxiety and stress, build confidence, improve productivity, reduce boredom, heighten interest, and encourage divergent thinking and the creation of new ideas (Chauvet & Hofmeyer, 2007; Dormann & Biddle, 2006; Weber, 2000; Ziegler, 1998).

The affective component of humor engages the limbic system thereby enhancing short- and long-term memory, and increasing the willingness of the learner to apply knowledge and skills (Flournoy et al., 2001; Hillman, 2001; Southam & Schwartz, 2004). The expression of feelings, such as empathy and anger, can be more constructive when approached in a witty manner (Hillman, 2001). Both sides of the brain are actively engaged during laughter and the perception of humor (Southam & Schwartz, 2004). The right side of the brain involves reading and interpreting the visual, nonverbal information of humor while the left side of the brain interprets the language nuances of humor. Novelty, imagination, and visualization help move information into long-term memory through the engagement of multiple brain cells firing simultaneously (Southam & Schwartz, 2004; Weber, 2000; Wild et al., 2003; Wrench & McCroskey, 2001). However, there is still much research to be done about the neuroscience related to humor and the perceptions about what is humorous (Wild et al., 2003).

TYPES OF LEARNERS

Humor is a type of playfulness that spans multiple ages and venues. Developmentally and intellectually appropriate humor can be employed with all levels of learner. Classroom humor relevant to course content is more appreciated by the adult learner than random humor. It is also necessary to be aware of students' cultural backgrounds as words and concepts may have different meanings and be misperceived, or worse, be taboo to discuss (Axtell, 1999). Studies have provided mixed reviews about students' acceptance and appreciation of humor used by the teacher. Some studies have shown that gender impacts the acceptance and use of humor, as does the match between the educators' and students' sense of humor (Martin, Puhlik-Doris, Larsen, Gray, & Weir, 2003). The associations found between intellectual ability and sense of humor suggest that educators need a firm check on the cognitive status of their students when employing wit or they risk offending rather than amusing them (Boyd, 2004; LaFarge, 2004; Wild et al., 2003). Gorham and Christophel (1990, as cited by Southam & Schwartz, 2004) found that learning outcomes of female students were not as influenced by teacher humor as were outcomes in male students whose achievement was enhanced through the use of humor. Females, while not appreciably influenced by humor in that study, did prefer personal stories that illustrated pertinent points related to course content. Student reaction to humor has been differentially related to the gender of the educator as well, with female educators eliciting less overall appreciation of their efforts to be humorous (White, 2001). Acceptance of humor in the classroom has been shown to be positively associated with a student's psychological health (Dziegielewski, Jacinto, Laudadio, & Legg-Rodriguez, 2003; Kuiper, Grimshaw, Leite, & Kirsh, 2004).

CONDITIONS FOR LEARNING

Humor can be used judiciously throughout a class session or course and in all types of classroom situations: lecture, lab, fieldwork, and various course assignments. Mood can enhance or inhibit the reception of humor (Wild et al., 2003), making it imperative to read the class members accurately and create a positive and pleasant classroom experience. Positive and constructive humor can be used to put the learner and the teacher at ease with the subject matter (Garner 2005, 2006; Hellman, 2007). Humorous activities, or icebreakers, that relate to the class session topic might begin a class. These activities can also be inserted at intervals to reaffirm the open, relaxed atmosphere that is most conducive to learning. Tension relievers before exams are usually helpful. As long as the humor remains embedded in the content, learners will internalize the new knowledge, otherwise the flow of the lesson can be lost or misdirected (Weaver & Cotrell, 2001). Humor can be used to facilitate creativity and retention of material at any point in a lesson—from initial setup, through final review (Chauvet & Hofmeyer, 2007; Garner, 2006; Hellman, 2007).

Relationship between class size and classroom size may impact the effective use of humor. Berk (2002, as cited by Torok et al., 2004) noted that laughter is likely to be greater in larger, more crowded classes, than in smaller classes in larger rooms. Laughter, like yawning, is contagious; so once a large group gets going it may take time to bring them back to focus. Dziegielewski and colleagues (2003) encourage the group leader, educator in this case, not to stop the laughter but to let it stop on its own accord. They perceive that this laughter helps reduce anger and tension, and may build cohesion and well-being—both of which are essential to productivity and learning.

Humor is a part of communication and not dependent on the natural comedic ability of an instructor. It is an attitude and permission for enjoyment of the educational process (Adamle et al., 2007; Chauvet & Hofmeyer, 2007; Joyner & Young, 2006; Weaver & Cotrell, 2001). It can be spontaneous or planned. Weaver and Cottrell recommend inserting humorous breaks every 15 minutes. Essential to creating open communication and allowing humor within the classroom is the teacher's nonverbal communication and voice tone, as these can convey openness or constrict enjoyment of learning. If the humor style of the teacher and that of the class do not mesh, then the use of humor in the learning process will not be effective. It is important to understand your audience, which, in this case is the class and to know one's own sense of humor and be willing to experiment with others (Garner, 2006; Girdlefanny, 2004; Hellman 2007; Wild et al., 2003).

Humor is not necessarily universally appropriate. McMorris, Boothroyd, and Pietrangelo (1997) summarized studies that used humor in testing situations with mixed results. Positive results depended on the type of humor used. Some studies found humor to reduce tension, but others found it to be distracting in a testing situation. Humor with a strong linguistic base may also disadvantage international students. Likewise, as mentioned previously, any use of sarcasm was seen to be detrimental to learning (Garner, 2006; Hellman 2007; Meyer, 1997; Torok et al., 2004).

Humor can be very useful in the enculturation of novices into one's profession, especially when dealing with elements of embarrassing intimacy and reality shocks that may occur in healthcare provision (Adamle et al., 2007; Southam & Schwartz, 2004). According to Sultanoff (1995), a lack of sense of humor is related to lower self-esteem. On the other hand, a healthy sense of humor is related to being able to laugh as one's self and one's life without degrading oneself. Those who enter the health professions must be able to cope with adversity and be able to help others cope as well (Adamle et al., 2007). The development of a healthy sense of humor, beginning in preservice classes and continuing through professional in-services, benefits everyone.

RESOURCES

As with any teaching strategy, the effective use of humor needs to be learned and refined. Before using humor in teaching situations, educators may want to assess their own sense of humor using a humor profile such as the one developed by Richmond, Wrench, and Gorham (2001) (Please see Appendix 7-1 on the Web site that accompanies this book). The score obtained on the humor profile reflects one's use of humor during communications. Completion of a humor profile is a preliminary step to learning one's current facility with humorous content.

Some ways to increase one's use of humor is by exposing oneself to and collecting humorous experiences, such as reading comics, sitcoms, joke books; visiting comedy clubs; and even looking for the humor around oneself. This may include viewing the world through exaggeration or broad, silly perspectives. Using exaggeration is a method to clarify concepts—the contrast assists understanding. Incongruity is another technique for promoting humor in the classroom. One such example is comparing a stripper and a corporate CEO regaining work skills (see applied example later). Creating a top 10 list of teacher pet peeves or preferred learning behaviors can be a humorous way to share class performance expectations (Kher, 2003; Kher et al., 1999). Using props in the classroom for role playing may also enhance the humor of a lesson (Joyner & Young, 2006; Polek, 2007; Priest, 2007; Sultanoff, 1995). The cinema or YouTube are treasure troves of humorous situations waiting to be tapped by the healthcare professional looking for examples of exaggeration, incongruity, or basic fun (Polek, 2007).

Articles about infusing humor into online courses have suggested a number of techniques to promote a positive learning environment in the virtual classroom that mirror applications of humor in the regular classroom. Primary among these techniques is the use of humor to project an authentic representation of the educator. The humor used, by necessity, is primarily linguistic, although cartoons are readily available (James, 2004). Being humorous online requires extensive commitment, time, and effort as it needs to be planned, personalized to the students, and monitored for receptivity (Boynton as cited by James, 2004).

1. Web resources

   Humor Matters Bibliography and Resources, retrieved from http://www.humormatters.com/bibindex.htm

   Listing of potentially relevant films (primarily on mental illness), retrieved from http://www.disabilityfilms.co.uk/mental1/men1dex.htm

2. Sources for cartoon humor

   Cartoons from the *New Yorker* magazine, retrieved from http://www.cartoonbank.com
   Single cartoons by Randy Glasbergen, often about business or family, retrieved from http://www.glasbergen.com/
   Variety of popular newspaper cartoon serials, retrieved from http://www.gocomics.com/explore/comics

3. Print Resources

   Print versions of cartoons (*Far Side, For Better or Worse, Calvin and Hobbes,* etc.), local newspapers, bookstores
   Desk calendars such as "A Little Bit of Oy;" "The Far Side," and "Charlie Brown"
   Cathcart, T., & Klein, D. (2007). *Plato and a platypus walk into a bar: Understanding philosophy through jokes*. New York: Penguin Group, Inc.
   Tibballs, G. (2000). *The mammoth book of humor*. New York: Carroll & Graf

Check the humor section of any bookstore.

USING THE METHOD

The use of humor can be learned, and has a growing evidence base, yet remains highly individualized. Gender, culture, ethnicity, mood, and context impact the acceptance or rejection of this teaching strategy (Garner, 2005, 2006; Wild et al., 2003; Ziegler, 1998). Wanzer and Frymier (1999) found that witty, rather than funny, professors were considered interesting, entertaining, and motivating by adult learners. Robinson is often cited (Hillman, 2001; Southam & Schwartz, 2004) as proposing four interrelated aspects to be considered in the area of education and humor: (1) enhancing the learning process itself through humor; (2) using humor to facilitate the process of socialization; (3) teaching the concept of humor as a communication and intervention tool; and (4) modeling the use of humor as a vehicle for facilitating the other three. Using humor in the classroom is not attempting to become a comedian. It is assuming an attitude of authenticity and comfort within the classroom (Garner, 2005, 2006; Hellman, 2007; Lottes, 2008; Polek, 2007). The ability to learn to use humor has been questioned by a few authors (Wrench & McCroskey, 2001). These authors distinguish sense of humor, a culturally taught trait, from the act of being humorous, which may be a genetic trait. However, most authors promote the idea that the use of humor not only can be learned, but ought to be learned by educators to enhance the teaching–learning process (Adamle et al., 2007; Chauvet & Hofmeyer, 2007;

Dormann & Biddle, 2006; Flowers, 2001; Garner, 2006; Girdlefanny, 2004; Priest, 2007; Yura-Petro, 1991). Employing humorous methods is within every educator's reach and will enhance the educational experience for students.

Using humor in the learning process can take several forms (Fig. 7-1). It is easy for most faculty to use spontaneous storytelling by relating their own experiences to enhance the learning process. Other faculty may need to collect jokes, cartoons, movie excerpts, and humorous exercises to insert into their regular teaching activities to enhance the learner's receptivity to information and participation during content presentations. Tamblyn (2003) highly recommends the frequent use of visuals such as cartoons, posters, and other images throughout an educational presentation to enhance the impact of the content. From a cognitive load perspective, the use of cartoons may enhance recall and retention due to the complimentary effect of visual and verbal information processing, as long as the cartoon/text match is consistent with the course content and learning level of the student (Khalil, Paas, Johnson, & Payer, 2005). As has been mentioned, faculty must realize that what works for some people does not necessarily work for others (Boyd, 2004; Hillman, 2001; Tamblyn, 2003; Wild et al., 2003).

Some specific techniques for including humor in a class situation include posting humorous situations on a bulletin board to teach interactive concepts (Flournoy et al., 2001). Using irony to contrast expected outcomes and actual occurrence enhances remembrance because of incongruity (Thorne, 1999). Case studies with funny names related to topical content also enhance memory of the examples. (Example: Petunia Potter liked working in her garden. She needed some ergonomic changes to facilitate her participation in this avocation; how would you adapt this occupation for her?) Use of exaggerations and unusual professions increases awareness of people's needs in the healthcare arena. Personal stories

Figure 7-1 Tips for using humor in the classroom.

1. Create a casual (and safe) atmosphere
2. Smile; adopt a laugh-ready attitude
3. Relax, use open, nonverbal posture; increase interpersonal contact through eye-to-eye and face-to-face contact
4. Remove social inhibitions; establish nonjudgmental forum for discussion
5. Begin class with a humorous example, cartoon, anecdote, or thought for the day
6. Use personal stories, anecdotes, current events related to class content
7. Plan frequent breaks in content for application, humorous commercials, or exaggerated examples; provide humorous materials
8. Encourage give and take with students; laugh at yourself occasionally

Source: Adapted from Weaver & Cotrell, 2001; Provine, 2000.

about real life experiences and challenges in one's role as a new professional, or unexpected circumstances (or embarrassing moment) can have teaching value. Sometimes when students are called on to do group presentations on a given topic they will use humor (often in the form of mimicry or parody of the instructors) to engage their classmates and, possibly, to alleviate their own stress. Humor usage will be as variable as those using it, which can be quite diverse (Chauvet & Hofmeyer, 2007; Garner, 2006; Hellman, 2007; Priest, 2007).

A picture's meaning can express ten thousand words —often misquoted Chinese proverb

POTENTIAL PROBLEMS

Not everyone gets a joke (Boyd, 2004; Wild et al., 2003). Some people are too serious. Some do not value humor in the educational process. Some find it too distracting to their learning. Using sarcasm, ridicule, and put-down humor can be counterproductive. Humor has the potential to be offensive, especially with ethnic, cultural, or gender issues. Incongruence between innate or cultural humor perceptions can be disruptive to the coordination of the learning environment. Besides potentially offending some members of a class, the use of deprecatory humor may affect student's perceptions of the faculty and undermine their effectiveness. Class clowns, who use humor for personal gain, also abuse the strategy and detract from the learning environment (Martin et al., 2003).

Figure 7-2 An example of a joke that may be appropriate for a class on clinical reasoning.

Sherlock Holmes and Dr. Watson went camping. After a good meal and an excellent bottle of wine, they lay down and went to sleep. A couple of hours later, Holmes woke up and nudged his faithful friend.

"Watson, Watson," he said. "Look up at the sky and tell me what you see?"

"I see millions and millions of stars," replied Watson.

"And what does that tell you?" inquired the master detective.

Watson thought for a moment, "Well, Holmes, astronomically, it tells me that there are millions of galaxies and potentially billions of planets. Astrologically, I observe that Saturn is in Leo. Horologically, I deduce that the time is approximately 2:25. Theologically, I can see that god is all powerful and that we are small and insignificant. Meteorologically, I believe we will have a glorious day tomorrow. What does it tell you, Holmes?"

"Watson, you imbecile! Some thief has stolen our tent!"

Source: Tibballs, G. (2000). *The mammoth book of humor*. New York: Carroll & Graf; joke 2470.

CONCLUSION

It has been said that Plato believed one could discover more about a person in an hour of play than in a year of conversation. The same could be said about the culture of a classroom, cohort, or department. Teaching–learning communities are built on engagement and communication amongst students and faculty. The development of respect and desire to learn can be facilitated with the thoughtful use of humor. All involved will find their creativity, enjoyment, and problem solving boosted by this cognitively stimulating and emotionally safe learning environment.

APPLIED EXAMPLE(S)

At the beginning of a class, in this case a pediatrics class on toddler development, cartoons that related to the lecture topic were used as a starting point for discussion. The cartoons had been selected from the daily newspaper over a span of years, and so there were many examples of toddler behaviors to choose from. Students who had their own children, or younger siblings, were able to immediately relate to the cartoon situations and discuss the behaviors depicted as well as other toddler behaviors and observations they had seen. Students without children and siblings participated in the discussion by asking questions of those with more experience. A lively discussion ensued. When presented with the accompanying reading material or tested on the material at a later date students exhibited better retention and recall of the information and the discussion that occurred around the visual cue of the cartoon.

Another example of a humor-enhanced class discussion related to client-centered evaluation by using exaggerated comparison and contrast of a stripper and a CEO's daily activity routines, expectations, and needs. Students started discussing their perceived stereotypes of these exaggerated individuals and, as new elements of typical activities of daily living were tossed out to the students to analyze for these individuals, another lively discussion occurred. When assessed for their understanding of activities of daily living evaluations, analyses, and syntheses for treatment plans, students exhibited a greater understanding of these processes related to individualized care with attention to details.

REFERENCES

Adamle, K., Chiang-Hanisko, L., Ludwick, R., Zeller, R. & Brown, R. (2007). Comparing teaching practices about humor among nursing faculty: An international collaborative study. *International Journal of Nursing Education, Scholarship, 4*(1), Article 2.

Axtell, R. (1999). *Do's and taboo's of humor around the world*. New York: John Wiley and Sons, Inc.

Boerman-Cornell, W. (2000). Humor your students. *English Journal, 88*, 66–69.

Boyd, B. (2004). Laughter and literature: A play theory of humor. *Philosophy and Literature, 28*(1), 1–22.

Cathcart, T., & Klein, D. (2007). *Plato and a platypus walk into a bar: Understanding philosophy through jokes*. New York: Penguin Group, Inc.

Chauvet, S., & Hofmeyer, A. (2007). Humor as a facilitative style in problem-based learning environments for nursing students. *Nurse Education Today, 27*, 286–292.

Ciesielka, D., Conway, A., Penrose, J., & Risco, K. (2005). Maximizing resources: The S.H.A.R.E. Model of collaboration. *Nursing Education Perspectives, 26*(4), 224–226.

Dormann, C., & Biddle, R. (2006). Humour in game-based learning. *Learning, Media and Technology, 31*(4), 411–424.

Dziegielewski, S. F., Jacinto, G. A., Laudadio, A., & Legg-Rodriguez, L. (2003). Humor: An essential communication tool in therapy. *International Journal of Mental Health, 32*(3), 74–90.

Flournoy, E., Turner, G., & Combs, D. (2001). Critical care: Read the writing on the wall. *Nursing, 31*(3), 8–10.

Flowers, J. (2001, May/June). The value of humor in technology education. *Technology Teacher*.

Garner, R. (2005). Humor, analogy, and metaphor: H.A.M. it up in Teaching. *Radical Pedagogy, 6*(2).

Garner, R. (2006). Humor in pedagogy: How ha-ha can lead to aha! *College Teaching, 54*(1), 177–180.

Girdlefanny, S. (2004). Using humor in the classroom. *Techniques: Connecting Education & Careers, 79*(3), 22–26.

Hellman, S. V. (2007). Humor in the classroom: Stu's seven simple steps to success. *College Teaching, 55*(1), 37–39.

Hillman, S. M. (2001). Humor in the classroom: Facilitating the learning process. In A. J. Lowenstein & M. J. Bradshaw (Eds.), *Fuszard's innovative teaching strategies in* nursing (3rd ed.). Sudbury, MA: Jones and Bartlett.

Hurren, B. (2006). The effects of principals' humor on teachers' job satisfaction. *Educational Studies, 32*(4), 373–385.

James, D. (2004). Commentary: A need for humor in online courses. *College Teaching, 52*(3), 93–94.

Joyner, B., & Young, L. (2006). Teaching medical students using role play: Twelve tips for successful role plays. *Medical Teacher, 28*(3), 225–229.

Khalil, M. K., Paas, F., Johnson, T. E., & Payer, A. F. (2005). Interactive and dynamic visualizations in teaching and learning of anatomy: A cognitive load perspective. *Anatomical Record, 286B*, 8–14.

Kher, N. (2003). Using humor in the college classroom to enhance teaching effectiveness in "Dread Courses". Nova Southeastern University, H Wayne Huizenga School of Busingess and Entrpereneurship, July 2003. Proquest Information and Learning Company.

Kher, N., Molstad, S., & Donahue, R. (1999). Using humor in the college classroom to enhance teaching effectiveness in "Dread Courses." *College Student Journal, 33*, 400–406.

Kuiper, N.A., Grimshaw, M., Leite, C., & Kirsh, G. (2004). Humor is not always the best medicine: Specific components of sense of humor and psychological well-being. *Humor, 17*, 135–168.

LaFarge, B. (2004). Comedy's intention. *Philosophy and Literature, 28*(1), 118–136.

Lottes, N. (2008). FIRE UP: Tips for engaging student learning. *Journal of Nursing Education, 47*(7), 331–332.

Martin, R. A., Puhlik-Doris, P., Larsen, G., Gray, J., & Weir, K. (2003). Individual differences in uses of humor and their relation to psychological well-being: Development of the Humor Styles Questionnaire. *Journal of Research in Personality, 37*, 28–75.

McMorris, R. F., Boothroyd, R. A., & Pietrangelo, D. J. (1997). Humor in educational testing: A review and discussion. *Applied Measurement in Education, 10*(3), 269–297.

Meyer, J. (1997). Humor in the member narratives: Uniting and dividing at work. *Western Journal of Communication, 61*(2), 188–208.

Polek, C. (2007). The podium as a stage: A one woman act. *Nurse Educator, 32*(1), 8–10.

Priest, A. (2007). Learning through laughter. *Nursing BC, 39*(5), 8–11.

Provine, R. R. (2000). *Laughter: A scientific investigation*. New York: Viking Penguin.

Richmond, V. P., Wrench, J. S., & Gorham, J. (2001). *Communication, affect, and learning in the classroom*. Acton, MA: Tapestry Press.

Shibles, W. (1989) Humor reference guide. Retrieved November 30, 2009, from http://www.drbarbaramaier.at/shiblesw/humorbook/index.html

Southam, M., & Schwartz, K. B. (2004). Laugh and learn: Humor as a teaching strategy in occupational therapy education. *Occupational Therapy in Health Care, 18*, 57–70.

Sultanoff, S. (1995). What is humor? Retrieved January 3, 2006 from http://www.aath.org/articles/art_sultanoff01.html

Tamblyn, D. (2003). *Laugh and learn: 95 ways to use humor for more effective teaching and training*. New York: American Management Association.

Thorne, B. M. (1999). Using irony in teaching the history of psychology. *Teaching of Psychology, 26*(3), 222–224.

Torok, S. E., McMorris, R. F., & Lin, W-C. (2004). Is humor an appreciated teaching tool? Perceptions of professors' teaching styles and use of humor. *College Teaching, 52*, 14–20.

Wanzer, M. B., & Frymier, A. B. (1999). The relationship between student perceptions of instructor humor and students' reports of learning. *Communication Education, 48*, 48–62.

Weaver, R. L., & Cotrell, H. W. (2001). Ten specific techniques for developing humor in the classroom. *Education, 108*(2), 167–179.

Weber, A. (2000). Playful writing for critical thinking. *Journal of Adolescent & Adult Literacy, 43*(6), 562–568.

White, G. W. (2001). Teachers' report of how they used humor with students perceived use of such humor. *Education, 122*(2), 337–347.

Wild, B., Rodden, F., Grodd, W., & Ruch, W. (2003). Neural correlates of laughter and humour. *Brain, 126*, 2121–2138.

Wrench, J., & McCroskey, J. (2001). A temperamental understanding of humor communication and exhilaratability. *Communication Quarterly, 49*, 142–159.

Yura-Petro, H. (1991). Humor: A research and practice tool for nurse scholar-supervisors, practitioners, and educators. *Health Care Supervisor, 9*(4), 1–8.

Ziegler, J. B. (1998). Use of humour in medical teaching. *Medical Teacher, 20*(4), 341–348.

SECTION II

Teaching in Structured Settings

Section II presents concept-based topics that are applicable in a myriad of situations, regardless of the level of the learner, the topic, or the class size. This section focuses on the structured (i.e., traditional) classroom setting. Yet the universal concepts evident in each chapter include the importance of planning and preparation on the part of the teacher, the manner in which information is conveyed, and the importance of active student involvement and responsibility for learning.

The principles presented in Section I, the Introduction, are used in the traditional classroom environments addressed in these chapters. Application of teaching and learning theories and planned activities directed toward critical thinking are apparent. Educators can use creative innovations with time-honored strategies, such as lecture, to bring a refreshing approach to teaching.

CHAPTER 8

Lecture: Reclaiming a Place in Pedagogy

Barbara C. Woodring and Richard C. Woodring

A common characteristic found in all great teachers is a love of their subject, an obvious satisfaction found in arousing this love in their students, and an ability to convince them that what they are being taught is deadly serious.

—*J. Epstein*

INTRODUCTION

I recently read a report dealing with the evolution of the chief learning officer (CLO) within major industries (Huntley, 2009). I was reminded just how important it is to be an educator regardless of the setting, how important it is to know your students (the audience), and how critical it is to know the best strategies to help a student/participant to learn. I was also introduced to a new term, one to which I could immediately attach meaning: ***edutainment***. (Huntley, 2009). Ms. Huntley, a global CLO for an international corporation, believes:

> Education is no longer enough. Learners expect to be engaged and entertained more than ever . . . [learners] are exposed to a variety of stimulating and on-demand media sources daily . . . learning modes need to be equally engaging (Huntley, 2009, p. 32).

And yet, I am reminded that the methodology that remains the backbone by which knowledge is conveyed in most educational settings is the lecture. How, then, can educators merge the need for interactive variety, edutainment, while implementing the most commonly utilized teaching method? Hopefully the information in this chapter will assist in addressing that question.

The authors of other chapters in this text provide insight into creative and innovative teaching approaches that are currently used in higher education. The implementation and refinement of these strategies/methods during the last decade tends to relegate the use of the lecture methodology to a lesser stature. Rather than revere what had previously been considered the educational gold-standard, it became trendy to "lecture bash," to describe colleagues who used lecture techniques as old-fashioned and out of step with educational trends. Many educators added the term "lecture" to their list of unspeakable, four-letter words. But a lecture is only a means to an end. Intrinsically, it is neither good nor bad; its success depends on how it is delivered.

In practice, the lecture format is alive and well and remains one of the most frequently utilized teaching methods in the repertoire of postsecondary educators. When the objective is to communicate basic facts, introduce initial concepts, or convey passion about a topic, a well prepared lecture is very useful (Cox & Rogers, 2005; Gleitman, 2006). In this chapter, readers will find rationale for the long-term popularity of this teaching strategy, suggestions regarding how to improve its utilization, and tips on ways to become a better lecturer.

DEFINITION AND PURPOSES

By definition, the lecture is one method of presenting information to an audience. Cox and Rogers (2005) described a well-designed lecture as "an instructor-led, interactive experience that actively engages students in the process of learning and can support diverse student learning" (p. 1). This recent definition indicates how far the educational process has come. Prior to the invention of the printing press, when only scholars had access to handwritten information sources, the lecture was the primary means of transmitting knowledge. Learners would gather around the master-teacher and take notes related to what was said. The lecture remained the common mode of disseminating information until printed resources and technological advancements became more available and affordable.

It would appear that when students were able to purchase their own textbooks, and then computers, methods of presenting information would have changed. Interestingly, change has occurred slowly. Today, with e-books and technology galore, the lecture remains a commonly used technique. It is suggested that there are two major reasons for this longevity: (1) most current educators learned via the lecture format, and it is well known that individuals teach as they were taught unless they make a specific effort to alter their approaches; and (2) the lecture is the safest and easiest teaching method, allowing the teacher the most control within the classroom setting. Some of the common advantages and disadvantages of using the lecture method are listed in Tables 8-1 and 8-2. Whatever the rationale, positive outcomes can still be achieved by using the lecture, especially when the lecture and lecturer are well prepared.

THEORETICAL RATIONALE

Few lecturers take time to contemplate the theoretical basis of their practice, but the lack of a theoretical or organizational framework may be one reason that learners perceive some lectures to be disorganized and/or difficult to follow.

Table 8-1 Advantages of Using Lectures as a Teaching Strategy

Advantages of a Lecture	Secondary Gain in Use of Lecture
Permits teacher maximum control of class	Relieves teacher anxiety of handling unexpected questions
Creates minimal threats to students or teacher	Lack of interaction or student participation may be desired
Clarifies and enlivens information that seem tedious in text	Highlights enthusiasm/personality of teacher for topic
Enables clarification of confusing/ intricate points immediately	Avoids frustration of time delayed responses or clarification
The teacher knows what has been presented	Diminishes the "I never heard that before" comment by students
Lecture material can become basis of publication	Contributes to academic scholarship
Students are provided with a common core of content	May help student to prepare for testing
Accommodates larger numbers of listeners at one setting	High priority in weak economy and/or teacher shortage
Saves time	Teacher can present key points in much less time than it takes to elicit from text or extensive list of references
Provides venue to become known as an expert in specific topic	Contribute to the scholarship of teaching
Encourages and allows deductive reasoning	Can support principles of critical analysis if desired
Enthusiasm of teacher motivates students to participate and learn more	Reinforces professional role modeling

(continued)

Table 8-1 Advantages of Using Lectures as a Teaching Strategy *(Continued)*

Advantages of a Lecture	Secondary Gain in Use of Lecture
Allows addition of the newest information on a moment's notice	Can support concept of evidence-based practice with "just-in-time" data
Permits auditory learners to receive succinct information quickly	Encourages higher level learner, not rote memorization
Enables integration of pro and con aspects of topic	

Source: Adapted from Woodring, B., & Woodring, R. (2007). Lecture is not a four-letter word. In M. Bradshaw & A. Lowenstein (Eds.), *Innovative teaching strategies in nursing and related health professions* (4th ed., p. 111). Sudbury, MA: Jones and Bartlett.

Foundational principles for a lecture presentation may be derived from a variety of philosophical and theoretical processes. Three common approaches flow from theories related to communication, cognitive learning, and pedagogical/andragogical approaches to teaching and learning. The theories supporting effective communications should be common knowledge to all healthcare providers; therefore, they are not discussed here. Healthcare educators should have an understanding of cognitive learning theory since it is the underpinning of developmental concepts found in most health-related courses. Pedagogical/andragogical approaches may not be as well understood and are addressed briefly.

Over the past few decades, graduate education for many health professionals has emphasized disciplinary skills. Nursing and physical therapy, for instance, have focused on advanced practice skills resulting in clinical specialization (CNS), nurse practitioners (NP), and the professional doctorate degrees (DPT/DNP). This change has resulted in limited numbers of newer faculty members who are prepared in areas of curricular design and learning theory. Pedagogy is a portion of learning theory that loosely refers to educating the chronologically or experientially immature. In a pedagogical approach, someone external to the learner decides who, what, when, where, and how information will be taught; the learner becomes a passive recipient of knowledge. Historically, professionally health-related content and practice has been taught from a framework and has been based upon the medical model. Within the pedagogical context, the lecture strategy establishes the teacher as the one in command, the authority from whom answers come. This approach may provide a rationale for lecturing being viewed

Table 8-2 Disadvantages of Using Lectures as a Teaching Strategy

Disadvantages of a Lecture
Teacher may attempt to cover too much material in abbreviated time frame
Less effective when not accompanied by another teaching strategy
Eighty percent of lecture information is forgotten 1 day later and 80% of remainder fades in 1 month
Presumes that all students are auditory learners and learn at the same rate
Alone, the lecture is not suited to higher levels of thinking
Not conducive for personalized instruction
Encourages passive learners
Provides little feedback to learners
Student attention wavers in 30 minutes or less
Not appropriate for children below 4th grade level
Consistent use inhibits development of inductive reasoning
Poorly delivered lecture acts as a disincentive for learning
Viewed by students as a complete learning experience; think lecturer presents all they need to know
Affective learning seldom occurs in a lecture-only format

Source: Adapted from Woodring, B., & Woodring, R. (2007). Lecture is not a four-letter word. In M. Bradshaw & A. Lowenstein (Eds.), *Innovative teaching strategies in nursing and related health professions* (4th ed., p. 112). Sudbury, MA: Jones and Bartlett.

as "traditional" and out of step with innovation and creativity in the academy. Over the years, both the age and experiential backgrounds of "traditional" college students have shifted, causing scholars to question the appropriateness of the previously used pedagogical methods. In response, educators such as Knowles (1970), Kidd (1973), and Cross (1986) introduced and refined the concept of andragogy. The principles previously utilized in teaching the young (pedagogy) were adapted and applied to "mature" learners (andragogy).

Those educators who ascribe to andragogical theory treat the learner as a mature individual who brings a variety of rich, valuable experiences to every learning situation. The who, what, when, and where of learning emanate from within the learner. Each model has value and the needs of the learner should determine the singular or blended approach utilized. Table 8-3 illustrates the comparison of andragogy and pedagogy within the educational process.

TYPES OF LEARNERS

The information included in Table 8-3 emphasizes that the teacher must know as much as possible about both the learners and the topic before deciding on a specific theoretical approach/model and/or teaching strategy. The concept of know-thy-student has always been important; however, now it is not only important, it is critical. Many classrooms are filled with students born after 1980 who have been raised in the wireless, techno age while the faculty may be uncomfortable even communicating electronically. This means that in order to bridge this generation gap, the teacher must understand and acknowledge that the new learner has a very short attention span, an arsenal of electronic devices at their finger tips (and in your classroom), is used to multitasking (answering text messages and listening to electro-tunes while reading about neuroanatomy), and is used to handling a rapid barrage of information. In order to address these different learning needs, the proficient teacher will accompany the lecture with other adjuncts, such as electronic innovations (e.g., Second Life), video clips, lecture–discussion (addressed later in this chapter), case studies, and questions/answers accompanied by automated audience response systems (the "clicker"), to accommodate the new and/or adult learner.

A lecture can be used effectively with learners who represent a variety of developmental and cognitive levels. Adaptability is one of its most positive aspects. A teacher may, at a moment's notice, alter the teaching style, depth, sophistication, and level of the material being presented. These alterations can be made based on the needs, interests, and/or responses of the learners; new scientific revelations; or breaking news from the media. It is assumed that the lecturer has a sufficient command of the subject matter, the presence of mind, and the

Table 8-3 Comparison of Characteristics: Andragogy vs Pedagogy

Characteristic	Pedagogy	Andragogy
Concept of learner	Dependent Passive learner Needs someone outside self to make decisions about what, when, and how to learn	Independent/autonomous Self-directed Wants to participate in decisions related to own learning Students will increase effort if rewarded rather than punished
Roles of learner's experiences	Past experiences given little attention Narrow, focused interest Focuses on imitation	Wide range of experience, not just in nursing, that impacts life/learning Broad interests; likes to share previous experience with others Focus on originality
Readiness to learn	Determined by someone else (society, teachers) Focus on what is needed to survive and achieve Tends to respond impulsively	Usually in the educational process because they have chosen to be Wants to assist in setting the learning agenda Tends to respond rationally
Orientation of teaching/learning	Looks to teacher to identify what should be learned and to provide the information/process to learn Focuses on particulars concerned with the superficial aspects of learning (grades, due dates) Evaluation of learning done by teacher or society (grades, certificates) Needs clarity/specificity	Teachers are facilitators, providing resources and supports for self-directed learners Likes challenging, independent assignments that are reality based Evaluation is done jointly by teacher, learner, and/or peers Tolerates ambiguity

Source: Adapted from Woodring, B., & Woodring, R. (2007). Lecture is not a four-letter word. In M. Bradshaw & A. Lowenstein (Eds.), *Innovative teaching strategies in nursing and related health professions* (4th ed., pp. 114–115). Sudbury, MA: Jones and Bartlett.

flexibility to alter the content and teaching plan; however, these assumptions may not be accurate with novice educators, or when material is being presented the first time.

Combining the lecture with pedagogical approaches can be especially useful in basic and/or beginning courses in a sequence, as well as in orientation to new clinical areas or agencies. Novice learners of any age tend to prefer the structure of pedagogy, rather than the more flexible andragogical approach; however, the more mature and secure teachers and learners become, the more they enjoy the flexibility and challenge of integrating andragogical concepts into the lecture format.

Types of Lecturers

Lectures survive because, like bullfights and "Gone With the Wind," they satisfy the need for dramatic spectacle and offer an interpersonal arena in which important psychological needs are met (Lowman, 1995). A teacher may vary a lecture from a very formal presentation to a much less formal monologue. Lowman described three types of lectures commonly used: formal, expository, and provocative. The *formal lecture* is sometimes referred to as an oral essay. In the formal setting, the lecturer delivers a well organized, tightly constructed, highly polished presentation. The information provided primarily supports a specific point and usually is backed by theory and research. The presentation may be written and read to the audience, although recent data indicates that most learners do not like lecture materials to be read to them (Masie, 2006). Preparation of a formal lecture is time consuming; therefore, is not used for every class period during a school term. It may, however, be appropriate to tie things together either at the beginning and/or end of a course, or to address specified topical area. One of the major problems with a formal lecture is that it ignores the interactive dimension and sometimes fails to motivate learners.

A variation on the formal lecture is *lecture-recitation*. This process is an integration into the formal lecture: The lecturer stops and asks a student to respond to a particular point or idea by reading/presenting prepared materials. An example of this approach may be a formal lecture related to the pathophysiology of sickle cell anemia (SCA), followed by a student-presented case study about a patient with SCA.

The *expository lecture* is considered the most typical type of lecture. It is much less elaborate than the formal oral essay. Although the lecturer does most of the talking, questions from learners are entertained.

In the *provocative lecture*, the instructor still does most of the talking, but provokes students' thoughts and challenges their knowledge and values with questions. This method, well suited for integration with evolving technology such as video streaming and lecture-capturing, is becoming more popular in today's college classrooms. Included in this category are *lecture practice* which utilizes props, illustrates the subject, and may include lectures with simulations, computer, or video integration; *lecture-discussion*, where the instructor speaks for 10 to 15 minutes and then stimulates student discussion around key points (the lecturer acts only as a facilitator to clarify and integrate student comments); *punctuated lecture*, the presenter asks the students to write down their reflections on lecture points and submit them; and *lecture-lab*, the lecture is followed by students conducting experiments, interviews, observations, etc., during the class period.

The recent introduction of automated audience response systems within the classroom has enhanced the interactivity, especially in large classes. Similar to a game show, each student has a synchronized response unit, a "clicker," similar to a TV remote control. This allows the students to reply to the lecturers questions and allows the presenter to immediately verify the connections and involvement of students (Harper, 2009; Mayer et al., 2009).

Keep in mind that a lecture, in and of itself, is neither a good nor a bad/inappropriate approach to teaching. It may be deemed the best method when dealing with certain groups; however, like any strategy, it is most effective when not used as the singular, exclusive technique. Eble (1982), in *The Craft of Teaching*, suggested that the lecture should be thought of as a discourse—a talk or conversation—not an authoritative speech. As a discourse, the lecture can be viewed as a planned portion of the art or craft of teaching. As such, lecturing becomes a learnable skill that improves with practice.

As the utilization of the lecture as a "best practice" in teaching has been called into question, numerous research studies have been undertaken. Amare (2006) studied the experiences of students in PowerPoint-enhanced versus non–PowerPoint-enhanced lectures. She found that, in 84 engineering, humanities, and education majors in a technical writing course, the performance scores were higher in the non-PowerPoint section. However, the students preferred the addition of PowerPoint slides. PowerPoint, pod casts, and other technological enhancements were found to support the lecture by (1) bridging direct and constructionist teaching methods (Clark, 2008; Read, 2005); (2) supporting class attendance (Dolincar, 2005); and (3) reinforcing difficult concepts (Guertin, Bodek, Zappe, & Kim, 2007; Young, 2008). However, Costa, van Rensburg, and Rushton (2007) compared group discussion to the lecture presentation method. Seventy-seven medical students found the interactive, group discussion style more popular, the retention of knowledge better, and the scores on written tests higher. Generally, however, educational research findings support the notion that the lecture is still a valid, effective teaching strategy that is most effective when accompanied by other thought-provoking interludes. In the thought-provoking article "Sage on the Stage in the Digital Age," Chung (2005) presents a number of very salient points but concludes that both graduate and undergraduate online education would suffer if the lecture component were absent.

PREPARING ONESELF TO LECTURE

Never underestimate preparation time, regardless of how well versed you may be with the topic. When presenting an oral essay or formal lecture, preparation must begin well in advance of the presentation date. Planning, organization, and written preparation are essential and time consuming. Less formal forms of lecture may take less time, but their preparation should not be procrastinated. If the lecture is one in a sequence (or within a course), the best time to add the finishing touches to the next lecture is at the completion of the preceding one. Significant ideas that need to be reemphasized are still fresh in the presenter's mind, as are the questions that were raised, or should have been raised, by the students. The lecturer can recall the presentation strategies that worked with this group of participants, and those that did not. Changes that might have made the lecture more effective can be identified. Most lecturers, however, do not heed this advice and lecture preparation is often relegated to a brief time immediately prior to the presentation.

In order to present an effective lecture, the speaker must invest in preparing for several crucial sections. Like the human body, a lecture is divided into specific parts, each with its own function: the first 5 minutes, the main portion or body of the lecture, and the last 5 minutes. Each "part" is reviewed briefly.

Lecture Introduction (First 5 Minutes)

During the first 5 minutes of the lecture, two significant things occur: (1) the speaker outlines the objectives, outcomes, and expectations held for the participants; and (2) the audience decides whether to trust the speaker to produce what was promised (objectives) and whether to invest energy in following the presentation.

> *"There is too much material to be covered within the time allocated, but I'll do the best I can."*

From a teacher's point of view, this statement is always true but it should **never** be said to an audience. If a lecturer opens a session with such a statement, the listener has already been conditioned to expect a less than top notch presentation.

The participant asks himself or herself, "Why should I bother to listen if I can't possibly learn what I need in this hour?" Once this statement has been made, the lecturer will have difficulty regaining the full attention of the listener. So, no matter how tempting it may be to use, eliminate the statement from your repertoire. Instead, begin by identifying what the learner should gain from this lecture: state the objectives in clear, interesting, pragmatic, and achievable terms. Then, make a solid connection with the listeners by using an example of how the lecture material can be (or has been) used in practice or life in general. Outline the key concepts that will be addressed, and use your expertise and clinical experience to provide some background and rationale for this lecture. The key points should be limited in number. Research on what is remembered following classes indicated that most students can absorb only three to four major points in a 50-minute lecture and four to five points in a 75-minute presentation (Lowman, 1995). Conclude the introduction by establishing an open atmosphere and describing the "rules of operation" (e.g., "feel free to ask questions at any time"; "I will be using the automated response system several times during class, have it ready"; "there will be time at the end of the lecture for questions"). An open atmosphere can be established by posing a question, making a bold statement, using a controversial quote, using humor, or using a visual aid or cartoon. The better one knows the audience, the easier and more successful the introduction becomes.

Body of Lecture

The main portion, or body, should begin with a definition of concepts or principles that are illustrated by pragmatic, personal/professional experiences. The speaker then conveys the critical information the learner needs to know. The body should be well organized, with smooth transitions between topics. The experienced presenter knows that a lecturer cannot carry the primary responsibility for conveying all information or imparting all skills. Readings or critical analysis assignments assist in accomplishing these goals, and students need to be appraised of this connection. The body of the lecture should contain (1) general themes that tie together related topics; (2) topics/concepts that are difficult for students to understand (e.g., fluid balance); (3) sufficient depth and complexity to retain the learners' interest; and (4) testimonies (e.g., quotes from cancer survivors), case-specific data (e.g., lab values from unusual patient diagnoses), and exhibits (e.g., charts/graphs of statistics) to support the outcome-related point being made.

The speaker's presentation style is most evident during the body of the lecture. Tips and suggestions made in Resources, the following section, will enhance presentation style.

Lecturer Conclusion (Last 5 Minutes)

The lecture needs a definite stopping point. Closing a notebook, running out of time, or simply dismissing the class is not an acceptable conclusion. An effective communicator knows that any interaction deserves closure—a lecture is no exception to that rule. By focusing the learners' attention during the last 5 minutes of class, the lecturer is able to establish finality and make a link between what was taught and what the learner will be able to use in life, practice, and/or an upcoming test. A good conclusion ties the introduction and the body together in a manner similar to that of an abstract that precedes a well-written manuscript.

The objectives and outcomes statements that were used as a portion of the introduction should be reiterated, assuming they have been accomplished. The conclusion should also contain a review of the key points or topics covered and allow time for elaboration, amplification, and/or clarification of issues presented. Offering suggestions related to the application and transfer of knowledge may be helpful to the participants and the use of summative "take-home" points may provide additional reinforcement. Using this approach allows the learner to quickly rethink the content, stimulate continued interest, and consider further action. The participants will leave the lecture hall feeling a sense of accomplishment because they can summarize what has been learned. Thus, each lecture should be carefully planned and presented with an introduction (first 5 minutes), a well-organized body, and a meaningful conclusion (last 5 minutes) (Woodring, 2001).

RESOURCES

The major resource needed to utilize the lecture techniques effectively is YOU, the lecturer. Since the introduction of podcasting, MP3 players, immediate lecture-capture techniques, etc., a number of faculty have opted to discontinue technological transmission of the last 5 minutes summarization at the end of the lecture. They reserve this summary and clarification for only those who attend class or are legitimately enrolled in distance transmission of the course (Young, 2008). That option, of course, is as faculty choice. Presenting an informative and interesting lecture is a craft and a learnable skill. Because the speaker is the key element for this strategy, the following points are presented to help polish your presentation skills—and, remember, participants want to believe that you are smart, interesting, and a good speaker (Germano, 2003)!

- ***Conveying enthusiasm is the key element in presenting an effective lecture.*** Enthusiasm is contagious and is demonstrated by facial expressions, excitement in the voice, gestures, and body language. A lack of enthusiasm on the part of the speaker is interpreted by the listener as a lack of self confidence, lack of knowledge, a disinterest in the learner, and/or disinterest in the topic. If you do not have an effusive personality, practice adding a smile and small hand gestures to each lecture. Once these movements are comfortable, add other interactive methods.

- ***Knowing the content***. Even a written, formal lecture will not hide the insecurity of being unprepared or underprepared. Be certain you clearly explain key points in a language understood by the audience.
- ***Using notes***. The use of notes is generally the option of the speaker; however, to avoid the distress of losing your train of thought or incorrectly presenting complex information, the use of some type of notes is highly recommended. For ease of handling, record the notes on the computer or on pages/cards that are all the same size and sequentially numbered. If you are using PowerPoint slides to accompany the lecture, you may wish to operationalize the notation section and have your lecture notes or outline appear on the screen in front of you, while remaining invisible to the participants. The depth and content of lecture notes should fit the lecturer's comfort level. Use of anything from a skeletal outline to a full manuscript is acceptable. Notes should be prepared leaving white space that is easy for the eye to follow.

  Major points should be highlighted so the eye can easily pick up a cue when scanning a page. Although the use of notes is perfectly acceptable, the verbatim reading of notes is *not* acceptable. Rehearse your presentation often enough to appear spontaneous and enthusiastic and to complete it within the allotted time frame.
- ***Speaking to an audience of 200 as if it were a single student***. Speak clearly and loudly enough to be heard in the back of the room. The use of a microphone may be necessary if you are presenting in a large room or auditorium. Always use the microphone if there is any doubt that your voice will not be heard in the last row. It is sometimes helpful to have a friend sit in the back and signal if your voice is not being heard during the presentation. A small clip-on microphone is preferable to using a handheld or stationary microphone because it allows the speaker the flexibility to move away from the podium and frees one's hands to handle notes and/or gesture. If a microphone is to be used, arrive in the assigned room early enough to try the equipment and to regulate microphone position and sound levels. If the lecture is being transmitted to multiple sites, as in distance/distributive education or videoconferencing settings, be certain to test the sound levels at all sites prior to beginning the lecture.
- ***Making eye contact***. Select a participant at each corner of the room with whom you plan to make eye contact. Slowly scan the audience until you have seen each of the designated participants. Smile at familiar faces. If needed, review information related to the process of group dynamics. If the

lecture is being transmitted to multiple sites, be certain to make eye contact via the monitors with participants in the distant sites. You may wish to make a concerted effort to look into each monitor or screen as you visually scan the lecture hall, and address participants at each site.

- ***Using creative movement.*** Movements of the speaker's head and hands in gesturing should appear natural, not forced. Be careful when standing behind a podium; do not grip the sides tightly with your hands or lock your (shaky?) knees. This action produces a circulatory response that could cause the speaker to faint. Occasionally step away from the podium and toward the listeners. This conveys an attitude of warmth and acceptance. Avoid distracting mannerisms such as pacing, wringing your hands, clearing your throat, or jamming your hands into pockets and jingling change.
- ***Avoiding barriers.*** The use of a stage or podium places an automatic barrier between the speaker and the listeners. This gulf needs to be bridged early and often during the lecture. Suggestions for bridging the gulf include (1) use note cards rather than a manuscript because they are more portable and allow freedom to move away from the podium; (2) step out from behind the podium, especially if you are short in stature—the audience does not wish to see a "talking head"; (3) walk toward the listeners, which is interpreted as a sign of warmth and reaching out to the audience; (4) address the right half of the audience, the left half of the audience, and then the audience at each distant site (each monitor or screen), do not turn your back to either side of the audience or transmitting cameras; (5) call on at least one participant in the audience and at each distant site by name; (6) use hand gestures to accentuate words, but be careful not to overdo this action (this is especially important if the lecture is being transmitted to multiple sites because large hand gestures are more distracting when seen on a monitor than when viewed in person); and (7) if given the opportunity to be seated on a stage/platform, be aware of the eye level of the audience.
- ***Creating a change of pace.*** An astute lecturer constantly assesses the audience and reads participants' signals. Facial cues indicate agreement/disagreement with what has been said and may express understanding/misunderstanding of content. Another signal is given when listeners begin having side conversations or squirm in their seats. These signals call for intervention, response, or a change of pace by the speaker. The change of pace can be as simple as turning off the computer/projector, shifting to a new slide, adding sound or animation to your visual, or changing the lighting—any of these actions will cause the listener to refocus attention on the speaker or back to the visual. Shifting the focus from the speaker to a handout, using a humorous example, altering the tone or inflection of your voice, using automated interaction with feedback from participants, dividing into small groups for a brief discussion

(Yazedjian & Kolkhorst, 2007), or taking a "stand and stretch" break also can provide a needed change of pace. Keep this rule of thumb in mind: an individual's optimal attention span is roughly 1 minute per year of age up to the approximate age of 45 (e.g., a 5-year-old has a 5-minute attention span; a 25-year-old, 25 minutes), and decreases among the younger, digitally minded. Therefore, plan a change of pace or break according to the average age of your audience. "The mind can only absorb as much as the seat can endure" is a fairly valid, reasonable guideline.

- ***Distributing a skeletal outline to help the learners identify key points***. Emphasize principles and concepts. Do not copy charts, graphs, and materials that are found in the learners' texts. Handout information should supplement the lecture. The lecture should not be a rehash of basic information from the learners' textbook. If handouts are used, they should be clear and contain a limited amount of information so the learner is not overwhelmed. Handouts printed on colored paper stand out and are more likely to be read than those printed on white paper. The reproduction or Web posting of the PowerPoint slides or lecture notes is a well debated topic. Germano (2003) declares technology to be a tool, but notes that tools are not friends and are often rivals. Stewart (2006) suggests the distribution of full-text class notes or slides that contain a significant proportion of the lecture content truly discourages class attendance.

Several publications that may be of assistance in keeping the lecture process fresh are *The Teaching Professor*, *Change*, *Masie's Learning TRENDS*, *The National Teaching & Learning Forum*, and *Survival Skills for Scholars* series. In addition, Web sites maintained by a number of universities offer assistance: Georgia State University, Master Teacher Program (http://www.masterteacherprogram.com/about/index.html), University of Chicago (http//teaching.uchicago.edu/handbook/tac06.html), University of Toledo (http://education.utoledo.edu/par/Adults.html), and Towson University (http://wwwnew.towson.edu/facultyonline/ISD/lectures.htm). Numerous online journals and listserves also can provide rapid access to information related to specific topics of interest.

POTENTIAL PROBLEMS

Nothing is perfect. As with any method or technique, some problems exist with the use of the lecture as a teaching strategy. A key question to be answered is "What makes lectures and lecturers unsuccessful?" Over the past decade, graduate nursing students have responded to that question, and each year student responses were consistent. The most frequently cited negative characteristics of lectures/lecturers focused on the person doing the presenting, *not* the method

(Woodring & Woodring, 2007). Examples of common negative factors associated with lectures and some suggestions for improvement are found in Table 8-4. The remainder of this section is devoted to dealing with negative perceptions, which are more generic than the characteristics in Table 8-4.

Student Boredom

Educators today face challenges that our predecessors did not even dream about! How can one obtain and retain the attention of the high-speed Internet, digital native, and MP3 player generation? This generation of learners is accustomed to fast-paced, action-packed, colorized entertainment at the flick of a finger. To compensate for this situational dilemma and still utilize the lecture technique effectively, the teacher should experiment with combining advanced technologies and the lecture within the classroom. Consider in-class use of a textbook on CD/DVD with capabilities of adding supplementary information during the lecture; the use of computer-linked electronic whiteboards to transfer information from e-boards to individual students laptop monitors; the appropriate and creative integration of PowerPoint-type visuals during the lecture; or integration of text/reference materials via a personal digital assistant (PDA) format. These electronic capabilities allow the lecturer to interject computer generated charts, graphs, diagrams, student input, and up-to-the-minute research findings into the lecture. Luck and Laurence (2005) validated that the use of videoconferencing technology used to present a lecture series for beginning college students. The lecture/videoconference was evaluated by the learners as encouraging "positive active participation" and allowing "prompt feedback."

Additionally, assignment of out-of-class computer-assisted instructional programs (such as ADAM/EVE, simulations, or patient-/disease-specific learning packages), communication packages (e.g., WebCrossings), and/or electronic/Internet-based assignments to complement the lecture will assist in gaining and maintaining the interest of more technologically savvy students.

Including many examples of electronic technologies would be a moot point. By the time this book is printed, newer modalities will have emerged. It might be wise to ask a 10-year-old what is "hot" (or "cool" or "rad" or whatever).

Institutional Barriers

Physical, political, and situational barriers exist within every institution—any or all of which may contribute to dissatisfaction with any instructional approach. The timing of a class offering cannot be overlooked. Traditionally, teachers have

Table 8-4 Perceived Negative Factors Associated with the Lecture Technique

Perceived Negative Factors	Suggestions for Improvement
Presentation disorganized or hard to follow Lack of outline or outline too detailed	Spend time in practice and preparation Prepare and follow brief outline for each lecture
Presenter lacks professional appearance	Dress as a professional role model. (If you do not care about wearing stripes and plaids together, enlist the help of a colleague who you consider to look professional.)
Speaker lacks facial expression Monotone voice or nervous/shaky voice Facial expression and/or voice lacks enthusiasm	Record one of your lectures; view recording with a friend/ colleague and establish goals for improvement.
Reads lecture material, eyes do not meet those of listeners	Practice your lecture in front of a mirror until you know the main points by memory. Use only as many written notes as are absolutely essential; place cues in the margin for yourself. (smile-walk-relax!)
Remains behind podium to lecture (referred to as the "talking head" because that is all that students see)	Do not stand behind a podium unless you are 6 feet tall; request a shorter, lower lectern or table.
Uses no visual aids or visuals of poor quality	Teachers tend to put too much information in small print on slides and/or handouts. Ask librarian, media center, or learning center personnel for assistance in preparing visuals.
Too many PowerPoint slides	Use visuals to support, not replace content.
Does not acknowledge that adult learners like to participate	Review techniques for keeping adult learners engaged. See references by Cross, Kidd, and Knowles
Inconsiderate of learners' needs	Schedule breaks and/or implement change-of-pace activities every 30–45 minutes.

(continued)

Table 8-4 Perceived Negative Factors Associated With the Lecture Technique *(continued)*

Perceived Negative Factors	Suggestions for Improvement
Distracting habits of presenter: pacing, staring out windows, playing with objects (paper clips, rubber bands, change), using non-words (ah, um) and repetitious phrases ("you know", "like", "well uh")	Use a video of your lecture to identify repetitive habits Repositioning hands or holding notes may help the "nervous hands" problem Make a list of alternate words that could be substituted for the frequently repeated pet phrases Non-words are a verbalization that allows your speech to catch up to what your brain is thinking; becoming aware of the use of non-words may or may not be all you need to eliminate them; when they occur, stop, take a deep breath, and then go on

Source: Adapted from Woodring, B., & Woodring, R. (2007). Lecture is not a four-letter word. In M. Bradshaw & A. Lowenstein (Eds.), *Innovative teaching strategies in nursing and related health professions* (3rd ed., pp. 124–125). Sudbury, MA: Jones and Bartlett.

disliked teaching, and students have disliked attending classes offered, at 7 AM or 9 PM. No one likes getting up that early or staying in class that late! Classes taught immediately after meal time are considered "sleepers" because blood leaves the brain and moves to the gastrointestinal tract, making everyone sluggish. Classes taught late in the afternoon or early evening are bad because the students and teachers are tired. Try as one may, short of one-on-one teaching, or totally online/asynchronous education, the perfect time to hold a class will probably never be found. Speakers must make their presentations stimulating and motivating at any time of the day!

Another institutional barrier to be considered is the number of students proportional to the size of the classroom and the number of students in proportion to the number of faculty (student:faculty ratio). Lecturers are often placed in small, crowded classrooms with large numbers of students or large, cavernous classrooms with smaller numbers of students. Often, geographical relocation of desks/tables could ease the space configuration and provide a more positive learning atmosphere. Should the lecturer have the option, it is most ideal to be able to clearly see and make eye contact with each participant. This may be accomplished by arranging seating in a semicircle around the lectern or angling tables/seats. But if seating is fixed within the classroom, then it becomes the responsibility of the speaker to move and make eye contact as often as possible.

The large student:faculty ratio within classes will probably not decrease in postsecondary education in the near future. Large classes, especially at the freshman and sophomore levels, are very cost effective. The bottom line will continue to impose restrictions that are exacerbated by the increase in distance and multisite class sessions and faculty shortage in many health-related professions. This disproportionate student:faculty ratio will require lecturers to implement the tips list under the previous Resources section, as well as utilize technological support, teaching assistants for smaller group interactions, and other creative strategies to enhance student learning for material presented in large lecture sections. The results of a study of undergraduate students (Long & Coldren, 2006) reinforced the need for the lecturer to make interpersonal connection with students in large classes. There was a positive correlation between the students' perception of interpersonal connection with the faculty and student success in the class.

Negative Press

The faculty member who consistently lectures may be subjected to student-generated negative comments, such as "This class is so boring, all he does is lecture"; "It's awful, she reads to us right out of her book"; or "I can't learn to think critically if all she does is lecture!" In fairness, it is generally not the method but the teacher who is at fault if such comments are disseminated. It is often said that lecturing is a poor teaching method, a kind of last resort for instruction. Many lecturers, in fact, do not know how to impart information or stimulate interest effectively; consequently, their lectures are often poorly presented, badly organized, dull, and uninspiring (Gleitman, 2006). In order to correct negative press, plan ahead, organize the content and introduce at least one additional teaching method (e.g., discussion, video, audience response system, small group interaction, role play) into each lecture session. This approach will increase student interaction and should increase student satisfaction. In addition, tell the students how you are attempting to improve the lecture setting and you will gain their respect because you have acknowledged their feelings and made an overt effort to respond to them.

Knowledge Retention

The problem of retaining information gained from a lecture should be acknowledged and addressed. Although those educators who enjoy using the lecture method hate to admit it, research conducted in the 1990s found that 80% of information gained by lecture alone cannot be recalled by students 1 day later, and that 80% of the remainder fades in a month. Since minimal research has been done to alter that perception, one must still heed the results. Educational data indicates the more a learner's senses (taste, touch, smell, sight, and hearing) are involved in the learning activity, the longer the knowledge is retained. Therefore, if certain types of equipment were used to illustrate a point (touch, sight), a video clip was inserted into the midst of the lecture (sight, hearing), or any other active learning process (gaming, lab experiments, audience response activities) was introduced, the student's knowledge retention would increase.

In recent years, the use of *punctuated lectures* has also been viewed as a method to increase retention of information. The punctuated lecture requires students and teachers to go through five steps: (1) **listen** (to a portion of a lecture), (2) **stop**, (3) **reflect** (on what they were doing, thinking, feeling during that portion of the lecture), (4) **write** (what they were doing, thinking, feeling during that portion of the lecture), and (5) **give** (the written feedback to the lecturer) (Cross & Steadman, 1996). This approach provides the lecturer and the students with an opportunity to become engaged with the learning process, as well as to self-monitor their in-class behaviors. In addition, Brookfield (2006) suggests that students cannot read the lecturer's mind. Students cannot be expected to know what teachers expect, stand for, or wish them to value unless it is explicitly and vigorously communicated to them. The reflective teacher, according to Brookfield, must continual work to build a case for learning, action, and practice rather than assume these values to be self-evident to the learner. Implementing these suggestions should enhance knowledge retention emanating from a lecture.

EVALUATION

An evaluation of the lecture/lecturer must be completed in a timely manner. The most useful time to obtain this data is at the completion of an individual lecture. Obtaining this information need not be laborious. Ask the listeners to respond to a few specific questions and then allow them to provide additional comments. This type of feedback is especially helpful for the novice lecturer. The evaluation process should aim to provide constructive criticism and comments for improvement. One means of accomplishing this is to allow the student to make any comments they wish; however, a negative comment cannot be made without offering a suggestion for its resolution. When this evaluation technique is used routinely, the learners become accustomed to it. The process can be completed in 5 minutes or less, especially if automated response systems are used. Often, teachers are so interested in assessing whether the course objectives have been met that they forget to evaluate the means by which they were met. Lecturers will not improve without suggested change, and suggested change can best be obtained via the use of a planned evaluation tool/method that is completed by peers and/or class participants. The evaluation of a lecture or lecturer should not occur in isolation—it must be viewed as a portion of an overall evaluation plan—and should be conducted only when there are plans for growth, follow-up, and change.

CONCLUSION

Presenting an effective lecture continues to be more than standing in front of a group and verbalizing information. The lecturer must be knowledgeable, well-spoken, and considerate of the learners' needs, abilities, learning styles, and cognitive/developmental level(s). The desired outcomes for the class and the individual objectives of the learners must be addressed. The lecture should be divided into three major segments: introduction (5 minutes), body, and conclusion (5 minutes). Each section should be planned and presented in an organized manner, never off the cuff. The prepared lecturer will be considerate, credible, and in control (not to be mistaken for rigid and controlling). Several factors enhance the presentation of a lecture, but none is more important than genuine enthusiasm. The lecture should not be considered a secondary teaching strategy. In many situations, it is the most appropriate methodology to be used. To elicit the best results, the lecture should be accompanied by at least one of the other effective strategies discussed in this text.

As we close this chapter on presenting a lecture, it is suggested that attention should be paid to the words of the wise elder: Select your words carefully, be sure your words are sweet, because you never know when you will be called upon them to eat! Happy lecturing.

REFERENCES

Amare, N. (2006). To slideware or not to slideware: Students' experiences with Powerpoint vs. lecture. *Journal of Technical Writing and Communication*, *36*(3), 297–308.

Brookfield, S. (2006). *The skillful teach* (pp. 100–101). San Francisco: Jossey-Bass Publishers.

Chung, Q. B. (2005). Sage on stage in the digital age: The role of online lecture in distance learning. *The Electronic Journal of e-Learning*, *3*(1), 1–14.

Clark, J. (2008). Powerpoint and pedagogy maintaining student interest in university lectures. *College Teaching, 56*(1), 39–45.

Costa, M., van Rensburg, L., & Rushton, N. (2007). Does teaching style matter? A randomized trial of group discussion versus lectures in orthopaedic undergraduate teaching. *Medical Education, 41*, 214–217.

Cox, J., & Rogers, J. (2005). Enter: The (well-designed) lecture. *The Teaching Professor, 19*(5), 1, 6.

Cross, K. P. (1986). A proposal to improve teaching. *AAHE Bulletin*, September, 9–15.

Cross, K., & Steadman, M. (1996). *Classroom research: Implementing the scholarship of teaching.* San Francisco: Jossey Bass Publishers.

Dolinicar, S. (2005). Should we still lecture or just post examination questions on the web?: The nature of the shift towards pragmatism in undergraduate lecture attendance. *Quality in Higher Education, 11*(2), 103–115.

Eble, K. (1982). *The craft of teaching.* San Francisco: Jossey-Bass Publishers.

Epstein, J. (1981). *Portraits of great teachers* (p. xiii). New York: Basic Books.

Germano, W. (2003). The scholarly lecture: How to stand and deliver. *The Chronicle of Higher Education, 50*(14), 14b.

Gleitman, H. (2006). Lecturing: Using a much maligned method of teaching. In *Teaching at Chicago: A handbook.* Chicago: The University of Chicago Center for Teaching and Learning.

Guertin, L., Bodek, M., Zappe, S., & Kim, H. (2007). Questioning the student use of and desire for lecture podcasts. *Journal of Online Learning and Teaching.* Retrieved November 12, 2009, from http://jolt.merlot.org/vol3no2/guertin.htm

Harper, B. (2009). I've never seen or heard it this way! Increasing student engagement through the use of technology-enhanced feedback. *Teaching Educational Psychology*, 3(2).

Huntley, J. (2009). Positioning the CLO. In B. Concevitch (Ed.), *The learning leaders fieldbook.* Saratoga Springs, NY: The Masie Center. Retrieved November 12, 2009, from http://masiewebcom/p7/learning-leaders-fieldbook-2.pdf

Kidd, J. R. (1973). *How adults learn.* New York: Association Press.

Knowles, M. (1970). *The modern practice of adult education: Andragogy versus pedagogy.* New York: Association Press.

Long, E., & Coldren, J. (2006). Interpersonal influences in large lecture-based classes. *College Teaching, 54*(2), 237–243.

Lowman, J. (1995). *Mastering techniques of teaching* (2nd ed.). San Francisco: Jossey-Bass Publications.

Luck, M., & Laurence, G. (2005). Innovative teaching: Sharing expertise through videoconferencing. *Innovate*, 2(1), 1–10.

Masie, Elliott. (2006). Learning TRENDS. Saratoga, NY: The MASIE Center. Retrieved December 11, 2009, from http://trends.masie.com/

Mayer, R., Stull, A., DeLeeuw, K., Almeroth, K., Bimber, B., Chun, D., et al. (2009). Clickers in college classrooms: fostering learning with questioning methods in large lecture class. *Contemporary Educational Psychology, 34*(1), 51–57.

Read, B. (2005). Lectures on the go. *The Chronicle of Higher Education, 52*(10), A39.

Stewart, E. (2006) Class-conscious: Teachers want tech to enhance-not replace-lectures. *Desert News (Utah)*, February 6, 2006. Retrieved November 12, 2009, from http://www.deseretnewscom/article/1,5143,635181866,00.html

Woodring, B. (2001). Preparing presentations that produce peace of mind. *Journal of Child and Family Nursing, 3*(1), 63–64.

Woodring, B., & Woodring, R. (2007). Lecture is not a four-letter word. In M. Bradshaw, & A. Lowenstein (Eds.), *Innovative teaching strategies in nursing and related health professions* (4th ed., pp. 109–130). Sudbury, MA: Jones and Bartlett.

Yazedjian, A., & Kolkhorst, B. (2007). Implementing small-group activities in large lecture classes. *College Teaching, 55*(4), 164–169.

Young, J. (2008). The lectures are recorded, so why go to class? *Chronicle of Higher Education, 54*(36), A1, A12.

CHAPTER 9

Problem-Based Learning

Patricia Solomon

INTRODUCTION

Problem-based learning (PBL) is an educational process where learning is centered around problems as opposed to discrete, subject-related courses. In small groups, students are presented with patient scenarios or problems, generate learning issues related to what they need to learn in order to understand the problem, engage in independent self-study, and return to their groups to apply their new knowledge to the patient problem. PBL is largely acknowledged as starting in the medical school at McMaster University in the mid-1960s in response to an educational environment that emphasized passive learning of large quantities of information that was quickly outdated and often appeared irrelevant. The emphasis is on learning all content in an integrative way through small group, self-directed study of a problem with the assistance of a faculty tutor who is a facilitator of learning rather than an expert lecturer (Walton & Matthews, 1989). While PBL is theoretically more effective in structuring knowledge, the most agreed upon advantage is that it is more enjoyable than traditional learning methods.

BACKGROUND AND DEFINITIONS

Since being introduced, PBL has been adopted by many health professional programs worldwide. Although many variants of PBL have been described, the essential elements remain: (1) students are presented with a written problem or patient scenario in small groups; (2) there is a change in faculty role from imparter of information to facilitator of learning; (3) there is an emphasis on student responsibility and self-directed learning; and (4) a written problem is the stimulus for learning with students engaging in a problem-solving process as they learn and discuss content related to the problem (Solomon, 1994).

While PBL may be viewed as an educational methodology, it is most often associated with an overall curricular approach. PBL was originally viewed as an "all or none" phenomenon in which an educational program had to commit entirely to the curricular philosophy to attain the most benefits (Barrows & Tamblyn, 1980). Programs that had individual problem-based courses and more traditional courses running concurrently were thought to produce mixed messages in the student and devalue the problem-based components (Walton & Matthews, 1989). While there is still concern that isolated problem-based courses will not be successful (Albanese, 2000), there is certainly greater acceptance of curricula that use mixed or partial PBL approaches.

There have been several attempts to define and classify PBL curricula. Barrows (1986) describes a taxonomy based largely on the problem design and role of the teacher. Charlin, Mann, and Hansen (1998) present an analytic framework to understand and compare PBL curricula that varies along 10 dimensions, such as the purpose of the problem and the nature of the task to be accomplished during study of the problem. Harden and Davis (1998) offer an 11-step continuum of PBL with theoretical learning and an emphasis on traditional lectures and textbooks at one end, and task-based learning (essentially learning in clinical practice settings with real patients) at the other. As one moves along the continuum, there is greater emphasis on the problem, activation of prior knowledge, contextual learning, and discovery learning. Solomon, Binkley, and Stratford (1996) provide a simple distinction between a problem-based curriculum, which they describe as "fully integrated" (with few or no subject-related courses), and a transitional PBL curriculum, which uses more traditional curricular elements early in the curriculum and incorporates increasingly larger components of PBL as the students progress through their program.

THEORETICAL FOUNDATIONS

Some of the original theoretical premises for PBL have not found strong support within the literature. Contextual learning was an appealing rationale for the superiority of PBL. The rationale was that by learning all content (including basic, clinical, and social sciences) within the context of a problem, a learner would be able to recall information better when he/she encountered a similar patient within the clinical setting. But there is weak empirical support and this theory is likely too simplistic to integrate the complexities associated with PBL (Colliver, 2000). The information processing theory (Schmidt, 1983) incorporates aspects of contextual learning theory and provides more comprehensive theoretical support for PBL as it also considers activation of prior knowledge and elaboration of knowledge as core elements (Albanese, 2000). However, one theory may be insufficient support for PBL. Albanese (2000) outlines three others that are salient to PBL: cooperative learning theory, self-determination theory, and control theory. Cooperative learning, in which individuals are dependent on other group members to achieve their goals, is used extensively in small-group PBL. Self-determination theory identifies controlled, more maladaptive motivators of behavior and autonomous motivators that the learner finds more interesting and enjoyable (Williams, Saizow, & Ryan, 1999). Controlled motivators, which include external demands under which people act with a sense of pressure and anxiety, are more characteristic of traditional curricula. Autonomous motivators, which involve a sense of volition and choice, would be more characteristic of a PBL curriculum. Control theory states that all behavior is based on satisfying the five basic needs of freedom, power, love and belonging, fun, and survival and reproduction (Glaser, 1985). Instruction can fail if it does not meet these basic needs of the learner. PBL may be superior at meeting these needs. For example, fun, or enjoyment of learning, has been frequently associated with outcomes of PBL (Albanese & Mitchell, 1993).

TYPES OF LEARNERS

PBL has been used extensively in many health professional programs. Health professional students at all levels can benefit from the use of PBL to simulate realistic clinical situations. It is important to note that students accustomed to more traditional ways of learning often experience stress and anxiety when adapting to this new student-centered style of learning (Solomon & Finch, 1998). Supports must be put in place to ease the students' transition to this type of learning.

RESOURCES

PBL requires different resources to support implementation. Contrary to more traditional programs in which one faculty member lectures to large numbers of students, learning occurs in small groups, necessitating additional faculty to support PBL. There is also a need for numerous small group tutorial rooms and extensive library and other learning resources that enable self-directed learning. As elaborated upon next, there is an additional need for faculty who are well trained to assume the role of facilitator.

ROLE OF FACULTY

There has been significant debate in the PBL literature as to whether expert or nonexpert tutors are preferable. Content experts are thought to be more likely to revert to "lecture type" of behaviors and be less facilitatory. Although some debate remains (Kaufman & Holmes, 1998), it is generally recognized that a combination of content and process expertise is preferable.

Dolmans, Wolfhagen, Scherpbier, and Van Der Vleuten (2001) provide an excellent summary of issues related to tutor expertise. Not surprisingly, they conclude that tutors initiate activities with which they are most familiar. Hence, content experts use their expertise to direct tutorial performance and noncontent experts use their process facilitation skills to direct group dynamics. However, this relationship is not as simple as once believed. A tutor's performance is not likely to be stable and is influenced by contextual circumstances such as the quality of the written cases, the structure of the course, and students' prior knowledge. Thus, tutor expertise may compensate if the structure of the problem is low and/or the students have little prior knowledge of the case.

While the evidence suggests that it is not a simple distinction between expert and nonexpert tutors, the implications for faculty development are clear; faculty require training to assume more facilitative roles. Hitchcock and Mylona (2000) note that there has been little systematic study on effective ways to train faculty to assume PBL roles, although there have been many descriptions in the literature. They emphasize that while the most obvious training is in tutor facilitation skills, there are many other roles and skills that need to be developed. They quote Irby's sequence of steps of skill development: (1) challenging assumptions and developing understanding of PBL, (2) experiencing and valuing the tutorial process, (3) acquiring general tutor skills, (4) developing content-specific tutor knowledge and skills, (5) acquiring advanced knowledge and skills, (6) developing leadership and scholarship skills, and (7) creating organizational vitality.

It is clear that faculty who possess a level of content expertise in the area under study are the preferred small group facilitators. However, there is an equally important need for faculty who are well trained in PBL and the tutorial process. The skills needed to facilitate and evaluate small group process, to promote metacognitive skills such as self-monitoring of one's reasoning and decision-making skills, and to design curriculum and develop problems and other instructional materials to support self-directed learning are very different than those skills required in a traditional curriculum and require long-term faculty development initiatives.

USING PROBLEM-BASED LEARNING METHODS

There appears to be no one "best way" to implement PBL. Although some maintain that fully integrated PBL is preferable, this curricular design may not be feasible for many institutions. Diversity in curricular design and approach is to be expected because different institutional structures and philosophies and faculty knowledge and skill development will influence the extent to which PBL can be incorporated into the curriculum.

Typically the process is as follows. Students are presented with a written problem as a stimulus for learning. Problems are carefully designed to facilitate discussion related to specific learning objectives. In groups of six to eight, students read the problem (either aloud or to themselves) and brainstorm about what they need to learn in order to better understand the problem or hypothesize potential causes of the problem. During this initial process, students generate learning issues or questions for self-study. Learning issues can range from factual knowledge (e.g., what nerves innovate the upper extremity?), to more complex physiological questions (e.g., what is the process of inflammation?), to questions that include broader psychosocial issues (e.g., how would I apply a model of ethical decision making to this patient?), or questions that require evaluation of the literature and integration of evidence-based practice (e.g., what is the effectiveness of ultrasound in the treatment of lateral epicondylitis?). The process of developing a high-quality learning issue that is researchable may be quite time consuming for the learner who is new to PBL. Generation of the final list of learning issues that will be researched and discussed at the next tutorial constitutes the end of the first stage of the PBL process. Students can choose to independently research all learning issues that have been generated for that session or to divide up the learning issues amongst themselves for self-study. When students return for the next tutorial, they discuss their findings and the implications for patient care. At the end of the tutorial, students engage in a structured evaluation of the tutorial process and their performance. Each student provides a verbal self-evaluation of their performance that day and their peers and the faculty tutor provide feedback.

During the tutorial, the faculty tutor does not provide expert content information. Rather his/her role is to establish the climate for learning, encourage problem solving, and promote debate and discussion within the group. The tutor also role models effective self-evaluation and provision of feedback. Barrows (1988) describes the faculty tutoring role as going through three stages: (1) *modeling*, the thinking process for the students by questioning and challenging them; (2) as the group becomes more comfortable with the process the faculty role shifts to one of *coaching* when the students are off-track or confused; (3) as students progress further and develop into a well functioning and effective learning group, the role of the tutor *fades*, leaving the group to work more independently. Barrows suggests that groups should meet for at least 8 weeks to allow for progression of these three stages.

POTENTIAL PROBLEMS

The costs associated with the number of faculty required to deliver education in small groups is a key concern and potential barrier to implementation

(Albanese & Mitchell, 1993). Other costs related to space requirements for small group tutorial rooms and development of self-directed learning resources may also pose barriers (Solomon, 1994). Without institutional support for curricular change, many programs may find it difficult to engage successfully in curriculum reform.

An additional barrier to the implementation of innovative problem-based curricula relates to the lack of rigorous long-term data that demonstrate significant differences between more traditional and PBL curricula. The lack of evidence reinforces the concerns of critics who ask "Why bother?" Some argue that PBL is worth implementing even if the only benefit of PBL is its more personal, humane, and enjoyable approach. Federman (1999) noted advantages of PBL that are not amenable to measurement and relate more to the personal and interpersonal aspects of practice. Even the most ardent of critics would agree that these are desirable in health professional education. Some of these include (1) the person-to-person contact inherent in a small group tutorial process; (2) the positive regard that is fostered by the respect afforded to the beginning student; (3) the focus on patients that promotes relevancy of the curriculum from early days; (4) increased opportunities to discuss moral and ethical issues and for the tutor to share his or her values; and (5) the positive effect on lectures because, with only a few lectures in the timetable, students are more committed to these lectures and this, in turn, has a stimulating effect on the faculty.

Recently, with the rise in popularity of online and Web-based learning, there has been an interest in doing PBL online. Increased accessibility and opportunities for asynchronous learning are obvious advantages for distance and continuing education courses. In health professional educational programs, PBL online has inherent appeal as the number of facilitators required could be reduced, thus making it possible to implement in programs without sufficient resources to do face-to-face PBL. Although there have been a few descriptive articles (Bresnitz, 1996), few have examined the effectiveness of computer-based PBL. Some of the characteristics of PBL, such as using patient problems, sharing learning, promoting integration of knowledge, and self-directed learning, are relatively easy to transfer to online formats. However, the advantage of flexibility, related to the ability to access the course in an asynchronous manner, may not be realized in an intensive, integrated professional curricula in which the students' timetables are more restricted. Face-to-face PBL allows for the development of communication and verbal skills related to the ability to clearly articulate and present information, provide feedback to others, and develop and evaluate group skills. The communication skills that are central to professional practice would clearly not be developed in the same way as they would in a small group face-to-face PBL as opposed to online PBL.

CONCLUSION

PBL is an increasingly popular teaching and learning strategy within the health professions. The clinical relevance, small group interactions, and active learning provided make PBL an appealing curricular alternative. Faculty training and expertise are essential for successful outcomes.

APPLIED EXAMPLE

An Interprofessional Problem-Based Learning Course on Rehabilitation Issues in HIV

Problem-based learning (PBL) was chosen as the educational model for an interprofessional course for teaching health profession students about rehabilitation issues in HIV/AIDS. PBL was determined to be ideal for promoting appreciation and respect for the roles of other professions. In this course, students from occupational therapy, physiotherapy, medical, nursing, and social work programs participated in an 8-week tutorial course. Students met once weekly for a 3-hour session. The objectives of the course were broad and included:

1. understanding the basic principles of the biology of HIV disease, its progression, and its transmission from person to person
2. becoming familiar with the types of medical and nonmedical interventions commonly used to maintain health in people living with HIV
3. understanding the management of HIV as a chronic—as opposed to terminal—illness
4. understanding how models of rehabilitation may be applied to the management of clients with HIV
5. developing an appreciation of the psychological, social, political, and ethical issues that have an influence on the experiences of a person living with HIV
6. understanding the various roles and contributions of health care and social service professionals in the rehabilitation of clients at different stages of HIV disease
7. developing skills in communicating, planning, and decision making with an interprofessional group of health professional students

In PBL, the learning stems from a problem itself. Students are expected to learn all content related to the stated objectives within the context of the healthcare problem. Typically, students are provided with a patient problem that is written; however, the problem may take the form of a standardized patient, a video, or other formats. In this course, students were provided with written patient problems. Students were directed to discuss their previous knowledge related to the patient problem. After students discussed their background knowledge and specific professional perspective, they then proceeded to a discussion on what would be a priority for learning in order to better understand the patient scenario. The learning issues were diverse, reflecting a range of content areas. For example, within the context of one problem, students' learning issues ranged from physiological issues (How is HIV transmitted?), to social issues (What are government and private options for short-term and long-term disability?), to ethical issues (What is the health professional's role in encouraging a newly diagnosed HIV-positive person to inform his/her partner about his/her status?). An important step was for the students to refine the learning issues or learning questions for further study. Neophytes to PBL often struggle with this portion of the process and need guidance to articulate a question that is clear and researchable. Students then engaged in self-directed study, sought appropriate resources to address the learning issues, and then returned to share their findings within the group setting.

Typically in PBL, students will choose to engage in self-directed study around all the learning issues that are generated by the group. This is important because if students select separate and individual learning issues, there can be a tendency for them to present their information in a didactic way when they return to the second tutorial session. If each student pursues all learning issues for self-study, the tutorial discussion is much richer and interactive as students share resources, challenge each other, and debate their findings. In this course, there was an additional individual learning issue related to students having to share their professional perspective. The complexities and interdisciplinary nature of HIV/AIDS provided the basis for diverse and broad-based discussions.

After engaging in self-study during the week, students returned to the tutorial and discussed and debated their findings. Students consulted both personal and written resources, which included texts, videos, journal articles, and Web sites. Students then related the information back to the patient problem and provided their perspective on what their professional role would entail (e.g., What would be the priority for the social worker in this scenario? Is there a role for the occupational therapist? What would be the role of the nurse in community care of the patient?). The final stage was evaluation of the tutorial process, the interprofessional learning that occurred, and the performance of the group members. The interprofessional makeup of the tutorial groups simulated a health care team environment. The course was designed with the hope that the sharing of information, discussion, and debate that occurred in the tutorial would promote understanding of roles and teamwork. This element was evaluated weekly by the tutorial group members.

PROBLEM DESIGN

Problem design is an important element of the overall PBL process. Problems are not simply a restatement of all salient clinical information. Rather, the problems are carefully designed to elicit discussion and lead to student identification of the learning issues for which the problem was designed. There is evidence that even small changes to a problem can influence the students' discussions (Solomon, Blumberg, & Shehata, 1992). For example, in this course a change in the gender or sexual orientation of the person living with HIV can lead to very different learning issues. If the problem was based on a heterosexual woman living with HIV, students might generate issues related to the prevalence of HIV in women, the differing risk factors and manifestations in women, and the influence of HIV on gender-related roles. In contrast, if the problem centered around a gay man, students might have discussions related to their values, beliefs, and prejudices.

EVALUATION

Students evaluated this course very positively. In addition to gaining factual knowledge related to HIV/AIDS, students gained increased knowledge and understanding of the roles of other disciplines. They also recognized that they came to the table with preconceived ideas and stereotypes of other professions and were able to gain a greater respect and appreciation of the contribution of others to their tutorial course. Through their discussion, students became aware of the increased breadth of learning that occurs when interacting with students from other disciplines. In having to explain and advocate for their role, students also learn more about what their particular profession could offer to the emerging need for rehabilitation in persons living with HIV/AIDS.

REFERENCES

Albanese, M. (2000). Problem-based learning: Why curricula are likely to show little effect on knowledge and clinical skills. *Medical Education, 34,* 729–738.

Albanese, M. A., & Mitchell, S. (1993). Problem-based learning: A review of literature on its outcomes and implementation issues. *Academic Medicine, 68,* 52–81.

Barrows, H. S. (1986). A taxonomy of problem-based learning methods. *Medical Education, 20,* 481–486.

Barrows, H. S. (1988). *The tutorial process.* Illinois: Southern Illinois University of Medicine.

Barrows, H. S., & Tamblyn, R. (1980). Problem-based learning. New York: Springer.

Bresnitz, E. (1996). Computer-based Learning in PBL. *Academic Medicine, 71*(5), 540.

Charlin, B., Mann, K., & Hansen, P. (1998). The many faces of problem-based learning: a framework for understanding and comparison. *Medical Teacher, 20,* 323–330.

Colliver, J. A. (2000). Effectiveness of problem-based learning: research and theory. *Academic Medicine, 75,* 259–266.

Dolmans, D., Wolfhagen, I., Scherpbier, A., & Van Der Vleuten, C. (2001). Relationship of tutors' group-dynamics skills to their performance ratings in problem-based learning. *Academic Medicine, 76,* 473–476.

Federman, D. D. (1999). Little-heralded advantages of problem-based learning. *Academic Medicine, 74,* 93–94.

Glaser, R. (1985). Control theory in the classroom. New York: Harper and Row.

Harden, R. M., & Davis, M. H. (1998) The continuum of problem-based learning. *Medical Teacher, 20,* 317–322.

Hitchcock, M. A., & Mylona, Z. (2000). Teaching faculty to conduct problem-based learning. *Teaching and Learning in Medicine, 12,* 52–57.

Kaufman, D. M., & Holmes, D. B. (1998). The relationship of tutors' content expertise to interventions and perceptions in a PBL medical curriculum. *Medical Education, 32,* 255–261.

Schmidt, H. (1983). Problem-based learning: rationale and description. *Medical Education, 17,* 11–16.

Solomon, P. (1994). Problem-based learning: A direction for physical therapy education? *Physiotherapy Theory and Practice, 10,* 45–52.

Solomon, P., Binkley, J., & Stratford, P. (1996). A descriptive study of learning processes and outcomes in two problem-based curriculum designs. *Journal of Physical Therapy Education, 10,* 72–76.

Solomon, P., Blumberg, P., & Shehata, A. (1992). The influence of patient age on problem-based learning discussion. *Academic Medicine, 67*(10), 531–533.

Solomon, P., & Finch, E. (1998). A qualitative study identifying stressors associated with adapting to problem-based learning. *Teaching and Learning in Medicine, 10,* 58–64.

Walton, H., & Matthews, M. (1989). Essentials of problem-based learning. *Journal of Medical Education, 23,* 542–558.

Williams, G., Saizow, R., & Ryan, R. (1999). The importance of self determination theory for medical education. *Academic Medicine, 74,* 992–995.

CHAPTER 10

In-Class and Electronic Communication Strategies to Enhance Reflective Practice

Lisa A. Davis, Traci D. Taylor, and Deborah Casida

Knowledge emerges only through invention and re-invention, through the restless, impatient, continuing, hopeful inquiry human being pursue in the world, with the world, and with each other.
—*Paulo Freire*

INTRODUCTION

The purpose of this chapter is to explore reflective practice models for nursing education. Increasingly, electronic communication strategies have been used by nurse educators as a teaching tool. Teaching strategies based on reflective practice can be modified for both traditional classroom activities and for computer-based learning opportunities.

DEFINITION AND PURPOSE

A goal of nursing education is to promote critical thinking, which is a process of reflecting that involves more than just analysis of the facts (Forneris & Peden-McAlpine, 2007; Idczak, 2007) in a way that emphasizes principles or patterns over "coverage" of material (Walsh & Seldomridge, 2006). Nursing students must learn to develop practical knowledge that augments textbook knowledge in order to learn clinical judgment in increasingly complex nursing situations (Tanner, 2006) by engaging in reflective activities.

More than ever, higher education has embraced teaching strategies that extend beyond the traditional classroom. Distance learning programs are proliferating. Today's learner expects technology and uses technology in all aspects of life, including formal learning. There is now a plethora of software to encourage both synchronous and asynchronous learning opportunities via Webcams, chat rooms, discussion forums, blogs (Web logs), vlogs (video logs), and virtual clinical learning situations. Internet, intranet, electronic databases, and "clicker" technology is available both outside the traditional classroom and in the traditional classroom, now termed "smart" classrooms because of the extensive electronic enhancements.

"Enhancement" is the operative word. While electronic communication strategies are important, they do not take the place of the teacher. In fact, because of the tremendous explosion of both knowledge and ways to retrieve knowledge, the teacher is even more important. Students can easily become overwhelmed by the sheer volume of information and ways to retrieve and integrate information. The crucial role of the teacher is to design learning opportunities that incorporate electronic learning strategies that enhance learning by addressing the integration of the four fundamental patterns of knowing (Carper, 1978) in a learning-centered environment (Candela, Dalley, & Benzel-Lindley, 2006; Palmer, 2007) in order to achieve the learning outcomes. Reflective activities should be incorporated in nursing education to facilitate critical thinking (Epp, 2008) and clinical reasoning using a variety of strategies.

In 2005, the National League for Nursing (NLN) published a position statement regarding standards for nursing education. Included in this position was the expectation that nursing educators should incorporate new technology into teaching that is supported by evidence-based practice. This same statement included a call for innovation in teaching strategies that promote student learning and nursing practice based on research (NLN, 2005).

THEORETICAL RATIONALE (FOUNDATIONS)

Carper (1978) identified four fundamental patterns of knowledge in nursing: empirics, esthetics, personal knowledge, and ethics. Empirics include both theoretical and research-based information geared toward development and evaluation of facts. Esthetics encompasses more than the art of nursing; it relates to the subjective appreciation that leads to understanding. Carper distinguishes esthetic knowing in terms of "knowing of a unique particular rather than an exemplary class" (p. 18). Personal knowledge involves more than just knowing *about* the self, it is knowledge *of* self both as a unique individual and in relation to others. Finally, ethical knowing is the moral component, focused on the deliberation of right and wrong.

While each pattern of knowledge is unique and indeed fundamental in understanding nursing, none are sufficient, independently or exclusively. The integration of these patterns of knowing require reflection. This reflection, as Schön (1983) reminds us, is both reflection *in action* and reflection *on action*. For nursing, this means reflection while in the act of caring for another and also reflection on the effect of that care after it has been rendered. Implicit in reflection is mindfulness—continuous appraisal, openness to new information, and awareness of multiple perspectives (Johns, 1995, 2004; Langer, 1997). It is important to note, from both the teacher and student perspective, critical reflection is tantamount to action (Freire, 2001). Therefore, reflection is both an ongoing process and a critical evaluation of what has already been done. Reflection involves both thinking and evaluation, creatively and systematically, in order to come to a deeper understanding and to develop praxis (Freire, 2001).

Benner (2001) identifies expert nurses as those who are able to understand, tacitly, a complex nursing situation using current knowledge and intuition gained from experience. This tacit knowledge results from reflection in clinical practice and is an example of reflection *in action*. The goal, in the development of novice nurses, is to develop this reflection *in action* by fostering learning situations that require reflection *on action*.

TYPES OF LEARNERS

Reflective practices integrate the fundamental patterns of knowing. Nursing students, as novices, all need experience in reflective practices. Most students come to higher education with a great working knowledge of computer-based technologies. Therefore, engaging in reflective activities using electronic communication strategies is appropriate to all levels of nursing students.

Because electronic communications transcend the boundaries of the classroom or clinical setting, it is possible to foster relational knowing between levels of nursing students. For instance, first semester students could interact with fourth semester students in reflective activities, allowing the more experienced students to model both reflective learning and relational learning. In the same vein, teaching/learning strategies of nursing faculty could be enhanced by relational learning via electronic communications. Here again, experienced faculty could mentor junior faculty in an ongoing discussion thread, sharing classroom experiences with new teaching/ learning strategies.

In addition, these strategies could be used effectively in staff development activities. Online blogs, for example, could provide a forum for expert nurses to model reflective practices for more novice nurses. This relational learning enhances reflection, particularly in personal knowledge. It is important to remember that nurses are developing, not only as practitioners of care, but as individuals (Newman, 2008; Silva, Sorrell, & Sorrel, 1995).

CONDITIONS FOR LEARNING

Reflective learning opportunities via electronic communications rely on trust, and a safe environment for disclosure. Because it is an ongoing process, interaction between members enhances appreciation and learning from various perspectives. The facilitator role is essential, first, to frame reflective questions for the learners and, second, to monitor the quality and collegiality of the discussions. While there are philosophical differences between faculty members regarding whether or not reflective activities should be graded, it is important, if graded, to provide students with both the grading rubric and objectives for reflective activities.

Finally, because of the nature of discussions and the need to maintain confidentiality, the Health Insurance Portability and Accountability Act (HIPAA) requirements should be meticulously kept. Most electronic communications, even those password protected, are not considered secure. Any discussion of specific patient information is not appropriate, which could limit discussion of actual clinical incidents. Additionally, if access is not limited to the class and faculty (such as with the use of Blogspot), outside influences such as other nurses responding to postings could become distracting for the student and overwhelming for the instructor to address. It is important for faculty to develop guidelines for discussion and strictly monitor for issues of confidentiality. Many of these particular issues are minimized or eliminated with the use of authorware commonly utilized by nursing schools and universities, such as *Angel*, *WebCT*, or *Blackboard*.

RESOURCES

In a traditional classroom setting, reflective activities can be facilitated by small group discussion. Classroom arrangement needs to be nontheatre in style (rows of desks facing a podium). Optimally, the classroom can be arranged so that students can face each other, or the desks can be rearranged to allow for several small discussion groups.

For any computer-assisted teaching strategies, technological support is an imperative. Ensure that whatever Web-based instructional strategy or software you intend to use is supported by the technical support of your institution. Both faculty and students involved in computer-enhanced learning activities need to be familiar with the equipment. Faculty need to have access to appropriate software, and the time and support to develop expertise with any new software or programs. Specific computer requirements should be conveyed to the students as required so student financial aid can help defray the cost of the equipment/software, or students should have access to computers at school.

USING THE METHOD

This discussion will be primarily focused on blogs and asynchronous discussions; however, there are increasingly diverse methods of electronic communication technologies available that could be equally useful at enhancing learning opportunities. Some of these are identified as additional resources at the end of the chapter.

As with any teaching strategy, use of specific technology depends on expected learning outcomes. Expectations regarding participation should be clearly indicated to students. Case studies, clinical observations, critical incidents from clinical experiences, narrative pedagogy (Diekelmann, 2003; Diekelmann & Lampe, 2004; Ironside, 2003; Scheckel & Ironside, 2006), logic models (Ellermann, Kataoka-Yahiro, & Wong, 2006), problem-based learning, and context-based learning can be developed for both traditional classroom and Web-based courses to support reflective activities.

The significant increase in online learning has changed the way students learn and has prompted a necessary change in the teaching focus and methods of faculty (Ryan, Carlton, & Ali, 2004). This paradigm shift results in the need for faculty to adopt new pedagogies or adapt conventional ones, such as changing to become a facilitator of learning rather than sole subject authority (Ryan et al., 2004). The use of interactive technology within a course encourages this student-centered focus, allowing the learner to actively engage in discussions, reflective journaling, peer review, and other methods that encourage critical thinking; however, nursing faculty often do not have adequate knowledge of the various roles that technology can play within their class.

Advantages of using technology are many. This benefits the educator by encouraging more objective scoring, rather than subjective, as he/she is able to better evaluate responses. There is more time to be with students. Students perceive that there is more interaction with the instructor. It allows freedom of expression within a professional context; all students are given the opportunity to respond even if they are reticent to actively participate in a traditional classroom. The student has the time to reflect rather than simply coming up with a quick answer.

Content of Blogs, Asynchronous or Synchronous Discussion Forums, and Other Methods

Blogs and other technology formats can incorporate multiple methods of learning, such as case studies, reflective journals, and postconference-type information. This would be directed by the project objectives and goals. Any of these methods can additionally help with professional writing and communication as well as application of previous knowledge, such as from prenursing courses. Students are able to develop insights into learning and nursing concepts if they routinely engage in critical thinking, enhancing their decision-making skills.

Questions used for any format should allow for more than one correct answer, thus facilitating a richer discussion. It should be clearly articulated to the students that substantive, constructive, and original responses are expected. It is incumbent upon the faculty develop a scoring rubric that reflects substantive and original thought.

Maag (2005), from the University of San Francisco School of Nursing, discussed the use of blogs in nursing education and proposes several advantages of incorporating blogs into learning. The opportunity to write and publish, after reflection and thought, provided an opportunity for students to connect with the topic. Skills such as those required for communication, good writing skills, and computer literacy are all promoted with the use of blogs. Suggestions for the use of blogs include as a discussion board, area for journal posting, electronic portfolios, or for reflective journaling.

SCORING

As previously mentioned, the merits of scoring of any type of reflective journal written by the student are avidly discussed among educators. However, if this is to be accomplished based on the objectives of the activity, a clear, simple scoring rubric should be utilized. This effectively eliminates questions regarding fairness; and although still subjective, is more objective than not. It should be emphasized that the rubric should be simple for the faculty to grade from as well (Table 10-1).

Smaller groups, such as those with 6 to 12 participants, tend to work better both in terms of scoring and in regard to student participation. This makes it easier for faculty to note repeated or unoriginal responses as well as respond in a manner specific for the student. Students do perceive faculty participation in discussion forums as crucial to the success of the forum; however, it does encourage more reflection on the part of the student if he/she is aware that the educator will respond (Mazzolini & Maddison, 2007). Educators are able to monitor responses as well as ask further critical thinking-type questions that, in turn, facilitate more discussion (Table 10-2).

Although scoring sounds time intensive, and it can be, this can be avoided if the students do not expect the instructor to respond to every posting. Faculty can elect to grade a representative sample of the students' work, noting this in the syllabus (e.g., "at least 5 blog postings will be graded"). This allows the faculty to provide formative feedback without the time-consuming task of scoring each blog. By indicating "at least," the faculty reserves the right to grade more if necessary. Also, if the educator clearly defines the expectations of the blogs, she/he may decide to post only at the end of the discussion, using a "wrap-up" format.

Table 10-1 Evaluation Rubric

Learning Outcome	Unsatisfactory (0)	Satisfactory (1)	Good (2)	Excellent (3)	Weight	Score
Participation	No posting, or posting 24 hours or more late	Posting is on time and engages with at least one classmate	Posting is on time and engages with more than one classmate	Posting(s) on time; engages with more than one classmate substantively	× 1	
Collegiality	Posting is not collegial			Posting is collegial	× 1	
Empirics	Posting does not reflect factual knowledge	Reflects minimal factual knowledge or some knowledge is not relevant	Reflects factual relevant knowledge	Reflects factual relevant knowledge with accurate interpretation; relates new knowledge to that already known	× 2	
Esthetics	Does not incorporate subjective information or feelings	Minimal incorporation of subjective information or feelings	Incorporates subjective information and feelings	Incorporates subjective information, esthetic appreciation and holism	× 2	

(continued)

Table 10-1 Evaluation Rubric ***(continued)***

Learning Outcome	Unsatisfactory (0)	Satisfactory (1)	Good (2)	Excellent (3)	Weight	Score
Personal	Does not reflect interpersonal relational knowing	Reflects knowing about self	Reflects knowing self; considers other perspective	Appreciates reciprocity of knowing self; authentic; considers all other perspectives	× 2	
Ethics	Does not reflect ethical considerations	Reflects awareness of ethical considerations	Discusses ethical considerations	Analyzes ethical considerations	× 2	
Reflective	Does not integrate ways of knowing	Develops integrated response or evaluated response	Reflects on past action and proposes future action	Reflects on past action and proposes future action demonstrating excellent integration of knowledge	× 3	
					Total	

POTENTIAL ISSUES

Diverse Methods of Learning

Students represent disparate ages and life experiences in a typical nursing program, increasing the need for accommodation for various methods of learning (Billings, Skiba, & Connors, 2005). Undergraduate students, up to about 40 years of age, tend to view the use of technology in education in a positive manner, as they routinely communicate via several methods of electronic communication and are comfortable with different types of technology (Billings et al., 2005). Graduate students, primarily from the generation that includes people over 40 years old, often prefer more traditional classroom settings that involve passive learning. However, this generation generally has increased need for accommodation in terms of flexibility of class times and locations; online or blended learning classes can address this need through increased use of technology (Billings et al., 2005).

Academic Misconduct

A prime concern that emerges when instructional technology is initiated in a course is concerns from faculty regarding the possibility of plagiarism. An initial approach to the problem may simply be to provide clarity to students regarding examples of plagiarism and consequences of it may deter some students (Embleton & Helfer, 2007). Several sources addressed this issue by encouraging the use of questions that require higher level thinking and analysis rather than simple knowledge-based answers (Teeley, 2007). Another proposal, for lengthier assignments, is to submit questionable works to antiplagiarism software that evaluates phrases or papers for plagiarism (Embleton & Helfer, 2007). Although these sites are not foolproof, they are a way to manage a problem. In addition, requesting that students submit rough drafts of works in progress, research articles, and outlines can prove that they are presenting original work (Embleton & Helfer, 2007).

Faculty Perceptions

Technology applications for learning, such as blogs and online discussion forums, are a fairly new phenomenon in education despite the general use by the public and are not readily appreciated by many educators for the great potential

Table 10-2 Sample Questions to Elicit Ways of Knowing and Reflection

Empirics	The patient is transitioning from peritoneal to hemodialysis dialysis. What is the most important thing to teach regarding that transition? Support or justify your answer. What is your priority nursing diagnosis for this client?
Esthetics	The patient is concerned about their ability to continue their work as an accountant. Discuss how this transition might affect their ability to continue to work. How would you respond to their concern? Is this the same issue as ________?
Personal	If you were in the position of receiving hemodialysis 3 days a week, what would you personally have to give up to accommodate this schedule? What are your assumptions?
Ethics	The patient has now been on hemodialysis for a month and has now decided to discontinue it due to "I just feel too bad." His wife has asked you about a Power of Attorney so that she can force him to continue dialysis, as she believes "he will be killing himself." How do you respond? His 16-year-old son is a perfect (and only) match for a transplant. He says, "I'm not going to donate the kidney and you can't make me." How do you respond?
Reflective	Identify a time in your life when you felt helpless. What helped you cope with that situation? Would you respond in the same way today? Identify a patient you have taken care of who has had to make life-altering decisions based on their new healthcare condition. Reflect on their response to this new condition. How did you respond? If you could do it again, what would you change about that response? Would you respond in the same way?

they have for education and promotion of critical thinking (Sanders, 2006). Educators must learn how to use this resource as one way to effectively engage learners in the nursing educational process. Although blogs and discussion forums can be implemented easily into a traditional class format or as an addition to online-based learning, faculty is often not comfortable with teaching in a learning style different from their own; developing an understanding of the differences in learning is crucial to providing a student-centered learning environment (Billings et al., 2005).

One suggestion from the literature is to use learning technology as a method of nursing faculty development to become comfortable with the technology before classroom implementation. Blogs can be established quickly, at no expense, and can be a way to communicate topics to educators both experienced and new to teaching (Shaffer, Lackey, & Bolling, 2006). Online discussion forums can be utilized as a communication tool for nursing departments and schools, not only facilitating communication between faculty members, but also raising the comfort level of that same faculty with the method.

Faculty, in our experience, perceived an increased time involvement for the students when using blogs as an alternative clinical postconference activity. However, one could use synchronous or asynchronous learning activities to take the place of postconference or simply augment clinical learning—the advantages are many. The students are able to rest after clinical and gather their thoughts, then "meet" online for conference when they are not as tired or overwhelmed. This has the advantage of allowing reticent students to actively participate in discussions, engaging them in a way that face-to-face discussions may not. Anecdotally, one student stated "[blogs] allow for 'extra' learning outside [the classroom] and it is not perceived as extra work." Even students of the older generations easily learn to use the technology, as most have experience with it through previous university courses. It prepares them as well for the new informatics-centered culture of the day.

CONCLUSION

In this chapter, reflective learning activities specifically using electronic communications (blogs) were explored as a way to promote critical thinking and enhance professional practice. Reflective activities are imperative to developing clinical judgment in increasingly complex nursing situations. The theoretical framework was Carper's fundamental patterns of knowing: empirics, esthetics, personal knowledge, and ethics, which is reflected in the grading rubric. Today's learner uses technology and expects it in all aspects of life, including formal education. Reflective learning activities using electronic communication are appropriate for all learners at all levels of nursing education. It is appropriate and supported by nursing organizations, such as the NLN, which calls for innovations in teaching strategies to promote learning, practice, and research.

EXAMPLE OF THE RESULT OF BLOGS

Blogs were instituted in a junior-level medical–surgical nursing class with the intent of increasing application and synthesis of the class content and providing an alternative to traditional post-conference. The rationale was that students were tired at the end of 2-day clinical and not actively participating in postconference. In addition, the students were failing the end-of-course case study exam. The faculty believed that more rested students in an environment that required active participation from all students would be more successful. Also, observation of the ease with which students routinely used various electronic communications outside the classroom indicated that blogs would provide an appropriate learning activity. When initiated, scoring rubrics and expectations (including collegiality, time frame, substantive remarks, and objectives) were provided in writing and communicated to students during orientation to the course.

While this was a significant learning experience for both students and faculty, the direct, immediate result was the substantial improvement of final examination scores. On average, students who participated in blogging scored 15% higher on the course case study examination than students who previously took the class. No other change in course delivery was initiated. Initially, the blogs were in a case study format with very directed, knowledge-based questions. As the semesters progressed, the questions regarding the case studies were modified to include more application-type questions, decreasing ability of students to copy and paste responses. In addition, ethical issues were discussed more fully. The scoring rubrics were also simplified to decrease grading time for faculty and allow for increased time for participation in discussions. The format then became more reflective, requiring students to use more resources than just the textbook. Students were required to give more original, substantive responses. That went beyond the empirics and included all of Carper's ways of knowing.

Initially, all students enrolled in the course were included in one blog, which became too cumbersome. Some faculty were skeptical of the efficacy of using blogs in place of traditional post-conference and time required to grade responses. As the grading tool was refined, this became less of an issue. Also, students were divided into smaller groups of 10–12, creating a more intimate learning environment that benefited both the student and faculty. This size of a group seems to be optimal, allowing for increased responses from students and more discussion from faculty. As the process evolved, students began to ask questions that they would not have asked in the didactic and clinical environments, also allowing for substantive responses from peers and anecdotally encouraging empathy and collegiality (esthetic knowing) among peers. This gave opportunity for faculty to have a "teachable moment."

STUDENT COMMENTS AT END-OF-COURSE EVALUATION

Responses to Supplemental Evaluation Question, "Do you prefer traditional postconference or blogs?"

"Blog, the student is able to think on their own and use critical thinking which promotes better understanding of the disease or condition the patient is in."

"Blog helps with clinical exams and real life experience with what we learned—application."

"Blogs—I found it to be most beneficial. It gave me time to think about my responses and was interesting to read other responses."

"Blogs, by the time postconference comes most of us are tired and ready to go home and don't pay attention, plus, the blog gives us another opportunity to apply what we've learned to an actual clinical problem."

"Blogging was good, and I learned more because I actually had to look things up."

"Blog are a better learning experience and we tend to remember more."

Additional Feedback

" . . . having to look up the info helped to engrave into my mind why things occur and what can be done."

" . . . it helps to wrap everything we have learned into one package and . . . helps you to analyze the problem."

" . . . it encourages all of us to think . . . sometimes in postconference, one person runs the show . . . now everyone else has a chance to come to conclusions on their own."

"They allow for "extra" learning outside [the classroom] and it is not perceived as extra work."

TEACHING EXAMPLE

Student Use of Reflective Practice Journal

Using the format for clinical supervision outlined earlier in the Using the Method section, a student submitted a journal entry for discussion in seminar. The journal topic was her clinical encounter with a woman regarding a sexual health issue. The student was aware of a barrier between herself and the client but was unable to identify the origins of the barrier. In the reflective process of describing the encounter in writing, the student started to uncover a reoccurring theme for herself. The student noted that the large age discrepancy between the client and the client's significant other had been an issue for the student.

The writing process gave the student the time and context in which to sort and organize her thoughts regarding the experience in order to be able to present them in a systematic manner. This in turn helped the student to uncover the reoccurring issue of age discrepancy that kept surfacing during her reflections. Once the underlying issue of age discrepancy was identified, the seminar leader was able to direct the group discussion around the student's knowledge, personal beliefs, and feelings concerning age discrepancies within intimate relationships. The student's and the other seminar participants' personal experiences and views were shared and examined using Johns's framing perspectives and reflective cues.

As a result of the discussion, the student became more aware of her own biases regarding age discrepancies within intimate relationships. She was able to identify some misconceptions and identify some beliefs and values that were important to her. There was a shift in the student's level of acceptance of such relationships without a complete revision of her underlying belief system. The shift was related to her becoming more aware of her own personal biases and the impact that they had on her interactions rather than a shift in her own personal value system. However, awareness of one's biases and being able to partially or completely bracket them off within the context of an interaction may represent a subtle shift in the intensity of one's value system with regard to the issue at hand.

REFERENCES

Benner, P. (2001). *From novice to expert: Excellence and power in clinical nursing practice.* Upper Saddle River, NJ: Prentice Hall.

Billings, D., Skiba, D., & Connors, H. (2005). Best practices in web-based courses: Generational differences across undergraduate and graduate nursing students. *Journal of Professional Nursing, 21*(2), 126–133.

Carper, B. (1978). Fundamental patterns of knowing in nursing. *Advances in Nursing Science, 1*(1), 13–23.

Candela, L., Dalley, K., & Benzel-Lindley, J. (2004). A case for learning-centered curricula. *Journal of Nursing Education, 45*(2), 59–66.

Diekelmann, N. (2003). Thinking-in-action journals: From self evaluation to multiperspectival thinking. *Journal of Nursing Education, 42,* 482–484.

Diekelmann, N., & Lampe, S. (2004). Student-centered pedagogies: Co-creating compelling experiences using the new pedagogies. *Journal of Nursing Education, 43,* 245–247.

Ellermann, C. R., Katahka-Yahiro, M. R., & Wong, L. C. (2006). Logic models used to enhance critical thinking. *Journal of Nursing Education, 45*(6), 220–227.

Embleton, L., & Helfer, D. (2007). The plague of plagiarism and academic dishonesty. *Searcher, 15*(6), 23–26.

Epp, S. (2008). The value of reflective journaling in undergraduate nursing education: A literature review. *International Journal of Nursing Studies, 45,* 1379–1388.

Forneris, S., & Pedan-McAlpine, C. (2007). Evaluation of a reflective learning intervention to improve critical thinking in novice nurses. *Journal of Advanced Nursing, 57*(4), 410–421.

Freire, P. (2001). *Pedagogy of the oppressed* (30th anniversary ed.). New York: Continuum.

Idczak, S. (2007). I am a nurse: Nursing students learn the art and science of nursing. *Nursing Education Perspectives, 28*(2), 66–71.

Ironside, P. (2003). New pedagogies for teaching thinking: The lived experiences of students and teachers enacting narrative pedagogy. *Journal of Nursing Education, 42,* 509–516.

Johns, C. (2004). *Becoming a reflective practitioner* (2nd ed.). Malden, MA: Blackwell.

Johns, C. (1995). Framing learning through reflection within Carper's fundamental ways of knowing in nursing. *Journal of Advanced Nursing, 22*(2), 226–234.

Langer, E. (1997). *The power of mindful learning.* Cambridge, MA: Perseus Books Group.

Maag, M. (2005). The potential use of "blogs" in nursing education. *Computers, Informatics, Nursing, 23*(1), 16–24.

Mazzolini, M., & Maddison, S. (2007). When to jump in: The role of the instructor in online discussion forums. *Computers & Education, 49,* 193–213.

National League for Nursing.(2005, May). *Postition statement: Transforming nursing education.* Retrieved October 2007, from http://www.nln.org/aboutnln/PositionStatements/transforming052005.pdf

Newman, M. (2008). *Transforming presence: The difference that nursing makes.* Philadelphia: F.A. Davis.

Palmer, P. (2008). *Courage to teach: exploring the inner landscape of a teacher's life* (10th ed.). San Francisco: Jossey-Bass.

Ryan, M., Carlton, K., & Ali, N. (2004). Reflections of the role of faculty in distance learning and changing pedagogies. *Nursing Education Persectives, 25*(2), 73–80.

Sanders, J. (2006). Twelve tips for using blogs and wikis in medical education. *Medical Teacher, 28*(8), 680–682.

Scheckel, M., & Ironside, P. (2006). Cultivating interpretive thinking through enacting narrative pedagogy. *Nursing Outlook, 54*(3), 159–165.

Schön, D. (1983). *The reflective practioner: How professionals think in action*. New York: Basic Books.

Shaffer, S. Lackey, S., & Bolling, G. (2006). Blogging as a venue for nurse faculty development. *Nursing Education Perspectives, 27*(3), 126–128.

Silva, M., Sorrell, J., & Sorrell, C. (1995). *From Carper's patterns of knowing to ways of being: An ontological philosophical shift in nursing. ANS Advances in Nursing Science, 18*(1), 1–13.

Tanner, C. (2006). Thinking like a nurse: A research-based model of clinical judgment in nursing. *Journal of Nursing Education, 45*(6), 204–211.

Teeley, K. (2007). Designing hybrid web-based courses for accelerated nursing students. *Journal of Nursing Education, 46*(9), 417–422.

Walsh, C., & Seldomridge, L. (2006). Critical thinking: Back to square two. *Journal of Nursing Education, 45*(6), 212–219.

ADDITIONAL RESOURCES

Betts, J., & Glogoff, S. (2004). *Instructional models for using weblogs in elearning: Case studies from a hybrid and virtual course*. Retrieved October 2007, from http://www.syllabus.com/news_article.asp?id=9829&typeid=156

Billings, D., Connors, H., & Skiba, D. (2001). Benchmarking best practices in Web-based nursing courses. *Advanced Nursing Science, 23*(4), 41–52.

Chirema, K. (2007). The use of reflective journals in the promotion of reflection and learning in post-registration nursing students. *Nurse Education Today, 27*, 192–202.

Distler, J. (2007). Critical thinking and clinical competence: Results of the implementation of student-centered teaching strategies in an advanced practice nurse curriculum. *Nurse Education in Practice, 7*, 53–59.

Garon, M. (2002). Science of unitary human beings: Martha E. Rogers. In J. George (Ed.), *Nursing theories: The base for professional nursing practice* (pp. 269–289). Upper Saddle River, NJ: Prentice Hall.

Kaas, M., Block, D., Avery, M., Lindeke, L., Kubik, M., Duckett, L., et al. (2001). Technology-enhanced distance education: From experimentation to concerted action. *Journal of Professional Nursing, 17*(3), 135–140.

Mezirow, J. (1990). How critical reflection triggers transformative learning. In *Fostering critical reflection in adulthood: A guide to transformative and emancipatory learning* (pp. 1–20). San Francisco: Jossey-Bass.

Murray, T., Belgrave, L., & Robinson, V. (2006). Nursing faculty members competence of Web-based course development systems directly influences students' satisfaction. *The ABNF Journal, 17*, 100–102.

Ornes, L., &. Gassert, C. (2007). Computer competencies ina BSN program. *Journal of Nursing Education, 46*(2), 75–78.

Rogers, M. (1994). Nursing science evolves. In M. Madrid (Ed.), *Rogers' scientific art of nursing practice* (pp. 3–9). New York: National League for Nursing.

Sanders, J. (2007). The potential of blogs and wikis in healthcare education. *Education for Primary Care, 18*, 16–21.

Skiba, D. (2005). The Millennials: Have they arrived at your school of nursing? *Nursing Education Perspectives, 25*(6), 370–371.

Utley-Smith, Q. (2004). Five competencies needed by new baccalaureate graduates. *Nursing Education Perspectives, 25*(4), 166–170.

VandeVusse, L., & Hanson, L. (2000). Evaluation of online course discussions: Faculty facilitation of active student learning. *Computers in Nursing, 18*(4), 181–188.

ELECTRONIC RESOURCES

E-learning Software

http://www.flextraining.com/default.asp?st=all&source=Goog

http://www.saba.com/products/centra/details.htm#virtual_classes

Create a Blog

Use resources on distance learning authorware such as WebCT and ANGEL.

http://moodle.com/

http://blackboard.com/products/Academic_Suite/index

http://www.angellearning.com/

https://www.blogger.com/start?utm_campaign=en&utm_source=en-ha-na-bk&utm_medium=ha&utm_term=blogger&gclid=CM_ug4Gyw5c-CFQsQagodoFKrRA

https://www.blogger.com/start

http://www.bloghelp.org/

Twitter

http://googleblog.blogspot.com/

Virtual Media

http://www.massively.com/2008/02/25/cisco-opens-virtual-hospital-in-second-life-and-ibm-doesnt/

http://secondlife.com/

Anti-plagiarism Software

http://www.turnitin.com (also available through many universities)

CHAPTER 11

Debate as a Teaching Strategy

Martha J. Bradshaw and Arlene J. Lowenstein

The debate is a strategy long recognized as a means by which to address a topic in which there may be more than one viewpoint. The value of a debate is not necessarily in the resolution of a topic or persuasive results, but the value as a teaching strategy lies more in the process and presentation of the viewpoints.

DEFINITION AND PURPOSES

A traditional view of debate may be that of argument for the purpose of persuading the audience toward a clearly identified position. To debate an issue is to consider or discuss it from opposing positions or arguments (Berube & DeVinne, 1982). Political debates are used as opportunities for candidates to make their perspectives known on key issues. This form of structured argument has long been used in philosophy, theology, law, and the sciences (Tumposky, 2004). Debate has been defined as "a systematic contest of speakers in which two points of view of a proposition are advanced with proof"(Barnhart, 1966, p. 311). Wikipedia's definition states that debating is a formal method of interactive and representational argument which has rules and a framework for participants to discuss and decide on differences as they interact (Wikipedia, 2009). Koklanaris, MacKenzie, Fino, Arslan, and Scubert (2008) noted that debate is useful to promote active learning because "debating inherently involves a variety of positive features: the impetus for intense preparation, active participation, and a forum ideally suited to controversial topics" (p. 235). Based on these definitions, debate becomes a useful teaching strategy.

Debate provides opportunities for students to analyze an issue or problem in depth and to reach an informed, unbiased conclusion or resolution. Debate encourages participants to identify quickly the essential nature of the issue as substantiated by evidence; to establish criteria for judging its successful resolution; and to weigh, compare, and contrast the merits of alternative strategies for resolution (Simonneaux, 2002). Debate is especially useful strategy for students who need to cultivate analytical thought processes (Vo & Morris, 2006). In addition, presentation of the debate allows students to practice oral communication skills, express professional opinions, and gain experience in speaking to groups and in working in groups when preparing the debates.

THEORETICAL RATIONALE

Two important components of the professional role are the analysis of significant issues and the ability to communicate in efficient and effective ways. Professional communication is seen in many forms; scholarly publication, oral presentations, and electronic networking are a few examples. Similar to other skills, the development of effective communication skills must be fostered by faculty. The ability to communicate one's thoughts clearly and concisely evolves from the formulation of a perspective on a topic, analysis of that perspective and other views, and development of sound conclusions. Debate enables students to participate actively in a meaningful communication exercise.

DeYoung (1990) differentiates debate from general discussion by pointing out that general discussion is based on open mindedness and a free flow of ideas. Discussion usually aims toward some sort of conclusion and often is a cooperative compromise. Debate, on the other hand, is argumentative, with each team competing to establish its position as the most correct one or the one that should be upheld.

The college environment is one that should develop the student's inquisitiveness and discriminating attitude (Vo & Morris, 2006). The debate is particularly helpful at causing a student to examine the position juxtaposed to a personally held view. One of the purposes of debate is for the learner to go beyond merely identifying an issue. Learners must analyze the issue: What are its key elements? What historical precedents have contributed to the issue? Who are the key proponents and opponents of the issue? What is the future of the issue? Students can learn how personal values or emotions influence thinking and responses to issues. Students also can identify what factors influence their thinking, such as the views of news analysts, popular literature, or peers (Simonneaux, 2002). Analysis on this level leads to powerful learning, calling for the use of reasoning and other forms of higher order thinking. The learner first becomes more aware of their own thinking, then broadens and purposefully adapts their thinking (Tumposky, 2004). A study by Koklanaris et al. (2008) found that when the objective was learning about a controversial topic, resident physicians who prepared for and participated in a debate achieved higher test scores and retained information better than those who attended a lecture. They concluded that organizing a debate may be more effective than giving a lecture about a controversial topic.

CONDITIONS FOR LEARNING

Debate is most useful as part of a course or seminar in professional and academic settings. Because of the nature of this strategy, it should be employed in a course that centers on issues or topics that raise debatable questions. Debate also is a means to validate and deepen content knowledge (Martens, 2007). This strategy can be used to facilitate students' ability to implement analytical skills, to systematically research and critique an issue, to arrive at salient points, and to demonstrate more professional development related to group process (Candela, Michael, & Mitchell, 2003). The learning goals for the debate strategy include improving oral communication and research referencing skills, structuring and presenting an argument, and exercising analytical skills. The process for formulating and presenting the debate should facilitate these goals as much as possible; therefore, the faculty should provide as much freedom as possible for the students to reach these learning goals independently. Students should be given enough structure or direction to help them plan and organize their work, but they also should understand the responsibility they must take for researching debate positions, analyzing key issues, and practicing speaking skills. In the debate strategy described by Lowenstein and Bradshaw (1989), students were encouraged to take the viewpoint opposite the one they (personally) held. This approach promoted an understanding of existing oppositional perspectives and enhanced the ability to respond to opposing views (Lowenstein & Bradshaw, 1989).

Preparation for the debate should begin early in the course to provide adequate opportunity for library research and exploration of issues. Faculty facilitation is an essential part of the learning process. Conditions central to use of debate as an effective strategy include the following:

- Students need to be introduced to key issues in the course and have to be able to identify controversial points suitable for debate.
- Students need to be familiar with one another in order to form working groups.
- Students need knowledge of existing resources to use in formulating debate. This includes increased familiarity with the faculty member(s) as a source of support and information.

TYPES OF LEARNERS

Debate can be used with all levels or types of learners, including undergraduate students, graduate students, and practitioners, because the learning goals of debate are suitable for all groups. Lowenstein and Bradshaw (1989) used debate with registered nurse students who were completing their BSN courses. Debate is a particularly successful strategy with this group because these students combine personal experience with actual patient or practice problems with the need to refine communication and analytical skills.

Swu-Jane and Crawford (2007) used debate as a new component to an introductory core course for pharmacy students who were in their first-professional year. Objectives were to facilitate the group process, improve critical thinking and communication skills, introduce controversial issues related to the US healthcare system, enable students' ability to analyze and evaluate evidence, help develop skills in formulating written arguments, and encourage tolerance of diverse points of view. Thus, debate provides a true opportunity for professional growth in this type of student. By immersing in the topic, students have a better understanding of it than they would through other means of study.

By creating the need to objectively analyze an issue, debate is useful for a student who is strongly influenced by personal values or certain work experiences. An undergraduate who has not formed a world view about sensitive ethical dilemmas, for example, can have the opportunity to examine the issues and how decisions are made. A practitioner who has been receiving negative influence in the work environment has the opportunity for objective analysis of the situation.

Debate is a strategy to be used when the instructor wishes to bring about active rather than passive learning, critical thinking, creativity, and introduce the learners to the role of conflict in professional endeavors. This last advantage, conflict, is an advantageous strategy in that it not only engages learners who tend to "drift," but also introduces students to how to effectively converse with those in opposition to their own view and be comfortable in holding onto and supporting own position (Vo & Morris, 2006).

RESOURCES

Faculty members serve as an important resource by assuming the role of facilitator. Formal debate questions and positions can emerge from class discussion about important issues. Faculty members can assist students in formulating the debate question and can direct them to resources related to the issue. Clinical experiences and current issues in health care offer a wide range of debate topics. Faculty may wish to prepare the students early in the course by encouraging them to be alert to ethical dilemmas or patient care problems that are suitable for debate (Candela et al., 2003).

The electronic and traditional libraries offer many resources for debate preparation. By using the professional literature to support the debate position, students are introduced to a wide range of journals, books, and other printed material. Electronic information systems are extremely helpful to students as they identify debate issues and develop related positions. Database searches enable students to consider related topics and sources, outside of their own professional field, which may generate additional support for a position. The electronic media access most current information, which may be particularly helpful for students who have timely political topics. Electronic bulletin boards and other communication networks provide students with the opportunity to interact with individuals outside their own institution who are involved with the issue.

The debate can be presented in any planned classroom setting. The environment should be such that the debate teams can be seen and heard by the audience. The debate process can be used in online courses as well (Swu-Jane & Crawford, 2007). Through a process of informal forum, students use critical thinking skills to research and retrieve information, then compile it in a manner by which they can make informed decisions or develop opinions on the issue under discussion (Huang, 2006). Just as with the traditional debate method, the informal forum is interactive between students, rather than being teacher directed. However, when conducted online, this approach does not provide the opportunity for face-to-face interaction and development of oral communication skills.

USING THE METHOD

In the Lowenstein and Bradshaw method, faculty members define broad (topical) areas from the course outline and identify an advisor for each area. Students choose the general area in which they are interested and form groups of four or five members. At least one group is formed for each topical area to guarantee that course objectives or topics are addressed. Depending on student interest and enrollment, a second group may be formed in certain areas. For example, two groups may choose to address the area of professional roles and responsibilities. Specific debate questions are formulated by the group in keeping with the objectives or broad topics of the course and personal interests of group members. Many of the topics are those currently being debated by our colleagues in all areas of health care. Patient care delivery systems, healthcare reform, genetic screening, and euthanasia are a few examples.

Each group should meet with the faculty advisor as needed to organize the debate presentation, gain insight into the points being presented, and receive assistance with resources. The instructor may assist the groups by refining their reasoning approaches. Martens (2007) identifies several types of reasoning as part of the argument:

Reasoning by: example, analogy, causal, cost–benefit, evidence

Students are guided to consider the perspectives of all individuals or interest groups (Simonneaux, 2002). For each debate group, two students select the affirmative position, two select the negative, and the fifth serves as moderator. In groups of four, the faculty advisor serves as moderator. Each group develops a reading list of significant articles related to the issue under debate. The list is circulated to the entire class at least 1 week prior to the debate. Students not involved in the presentation are expected to be prepared to discuss the issues under consideration.

The debate consists of opening remarks by a moderator, two affirmative and two negative presentations, rebuttal, and summary. Following the presentation, the floor is opened to the class for discussion. Questions and comments based on the presentations and readings are generated by the class. The debate moderator facilitates discussion and provides a final summary of the issues and discussion. In most situations, the burden of supporting the affirmative view is the more difficult position to hold (Law, 1998). With some issues, it may be appropriate to develop a resolution plan upon conclusion of the formal debate. This plan can incorporate some ideas from both positions to encourage win–win negotiation. This process gives students experience in developing workable solutions to practice-related issues. Class members not participating in the debate are asked to evaluate each presenter based on a rating scale. Students evaluate the analysis of the issue, the evidence presented, supporting resources, organization of the presentation, the argument presented, interaction with the audience and opponents, and response to questions (Fig. 11-1). An overall effectiveness score is given, and the evaluators indicate if their stand on the issue changed as a result of the debate. All faculty members participating in the seminar also evaluate the presenters. Debate grades are based on preparation, individual performance, and group efforts that were reflected in the effectiveness of the debate.

Figure 11-1 Grading tool: Debate.

Date: ____________________ **Subject/topic:** ____________________

Evaluate each speaker using the following scale:

Superior = 5; Excellent = 4; Good = 3; Fair = 2; Below standard = 1

***Team* A**		***Team* B**
1 2 3 4 5	Bibliography (4 max)	1 2 3 4 5
1 2 3 4 5	Overview of problem (1–2)	1 2 3 4 5
1 2 3 4 5	Representing side of debate (1–2)	1 2 3 4 5
1 2 3 4 5	Opening remarks, Debater 1	1 2 3 4 5
1 2 3 4 5	Opening remarks, Debater 2	1 2 3 4 5
1 2 3 4 5	Resolution plan, Debater 1	1 2 3 4 5
1 2 3 4 5	Resolution plan, Debater 2	1 2 3 4 5
1 2 3 4 5	Response to opposing team, Debater 1	1 2 3 4 5
1 2 3 4 5	Response to opposing team, Debater 2	1 2 3 4 5
1 2 3 4 5	Closing remarks	1 2 3 4 5

Comments: ____

____

____

To reinforce the learning from the debate, students may be asked to write a formal paper on one of the professional issues discussed in the course. The paper can be evaluated on the presentation of the issue, arguments for both sides of the issue supported by literature, the student's position and rationale for selection of the position, application of ideas to practice, and use of references and format.

In the online format, Swu-Jane and Crawford developed a series of three debates over a 12-week term. Teams of four to five members were established and paired as pro (affirmative) or con (negative). Teams were encouraged to appoint a team leader to coordinate the work and communicate with an assigned teaching assistant. A forum was set up for discussion posts for the paired teams. Students were expected to post three arguments in an online forum that included two constructive arguments and one rebuttal and summary argument. Each group posted in 1-week intervals beginning with affirmative followed by negative, a second affirmative followed by negative, and the final argument started with negative first and then positive. A word limit of 400 to 600 words, excluding references, was set to correspond to a speaker's time limit in an oral debate. Students were encouraged to read articles recommended by the instructors to provide an overview for both sides of the debate topic and to search, use, and cite additional reference sources. An orientation to the debate process was provided with written materials to assist the students in understanding the expectations and flow. Three judges were appointed by the instructors to decide the winners of the debate.

POTENTIAL PROBLEMS

The debate strategy calls for significant student responsibility and preparation, for both debaters and the audience. Debaters are required to thoroughly research the issue and the position taken for the argument. From this preparation, they formulate a succinct and effective presentation. Debaters are expected to practice speaking skills and to prepare supporting materials for the oral presentation. The debate group provides an appropriate reading list for the other class members. Those students take the responsibility to read about the issue prior to the presentation in order to understand the issue and participate effectively in discussion. Lack of preparation on the part of the team members leads to inadequate presentation of the issue and superficial discussion. On the other hand, students who are acquainted with the opposing team members may collaborate and develop a "planned" debate in order to maximize opportunity for a successful outcome. While this may be difficult to discover on the part of the instructor, it clearly is an example of academic dishonesty.

The debate causes students to clearly classify an issue as one that is right or wrong, or answered "yes" or "no." Many topics have no conclusions or answers, and thus may impose a false dualism (Tumposky, 2004). Students may have to defend a position to which they are not clearly committed. Students with strong moral beliefs about an issue may have difficulty defending a specified position or accepting the views of others. Faculty may have difficulty presenting a neutral position when moderating the debate and guiding discussion (Simonneaux, 2002). At some point during the presentations, it must be made very clear that there is no right or singular answer to most issues.

Nervousness about speaking in public can be a major concern. Some students have had little or no public speaking experience, or they may have had negative experiences that generated anxiety. Tumposky (2004) asserts that female students may be more uncomfortable with the adversarial nature of this strategy than their male peers. In addition, students of certain cultural groups may have difficulty with open debate as a way to learn. Students need encouragement and need to view the debate as an opportunity to speak to an open, receptive group in order to gain experience. What some students look upon with apprehension often results in being uplifting and beneficial. For example, one student was timid about speaking in groups and was extremely nervous before and during her debate presentation. Her nervousness was manifested in physical symptoms, such as sweating, flushed face, tremulous voice, shaking hands, and rapid blinking. She received appropriate support from faculty and students, which encouraged her to work on this problem during the rest of her academic work. Three years later, she successfully defended her master's project in a dignified and professional manner. Her public speaking skills have now advanced to the point that she is able to address both groups and individuals effectively in her current employment as a clinical specialist.

The argumentative or confrontational nature of the debate may create anxiety. In addition, debate or public speaking may be a new strategy on which students are graded, thus heightening anxiety. Faculty and students must continually place emphasis on the debate as a learning experience. The excitement of defending a position, stressing key points, and deriving a workable solution should be presented as positive outcomes of the debate. Faculty members should stress that students will not be condemned or inappropriately criticized for taking unpopular viewpoints during the debate. Faculty members are prepared to handle strong emotional viewpoints and to help students understand that there is room for conflicting opinions in our society. In using debate as a teaching strategy, Candela et al. (2003) discovered that students liked the strategy and found it challenging, but did not see how they would use the skill or strategy in their professional careers. It is possible that, as novices, students are not aware of potential situations in which there will be a need to defend a position regarding health care. Students also need to be encouraged to see the benefit of the opportunity to practice speaking skills, research skills, and group work. As a teaching strategy, Tumposky (2004) points out that use of debate is widespread despite lack of evidence to validate its effectiveness.

CONCLUSION

Debate is a strategy that promotes student interaction and involvement in course topics. There are many advantages to using this strategy. Debate expands the student's perspective on a given issue, creates doubt about the existence of one clear answer, and requires much thought and further evidence before deriving a solution. Debate also increases awareness of opposing viewpoints. As an interactive strategy, debate develops techniques of persuasion, serves as a means by which students confront a controversial issue, and promotes collaborative efforts and negotiation skills among peers. This strategy promotes independence and participation in the decision-making process, as well as enhancing writing and organizational skills. Debate allows for examination of broad issues that influence professional practice. Critical thinking is enhanced by the scrutiny of more than one position on the issue. Debate allows the student a wider forum than writing a paper does, and it may give a greater sense of accomplishment (DeYoung, 1990).

Selection of debate as a teaching strategy requires a strong commitment to preparation and guidance from faculty. Faculty members will have to deal with emotions that can be elicited by the arguments. Faculty members will need to provide support for students who take minority or unpopular positions and for those who have limited public speaking skills. Following the debate, those students whose ideas are not accepted by the majority should be encouraged to recognize those parts of their work that were of value, even if others disagreed with their position. Those students whose ideas reflected the majority view should also recognize that public consensus can change quickly, and, as more information becomes available, opinions may be swayed. Finally, faculty members can help students to recognize that the debate is just a start to exploration of professional issues. Students will need to be encouraged to incorporate their newly learned and practiced skills into their professional practice.

REFERENCES

Barnhart, C. L. (Ed.) (1966). *The American college dictionary*. New York: Random House

Berube, M. S., & DeVinne, P. B. (Eds.) (1982). *The American heritage dictionary*. Boston: Houghton, Mifflin.

Candela, L., Michael, S. R., & Mitchell, S. (2003). Ethical debates: Enhancing critical thinking in nursing students. *Nurse Educator, 28*, 37–39.

DeYoung, S. (1990). Teaching nursing. Redwood City, CA: Addison-Wesley.

Huang, G. H-C. (2007). Informal forum: Fostering active learning in a teacher preparation program. *Education, 127*(1), 31–38.

Law, C. F. (1998). Using argumentation to teach literature. *Exercise Exchange, 43*, 10–11.

Lowenstein, A. J., & Bradshaw, M. J. (1989). Seminar methods for RN to BSN students. *Nurse Educator, 14*(5), 27–31.

Koklanaris, N., MacKenzie, A. P., Fino, M. E., Arslan, A. A., & Scubert, D. E. (2008). Debate preparation/participation: An active effective learning tool. *Teaching and Learning in Medicine, 20*(3), 235–238.

Martens, E. A. (2007). The instructional use of argument across the curriculum. *Middle School Journal, 38*(5), 4–13.

Simonneaux, L. (2002). Analysis of classroom debating strategies. *The Journal of Biological Education, 37*, 9–12.

Swu-Jane, L., & Crawford, S. Y. (2007) An online debate series for first-year pharmacy students. *American Journal of Pharmaceutical Education, 71*(1), 1–8.

Tumposky, N. R. (2004). The debate debate. *Clearing House, 78*, 52–55.

Vo, H.X., & Morris, R. L. (2006). Debate as a tool in teaching economics: Rationale, technique, and some evidence. *Journal of Education for Business, 81*(6), 315–330.

Wikipedia. (2009). Debate. Retrieved September 1, 2009, from http://en.wikipedia.org/wiki/Debates

SECTION III

Simulation and Imagination

The teaching-learning strategies presented in Section III promote the use of imagination as a way of encouraging students to stretch their thinking and explore their understanding of concepts in different ways. Simulation and imagination techniques encourage students to avoid being locked in to one solution to a problem and provide an opportunity to learn to develop different approaches to the problems they face. Effective learning requires active participation. When students use their imagination to play a role, take an opposing viewpoint to their held view, learning to express themselves in new and different ways, or are involved in games as a learning strategy, they become involved in their learning. The role of faculty is a facilitating one, helping students interact with each other to bring out other possibilities, to reinforce learning objectives, and, in a safe, less stressful setting, help students develop insight into the translation of classroom to the clinical environment.

Clinical experience has been a mainstay of a health professional's education. However, it is more and more difficult to find student clinical experiences in today's managed care world, when providers are under the gun to reduce patient length of stay and restrict the time and amount of ambulatory care visits. The requirement for increased provider productivity does not allow time for teaching. In addition, the informed healthcare consumers of today may or may not be willing to allow neophyte students to practice their skills.

Students can be encouraged to use simulation and imagination to learn how to adapt their clinical knowledge to the practical world. Simulation used in conjunction with role-playing clinical situations involving patients, families, and staff may provide an orientation to situations they may face in the clinical area, and allows students to problem solve in a safe environment. They can learn to make decisions and correct their mistakes without causing injury to a patient. Participation in simulation activities can make learning a fun, enjoyable, and memorable learning experience. Through simulation, they can be prepared to gain experience that may not be available in the immediate clinical area, but will be part of their practice in the real world of health care.

CHAPTER 12

Games are Multidimensional in Educational Situations

Lynn Jaffe

Games are central to human experience and an important way in which it is made meaningful.
—*Dormann & Biddle (2006)*

Today's college students and adult learners seek more from academics and in-services than lecture formats (University of North Carolina, 2009). Current technology has fostered reduced attention spans and reinforced students' reliance on instant gratification and immediate feedback, as well as innovation and novelty to sustain interest in learning situations (Greenfield, 2009; Oblinger, 2006a; Reiner & Siegel, 2008; Sauve, Renaud, Kaufman, & Marquis, 2007). Games can address these needs because they are experiential and can provide frequent feedback. Games used for educational purposes, or serious games, are a way to motivate, reinforce skills, and promote collaboration through their experiential format. There is extensive literature on games theory and gaming in multiple disciplines. This chapter is an introduction to the use of games as a teaching/learning tool within the classroom or clinical setting. Definitions, evidence regarding practice, and the types of learning that will fit most easily within the various game structures will be described, as will the limitations of game use within the educational or clinical environment.

DEFINITION AND PURPOSE

A game is an activity often classified as fun, governed by precise rules that involve varying degrees of strategy or chance, and one or more players who cooperate or compete (with self, the game, one another, or a computer) through the use of knowledge or skill in an attempt to reach a specified goal (Beylefeld & Struwig, 2007; Sauve et al., 2007). Educational or serious games expect learning benefits for all participants that last beyond the game itself. There are three major categories within the genre: games, simulations, and simulation games.

Game is the generic that includes board, card, and skilled activities. Many simple educational games have popular formats, such as Bingo, Jeopardy, Trivial

Pursuit, Monopoly, and Who Wants to Be a Millionaire?, that provide frameworks for inserting content and creating learning activities. These games typically involve a set of rules for player moves and termination criteria so that winners may be determined. The frameworks are easily adaptable to a wide variety of content and instructional objectives usually in the lower cognitive domain areas. These games have been described in the literature and examples are listed under Additional Resources. Also see Electronic Resources for templates of popular game shows for educational use.

Simulations, in this context, are role playing games and discussed in Chapters 14 and 16. Simulation games are contrived reality-based conflicts that must be resolved within the constraints of the game rules and have been shown to enhance competency development among health professionals (Allery, 2004; Graham & Richardson, 2008; Sauve et al., 2007). They have the potential to attain new heights of efficacy in digital game formats where they can be used to enhance other aspects of the educational experience than mere review of content. Within authentic contexts, students have the opportunity to get immersed in the game and call on past knowledge and experience to problem solve and make decisions about clients (Oblinger, 2006b; Skiba, 2008).

Debriefing is an important aspect of the learning process that occurs after the game. It is a discussion about the concepts, generalizations, and applications of the topics covered within the game (Gee, 2008; Graham & Richardson, 2008). This process assists learners in recognizing the learning that has occurred within the fun experience of the game and contributes to the learners' ability to use self-reflection (Allery, 2004). Effective debriefing requires a good deal of skill and experience in the facilitator and should be allotted as much time as was spent actually playing the game.

THEORETICAL FOUNDATIONS

The use of games for educational purposes is a very old idea. The earliest recorded use was for war games 3000 years ago in China, in the 18th century in Europe, and, within this century, by the US military. Game use was brought to the business community by ex-officers to provide training in problem solving and decision making. It was considered a bridge between academic instruction and on-the-job training. In the 1950s and 1960s, as the theoretical focus of learning shifted from the instructor to the student, experience-based learning became prominent and games were used to meet this goal. In health-related areas, psychologists and nurses made numerous contributions to the literature on game use in both academic and clinical education, although the research is still inconclusive when judging their effectiveness primarily due to small sample sizes, poor operational definitions, and other design flaws (Akl et al. 2008; Beylefeld & Struwig, 2007; Blakely, Skirton, Cooper, Allum, & Nelmes, 2009; Bochennek, Wittekindt, Zimmermann, & Klingebiel, 2007; Royse & Newton, 2007).

Game use falls under the theoretical umbrellas of active learning strategies and cooperative learning described in Chapter 1 and under the concept of flow coined by Csikszentnikhlyi, which refers to a psychological state achieved when learning and enjoyment coincide (Beylefeld & Struwig, 2007). The focus is on actual engagement with both the educational material and classmates, engendering positive attitudes that promote deep processing of the learning experience. It can be intense, absorbing, and motivating (Dormann & Biddle, 2006).

TYPES OF LEARNERS

Games are being used throughout the educational continuum, from preschool through graduate education. They can be used for students who like to compete or for those who prefer to cooperate. For learners with achievement needs games motivate through competitiveness. Games may also be motivating for those with strong affiliation needs because games can require team play and cooperation for completion. The element of luck within an educational game gives all students, not just the studious ones, a chance at winning and thereby keeps engagement higher. Educators must appreciate the different maturational stages students pass through. Adult learners have a particular need to engage meaningfully with content and apply it in a variety of methods, which can be accomplished through the interactive, immediate, and diverse format of gaming.

Games can be structured to require a degree of flexibility on the part of the student to adapt to changing circumstances, especially when addressing the development of interdisciplinary awareness, problem solving, cultural sensitivity, and empathy with clients (Graham & Richardson, 2008; Jarrell, Alpers, Brown, & Wotring, 2008). Finally, particularly with the use of digital simulation games, some degree of computer/technology comfort is required on the part of both the students and the faculty/trainer. Most millennial and postmillennial students arrive on campus equipped to use Web 2.0 technologies, some faculty need to increase their comfort level.

CONDITIONS FOR LEARNING

Games can be used to address all levels of cognitive objectives, from reinforcing the learning of basic facts, through developing application and analysis skills, and culminating in promoting synthesis and evaluation. They do this through the promotion of initiative, creative thought, and affective components within a safe forum for listening to others. Games are credited with supplementing rote memorization, providing useful organization of material, encouraging application of ideas, and providing comic relief from the otherwise anxiety-provoking task of preparing for exams.

Games are inherently student-centered and interactive, generating enthusiasm, excitement, and enjoyment. When new students are asked what their preferred learning style is the predominant answer is usually hands on/experiential. An experiential learning method, such as gaming, creates an environment that requires a participant to be involved in a personally meaningful activity. Fostering a match between teaching strategies and student needs is one of the key factors in effective education. In addition, learning has greater impact when it has an element of emotional arousal, takes place within a safe environment, and has a period of debriefing to provide a cognitive map for understanding the experience (Allery, 2004).

Board or card games tend to be most appropriate for skill-based knowledge and practice in the cognitive domain, such as memorizing or concept matching (Bochennek et al., 2007; Van Eck, 2006). Jeopardy and Trivial Pursuit are quite popular in many disciplines for reviewing course information in such subjects as abnormal psychology and research methods because of the quick mobilization of facts or labels required. In health care, both would lend themselves to reviews in human development, clinical conditions, or other primary knowledge topics. These games are used to review facts, reinforce or test knowledge and understanding, and foster application (Patel, 2008). The games can be adapted in multiple ways—through the content and through the external attributes of the game itself, such as time limits and the degree of luck built into the format. Crossword puzzles, word searches, and bingo-style games have been used in nursing in-service training to review required materials as well as increase staff attendance and compliance. Games can also be created for the psychomotor domain; speed of manipulation, safety in transfers, and knowledge of intervention techniques could all be addressed through a game format that would reward an individual or a team.

Simulation games, referred to as adventure games when in digital format, are more adapted to teaching problem solving, hypothesis testing, and the affective domain outcomes. Problem solving is best taught through practice and reflection. Within the format of the simulation game, especially in a computer or video game format, there is more opportunity for such repetition and practice than available during limited classroom or clinical time (Reiner & Siegel, 2008). Video games may also offer consistent assessment of clinical reasoning skills in case study situations of home or clinic visits (Duque, Fung, Mallet, Posel, & Fleiszer, 2008). The potential is there for multiple users in these virtual environments and professional exploration may be accomplished through digital simulation games. Serious game design works best when communication is built in through blogs,

Wikis, and other Web 2.0+ technologies (Derryberry, 2007). The time/effort involved in creating such environments becomes more feasible when faced with overloaded clinical placements (Oblinger, 2006b; Skiba, 2008).

RESOURCES

Creating games for the classroom usually takes time, imagination, and desire. The rewards can be great, although in our productivity-driven age the tradeoffs must be considered. As has been described, the quickest resources are based on those games that are currently available in toy stores or on television. Using the frames of these games requires loading in course material and then it is easy to introduce to the students because of their familiarity with the format.

Web sites that offer templates for such games include:

PowerPoint games at http://jc-schools.net/tutorials/PPT-games/

Game boards at http://jc-schools.net/tutorials/gameboard.htm

Crossword puzzles or word games at http://www.crossword-puzzles.co.uk/ or GreenEclipse Crosswords at http://www.eclipsecrossword.com/

Digital games can be explored at ZaidLearn at http://zaidlearn.blogspot.com/2008/05/75-free-edugames-to-spice-up-your.html

WebQuests has http://www.webquest.org/index.php as a good starting point

A more challenging approach is developing the entire game from your imagination, although if you engage small groups from a class to create the game using some of the guiding principles in the next section, this may become more doable (Patel, 2008). Digital game developers have been creating structures that may be available as frameworks for cognitive and affective domain objectives. These frameworks range from addressing the lower/moderate end of knowledge/awareness, as in a WebQuest search for specific information, through to the high-end evaluating/internalizing found in The Pod Game (ZaidLearn) where one is making judgments and decisions under a time constraint. The challenge for the educator is in finding and then using such formats because of the technological knowledge required on top of the content application (Van Eck, 2006). Currently there are only a few such games that are directly applicable to health care. It has been recommended that it is better to make teaching practices more gamelike rather than trying to develop whole games that may actually detract from the educational intent because of the novelty or the development time involved (Begg, 2008).

Additional Resources has a variety of articles describing gaming used in classroom education and in-service training. Some articles specifically target a greater use of technology, such as computer or Web-based games. The references that describe active learning and cooperative learning are excellent background information for the new academician and are available online.

USING THE METHOD: BASIC HOW-TO

Many authors have described the methodology behind using games in the classroom and their advice is summarized in Table 12-1. To begin, games rarely succeed as add-ons, they must be integrated into the overall educational strategy (Ridley, 2004). A game pulled out of nowhere, just to be novel, will have no effect on outcome measures. In essence, when developing a game, the educator must determine the content area, statement of the problem, and objectives of the game. After this, determine the game format, number of players, time frame, and rules. If using a frame game, the generic rules already exist and can be adapted for the topic within health care. The next decisions regard roles players assume and scenarios in which play occurs. These can be simple adaptations for frame games, or more complex if setting up a simulation game of a clinic. The scoring system and physical elements of a frame game tend to remain consistent with the original game; for simulation games they need to be created outright. The media used, whether common materials or specially constructed components, are chosen by the designer based on available time and resources. The game needs to be piloted, critiqued, and possibly revised. Finally, it is beneficial to the community of healthcare educators if the game is then disseminated (Blakely et al., 2008).

Overarching elements that must be considered when using instructional games include the layout and amount of space in the classroom or availability of technology, to ensure equal opportunity to play. Time to be spent during the game with enough time for the debriefing must be planned. Also essential in planning are the method by which the students will become aware of the rules of the game and rewards for results, including whether the rewards are intrinsic or extrinsic. Remember that for best effect, the game must be integrated into the instructional strategy of the course and directly related to the subject. It must be challenging enough and not feel like work.

POTENTIAL PROBLEMS

Effective use of games in the classroom can be undermined in the ways most strategies fail: poor planning, lack of attention, and lack of follow-up. One example of inappropriate game use stemming from each of these obstacles was the use of a simulation game to evaluate treatment skills. There was a specific scoring sheet to test students on the use of a computer program for cognitive rehabilitation. The students were *therapists* with faculty *clients*. This experience

Table 12-1 Process for Game Development

Step	Element	Probes
1	Specific objectives for game	Do they parallel and/or facilitate the course objectives?
2	Fit within the curriculum and the environment	Are the concepts relevant? Is this for review or to move understanding forward? Is there adequate functional space for implementation? If digital, are there enough computers and technical support?
3	Employs conflict	This could be a time limit, competition between teams, or competition with manager, depending on the objectives. Does it provide a just-right challenge? Can the student alter the level of challenge?
4	Rules of play and criterion for closure are easily communicated	Are all the rules known up front, or are they learned over time? If there are deadends or eliminations, what happens next?
5	It is fun	If not, stop right here and rework or discard
6	Provides immediate feedback to the participants	Do students know how they are doing at all times? Is uncertainty part of the game? Does the feedback assist the student in modifying beliefs or performance in order to improve?
7	Meets the needs of the students	Does the game help organize the course material? Is it a reliable measure of their comprehension, or will it mislead them? Does the game encourage the players to "laugh with" as opposed to "laugh at" one another? Is it inclusive in nature?
8	Field-test to eliminate bugs	Did it go as planned, or are there needed revisions?
9	Mechanism (such as pretesting and posttesting) that allows measurement of learning	Other than student satisfaction, check to see if actual learning occurs.
10	Share it with colleagues	Publish or post—there are many educational game Web sites.

was to provide feedback on the student's knowledge of the computer program, as well as provide valuable lessons on therapist–client interaction and use of the environment (e.g., paying attention to the physical environment even though they were intervening for a cognitive task). The main drawbacks to this experience were neglecting to emphasize the game nature of the simulation to reduce trepidation and having faculty be the clients, which increased anxiety. More planning would have improved the introduction of the activity. More faculty attention during the experience may have provided the impetus to revise the format so that there could have been *peer* clients. More knowledge about the use of educational games could have made this a more relaxed and appreciated learning experience.

Other potential pitfalls of game use require the instructor to be aware of:

- Timing: monitoring play, termination, and transition to the next learning activities. Fun activities can take on a life of their own. Simulations (especially) and games reduce control of the timing of the class period, the instructor must be comfortable with that reduced control or it will not work. While spontaneity and flexibility are admirable, there is also a need for planned sequences of activities and firm timekeeping.
- Competition: motivation may be limited to those who win; losing may produce a failure experience that decreases self esteem. Be conscious of all class members and monitor the degree of competition and cooperation required to achieve educational goals.
- Costs of developing and running a game may be high initially: it is quite time-consuming to create or flesh-out even a frame game. In some instances it is no more than developing more test questions (as in Jeopardy or Trivial Pursuit games), but that is often easier said than done. In the case of simulation games, a lot of thought is necessary to create an adequate situation and produce a complete cast of characters with goals and belief systems.
- Needs of all participants may not be met within a simulation or game: Therefore, do not depend on these strategies as solo teaching approaches.
- Closure: Facilitate appropriate debriefing by allowing adequate time for this phase of the learning experience and being an active listener.

CONCLUSION

Games are a suitable supplement for a variety of academic and clinical situations. They are a method of helping students recognize how much they know, or how much they still need to study. Different types have been described, as has the appropriate usage within the wide variety of instructional objectives and

Applied Examples: Descriptions of Strategy in Use

The format of Jeopardy lends itself for review of lots of material. One example was for pre-exam reviews in an undergraduate mental health class for occupational therapy students with categories covering such areas as theories, Diagnostic and Statistical Manual of Mental Disorder (DSM-IV), defense mechanisms, leadership techniques, and pharmaceuticals. The class was divided into three teams. The regular Jeopardy and Double Jeopardy were employed, although Final Jeopardy was not. Each team had a person designated as the "beeper" and they could collaborate within the team to come up with the question that matched the answer on the overhead projector. Most of the class engaged in the spirit of the game. During the process there was time for discussion and clarification of the topic areas. There were errors made on the exam itself, despite the review, so the game did not lead to the degree of achievement expected. However, it was not formally evaluated nor compared with other methods. The participation and apparent enjoyment of that review class was clear though.

An example of a simulation game used in a class on life span development employed the use of percentage dice rolls that each pair of students used to create families and newborns that would function across the semester to demonstrate typical human development from birth through adolescence. Each newborn had characteristics (motor skill, cognitive level, appearance, longevity, social environment, financial environment, etc.) that would be based on a limited number of dice rolls. The higher the dice roll, the better the performance or status of the attribute to which it was assigned. The students' first objective was to determine which combination of attributes would lead to the best life outcomes for their children. Was it more important to be very smart, or very attractive? Could you be successful in life with poor motor skills? After these decisions, there were journaling assignments regarding the development of the children and lots of negotiation between the partners regarding a series of developmental issues, culminating in special dice rolls in adolescence that determined whether the adolescent engaged in smoking and/or sexual activity, was involved in violence, etc. Student feedback on this experiential assignment was mostly positive, although some did report that it was quite time consuming. The expected degree of learning regarding human development was demonstrated in the journals. However, the greater learning experience was attitudinal change based on the discussions between partners of differing backgrounds and how they managed to cope with some of the unexpected events of these simulated lives.

content in healthcare curriculums. The choice and time management required may seem daunting, but educators have found they enjoyed the respite from standard classroom practice while developing and implementing an educational game. It is well worth the effort.

REFERENCES

Akl, E. A., Sackett, K.M., Pretorius, R., Bhoopathi, P.S., Mustafa, R., Schünemann, H., et al. (2008). Educational games for health professionals. *Cochrane Database of Systematic Reviews, (1)*, CD006411.

Allery, L. A. (2004). Educational games and structured experiences (Commentary). *Medical Teacher, 26*(6), 504–505.

Begg, M. (2008). Leveraging game-informed healthcare education. *Medical Teacher, 30*, 155–158.

Beylefeld, A. A., & Struwig, M. C. (2007). A gaming approach to learning medical microbiology: students' experiences of flow. *Medical Teacher, 29*, 933–940.

Blakely, G., Skirton, H., Cooper, S., Allum, P., & Nelmes, P. (2009). Educational gaming in the health sciences: systematic review. *Journal of Advanced Nursing, 65*(2), 259–269.

Bochennek, K., Wittekindt, B., Zimmermann, S., & Klingebiel, T. (2007). More than mere games: A review of card and board games for medical education. *Medical Teacher, 29*, 941–948.

Derryberry, A. (2007). *Serious games: online games for learning* (White Paper). Retrieved June 20, 2009, from http://www.adobe.com/resources/elearning/pdfs/serious_games_wp.pdf

Dormann, C., & Biddle, R. (2006). Humour in game-based learning. *Learning, Media and Technology, 31*(4), 411–424.

Duque, G., Fung, S., Mallet, L., Posel, N., & Fleiszer, D. (2008). Learning while having fun: The use of video gaming to teach geriatric house calls to medical students. *Journal of American Geriatric Society, 56*, 1328–1332.

Gee, J. P. (2008). Learning and games. In K. Salen (Ed.), *The ecology of games: Connecting youth, hames, and learning* (pp. 21–40). Cambridge, MA: MIT Press.

Graham, I., & Richardson, E. (2008) Experiential gaming to facilitate cultural awareness: its implication for developing emotional caring in nursing. *Learning in Health and Social Care, 7*, 37–45.

Greenfield, P. M. (2009). Technology and informal education: What is taught, what is learned. *Science, 323*, 69–71.

Jarrell, K., Alpers, R., Brown, G., & Wotring, R. (2008). Using BaFa' BaFa' in evaluating cultural competence of nursing students. *Teaching and Learning in Nursing, 3*, 141–142.

Oblinger, D. (2006a). Games and learning. *EDUCAUSE Quarterly, 29*(3), 5–7.

Oblinger, D. (2006b). Simulations, games, and learning. *EDUCAUSE Learning Initiative*. Retrieved June 24, 2009, from http://www.educause.edu/ELI/SimulationsGamesandLearning/156764

Patel, J. (2008). Using game format in small group classes for pharmacotherapeutics case studies. *American Journal of Pharmaceutical Education, 72*(1), 1–5.

Reiner, B., & Siegel, E. (2008). The potential for gaming techniques in radiology education and practice. *Journal of the American College of Radiology, 5*, 110–114.

Ridley, R. T. (2004). Classroom games are COOL: Collaborative opportunities of learning. *Nurse Educator, 29*(2), 47–48.

Royse, M. A., & Newton, S. E. (2007). How gaming is used as an innovative strategy for nursing education. *Nursing Education Perspectives, 28*(5), 263–267.

Sauve, L., Renaud, L., Kaufman, D., & Marquis, J. (2007). Distinguishing between games and simulations: A systematic review. *Educational Technology & Society, 10*(3), 247–256.

Skiba, D. J. (2008). Nursing education 2.0: Games as pedagogical platforms. *Nursing Education Perspectives, 29*(3), 174–175.

University of North Carolina. (2009). Eshelman School of Pharmacy learning & teaching resources. Retrieved June 20, 2009 from http://www.pharmacy.unc.edu/labs/teaching-resources/nuts-and-bolts-for-teaching-and-learning/students-and-learning-styles/millennial-students

Van Eck, R. (2006). Digital game-based learning: It's not just the digital natives who are restless. *EDUCAUSE Review, 41*(2), 16–30.

ADDITIONAL RESOURCES

Cowen, K. J., & Tesh, A. S. (2002). Effects of gaming on nursing students' knowledge of pediatric cardiovascular dysfunction. *Journal of Nursing Education, 41*(11), 507–509.

Dologite, K. A., Willner, K. C., Klepeiss, D. J., York, S. A., & Cericola, L. M. (2003). Sharpen customer service skills with PCRAFT Pursuit©. *Journal for Nurses in Staff Development, 19*(1), 47–51.

Flanagan, N., & McCausland, L. (2007). Teaching around the cycle: Strategies for teaching theory to undergraduate nursing students. *Nursing Education Perspectives, 28*, 310–314.

Gifford, K. E. (2001). Using instructional games: A teaching strategy for increasing student participation and retention. *Occupational Therapy in Health Care, 15*, 13–21.

Jones, A. G., Jasperson, J., & Gusa, D. (2000). Cranial nerve wheel of competencies. *Journal of Continuing Education in Nursing, 31*(4), 152–154.

Masters, K. (2005). Development and use of an educator-developed community assessment board game. *Nurse Educator, 30*(5), 189–190.

Morton, P. G., & Tarvin, L. (2001). The pain game: Pain assessment, management, and related JCAHO standards. *Journal of Continuing Education in Nursing, 32*(5), 223–227.

Pearce-Smith, N. (2007). Teaching tip: Using the "Who wants to be a millionaire?" game to teach searching skills. *Evidence Based Nursing, 10*, 72.

Persky, A.M., Stegall-Zanation, J., & Dupuis, R. E. (2007). Students perceptions of the incorporation of games into classroom instruction for basic and clinical pharmacokinetics. *American Journal of Pharmaceutical Education, 71*(2), 1–9.

Smith-Stoner, M. (2005, September/October). Innovative use of the Internet and Intranets to provide education by adding games. *CIN: Computers, Informatics, Nursing*, 237–241.

Stringer, E. C. (1997). Word games as a cost-effective and innovative inservice method. *Journal of Nursing Staff Development, 13*(3), 155–160.

Terenzi, C. (2000). The triage game. *Journal of Emergency Nursing, 26*(1), 66–69.

Ward, A. K., & O'Brien, H. L. (2005). A gaming adventure. *Journal for Nurses in Staff Development, 21*(1), 37–41.

CHAPTER 13

Role Play

Arlene J. Lowenstein

DEFINITION AND PURPOSES

Role play is a dramatic technique that encourages participants to improvise behaviors that illustrate expected actions of persons involved in defined situations. A scenario is outlined and character roles are assigned. The drama is usually unscripted, relying on spontaneous interplay among characters to provide material about reactions and behaviors for students to analyze following the presentation. Those class members that are not assigned character roles participate as observers and contribute to the analysis.

Part of the category of simulation, role play allows participants to explore why people behave as they do. Participants can test behaviors and decisions in an environment that allows experimentation without risk. The scenario and behaviors of the actors are analyzed and discussed to provide opportunity to clarify feelings, increase observational skills, provide rationale for potential behaviors, and anticipate reactions to decisions. New behaviors can be suggested and tried in response to the analysis.

Role play is used to enable students to practice interacting with others in certain roles and to afford them an opportunity to experience other people's reactions to actions they have taken. The scenario provides a background for the problem and outlines the constraints that may apply. Defining the important characteristics of the major players establishes role expectations and provides a framework for behaviors and actions to be elicited. The postplay discussion provides opportunity for analysis and new strategy formation.

Although it is a dramatic technique, the focus is on the actions of the characters and not on acting ability. An actor plays to the audience; the role player plays to the characters in the scenario. The audience also has a role, that of observing the interplay among characters and analyzing the dynamics occurring. The instructor's role is that of facilitator rather than director. The impetus for the analysis and discussion belongs with the learners. The instructor's role is more passive, clarifying, and gently guiding.

Clinical simulations often incorporate role play. Although the simulation computer and mannequin provides the physiological issues in the scenario, students or faculty members may play the human roles, such as the doctor or family members. The computer operator may also provide a voice for the patient, to which the nurse needs to relate, and allows for better assessment of a patient's response to issues such as anxiety or pain. The use of role play allows the nurse providing care to the simulated patient to work in a more realistic environment, and requires reactions to more complexity in the situation. Smith-Stoner used high-fidelity simulation together with role play to provide a scenario where a student nurse, who was caring for a simulated patient who died during the scenario, needed to interact with the family member, who was in the room. The exercise allowed the students in the class to explore their attitudes toward death and caring for dying patients (Smith-Stoner, 2009).

Role play can also be used in online courses. Although there may be no person-to-person drama, a scenario can be set up, parts assigned, and the conversation could be carried out in a chat room or on the discussion board. Riddle (2009) noted that online educational role plays engage students in the learning, and can be an improvement over didactic teaching strategies alone. Online role play systems afford students the opportunity of acting and doing instead of only reading and listening.

Role play is a particularly effective means for developing decision-making and problem-solving skills (Hess & Gilgannon, 1985). Imholz (2008) studied clinical research on psychodrama practice of role play, looking at the therapeutic activity that has both cognitive and emotional outcomes of the role play as change agent, but also as a process that contributes to personal growth. Through role play the learner can identify the systematic steps in the process of making judgments and decisions. The problem-solving process—identification of the problem, data collection and evaluation of possible outcomes, exploration of alternatives, and arrival at a decision to be implemented—can be analyzed in the context of the role play situation. The scenario can include reactions to the implementation of the decision as well as the evaluation and reformulation process (Alden, 1999; Domazzo & Hanson, 1977). Role play has also been used to increase student cultural awareness, aiding in the development of cultural competence in patient care (Shearer & Davidhizar, 2003).

Role play provides immediate feedback to learners regarding their success in using interpersonal skills as well as decision-making and problem-solving skills. At the same time, role play offers learners an opportunity to become actively involved in the learning experience but in a nonthreatening environment. Role play is not limited to use in the classroom. Corless et al. (2004) successfully used role play as a student assignment that required the adoption of a persona of a person with HIV who was required to take a number of medications over a specific period of time. Students carried out the role play in their homes, taking placebos in place of medication over a specific time frame. Their experiences in following the HIV regime was then discussed in class, leading to an awareness of the difficulties patients faced in following the regime. Role play is also being used as a teaching strategy in online courses (Mar, Chabal, Anderson, & Vore, 2003).

THEORETICAL RATIONALE

Role play developed in response to the need to affect attitudinal changes in psychotherapy and counseling (Shaffer & Galinsky, 1974). Psychodrama, a forerunner of role play, was developed by Moreno as a psychotherapy technique. Moreno brought psychodrama to the United States in 1925 and continued to develop it during the 1940s and 1950s (Moreno, 1946). In psychodrama, players may be required to recite specific lines or answer specific questions and may represent themselves, whereas in role play players are encouraged to express their thoughts and feelings spontaneously, as if they were the persons whose roles they are playing (Sharon & Sharon, 1976).

Psychodrama provided a foundation for further development of role play as an educational technique. Corsini (1957) and other psychotherapists and group dynamicists began using role play to assist patients to clarify people's behavior toward each other. Further development led to the use of role play in sensitivity training, a technique that became popular in the 1970s. Human relations and sensitivity training events share a common educational strategy. The learners in the group are encouraged to become involved in examining their thought patterns, perceptions, feelings, and inadequacies. The training events are also designed to encourage each learner with the support of fellow learners to invent and experiment with different patterns of functioning (Gordon, 1970). Role play can be used to meet those educational objectives and is often used in human relations and sensitivity training but has many other uses as well. DeNeve and Hepner (1997), in a study comparing role play to traditional lectures, found that students believed that the use of role play was stimulating and valuable in comparison to the traditional lecture method, their learning increased, and they remembered what they had learned.

CONDITIONS

Role playing is a versatile technique that can be used in a wide variety of situations. One set of learning objectives might be role play dealing with the practice of skills and techniques, whereas another different group of objectives would use role play to deal with changes in understanding, feelings, and attitudes. Van Ments (1983) points out that role play is conducted differently for these two sets of learning objectives. The role play used for the practice of skills may be planned with the emphasis on outcome and overcoming problems. The second type of objective may be best met with an emphasis on the problems and relationships. This method explores why certain behaviors are exhibited and requires expertise from the instructor in dealing with emotions and human behavior. The teacher is responsible for helping the students to avoid the negative effects that could come from the exploration of their feelings and behaviors.

PLANNING AND MODIFYING

Teachers who are new to the technique need to plan before class, but they should monitor the needs of the group as the experience progresses and be able to modify those plans if necessary. The situation developed should be familiar enough so that learners can understand the roles and their potential responses, but it should not have too direct a relationship to students' own personal problems (McKeachie, 2002). It can also be effective to use two or more presentations of the same situation with different students in the roles if the objective is to point out different responses or solutions to a given problem. When that method is used, the instructor may choose to keep those students involved in the second presentation away from viewing the first presentation, to avoid biasing their reactions. The same role play scenario can be used throughout the semester to allow students to react to changing events within the same scenario (Rabinowitz, 1997).

Role play strategy qualifies as an adult-learning approach because it presents a real life situation and tries to stimulate the involvement of the student. It has special value because it uses peer evaluation and involves active participation. However, it must be carefully guided to be sure participants have an understanding of the objectives and that feedback received from other players is congruent with outcomes that would exist in the real world (Mann & Corsun, 2002).

TYPES OF LEARNERS

Role play is appropriate for undergraduate and graduate students. It is especially effective in staff development programs because of its association with reality. It is used effectively to reach affective outcomes. Role play can be simple or complex, depending on the learning objectives. Regardless of the simplicity of the play itself, it is important to allow adequate time for planning, preparing the students for the experience, and postplay discussion and analysis. The actual role play may be as brief as 5 minutes, although 10 to 20 minutes is more common. Van Ments (1983) suggests that the technique be broken into three sections: briefing, running, and debriefing. Equal amounts of time may be spent for each session for simple objectives, or a ratio of 1:2:3, with most time spent on the debriefing or analysis, for more complex learning objectives.

RESOURCES

Role play can be used in most settings, although tiered lecture rooms may inhibit the ability of the players to relate to each other and to the observing students. In that setting, the theatricality of the technique is likely to be emphasized over the needed behavioral focus (Van Ments, 1983). Special equipment or props may be simple or not used at all, again depending on the objectives. An instructor may choose to use video or audio taping. This can be especially helpful to review portions of the action during the debriefing and analysis section. Reviewing tapes may also be helpful for participating students who, because of their roles, were not in the room to hear and see some of the interaction that occurred in other role plays.

Outside resources are not usually needed for most role play situations, although additional instructors, trained observers, or specific experts may appropriately be used to meet certain objectives. The technique is best for small groups of students so that those not involved in the character parts can be actively involved in observing and discussing the action in the debriefing or analyzing portion. Van Ments (1983) found role play increasingly unsatisfactory as a technique in groups with more than 20 to 25 students, although there may be exceptions, depending on objectives and strategies for involving the audience.

USING THE METHOD

Planning is crucial to effective use of role play as a learning technique. It may be helpful to pilot the exercise before running it in the class situation to allow the instructor to anticipate potential problems and evaluate if the learning objectives can be met. Discussing critical elements of the role play with colleagues can be useful if full-scale piloting is not feasible. A small amount of time going through the plans with someone else may prevent a critical element from going wrong and disrupting the exercise (Van Ments, 1983).

Selecting a scenario and deciding on character roles is an important part of planning. McKeachie (2002) cautions that situations involving morals or subjects of high emotional significance, such as sexual taboos, are apt to be traumatic to some students. He found that the most interesting situations, and those revealing the greatest differences in responses, are those involving some choice or conflict of motives. Student input into planning can also be effective.

To implement the role play, the scenario and characters need to be described briefly but with enough information to elicit responses that will meet the learning objectives. This planning is extremely important for obtaining good results. Spontaneity should be encouraged, so it is preferable to avoid a script, other than bare outlines of the action. Although spontaneity is valued in character dialogue, students need to have a clear understanding of their characters and their basic attitude and/or thought patterns. In some instances, spontaneity in the character description area could compromise the objectives and results, but if students understand the expected character, they can still be spontaneous within the character parameters. Allowing students in the character roles to have a few minutes to warm up and relate to the roles they will be playing is often helpful. Observing students absolutely must be briefed on their role. Enough time must be allotted for discussion and analysis of the action. The debriefing following the role play also allows for evaluation of the success in meeting the learning objectives.

In addition to the development of learning objectives and planning, the instructor is responsible for setting the stage for the role play, monitoring the action, and leading the analysis. Students need a clear understanding of the objectives, the scenario, the characters they are to play, the importance of the role of the observers, and the analysis as a vital part of the process. On occasion, the instructor may take a character role, but usually character roles are given to students.

When planning a role play session, the instructor needs to be concerned with the amount of time students may be excluded from the room while waiting for their turn to participate. This issue is especially important when two or more presentations of the same situation are to be used, or the role play has characters that should not be exposed to the dialogue that occurs before they appear in their roles. It is important to avoid the need for the excluded students to roam the corridors with nothing to do for long periods.

In some instances, it may be appropriate to have students switch roles during the role play. This technique can be useful if the group is large and more students need to be involved in the action. This approach also may provide students with an opportunity to see and feel different reactions to similar situations. Another example of when to use this technique might be when the objective is to learn how to conduct a group. Students may benefit by playing group member and switching to leader or vice versa during the exercise.

The instructor needs to encourage students to respond to interactions in the role play in a spontaneous, natural manner, avoiding melodrama and inappropriate laughing or silliness. Effective use of role play focuses on student participation and interaction. The instructor, as facilitator, channels the discussion to meet the learning objectives but avoids monopolizing the play or discussion. The instructor must also be able to monitor and control the depth of emotional responses to the situation or interplay as needed; terminating the play when the objective has been met or the emotional climate calls for intervention.

Students need to understand the importance of playing the character roles in ways in which they believe those characters would act in a real life situation (Mann & Corsun, 2002). Students in the observer role must be strongly encouraged to present their observations and contribute to the discussion and analysis. Students can also take part in the developing role play scenarios; identifying their learning objectives, issues, and problems they feel need to be explored; and identifying scenarios that may provide that exploration.

Role play can be used in the online environment using the same basic principles, but with some differences, since the characters will not be visible to each other or to the audience (Mar et al., 2003). A synchronous environment, where all parties are online at the same time, will allow for a written dialogue flow between parties, with more similarity to an actual conversation (Phillips, 2005). An asynchronous environment, where parties log on at different times, will take longer to carry out the scenario, and may not have as much spontaneity, but can be as effective (Lebaron & Miller, 2005). As in all cases of role play, designing an online role play will depend on the learning objectives.

POTENTIAL PROBLEMS

Van Ments (1983) refers to the "hidden agenda" and warns that stereotyping may occur as roles are presented, often reflecting the expectations and values of the students or the teacher. This stereotyping may lead to unanticipated learning that can reinforce prejudices and preconceptions. Instructors need to be aware of this possibility and avoid writing in stereotypes. They should describe only functions, powers, and constraints of the role described. Roles should be rotated to avoid over-identification of one student with a specific role. In the debriefing session, the students are invited to question and challenge assumptions.

Students may not always make a distinction between an actor and a role. Criticism of the student playing the role must be avoided, while allowing for critique of the behavior of the role character. The instructor must be aware of the emotional tones involved in the role play and channel the emotions into activities that will lead to successful attainment of the learning objectives.

Planning and learning objectives should determine the course of the role play. Students may take the role play in an unexpected direction, possibly because they have a need to explore another issue or problem. If it is not appropriate to revise the learning objectives to accommodate student needs, then the play can be terminated. In that case, the postplay discussion can be used to assist students in recognizing why the technique was not effective. Students should advise how to improve the role play or develop a different teaching strategy. Repeating a scenario with the same or different characters can sometimes afford a more in depth examination and add to the experience.

The instructor and students need to be aware that this is not a professional drama. Some students, because of stage fright, shyness, or other reasons, do not like participating (Middleton, 2005; Turner, 2005). Although at times it may be appropriate to change actors, if the role play does not seem to be going well, it is important not to blame the students. In most cases, the teaching strategy needs changing, rather than the actors. If that is understood and addressed, role play can be an effective and creative strategy to provide active student participation to meet specific learning objectives.

Example Role Play

Shawna Patrick

BACKGROUND

The use of mock trials in nursing education has been an effective teaching method used to make nurses aware of the legal implications of nursing practice. In a lawsuit, nurses are typically charged with negligence. Negligence is defined as, "failure to act as a reasonably prudent person would have acted in specific circumstances" (Chitty & Black, 2007). There are six major categories of negligence that may result in malpractice lawsuits including failure to follow standards of care, failure to use equipment in a responsible manner, failure to communicate, failure to document, failure to assess and monitor, and failure to act as a patient advocate (Chitty & Black, 2007).

In a lawsuit, there are four elements of negligence that the plaintiff must prove by a preponderance of the evidence to demonstrate that a nurse was liable for a patient's injury. First, duty to treat, the nurse accepted the duty to care for and treat the patient. Second, breach of duty, the nurse breached that duty typically by failing to meet the standard of care. Third, causation, the breach of duty was the proximate cause of the patients harm. Fourth, damages, the injury and the nurse's negligence caused damage or losses to the patient. Consider these elements in the following mock trial role play.

Instructions

1. Read the mock trial role play and the standards of care for dehydration and hypokalemia (Box 13-1). Assign staff to play the roles of bailiff, attorney, witness, and judge and provide them with the script in advance so they can practice before class.
2. The day of class, review the following with jury members: standards of care in question (Box 13-1), courtroom procedure (Box 13-2), and hospital summary. Next, explain the

role of the jury, including instructions concerning how to prove negligence by the four elements, based on a preponderance of the evidence presented in court.

3. Finally, conduct the mock trial role play as described here and conclude the mock trial with jury deliberation and determination of a verdict. (Fig. 13-1 provides the layout for the classroom/courtroom.) Provide follow-up discussion with the class to talk about why and how the jury reached its decision.
4. Note: The education team is responsible for providing support to staff, educating staff as mentioned here, facilitating the mock trial, serving as a moderator for jury deliberation, and facilitating classroom discussion following the mock trial.

Role Key

J: Judge
B: Bailiff
DA: Defendant attorney
PA: Plaintiff attorney
MS: Martha Smith, widow
KJ: Kathy Jones, RN
DW: Amy Brown, defendant expert witness
PW: Mary Johnson, plaintiff expert witness

MOCK TRIAL ROLE PLAY

Hospital Summary

John Smith, age 55, arrived in the Emergency Department (ED) on January 10, 2009, at 11 PM. He complained of severe nausea and vomiting for the past 3 days and muscle weakness for the past 1 day. He presented with hypotension (blood pressure [BP] 90/60), tachycardia (heart rate [HR] 110), and decreased serum potassium (potassium [K+] 1.8 mEq). After evaluation by the ED physician, he was diagnosed with dehydration and hypokalemia. He was given 2 liters of normal saline intravenous (IV), 4-mg Zofran IV, and started on a continuous infusion of normal saline with 20-mEq potassium at 100 ml/hour. A Foley catheter was inserted with a 50 ml return of urine; and strict intake and output measurements were ordered every 2 hours. He was placed on continuous cardiac monitoring and admitted to the Medical-Surgical Telemetry unit at 1 AM. The admitting physician ordered 3 doses of 10-mEq potassium/100-ml normal saline IV over 1 hour per dose. The unit was extremely busy and understaffed. Kathy Jones, the admitting nurse, was assigned eight patients instead of the hospital's standard nurse to patient ratio of five patients per one nurse for the medical-surgical telemetry unit. No one was available to help Kathy, so she took it upon herself to mix the potassium infusion and administer the first dose. However, instead of mixing 10 mEq of potassium in 100-ml normal saline, she mixed 100 mEq of potassium in 100-ml normal saline. Fifteen minutes after the start of the infusion, Kathy returned to John's room to assess his tolerance of the potassium infusion. When she entered the room, she noticed that John was unable to arouse and the cardiac monitor showed ventricular tachycardia. A code blue was called and resuscitative measures were taken, but they were unsuccessful. John Smith was pronounced dead at 1:45 AM on January 11, 2009. The family is suing Kathy Jones for negligence.

Calling of the Case

Bailiff (B): All rise, the court of Mountain Valley Hospital is now in session. Honorable Judge X presiding. (The judge will be seated and will strike the gavel three times.)

Judge (J): You may be seated. We are assembled to hear the case of *John Smith* v. *Kathy Jones*. Are both attorneys ready to present opening statements? (Both answer, "Yes.")

Plaintiff Opening Statement

John Smith was a loving husband and dedicated father of four children. He was a caring man and diligent provider. His death was tragic and the direct result of negligent nursing care by Kathy Jones, who gave him 10 times the prescribed dose of potassium on the night of January 10. You will hear from his widow, Martha, how his premature death caused total devastation for her family. The defendant will try to convince you that Kathy Jones was not the cause of John's death. That, considering the circumstances, she acted as a reasonably prudent nurse would. They will encourage you to make a decision based on the poor management of her nursing unit and the number of patients she was assigned. Members of the jury, I will show you solid evidence that Kathy Jones was negligent and blatantly neglected to follow hospital policy. As a result, John Smith died from a totally preventable error.

Defendant Opening Statement

Kathy Jones is a competent, dedicated nurse committed to the safety of all patients. She has been a registered nurse (RN) for 20 years and has never been proven to have caused harm to any patient. Today, the plaintiff will try to disprove the competence of Kathy Jones and tell you that she was the direct cause of John Smith's death. They will tell you that she neglected to treat him appropriately. They will have his widow, Martha, testify to persuade you to make a decision based solely on emotions, not facts. I will prove that Kathy behaved in a manner consistent with the normal care of a patient diagnosed with dehydration and hypokalemia. I will prove that John's death was a tragic and utter mistake related to the mismanagement of Kathy's nursing unit and the unsafe number of patients assigned to her. Members of the jury, I urge you to look at the facts of the case and the diligent care that was given John. I ask you to put yourself in Kathy Jones' shoes so you can see that her only goal was to help John.

Plaintiff's Case

J: Is the plaintiff prepared to call its first witness?
Plaintiff Attorney (PA): Yes, your honor. The plaintiff calls Martha Smith to the witness stand.
B: Please state your name.
Martha Smith (MS): Martha Smith
B: Please raise your right hand (she does). Do you swear to tell the truth, the whole truth, and nothing but the truth? If so, answer "I do."
MS: I do.
B: Thank you, you may be seated.
PA: Hi, Mrs. Smith. Can you tell me about your relation to the patient in question, John Smith?
MS: John was my husband for the last 30 years.
PA: Do you have any children?
MS: Yes, we have four beautiful children; two boys, ages 10 and 12, and two girls, ages 14 and 16.
PA: Tell me about John's occupation, length of employment, and annual income.
MS: He was a stock broker for the last 25 years and made about $125,000/year.
PA: Tell me about your relationship with John.
MS: Amazing. He was the love of my life. We were high school sweethearts and kept the love growing for the past 30 years. I don't know what I will do without him.

PA: When you visited John briefly on the night of January 10, how did he appear to you?
MS: He had been sick for the previous 3 days but after he was given the medicine for nausea, he looked a little better.
PA: What has been the impact of this tragic event on your family?
MS: We are completely devastated. He was the breadwinner of the family and we counted on him for everything. I have never worked because I stayed home to raise the children. I don't know how we'll manage financially; I just don't know what we will do.
PA: Thank you Mrs. Smith, the plaintiff has no further questions for this witness.
J: Would the defendant like to cross-examine this witness?
Defendant Attorney (DA): Yes, your honor. Mrs. Smith, you said you are a homemaker, is that correct?
MS: Yes, that's correct.
DA: So you have no formal medical training, do you?
MS: No, I don't.
DA: So when you said that your husband, "looked a little better," you really didn't know that he was getting better, did you?
MS: No.
DA: Were you at the hospital at the time of John's death?
MS: No, I wasn't.
DA: So you don't specifically know what happened to cause his death, do you?
MS: No, I don't.
DA: The defendant has no further questions for this witness.

J: The witness may step down. Would the plaintiff like to call another witness?
PA: Yes, your honor. The plaintiff calls Mary Johnson to the stand.
B: Please state your name.
Plaintiff Expert Witness (PW): Mary Johnson
B: Please raise your right hand (she does). Do you swear to tell the truth, the whole truth, and nothing but the truth? If so, answer "I do."
PW: I do.
B: Thank you, you may be seated.
PA: Hi, Ms. Johnson, can you tell me about your professional experience?
PW: I have been an RN for 25 years. I worked on a medical-surgical unit for the first 15 years of my career and have been working as a legal nurse consultant for the past 10 years.
PA: What is your educational background?
PW: I have a Bachelor of Science degree in Nursing and certifications in Medical-Surgical Nursing and Legal Nurse Consulting.
PA: What is your background with caring for patients with dehydration and hypokalemia?
PW: I have cared for hundreds of patients with both of these conditions.
PA: Based on your experience with patients diagnosed with dehydration and hypokalemia, you are deemed an expert on these subjects?
PW: Yes, I am.
PA: Have you reviewed the facts of the case including the medical record and hospital policy?
PW: Yes, I have.

PA: Do you believe that you have a good understanding of the case?
PW: Yes, I do.
PA: Given the facts, did Kathy Jones comply with the standard of care for dehydration and hypokalemia?
PW: No, she did not. She neglected to follow hospital policy. She mixed the potassium independently without having a second nurse double check her. She also mixed 10 times the dose of potassium that was ordered and administered this to John.
PA: Could giving 10 times the dose of potassium cause death?
PW: Yes, giving that much can cause lethal cardiac dysrhythmias, which can lead to death.
PA: The plaintiff has no further questions for this witness.
J: Would the defendant like to cross-examine this witness?
DA: Yes, your honor. Ms. Johnson, are you a practicing nurse?
PW: I was for the first 15 years of my nursing career, but have been working as a legal nurse consultant for the past 10 years.
DA: So, you haven't cared for a patient with dehydration and/or hypokalemia for at least 10 years, is that correct?
PW: Yes, but . . .
DA: So, you don't know what the current standards of care are for dehydration and hypokalemia?
PW: I would imagine they haven't changed too much.
DA: Please answer either yes or no.
PW: No.
DA: So you don't know for a fact that Kathy Jones actions directly caused John to die, do you?
PW: No, I don't, but . . .
DA: No further questions for this witness.
J: The witness may step down.

Defendant's Case

J: Would the defendant like to call its first witness?
DA: Yes, your honor. The defendant calls Kathy Jones to the witness stand.
B: Please state your name.
Kathy Jones (KJ): Kathy Jones
B: Please raise your right hand (she does). Do you swear to tell the truth, the whole truth, and nothing but the truth? If so, answer "I do."
KJ: I do.
B: Thank you, you may be seated.
DA: Hi, Ms. Jones, how long have you been a practicing nurse?
KJ: For the past 20 years.
DA: Can you tell me about your professional experience, including where you currently work?
KJ: I have worked at Mountain Valley Hospital in the medical-surgical telemetry unit for the past 20 years.
DA: What was your initial assessment of John on the night of January 10? What was he being treated for?
KJ: When I assumed care of John, he was being treated for dehydration and hypokalemia. He was calm and he did not appear to be in any acute distress.
DA: What type of education did you receive at Mountain Valley Hospital in regard to treating a patient with hypokalemia?

KJ: We are required to read the policy for potassium administration and take a test every year to demonstrate competence.
DA: And did you complete this annual education?
KJ: Yes, I did.
DA: What type of education did you receive in regard to dehydration?
KJ: We are not required to complete this education annually because it is a basic condition that I am routinely exposed to and have learned about in nursing school.
DA: Tell me about the medical-surgical telemetry unit and your patient assignments on the night of January 10.
KJ: The unit was completely filled with patients. We had two nurses call in sick so we were severely understaffed. We are usually assigned five patients each, but because of understaffing, I was assigned to eight patients.
DA: Did you feel like you could safely accept the assignment of eight patients?
KJ: Well, no, but I didn't have a choice. I spoke with the house supervisor but there weren't any other nurses to pull from. The patients needed a nurse and I had to do the best I could.
DA: Is it a common practice at your hospital for nurses to mix potassium infusions for patients?
KJ: It is common on the night shift because there is not a pharmacist in the hospital at night. Pharmacists are only in the hospital during the day shift.
DA: So on the night of January 10, did you mix the potassium infusion yourself?
KJ: Yes, I did. I was worried about John because his potassium level in the ED was 1.8 mEq, which is considered critically low. The other nurses on the unit were also assigned eight patients and no one could help me at that time.
DA: If you did not give the potassium upon his arrival to your unit, what could have happened to John?
KJ: He could have died from a lethal arrhythmia.
DA: So you were acting in the best interest of John?
KJ: Yes, I was.
DA: The defendant has no further questions for this witness.

PA: Ms. Jones, isn't it true that your hospital policy dictates that a second nurse must double check any potassium infusion that is mixed by a nurse?
KJ: Yes.
PA: Isn't it true that potassium is considered a high-alert medication and can quickly cause lethal arrhythmias if mixed and administered incorrectly?
KJ: Yes.
PA: But, you stated that your unit was understaffed, so did you mix the potassium and give it without double checking it with another nurse?
KJ: Yes.
PA: So you neglected to follow your hospitals policy?
KJ: Yes, but . . .
PA: And what was the ultimate outcome for John after you administered the potassium infusion?
KJ: We tried to resuscitate him but he died.
PA: The plaintiff has no further questions for this witness.
J: The witness may step down.

DA: The defendant calls Amy Brown to the stand.
B: Please state your name.
Defense Expert Witness (DW): Amy Brown
B: Please raise your right hand (she does). Do you swear to tell the truth, the whole truth, and nothing but the truth? If so, answer "I do."
DW: I do.
B: Thank you, you may be seated.
DA: Ms. Brown, are you a practicing nurse?
DW: Yes.
DA: Tell me about your professional experience.
DW: I have been an RN for the past 18 years and have worked on a medical-surgical telemetry unit my entire career. I have also worked as a legal nurse consultant for the past 5 years on a part-time basis.
DA: What is your experience with the standards of care for dehydration and hypokalemia?
DW: I have cared for thousands of patients with these conditions as they are very common conditions seen on my nursing unit.
DA: Based on your experience with dehydration and hypokalemia, you are deemed an expert on these conditions?
DW: Yes, I am.
DA: Have you had a chance to review the facts of the case such as evaluating the medical record and hospital policies related to these conditions?
DW: Yes, I have.
DA: In your expert opinion, did Kathy Jones comply with the standards of care for dehydration and hypokalemia?
DW: Yes, she did.
DA: Were the actions of Kathy Jones the direct cause of John's death?
DW: No, they weren't. He could have died without the potassium.
DA: The defendant has no further questions for this witness.

J: Would the plaintiff like to cross-examine this witness?
PA: Yes, your honor. Ms. Brown, you stated that you reviewed the hospital policy for hypokalemia and potassium administration, is that correct?
DW: Yes, I did.
PA: Did you read that all potassium infusions mixed by a nurse must be double checked with a second nurse before administration?
DW: Yes.
PA: Isn't it true that Kathy just testified that she did not have a second nurse double check the potassium infusion prior to administration and this is reflected in the medication record?
DW: Yes.
PA: So Kathy Jones did not follow the hospital's policy regarding hypokalemia and potassium administration, did she?
DW: No, she didn't, but . . .
PA: And isn't it true that giving too much potassium quickly can cause lethal arrhythmias?
DW: Yes.
PA: And remind me again, what was the outcome for John?

DW: He was pronounced dead after aggressive resuscitative measures were taken.

PA: The plaintiff has no further questions.

J: The witness may step down. Are the plaintiff and defendant prepared to give their closing arguments? (Both say "Yes.")

Plaintiff Closing Argument

Today we have proven that Kathy Jones was negligent in the care of John Smith. We have demonstrated that Ms. Jones was knowledgeable of the policy regarding hypokalemia and potassium administration, but chose to breach hospital policy. She mixed potassium, a dangerous high-alert medication, and administered it to John without having a second nurse double check it. As a result, Ms. Jones gave 10 times the prescribed amount resulting in John's untimely death. The family is devastated both emotionally and financially. John was the breadwinner of the family and now they will have to struggle for food and shelter. Members of the jury, we urge you to make the right decision and find Kathy Jones liable for the death of John Smith.

Defendant Closing Argument

On the night of January 10, Kathy Jones' nursing unit was severely understaffed and poorly managed. Kathy was assigned to care for eight patients, three more than the hospitals standard nurse to patient staffing ratio, and no one was available to help her. We have told you how John could have died without the potassium infusion and how Kathy was doing her best to give it to him quickly in order to save his life. In her 20 years as a professional nurse, Kathy has never been proven to cause harm to any patient and this trend continues today. Members of the jury, we urge you to look at the facts of the case so you can see that John's death was a tragic mistake, and not the result of negligent care by Kathy Jones. We implore you to find Kathy Jones not liable.

J: We will now proceed with jury deliberation and determination of a verdict. If the jury determines that the defendant, Kathy Jones, deviated from the standard of care for dehydration and hypokalemia, the jury must find in favor of the plaintiff. If the jury determines that the defendant did not deviate from the standards of care for dehydration and hypokalemia, then the jury must find in favor of the defendant. The jury will now deliberate and determine a verdict of liable or not liable. If the verdict is liable, the jury will award compensation for damages incurred by the plaintiff.

Box 13-1 Standard of Care Summary for Dehydration and Hypokalemia

DEHYDRATION

Signs and Symptoms

Dry eyes and/or mouth, fever, vomiting, postural hypotension, change in mental status, pulse $>$ 100 beats/minute and/or systolic blood pressure $<$ 100 mm Hg, dizziness, and/or lethargy and weakness.

Diagnosis

The following criteria must be present to make a clinical diagnosis of dehydration:

- Suspicion of increased urinary output and/or decreased oral intake
- A minimum of two signs or symptoms of dehydration

- A blood urea nitrogen (BUN)/creatinine ratio of > 25:1; orthostasis defined as a drop in systolic blood pressure ≥ 20 mm Hg with a change in position; heart rate of > 100 beats/minute; or a change of 10 to 20 beats/minute above baseline heart rate with a change in position (National Guideline Clearinghouse, n.d.).

Monitoring

Fluid intake and output, blood chemistry including sodium and potassium, and urinalysis including osmolality and specific gravity.

Treatment

- If the patient is able, offer oral fluids by mouth. If the patient is unable to tolerate oral replacement, IV rehydration is necessary.
- For mild to moderate volume depletion, a safe regimen is to administer isotonic saline at 50 to 100 ml per hour in excess of continued losses.
- For severe volume depletion, 1 to 2 liters of isotonic saline should be given rapidly and continued at a rapid rate until clinical signs stabilize (Rose, 2008a).

HYPOKALEMIA

Diagnosis

- Mild to moderate hypokalemia is defined by serum potassium between 3.0 and 3.5 mEq/l and does not typically cause symptoms.
- Severe hypokalemia is defined by serum potassium less than 2.5 to 3.0 mEq/l or by symptoms including arrhythmias and marked muscle weakness (Rose, 2008).

Treatment

- If serum potassium is 3 to 3.5 mEq/l, administer 40 to100 mEq daily divided into 2 to 3 doses, with no more than 20 mEq given per dose.
- If serum potassium greater than 2.5 mEq/l, administer 10 to 15 mEq/hour IV, up to a maximum of 200 mEq/day.
- If serum potassium less than 2 mEq/l, administer 20 to 40 mEq/hour IV with continuous cardiac monitoring, up to a maximum of 400 mEq/day ("Potassium,"2009).

Box 13-2 Courtroom Procedure

1. Calling of the Case: Typically announced as, "All rise. The court of X is now in session. Honorable Judge X presiding." The judge will then be seated and will call the court to order by striking the gavel three times, and stating, "You may be seated."
2. Opening Statements: Used to present a story to the judge and jury about the facts surrounding the case and the evidence they will present during the trial. The plaintiff presents first, followed by the defendant.
3. Plaintiff's Case: The plaintiff's attorney presents testimony through examination of their witnesses with direct examination questions, followed by cross-examination questions

by the defendant's attorney, and completed with redirect examination questions by the plaintiff's attorney, if necessary. This process is repeated for each of the plaintiff's witnesses.

4. Defendant's Case: The process for examining witnesses is the same as for the plaintiff except the defendant's attorney calls their witnesses first, followed by the plaintiff's cross-examination, and completed with redirect examination by the defendant's attorney, if necessary.
5. Closing Arguments: Used by each side to summarize the testimony and evidence they presented during trial in order to sway the jury in their favor. The plaintiff's attorney presents first, followed by the defendant's attorney.
6. Jury Deliberations: The jury deliberates about the testimony and evidence among themselves and determines a verdict for the defendant. Note: Before the trial, the judge will provide the jury with instructions about how they should judge the case based on the claim.
7. Verdict Announcement: The verdict is announced and damages are awarded if the defendant is found liable.

Source: Patrick, S. (2008). *The mock trial method: An innovative approach to nursing education*. Aspen, Colorado: Nurses for Nursing.

Figure 13-1 Courtroom Layout: A, attorney; B, bailiff; D, defendant; J, judge; P, plaintiff; W, witness stand.

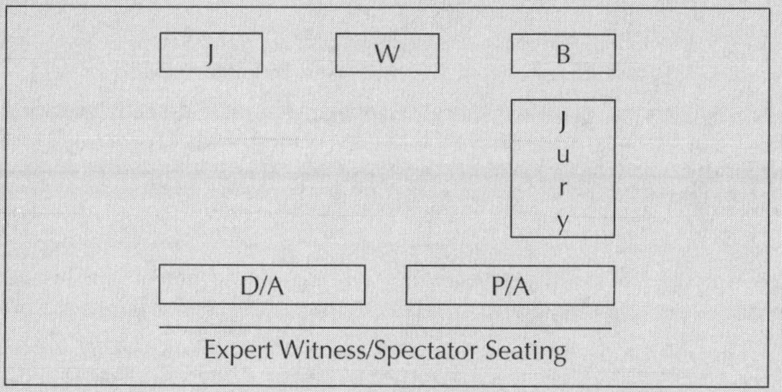

(*Source*: Patrick, S. (2008). *The mock trial method: An innovative approach to nursing education*. Aspen, Colorado: Nurses for Nursing.)

REFERENCES

Chitty, K., & Black, B. (2007). *Professional nursing: Concepts & challenges*. St Louis, MO: Saunders Elsevier.

National Guideline Clearinghouse (n.d.). *Dehydration and fluid maintenance*. Retrieved February 9, 2009, from http://www.guideline.gov/summary/summary.aspx?ss=15&doc_id=3305&nbr=2531.

Patrick, S. (2008). *The mock trial method: An innovative approach to nursing education*. Aspen, CO: Nurses for Nursing.

Potassium. (2009). In *Micromedex healthcare series*. Retrieved January 21, 2009, from http://www.thomsonhc.com/hcs/librarian/ND_T/HCS/ND_PR/Main/CS/72854B/DUPLICATIONSHIEL.

Rose, B. (2008a). *Clinical manifestations and treatment of hypokalemia*. In *UptoDate*. Retrieved January 27, 2009, from http://www.utdonline.com/online/content/topic.do?topicKey=fldlytes/13620&view=print

Rose, B. (2008b). *Maintenance and replacement fluid therapy in adults*. In *UptoDate*. Retrieved February 9, 2009, from http://www.utdonline.com/online/content/topic.do?topicKey=fldlytes/13345&view=print

REFERENCES

Alden, D. (1999). Experience with scripted role play in environmental economics. *Journal of Economic Education, 20*(2), 127–132.

Corless, I., Gallagher, D. Borans, R., Crary, E., Dolan, S. E., & Kressy, S. (2004). Understanding patient adherence. In A. J. Lowenstein, & M. J. Bradshaw (Eds.), *Fuszard's innovative teaching strategies in nursing* (3rd ed., pp. 128–132). Sudbury, MA: Jones and Bartlett.

Corsini, R. J. (1957). *Methods of group psychotherapy*. New York: McGraw-Hill.

DeNeve, K. M., & Hepner, M. J. (1997). Role play simulations: The assessment of an active learning technique and comparisons with traditional lectures. *Innovative Higher Education, 21*, 231–246.

Domazzo, R., & Hanson, P. (1997). Community health problems, apparent vs. hidden: A classroom exercise to demonstrate prioritization of community health problems for programs. *Journal of Health Education, 28,* 383–385.

Gordon, G. K. (1970). Human relations—sensitivity training. In R. M. Smith, G. F. Aker, & J. R. Kidd (Eds.), *Handbook of adult education* (pp. 427–440). New York: Macmillan.

Hess, C. M., & Gilgannon, N. (1985, April). Gaming: A curriculum technique for elementary counselors. Paper presented at the Annual Convention of the American Association for Counseling and Development, Los Angeles, CA (ERIC Document 267327).

Imholz, S. (2008). The therapeutic stage encounters the virtual world. *Thinking Skills and Creativity, 3*(1), 47–52.

Lebaron, J., & Miller, D. (2005). The potential of jigsaw role playing to promote the social construction of knowledge in an online graduate education course. *Teachers College Record, 107* (8), 1652–1674.

Mann, S., & Corsun, D. L. (2002). Charting the experiential territory: Clarifying definitions and uses of computer simulation, games and role play. *The Journal of Management Development, 21*(9,10), 732–745.

Mar, C. M., Chabal, C., Anderson, R. A., & Vore, A. E. (2003). An interactive computer tutorial to teach pain assessment. *Journal of Health Psychology, 8*, 161–173.

McKeachie, W. J. (2002). *McKeachie's teaching tips: Strategies, research,* and theory for *college and university teachers* (11th ed.). Boston: Houghton Mifflin.

Middleton, J. (2005). Role play is not everyone's scene. *Nursing Standard, 19*(24), 31.

Moreno, J. L. (1946). *Psychodrama*, Vol. 1. Boston: Beacon.

Phillips, J. M. (2005). Syllabus selections: Innovative learning activities. Chat role play as an online learning strategy. *Journal of Nursing Education, 44*(1), 43.

Rabinowitz, F. E. (1997). Teaching counseling through a semester long role play. *Counselor Education and Supervision, 36*, 216–223.

Riddle, M. D. (2009). The campaign: A case study in identity construction through performance authors. *Association for Learning Technology Journal, 17*(1), 63–72.

Shaffer, J. B. P., & Galinsky, M. D. (1974). *Models of group therapy and sensitivity training*. Englewood Cliffs, NJ: Prentice-Hall.

Sharon, S., & Sharon, Y. (1976). *Small group teaching*. Englewood Cliffs, NJ: Educational Technology Publications.

Shearer, R., & Davidhizar, R. (2003). Educational innovations: Using role play to develop cultural competence. *Journal of Nursing Education, 42*(6), 273–276.

Smith-Stoner, M. (2009). Using high-fidelity simulation to educate nursing students about end- of-life care. *Nursing Education Perspectives, 30*(2), 115–120.

Turner, T. (2005). Stage fright. *Nursing Standard, 19*(22), 22–23.

Van Ments, M. (1983). *The effective use of role play: A handbook for teachers and trainers*. London: Kogan Page.

ADDITIONAL RESOURCES

Alden, D. (1999). Experience with scripted role play in environmental economics. *Journal of Economic Education, 20*(2), 127–132.

Ashmore, R., & Banks, D. (2004). Student nurses' use of their interpersonal skills within clinical role plays. *Nurse Education Today, 24*(1), 20–29.

Chester, M., & Fox, R. (1996). *Role playing methods in the classroom*. Chicago: Science Research Associates.

Goldenberg, D., Andrusyszyn, M., & Iwasiw, C. (2005). The effect of classroom simulation on nursing students' self-efficacy related to health teaching. *Journal of Nursing Education, 44*(7), 310–314.

Greenberg, E., & Miller, P. (1991). The player and professor: Theatrical techniques in teaching. *Journal of Management Education, 15*(4), 428–446.

Griggs, K. (2005). A role play for revising style and applying management theories. *Business Communication Quarterly, 68*(1), 60–65.

Kane, M. (2003). Teaching direct practice techniques for work with elders with Alzheimer's disease: A simulated group experience. *Educational Gerontology, 29*, 777–794.

Loprinzi, C. L., Johnson, M. E., & Steer, G. (2003). Doc, how much time do I have? *Journal of Clinical Oncology, 21*(9), 5S-7S.

Northcott, N. (2002). Role play: proceed with caution! *Nursing Education in Practice, 2*(2), 87–91.

Silberman, M. (1996). *Active learning: 101 strategies to teach any subject*. Boston: Allyn & Bacon.room, she noticed that John was unable to arouse and the cardiac monitor showed ventricular tachycardia. A code blue was called and resuscitative measures were taken, but they were unsuccessful. John Smith was pronounced dead at 1:45 AM on January 11, 2009. The family is suing Kathy Jones for negligence.

CHAPTER 14

High-Fidelity Patient Simulation

Catherine Bailey, Judy Johnson-Russell, and Alfred Lupien

Patient simulators have been used by health professional educators for more than 50 years (Rosen, 2004, 2008). Computer software may be used to teach anatomy, physiology, pathophysiology, pharmacology, and clinical decision making. Technical skills associated with the practice of cardiopulmonary resuscitation (CPR), airway management, vascular catheter insertion, birthing, and various surgical procedures can be developed with the use of task trainers. Virtual reality devices combine computer-generated images and auditory and haptic (replicating kinesthetic and tactile perceptions) experiences to enable the learner to refine technical skills. High-fidelity simulators, the focus of this chapter, are computerized, life-sized mannequins with complex interrelated multisystem physiologic and pharmacologic models that generate observable responses from the mannequin and allow students to interact with the simulator as they would with an actual patient in the clinical environment.

DEFINITION AND PURPOSES

The first high-fidelity patient simulators (HFPSs) were developed in the 1960s and their use became widespread by the early 1990s when anesthesia educators and researchers began to use simulators to improve education and study clinical performances (Gaba & DeAnda, 1988; Good & Gravenstein, 1989). By the end of the 1990s, the use of human patient simulations for crisis management expanded to include other medical disciplines such as emergency medicine (Fritz, Gray, & Flanagan, 2008), armed forces medicine, pediatrics, surgery, trauma, cardiology, intensive care medicine, dentistry, and military medicine triage (Rosen, 2008). In 2005, computerized infant mannequins were introduced to assist neonatal resuscitation. Applications of HFPS use have included procedure training, evaluation of individual responses to critical incidents, equipment evaluation, task analysis, and team training (Lupien, 2007). Common educational applications of simulation have included theme-based workshops on ventilation, pharmacology, airway management, conscious sedation, disaster response, ongoing skills development, and practicing clinical decision making. The first nursing users of HFPSs were nurse anesthetists (Fletcher, 1995); however, since that time other nursing applications have expanded to include acute care, critical care, perioperative, and emergency nursing situations. According to Nehring's (2010) literature review, areas of focus have included the development of skills, critical thinking, patient safety, the development of safer patient and nurse environments, competency testing of skills, the development of effective healthcare teams, and comprehensive models for the development of the graduate nurse from novice to expert.

Depending on the sophistication of the specific HFPS, features may include a functioning cardiovascular system with synchronized palpable pulses, heart sounds, measurable blood pressures (by palpation or auscultation), electrocardiographic waveforms, and invasive parameters such as arterial, central venous, and pulmonary artery pressures that may be displayed on a physiologic computer monitor (Gaumard Scientific, 2009; Laerdal, 2009; METI, 2009). Respiratory system components include self-regulating spontaneous ventilation, measurable exhaled respiratory gases, and breath sounds. Other simulator features include bowel sounds, speech, pharmacologic systems capable of responding to administered drugs, a urologic system, blinking and reactive pupils, tongue swelling, bronchial occlusion, jugular vein distention, the ability to accept defibrillation, the use of a transthoracic pacemaker, needle cricothyroidotomy, jet ventilation, needle thoracentesis, chest tube insertion, IV fluid administration, intraosseous capability, and pericardiocentesis.

This chapter emphasizes automated patient simulators such as (1) the METI (Medical Education Technologies, Inc.; Sarasota, FL), adult human patient simulator (HPS), emergency care simulators (ECS), PediaSIM, BabySIM, iStan products, METIman, (2) the Laerdal (Laerdal Medical Corporation, Wappingers Falls, NY), SimMan, and (3) the Gaumard Scientific (Miami, FL) various models of Hal and Noelle simulators. Typically, simulators include four components: a lifelike mannequin, a freestanding enclosure that contains many of the simulator's components, a computer to integrate the function of the simulator components, and an interface that allows the user to control the simulation and modify physiologic parameters. Examples of some of the physiologic parameters, which are not exhaustive, include changes in heart rates or sounds, respiratory rates or breath sounds, or bowel sounds. Many of the simulators have both a portable interface allowing instructors to control simulations from either the mannequin's bedside or a remote location where changes can be made without the students' knowledge. To initiate a simulation the user selects a patient profile, such as a healthy adult male. If desired, a clinical scenario, such as anaphylaxis, can be superimposed on the physiology of the healthy adult male profile. Once the scenario has been initiated, the instructor may allow the simulation to run as preprogramed or make on-the-fly modifications to emphasize specific teaching points.

A well-planned simulated clinical experience allows the healthcare provider to practice nursing skills under realistic conditions in real time while using actual clinical supplies in a safe and controlled environment (Larew, Lessons, Spunt, Foster, & Covington, 2006). Observable practical advantages of simulation include the ability to replicate critical or common problems, to allow student driven management errors to develop, to provide multiple treatment options to be explored without injury or discomfort to a real patient, or to manipulate time as a factor in managing nursing care.

Educational advantages of simulation include opportunities for learners to improve skill performance and critical thinking, gain self-confidence, experience learner satisfaction (Jeffries, 2005; Monti, Wren, Haas, & Lupien, 1998), and gain feedback during debriefing or reflective sessions following the simulation (Fanning & Gaba, 2007). The simulated environment also provides a cost-effective strategy to translate the real world of nursing into a standardized setting for testing critical thinking and decision making.

Disadvantages of simulation include the investment costs associated with the initial set up (including the purchase of the simulators and their associated support systems), maintenance of the simulation laboratory, and additional supporting lab personnel (Good, 2003; Harlow & Sportsman, 2007; Parker & Myrick, 2008). Thus, the integration of patient simulations into the curriculum is resource intensive, as well as time intensive (Radhakrishnan, Roche, & Cunningham, 2007; Sittner, Schmaderer, Zimmerman, Hertzog, & George, 2009). Finally, the transfer of knowledge to actual clinical practice is not well documented because there remains a need to capture simulation's impact on nurses' knowledge and clinical judgement on actual patient outcomes.

THEORETICAL FOUNDATIONS

The landmark *Flexner Report to the Carnegie Foundation* in 1910 established the dominant paradigm for healthcare education in the 20th century (Beck, 2004). Two key components of the model were to practice scientific medicine while the learner was also engaged in laboratory experimentation and hands-on care at the bedside. The scientific curriculum had historically featured lecture-based instruction during the first 2 years of training where students were passive recipients of factual scientific knowledge (Papa & Harasym, 1999). Information was imparted by domain experts according to a predetermined timetable. Although the lecture format assured that the important educational material had been disseminated, the learner was at risk of lacking the conceptual links that were necessary for retention of the information. By contrast, the clinical practicum involved students more effectively as active participants with a contextual experience for the facts that they had learned.

Achieving a successful balance between academic and clinical education has challenged educators who must prepare graduates for healthcare institutions with both broad-based knowledge and technologically current specialty clinical skills (Manuel & Sorenson, 1995). These expectations have, in the past, created a sense of placing classroom learning, viewed as the foundation of academic priorities, in competition with the need for clinical experiences, a workplace priority. From the perspective of "situated cognition," both classroom and clinical experiences are equally necessary as knowledge is believed to be situated as a product of the activity, context, and culture in which it is used and not just something that happens inside the head of the person (Brown, Collins, & Duguid, 1989). With the synthesis of situated cognition principles and the characteristic needs of nursing education, three interacting components may be used to support learners in their quest for knowledge (Paige & Daley, 2009). The principles of the situated cognitive framework (see figure 14-1) include:

1. Thinking and learning as measures of knowledge make sense only within particular situations.
2. People act and construct meaning within communities of practice.
3. Knowledge depends on the use of a variety of artifacts and tools.
4. Situations make sense with a historical context (Paige & Daley, p. e99).

The interacting components may be viewed as people (including the community or, more specifically, patients, families, nurses, physicians, and ancillary personnel), ingredients or tools (including prior knowledge or concepts), and activity (including participation in real life events).

Learning that is structured within the situated cognition framework and the application of HFPSs offers nursing educators a strategy to bridge a student's advancement from theory-based knowledge to practice and to social integration into professional nursing (Paige & Daley, 2009). For explanation purposes, Paige and Daley described a case of the care of a patient experiencing unstable angina. An HFPS provided students with opportunities to transfer knowledge that was enhanced by an environment, in which they needed to page the physician, provide a status report, take verbal orders, and prepare a drug for administration. The construction of meaning within the community of practice was exemplified by the necessity to meet the needs of the simulated patient which included providing answers to the patient's questions about chest pain and interventions to reduce pain and anxiety. The ingredients or tools included the student's prior knowledge of the concept of pain that demanded more than an abstract understanding of pain, but one that was tailored to the unique needs of a patient with cardiac tissue ischemia. Finally, the principle of the historical context that encompassed

Figure 14-1 Situated cognition framework.

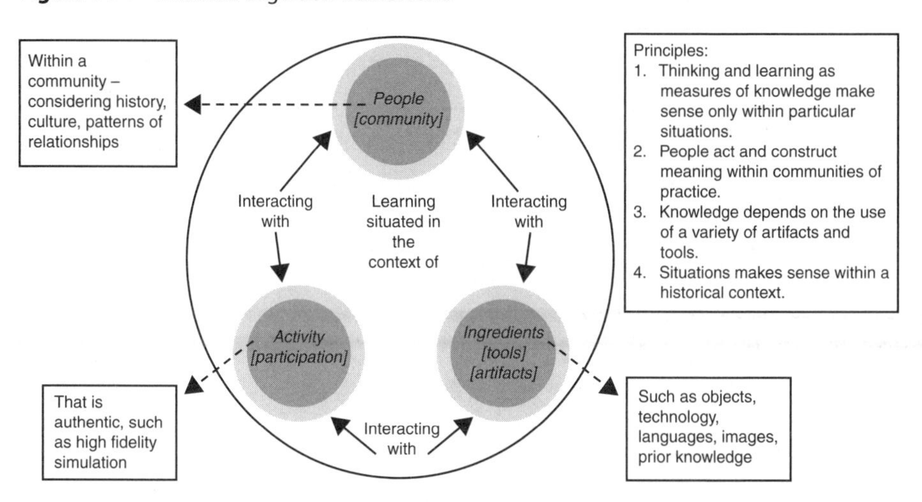

Source: From Situation cognition: A learning framework to support and guide high-fidelity simulation, by J. B. Paige, and B. J. Daley, 2009. *Clinical Simulation in Nursing, 5,* (*p.* e99) Copyright 2009 by Elsevier. Reprinted with permission.

cultural practices, values, and strategies of thinking and perceiving were viewed as inculturation into the healthcare environment with a review of the roles and responsibilities of professional nurses.

The simulated environment can promote the role of the teacher as an active participant and role model. Because clinical situations may be repeated as desired, the teacher can act initially as a role model by demonstrating a procedure or decision-making process, and then allow the student to practice in an identical or similar situation. By contrast, in the actual clinical setting, the faculty member who actively models a procedure, such as insertion of an intravenous catheter, often provides the demonstration at the expense of the student, who may not be able to repeat the process with another patient. The timing of simulated experiences can be scheduled to reinforce recently introduced material from the classroom, with the level of difficulty adjusted to match the student's capabilities. The ability to create an active learning environment that has been customized for each student is a compelling argument for the addition of HFPS to the instructional armamentarium of nurse educators.

There are a variety of conceptual frameworks that may be used to support the education of nurses who use HFPS. The critical incident nursing management (CINM), a nursing practice conceptual model derived from the concepts of the anesthesia crisis resource management (ACRM) model developed by Gaba, Fish, and Howard (1994), focuses on the nurse's responses to a patient's critical incident based on the characteristics of the patient, nurse, environment, and other members of the healthcare team (Nehring & Lashley, 2002).

Figure 14-2 The nursing simulation framework.

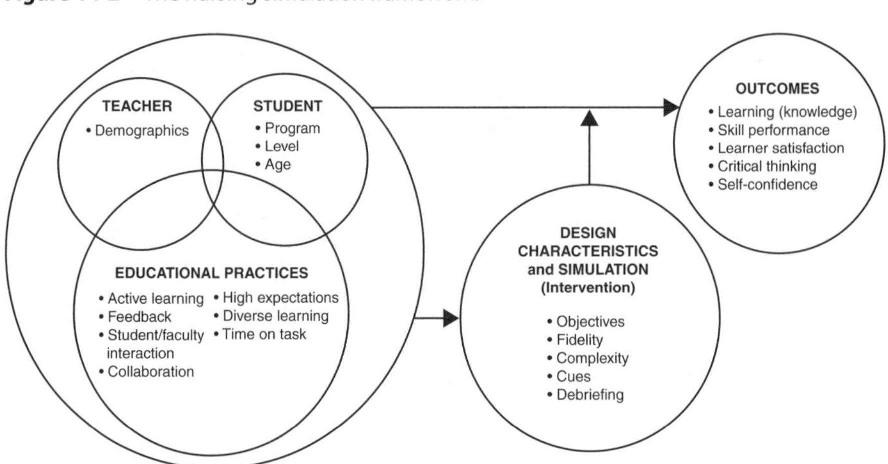

Source: The Nursing Education Simulation Framework. From Simulation in nursing education: From conceptualization to evaluation (p. 23), by P. R. Jeffries, 2007, New York: National League of Nursing.

Jeffries (2005, 2007) has also developed a simulation framework for nursing education (see figure 14-2). The model is intended to guide the design and implementation of simulations with expected outcomes as well. Accordingly, variables of the model include the simulation design characteristics, teacher, student, educational practices, and outcomes that include learning, skill performance, learner satisfaction, critical thinking, and self confidence.

The clinical judgment model (CJM) (Tanner, 2006) is an example of a conceptual framework that describes the variety of reasoning processes that nurses experience as they provide care in complex patient care situations (see figure 14-3). As clinical learning is one of the outcomes of clinical judgement, the model implies that nurses are continually learning as they develop their expertise through experiences and reflection. Components of the model include noticing, interpreting, responding, and reflecting. These components suggest that the nurse must be aware of the patient's needs, make sense of the situation, and respond with the best course of action that will be submitted to reflection after outcomes are realized and evaluated.

Lasater (2007) developed the Lasater clinical judgement rubric (LCJR) from the conceptual framework of the CJM (Tanner, 2006) in an attempt to provide a measure of clinical judgement skills. The four phases of the CJM of noticing, interpreting, responding, and reflecting provide the basis for the original rubric with 11 dimensions (Lasater, 2007). Effective noticing involves focused observations, recognizing deviations from expected patterns, and information seeking. Effective interpreting involves prioritizing and making sense of data.

Figure 14-3 Clinical judgment model.

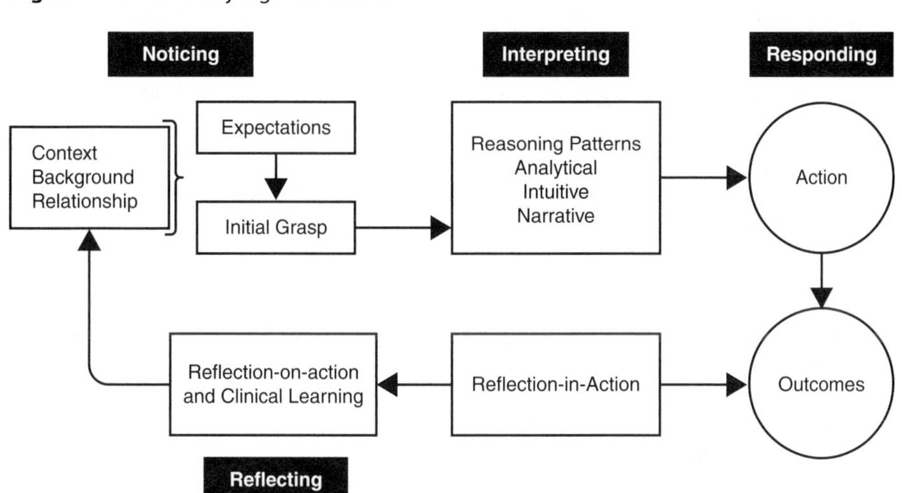

Source: Clinical judgement model. Reprinted with permission from Slack Incorporated, Copyright 2009. From Thinking like a nurse: A research-based model of clinical judgment in Nursing, 2006, Journal of Nursing Education, 45, p. 208.

Effective responding involves a calm, confident manner, clear communication, well-planned intervention/flexibility, and being skillful. Effective reflecting involves evaluation/self-analysis and commitment to improvement. The rubric offers students an opportunity to reflect on their performance for each dimension and rate themselves as exemplary, accomplished, developing, or beginning following a simulation experience.

TYPES OF LEARNERS

The Russian psychologist Vygotsky (1978) believed that learning was most effective when it occurred within the "zone of proximal development," where the content of learning was just beyond the current knowledge level of the student. Thus, each simulation session can be adjusted to the optimal level of difficulty for a particular student or group from beginner through expert and to technical levels by altering the delivery of care setting, patient history, clinical conditions, and patient sensitivity to therapeutic interventions. For example, beginning emergency and critical care students who are learning to recognize the signs of acute myocardial infarction may be asked to provide care for a patient with a robust cardiovascular system when signs of myocardial ischemia develop gradually without precipitating a cardiac arrest. A more advanced student would be expected to recognize subtle physiologic clues quickly and initiate prompt, effective interventions. Nurse anesthetists, acute care nurse practitioners, respiratory care, or emergency care students who are learning basic principles of airway management can use the simulator as a task trainer to refine fundamental skills such as insertion of pharyngeal airways and bag-valve-mask ventilation in an apneic patient using oxygen saturation and respiratory gas measurements to guide ventilation. Alternately, advanced students may be expected to perform sophisticated airway procedures to include tracheal intubation and needle cricothyroidotomy in simulated patients with an abnormal airway anatomy.

CONDITIONS FOR LEARNING

Because of the ability to create customized learning scenarios, HFPSs can be used in a wide variety of situations for all types of students. Simulation is useful to precede, complement, or replace actual clinical experiences.

Prior to clinical experiences, simulation can be used to orient students to care on an unfamiliar unit. Chatto and Dennis (1997) used HFPS to desensitize physical therapy students prior to their first critical care rotation. The simulation laboratory was configured to resemble a surgical intensive care unit. Students were introduced to types of monitoring equipment, life support devices, dressings, tubes, and drains that could be encountered during an actual clinical experience. As students performed physical therapy on the HFPS, common events were simulated, including sudden vital sign changes, gradually increasing intracranial pressure, cardiac alarms, and a ventilator disconnection. Together with the physical therapist and nursing faculty, students implemented safe and effective therapy, identified problems that were unique to the critical care environment, and practiced collaborative patient care.

In contrast to a one-time orientation session, simulation can also be used to allow students to practice technical skills and decision making before actual clinical experiences. For example, students in an anesthesia nursing program were permitted to accrue up to 100 hours of simulation practicing sequences of technical skills and decision making prior to their first clinical experience as a nurse anesthetist (Lupien, 1998; Monti et al., 1998). Students who have practiced using simulation prior to real clinical situations may be received more positively by clinical preceptors thus allowing the students to receive a more efficient and constructive clinical education.

Used concomitantly with clinical practice, simulation provides students and faculty the opportunity to replicate real clinical experiences and then use the simulator for reflection to explore alternative strategies for managing the situation. Students also have the opportunity to create customized patients based on their knowledge of physiology and pathophysiology to then compare the responses of their simulated patients to actual patients observed in clinical practices (Register, Graham-Garcia, & Haas, 2003).

Although the fidelity of HFPSs is not sufficiently developed to replace the practice of caring for human patients, simulation can be used to create learning opportunities that are not ordinarily available in most clinical environments. For example, students can practice high risk technical procedures such as defibrillation, using actual equipment in real time, or provide patient care during cardiopulmonary resuscitation or anaphylactic reactions on the simulator.

Simulation has also been used to develop higher order skills in ways that exactly parallel applications of simulation in commercial aviation. Aviation simulation has expanded beyond its use as a teaching/training tool for individual pilots to encompass team training through crew resource management (Helmreich & Foushee, 1993). Similarly, in the field of anesthesiology, programs such as ACRM (Gaba, Howard, Fish, & Smith, 2001) and team-oriented medical simulation focused on the actions of all members of a healthcare team with the goal of improving team performance (Baker, Gustafson, Beaubien, Salas, & Barach, 2005). Fletcher (1995) extended the concept of ACRM by developing ERR WATCH, a program focused specifically on the role of the nurse anesthetist in crisis management.

In addition to its uses as an instructional tool, simulation has the potential for formative and summative evaluation of student skills. Techniques for formative evaluation of student performances include using simulation as a mechanism for providing feedback on current skills and decision making processes or to observe progression of a student's competencies. Applications of simulation in summative evaluation are more controversial because the relationship between the performance of the student in a simulated environment and the actual clinical setting has not been demonstrated and descriptions of the psychometric properties to measure these relationships are limited. Devitt et al. (1997) reported estimates of internal consistency as high as 0.66 with their instruments for the evaluation of anesthesiology performance of beginning students, while Monti et al. (1998) described a rudimentary, weighted, scored checklist to evaluate the performance of beginning students in a limited clinical scenario with a moderately high reliability ($r = 0.83$). Devitt et al. (1997) and Gaba et al. (1998) reported excellent indices for inter-rater reliability for instruments to evaluate performance in simulated environments. While these reports suggest progress in measuring performance during simulation, it must be remembered that simulators do not provide an accurate representation of a patient to the learner. Additionally, the simulator environment may cause the learner to be overly vigilant or anxious (Hotchkiss, Biddle, & Fallacaro, 2002) and create a threat to the validity of the quality of observed performance.

RESOURCES

Perhaps the most critical aspect of a successful simulation program is the designation of dedicated physical space for the simulator and its support equipment. To accommodate the simulator, instructor, and to four to six students requires approximately 250 square feet of floor space. A sample floor plan for a simple simulation room is presented (see figure 14-4).

Simulators require both electricity and, in the case of student anesthetists, gas sources, which could include oxygen, carbon dioxide, and nitrogen. Nitrous oxide is optional for simulation of general anesthesia. Electricity requirements include two to four outlets for the simulator plus additional sources of power for patient care equipment.

Depending on the type of simulation selected, patient care equipment may include physiologic monitors, infusion pumps, ventilators, anesthesia machines, wall suction and oxygen, and a defibrillator. Support equipment includes airway devices, needles and syringes, dressings, chest tubes, urinary catheters, scrub wear, gloves, surgical masks, caps, and gowns.

The efficacy of simulation can be enhanced through a video recording of sessions with subsequent debriefing. Recording systems range from a single video camera to complex recording systems that allow multiple camera views,

Figure 14-4 Sample floor plan for a simple simulation room.

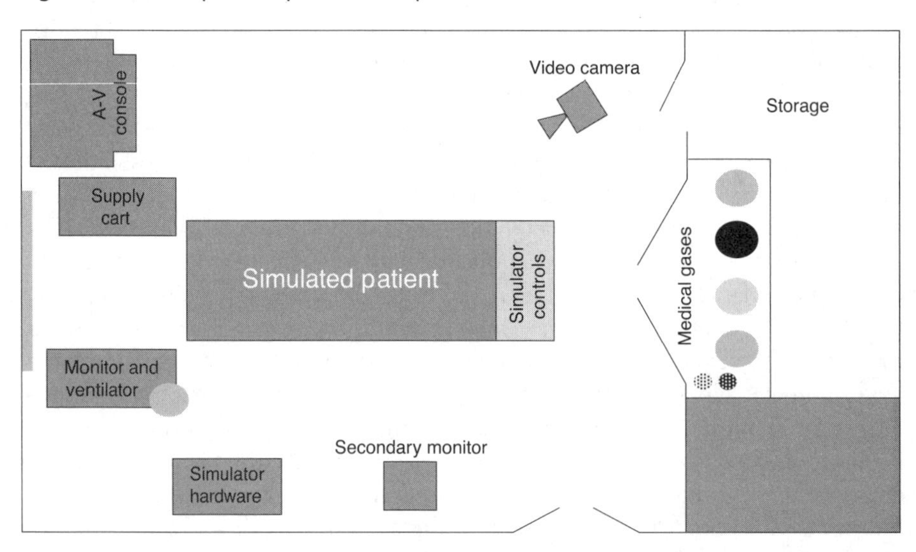

superimposed physiologic waveforms, logs and annotated notes, and audio recordings from participants and faculty. Dedicated simulation centers include a debriefing room where the video tapes can be reviewed. The debriefing room may also have the ability to receive live video and audio transmissions from the training room for the purpose of observation or simultaneous instruction of other students.

Some simulation centers also include a control room adjacent to the training room. One-way glass windows between the rooms allow individuals in a control room to observe simulation sessions as the operator and faculty communicate via headsets with microphones. In this type of room arrangement, a technician or faculty member in the control room is responsible for monitoring the simulation, making adjustments to the scenario as necessary, and selecting video and audio sources for recording.

Because simulation is so resource intensive, adequate personnel support is essential. Depending on the type of simulators and the selected scenario, key faculty with moderate computer skills may be adequately prepared to support simulation activities on an as needed basis, although many centers have found it beneficial to designate one faculty member or an associate to coordinate simulation activities and maintain the simulator.

USING THE METHOD

Successful simulation sessions depend on carefully planned scenarios and clearly defined roles for the participants. The primary instructor is responsible for selecting the scenario, guiding students through the simulation, providing important information and clinical cues that are not immediately available from the simulator, providing transition cues to a simulator operator, modeling behaviors, monitoring student performance, and troubleshooting in the event of an unexpected simulator issue. In some situations, the faculty may be assisted by another faculty member or technician who may serve as the simulator operator. In this case, the operator's responsibilities would include activating the simulation system, starting the patient software, overlaying the clinical scenarios, monitoring the progress of a scenario, and adjusting the scenario as it was intended to be by the primary instructor. Depending on the expertise of the faculty, the complexity of the scenario and the type of simulator, one individual may serve as both the faculty member and operator. A complex scenario, however, may require not only an instructor and operator, but additional faculty, students, or assistants to role play as members of the healthcare team and family.

To develop and implement a new simulation scenario, a seven-step process is recommended.

1. **Determine educational objectives or goals.** For example, the simulation may be intended to promote the advancement of technical, cognitive, or behavioral abilities or a combination of these competencies. The instructor should determine in advance whether the progression of the simulation will be constrained to unfold with a predetermined sequence or develop spontaneously.
2. **Construct a clinical scenario to facilitate attainment of educational objectives.** While the scenario should be clinically realistic, it should be customized to the student's level of expertise and designed to promote successful progression toward a higher level of decision making and demonstration of competencies.
3. **Define underlying physiologic concepts to be manifested throughout the scenario as they relate to the patient's responses to various events as they occur.** The primary instructor determines which essential elements of the clinical scenario are to be represented in the simulation experience, which elements may be absent or overlooked, and which missing elements need to be integrated into the experience. For example, as a patient develops progressive hypoxemia, tachypnea and decreasing hemoglobin saturation, as measured by pulse oximetry, are expected to occur. Although a real patient would also eventually become cyanotic, the instructor must decide whether the observation of skin color changes should be a necessary part of the educational objectives. When considering the accuracy of clinical situations, it is also essential to decide whether changes need to be technically accurate or sufficiently realistic and prominent to elicit the intended response from the learners.
4. **Modify programmed patients and scenarios, as necessary.** Program modification generally includes specifying the baseline physiology and clinical condition of the underlying patient, preparing the scenario to include optional modifiable states, and defining transitions between various patient states as the scenario evolves.
5. **Identify required equipment.** The instructor decides what devices will be displayed prominently or stored (as they might be in the clinical environment); whether learners will have the opportunity to inspect, assemble, and test equipment prior to the experience; and if the student will have options among multiple devices for use in the simulation. The instructor also determines whether additional personnel will be required to implement the clinical scenario, the qualifications (both actual and the role played) of the additional participants, and how primary learners will be able to access/involve the supplemental personnel resources.

6. **Run program and collect feedback.** Prior to use with students, the scenario should be run to establish that the simulation scenario unfolds as designed, with the intended levels of instructor and faculty participation.
7. **Reiterate steps until satisfied.** The simulation scenario is continuously refined until it unfolds as intended, without unintentional ambiguous details that distract from the attainment of the educational objectives, and the faculty is able to concentrate on observing and evaluating the student's performance while maintaining a positive effective learning environment.

Once the simulated scenario begins, the instructor may participate in a variety of ways. The instructor may function as a role model who demonstrates critical thinking, decision making, and therapeutic interventions; a coach who is available to help students when necessary; or as a passive bystander observing the scenario with minimal involvement. Regardless of the level of participation during the simulation, one of the instructor's key responsibilities is to facilitate the debriefing session afterward to reinforce the objectives of the scenario and to ensure that the intended learning occurred. During an ideal debriefing session, through reflective thinking, the students should have opportunities to describe and interpret the scenario, clarify their thoughts and actions as they occurred during the simulation, critique their performance in a nonthreatening way, and generate alternative decisions and plans of actions that would improve future performances.

POTENTIAL PROBLEMS

Perhaps the most significant potential problem with simulation is its dependency on faculty support and the time it takes to feel comfortable while using the technology for nursing teaching. Although issues revolving around the "learning curve" associated with faculty use of simulation have been recognized as barriers for the implementation of HFPSs, this has not been substantiated in the literature. However, the concern for the estimated amount of time faculty perceived it would take them to plan, implement, and evaluate the use of SimMan to teach clinical skills was studied by Jones and Hegge (2008). The results indicated that a majority of faculty respondents estimated that they would need a full-time equivalent (FTE) of 0.50 FTE release for one semester. Thus, the researchers recommended a need for administrative support to identify funding mechanisms for faculty training and planning sessions.

A second limitation to simulation is its incomplete presentation of reality. Although quite lifelike in representing human beings, simulators do not exhibit a complete range of signs and behaviors. Participants in a simulation are expected to suspend disbelief and respond to the patient according to what they observe.

In some cases, the instructor may need to provide missing cues that are necessary for appropriate use of the scenario. Although it is surprisingly easy to engage in a simulation, instructors need to be aware of critical cues that are absent or contradictory with the intended signs. Efforts to overcome some of these issues have been supported by the use of various moulage recipes to create realistic appearances of signs of disorders on the simulators.

Another potential problem with simulation is controlling the overgeneralization of findings to the real world. At least two types of generalization errors can occur. The first type is generalizing an observed response in one situation to all patients. For example, whenever the baseline healthy 70-kg patient receives an intravenous bolus of 20-μg epinephrine, the heart rate is raised approximately 20 beats per minute. Caution must be exerted to avoid the generalization that to increase a patient's heart rate by 20 beats, a dose of 20-μg epinephrine can be administered. To overcome this limitation, faculty can introduce the learners to a series of similar-appearing patients with slightly different physiologic parameters such as body weight, oxygen consumption, or baroceptor responses. By using these similar patients interchangeably, students may see variations in drug responses.

The second error of generalization is an incorrect attribution of simulation responses. As an incomplete representation of a human patient, simulators do not represent a completely accurate or comprehensive clinical portrait. For example, the simulator patient, when breathing spontaneously, cannot create high negative pressures like a human is capable of generating. Therefore, using the simulator to practice measuring inspiratory effort would lead to inaccurate results. Faculty who understand how simulators function will quickly recognize which clinical findings are authentic and which are artifacts. Simulation sessions can then be designed to take advantage of areas where the simulator provides a reasonable portrayal of a real human and avoid involving students in activities that are different than would be expected under actual clinical conditions.

Finally, participants are sometimes hypervigilant during simulation sessions because they anticipate the onset of a clinical problem. This has been demonstrated by students during a scenario related to the care of a patient with anaphylaxis following the administration of blood. Although hypervigilance cannot be avoided completely, its effect can be minimized by either mixing routine and critical event simulations or developing a series of potential events which evolve from a common scenario stem.

CONCLUSION

Simulation is an exciting application of advanced technology in healthcare professions education. Used correctly, whole-body HFPSs can effectively bridge the gap between static classroom-based instruction and the dynamic, unpredictable clinical environment. Although the use of simulation in healthcare education was, at one time, limited to adults receiving anesthesia, critical care, and emergency care, ongoing refinements in simulators, such as the introduction of pediatric and infant models and open architecture for the development of new simulation applications, have gradually allowed the introduction of high-fidelity simulation in settings not imagined even 10 years ago.

Jeffries (2009) has suggested that with evidence supported by quality outcomes, simulation may eventually be used for the majority of the clinical time for nursing education to overcome issues, such as "decreased numbers of clinical sites, patient safety issues, and the many rules and regulations required by clinical agencies' regulatory bodies and their effect on the amount and quality of education instructors can provide their students" (p. 71). From a broader perspective, Lashley (2010) anticipates greater opportunities of HFPS use as simulation centers become available to shared partnerships among the professions between educational groups and healthcare agencies. Aside from nursing education, the popular use of HFPS has potential application in the areas of nursing licensure, advanced practice nursing credentialing, orientation programs, and continuing education.

Applied Example

Using High-Fidelity Simulation in an Undergraduate Critical Care Nursing Course

This example[1] illustrates how simulation was used to reinforce concepts of respiratory assessment and nursing care as part of a critical care nursing elective for senior level undergraduate nursing students. The course included 40 didactic hours and was designed to complement a 200-hour clinical practicum. The course focused on pulmonary, cardiovascular, and neurological critical care; advanced hemodynamic monitoring; and critical care pharmacology. The respiratory care section of the course included lectures on respiratory gas exchange, advanced assessment techniques, arterial blood gas analysis, airway management, and ventilatory support. To complement the lectures, a seven-step process was used to develop a simulation session.

1. **Determine educational objective.** The simulation session was designed so that the student would be able to achieve the following objectives:
   - Complete and continuously revise the assessment of a patient who is acutely and dynamically ill.
   - Select appropriate oxygen therapy devices for a specified clinical situation.
   - Collect and prepare the appropriate equipment and medications for emergent tracheal intubation.

[1]Scenario developed by Beverly George-Gay, MSN, CCRN; Assistant Professor and Coordinator of Distance and Continuing Education; Department of Nurse Anesthesia; Virginia Commonwealth University; Richmond, VA.

- Administer appropriate medications to facilitate emergent tracheal intubation and assess the drug effects.
- Perform airway management procedures, as indicated, to include bag-valve-mask ventilation, tracheal intubation, and an endotracheal tube.
- Confirm appropriate placement of an endotracheal tube.
- Prepare an unstable patient for transport from an inpatient unit to a critical care unit.
- Initiate positive pressure ventilatory support for an acutely ill patient and adjust ventilatory parameters (to include mode, FiO_2, tidal volume, respiratory rate, and positive-end expiratory pressure) as indicated by patient condition, arterial blood gases, capnography, and spirometry.

  Although the scenario involved only nursing students, it can be easily expanded to include respiratory and emergency care providers. The instructor was actively involved in the session as a coach to students who provided interactive feedback and helped students clarify clinical observations.

2. **Construct a clinical scenario.** Students were told that they were going to evaluate a patient with pneumonia hospitalized on an inpatient medical unit. A brief patient history was provided.
   - Students were given the opportunity to assess the patient, including observation of respiratory effort, lung auscultation, estimation of arterial oxygenation by pulse oximetry, and measurement and analysis of arterial blood gases. At the time of initial contact, the patient demonstrated signs of moderate hypoxia to include rapid shallow breathing, mild oxyhemoglobin desaturation, and rales on chest auscultation. Upon a signal from the instructor to the simulator operator, the patient experienced significant oxyhemoglobin desaturation.
   - The scenario was designed so that the patient initially would require oxygen therapy and then require more aggressive treatment including tracheal intubation and positive pressure ventilation using a bag-valve device with both face mask and tracheal tube. Once transferred to the critical care unit, ventilatory support using various modes such as assist control, intermittent mandatory ventilation, positive-end expiratory pressure, and pressure support ventilation could be explored.
3. **Define underlying physiologic concepts to be manifest through the scenario: patient and events.** The physiologic concepts underlying pneumonia include decreased lung compliance and increased shunt. Manifestations of these alterations include an adaptive respiratory pattern with increased rate and smaller tidal volume, increased peak inspiratory pressure, hypoxemia, mild hypercarbia, rales, tachycardia, and cardiac dysrhythmias. Patient deterioration within the scenario results from progressive reductions in lung compliance and increases in shunt. For this exercise, it was determined that sufficient physiologic changes to induce learner critical thinking, decision making, and action were more important than technical accuracy.
4. **Modify programmed patient and scenarios, as necessary.** A geriatric model developed by faculty and master's level nursing anesthesia students was used.[2] To exhibit signs of

[2]Development of the geriatric model was supported, in part, by a grant from the Division of Nursing, US Department of Health and Human Services Bureau of Health Professions.

pneumonia, rales were introduced, lung compliance was decreased, shunt fraction was increased, and the CO_2 set point was increased slightly (to produce mild hypercarbia). Temperature was increased slightly to reflect an underlying infective process. As a result of these changes, tidal volume decreased automatically and respiratory rate increased to compensate for the reduced tidal volume. Physiologic alterations were also manifested automatically through changes in heart rate and arterial blood gases.

- So that the patient would initially appear to be stable and then deteriorate upon the instructor's command, baseline and decompensation states were created. Although an automatic transition could have initiated the decompensation at a predetermined time, a manual transition was selected to assure that the destabilization occurred when intended by the instructor.

5. **Assemble required equipment.** Because the patient is not physically transported from the medical unit to the critical care unit, the simulation lab was originally configured with equipment available to acute care personnel. Items included a resuscitation cart with a cardiac monitor and defibrillator, an oxygen source, oxygen therapy devices, various airway management devices such as a bag-valve-mask device, pharyngeal airways, endotracheal tubes, laryngoscopes, and suction equipment. Once the scenario shifted to the critical care unit, a positive pressure ventilator was also available for student use.
6. **Run program and collect feedback.** Prior to use with students, the scenario was run several times to observe the rate of change for physiologic variables and the effects of various therapeutic options.
7. **Reiterate steps 2 to 6 until satisfied.** Physiologic parameters were modified incrementally so that the patient would appear stable, but with sufficient respiratory compromise to entice the learner to initiate oxygen therapy. Once the deterioration sequence was initiated, the decompensation needed to be sufficient to warrant more aggressive therapy yet progress at a rate such that novice nurses with limited skills and therapeutic options could stabilize the patient.

   To implement the simulation, the instructor selects the customized geriatric patient from the patient options menu of the user interface and respiratory exercise from the scenario options menu. The simulator immediately begins emulating the pneumonia patient in the stable baseline state. Progression to the decompensation state requires only one additional keystroke or mouse click.

Careful pilot testing of the simulated patient and clinical scenario reduces the likelihood of unanticipated events during the educational session; however, the instructor should be prepared to help students with assembling and using unfamiliar equipment as well as performing advanced technical skills, such as effective bag-valve-mask ventilation and tracheal intubation. Careful coordination with the simulator operator will allow the patient to deteriorate at a rate appropriate for the experience of the learners with pauses in the deterioration, if desired during specific teaching moments or as technical maneuvers are performed.

For this exercise, evaluation of the learner achievement was formative and informal. After the simulated patient's condition was stabilized, the faculty and students reflected on the observed clinical signs and how the patient's condition, clinical setting, and events affected decision making and actions; medications, devices, and procedures used to stabilize the patient; and potential alternative solutions that would have led to more rapid or improved outcomes.

REFERENCES

Baker, D. P., Gustafson, S., Beaubien, J. M., Salas, E., & Barach, P. (2005). Medical team training programs in health care. In Agency for Healthcare Research and Quality, *Advances in patient safety. From research to implementation* (pp. 253–267). (AHRQ Publication No. 050021-4). Rockville, MD: Author. Retrieved June 1, 2009, from http://www.ahrq.gov/downloads/pub/advances/vol4/Baker.pdf

Beck, A. H. (2004). The Flexner Report and the standardization of American medical education. *Journal of American Medical Association, 291*(17), 2139–2140.

Brown, J. S., Collins, A., & Duguid, P. (1989). Situated cognition and the culture of learning. *Educational Researcher, 18*, 32–42.

Chatto, C., & Dennis, J. K. (1997). Intensive care unit training for physical therapy students: Use of an innovative patient simulator. *Acute Care Perspectives, 5*(4), 7–12.

Devitt, J. H., Kurrek, M. M., Cohen, M. M., Fish, K., Fish, P., Murphy, P. M., et al. (1997). Testing the raters: interrater reliability during observation of simulator performance. *Canadian Journal of Anaesthesia, 44*, 925–928.

Fanning, R. M., & Gaba, D. M. (2007) The role of debriefing in simulation-based learning. *Society for Simulation in Healthcare, 2*(2), 115–125.

Fletcher, J. L. (1995). AANA Journal Course: Update for nurse anesthetists - Anesthesia simulation: A tool for learning and research. *Journal of the American Association of Nurse Anesthetists, 63*, 61–67.

Fritz, P. Z., Gray, T., & Flanagan, B. (2008). Review of mannequin-based high fidelity simulation in emergency medicine. *Emergency Medicine Australasia, 20*, 1–9.

Gaba, D., & DeAnda, A. (1988). A comprehenisive anesthesia simulation environment: Recreating the operating room for research and training. *Anesthesiology, 69*, 387–394.

Gaba, D. M., Fish, K. J., & Howard, S. K. (1994). *Crisis management in anesthesiology*. New York: Churchill Livingston.

Gaba, D. M., Howard, S. K., Flanagan, B., Smith, B. E., Fish, K. J., & Botney, R. (1998). Association of clinical performance during simulated crises using both technical and behavioral ratings. *Anesthesiology, 89*, 8–18.

Gaba, D. M., Howard, S. K., Fish, K. J., & Smith, B. E. (2001). Simulation-based training in anesthesia crisis resource management (ACRM):A decade of experience. *Simulation & Gaming, 32*(2), 175–193.

Gaumard Scientific. (2009). *Simulators for health care education*. Retrieved May 31, 2009, from http://www.ism-tec.com/companies/gaumard/index.htm

Good, M. L. (2003). Patient simulation for training basic and advanced clinical skills. *Medical Education, 37*(Suppl. 1), 14–21.

Good, M. I., & Gravenstein, J. S. (1989). Anaesthesia simulators and training devices. *International Anesthesiology Clinics, 27*, 161–166.

Harlow, K. C., & Sportsman, S. (2007). An economic analysis of patient simulators for clinical training in nursing education. *Nursing Economics, 25*(1), 24–29.

Helmreich, R. L., & Foushee, H. C. (1993). Why crew resource management? Empirical and theoretical basis of human factors training in aviation. In E. L. Weiner, B. G. Kanki, & R. L. Helmreich (Eds.), *Cockpit resource management* (pp. 3–46). London: Academic Press.

Hotchkiss, M. A., Biddle, C., & Fallacaro, M. (2002). Assessing the authenticity of the human patient experience in anesthesiology. *AANA Journal, 70*, 470–473.

Jeffries, P. R. (2005). A framework for designing, implementing, and evaluating simulations used as teaching strategies in Nursing. *Nursing Education Perspectives, 26*(2), 96–103.

Jeffries, P. R. (2007). *Simulation in nursing education: From conceptualization to evaluations*. New York: National League for Nursing.

Jeffries, P. R. (2009). Editorial: Dreams for the future for clinical simulations. *Nursing Education Perspectives, 30*(2), 71.

Jones, A. L., & Hegge, M. (2008). Simulation and faculty time investment. *Clinical simulation in Nursing, 4,* e5–e9.

Laerdal. (2009). Patient simulators. Retrieved May 31, 2009, from http://www.laerdal.com/document.asp?docid=1022609

Larew, C., Lessons, S., Spunt, D., Foster, D., & Covington, B. (2006). Innovations in clinical simulation: Application of Benner's theory in an interactive patient care simulation. *Nursing Education Perspectives, 29(1)*, 16–21.

Lasater, K. (2007). Clinical judgement development: Using simulation to create an assessment rubric. *Journal of Nursing Education, 46*(11), 496–503.

Lashley, F. R. (2010). Using high-fidelity patient simulation: What does the future hold? In W. M. Nehring, & F. R. Lashley (Eds.), *High fidelity patient simulation in nursing education* (pp. 427–431). Sudbury, MA: Jones and Barlett.

Lupien, A. E. (1998). Simulation in nursing anesthesia education. In L. C. Henson & A. C. Lee. *Simulators in anesthesiology education* (pp. 29–37). New York: Plenum.

Lupien, A. (2007). High fidelity patient simulation. In M. J. Bradshaw, & A. J. Lowenstein (Eds.), *Innovative teaching strategies in nursing and related health professions* (4th ed., pp 197–214). Sudbury, MA: Jones and Bartlett.

Manuel, P., & Sorenson, L. (1995). Changing trends in healthcare: Implications for baccalaureate education, practice, and employment. *Journal of Nursing Education, 34*(6), 248–253.

METI. (2009). HPS. Retrieved May 31, 2009, from http://www.meti.com/products_ps_hps.htm

Monti, E. J., Wren, K., Haas, R., & Lupien, A. E. (1998). The use of an anesthesia simulator in graduate and undergraduate education. *CRNA: The Clinical Forum for Nurse Anesthetists, 9*(2), 59–66.

Nehring, W. (2010). History of simulation in nursing. In Nehring, W. M. & F. R. Lashley (Eds.), *High fidelity patient simulation in nursing education* (pp. 3–26). Sudbury, MA: Jones and Barlett.

Nehring, W. M. & Lashley, F. R. (2004). Using the Human Patient Simulators in nursing education. *Annual Review of Nursing Education, 2,* 163–181.

Paige, J. B., & Daley, B. J. (2009). Situation cognition: A learning framework to support and guide high-fidelity simulation. *Clinical Simulation in Nursing, 5,* e97-e103.

Papa, F. J., & Harasym, P. H. (1999). Medical curriculum reform in North America, 1765 to the present: A cognitive science perspective. *Academic Medicine, 74*(2), 154–164.

Parker, B. C., & Myrick, F. (2008). A critical examination of high-fidelity human patient simulation within the context of nursing pedagogy. *Nurse Education Today, 29,* 322–329.

Radhakrishnan, K., Roche, J. P., & Cunningham, H. (2007). Measuring clinical practice parameters with human patient simulators: A pilot study [Electronic Version]. *International Journal of Nursing Education Scholarship, 4*(1), Article 8.

Register, M., Graham-Garcia, J., & Haas, R. (2003). The use of simulation to demonstrate hemodynamic response to varying degrees of intrapulmonary shunt. *AANA Journal, 71*, 277–284.

Rosen, K. R. (2004). The history of medical simulation. In G.E. Loyd, C. L. Lake, & R. B. Greenberg (Eds.), *Practical health care simulations* (pp. 3–26). Philadelphia: Elsevier Mosby.

Rosen, K. R. (2008). The history of medical simulation. *Journal of Critical Care, 23*, 157–166.

Sittner, B. J., Schmaderer, M., Zimmerman, L., Hertzog, M., & George, B. (2009). Rapid response team simulated training for enhancing patient safety (STEPS). *Clinical Simulation in Nursing, 5*, e119–e127.

Tanner, C. A. (2006). Thinking like a nurse: A research-based model of clinical judgement in nursing. *Journal of Nursing Education, 45*(6), 204–211.

Vygotsky, L. S. (1978). Mind in society: *The development of higher psychological processes*. Cambridge, MA: Harvard University Press.

CHAPTER 15

The New Skills Laboratory: Application of Theory, Teaching, and Technology

Deborah Tapler and Judy Johnson-Russell

INTRODUCTION

Creating an effective skills laboratory can energize students and facilitate the transition from practice of required skills to delivery of direct care to clients. The skills laboratory, using multiple modes of teaching and learning, provides an atmosphere for students to acquire new skill knowledge and implement those new skills. With emerging restrictions of clinical placement of health-related students, the skills lab can be used as a learning environment without the presence of clients (Duffin, 2004). Nursing programs are debating proposals that would allow students to spend much more clinical time in practice labs instead of in actual hospital units. With unlimited hours of operation, the lab can provide needed opportunities to practice procedures, evaluate learning outcomes, and reinforce critical thinking objectives. As technology increases in complexity through the use of advanced human patient simulators, the skills laboratory can now provide almost true-to-life clinical situations.

DEFINITIONS AND PURPOSES

Acquisition of new knowledge and skills is an important component of the educational curriculum for healthcare professionals. Nurses must be able to perform procedures such as wound care, intravenous therapy, and endotracheal suctioning. Through the use of a skills laboratory, these and other integral patient care skills are learned and practiced before implementation on patients. The instructor educating students about skills uses several sources for instruction.

The roles and responsibilities of the skills lab have changed with time and advances in learning technology. The skills lab takes on various labels based on its broad offering of services or purposes (Childs, 2002). Schools of nursing across the country suggest the following names: Clinical Skills Laboratory, Clinical Resource Center, Learning Resource Center, Clinical Competencies Learning Laboratory, or, simply, Nursing Laboratory. Current laboratory facilities offer assessment labs, bed labs, static mannequins, simulation, training devices such as intravenous insertion simulators, video libraries, and computer services. Some universities support patient clinics associated with the skills lab for student experiences with actual patients. The skills lab offers a continuum of services depending on the school's interests, specific curriculum needs, and financial capability.

Theory-based practice guides the educator when preparing to teach new skills. Theory has a direct link to practice. Educational theories relate the instructor to students through the development of effective learning strategies appropriate for selected students. Theory also influences practice through theory-driven research that impacts patient care. For example, germ theory dictates the procedure of successful hand washing, which is a skill that every student must master to prevent infection. When learning in the skills lab, the student must progress beyond the "how" of a procedure to the more complex level of thinking to ask "why."

Evidence-based practice must also be used in the skills laboratory. Evidence-based practice is a systematic approach to problem solving that can be applied to patient care delivery as well as education (Pravikoff, Tanner, & Pierce, 2005). Teaching skills that are based on valid research provide students with state-of-the-art information for safe implementation of skills in actual clinical experiences. It is imperative to educate students about the process of accessing research evidence as part of a lifelong learning goal. Inviting students to participate in the evidence-based process is an important teaching opportunity to allow students to discover best practices regarding content reviewed in the skills lab. For example, students are assigned a particular topic, such as blood pressure monitoring or safe medication administration, to seek reputable best practice standards regarding the psychomotor skill. Elements of procedures and relevancy of skills change as knowledge and technology grow. The skills laboratory must reflect the most current information when educating nurses for the future.

The purpose of this chapter is to explore the roles, diverse uses, and effectiveness of a skills laboratory. Based on current theory, valuable teaching modalities, and advanced technology, the skills laboratory can be an effective tool of education for a wide range of health-related disciplines.

THEORETICAL RATIONALE

Knowles' theory of adult learning has shaped the way that educators present information to adult learners (Knowles, 1989). Adults approach a learning situation differently than children. With life experiences to color the acquisition of new knowledge and skills, adults thrive in a learning environment that is open to creativity, values personal knowledge, and is relevant to immediate learning goals. Adult learners desire to make individual choices and decisions. Education in the skills laboratory is hands-on and relevant to direct patient care. Students are allowed and encouraged to self-evaluate their competence prior to clinical placement (Clarke, Davies, & McNee, 2002). They develop self-confidence as they learn psychomotor skills without fear of failure. After the students attend traditional learning presentations, such as lecture, the adult learners are motivated to learn those things in the skills lab that they know will be necessary to accomplish course objectives. Practice in the skills lab allows the students to cope effectively with future patient interactions. The skills lab can also provide academic assistance when a student has difficulty integrating knowledge regarding a psychomotor skill.

Benner's theory of skill acquisition plays an important part in the nursing education curriculum (Benner, 2001). Benner proposed a model for the nursing profession based on the Dreyfus model explaining that nurses function at various levels of skill from novice to expert. The novice level is characterized by a lack of experience of the situations in which the person is involved and is expected to perform. The beginning nursing student functions at the novice level. The nursing curriculum gives students entry to nursing situations and allows them to gain the experience through skills development. The skills lab acts as an instrument to transfer knowledge and skills to novice nursing students so that they may progress to increasingly more complex levels of understanding. The skills lab can be used to teach about situations in terms of "objective attributes" such as intake and output, blood pressure, and temperature (Benner, 2001, p. 20). These features of the task world of nursing have to be learned before actual situational experiences with patients. The behavior of the novice is rule-governed and very limited and inflexible. Faculty members impart rules to guide performance before the information makes sense to students. Practice and rehearsal of new behaviors allow the students to gain confidence in their abilities despite little understanding of the contextual meanings of recently learned nursing concepts. Thus, the skills lab plays an important role in the learning process of new students who have no contextual cues. As the nursing student progresses through the nursing curriculum to graduation, the role of the skills lab can evolve and change to meet the expectations for learning dictated by the faculty and content objectives. According to Benner, students may progress from novice to advanced beginner then to the competent, proficient, and expert levels of nursing ability over the lifetime of a career.

CONDITIONS

The skills laboratory can be used effectively throughout the curriculum. According to Infante (1985), the purpose of a skills laboratory is to offer students the appearance of reality in an artificial environment where the setting is controlled and offers practical application. The students are encouraged to achieve a predefined level of skill competence (Clarke et al., 2002). As skills move from simple (such as bathing) to complex (such as suctioning), the skills lab can be a learning experience that provides for advancing levels of knowledge and abilities.

Faculty involved in undergraduate curricula should identify skills associated with each level of progression to ensure that all necessary content is reflected in the educational goals of the laboratory. In addition, identified skills should be appropriate to the skill level of the student. Typically, nursing education has utilized the skills lab to provide psychomotor skill acquisition at the beginning of the curriculum. However, with technologies used in the lab, such as computer-based interactive case studies and human-patient simulators, new modalities have provided unlimited opportunities for knowledge as well as skill development. Critical thinking scenarios are appropriate and can be facilitated by skills lab experiences.

Faculty members using the skills lab should strive to teach a diversity of skills to students. Even though the skills lab typically provides an environment that lends itself to the training of psychomotor skills, other cognitive and affective domain skills can be developed by students. Students learn therapeutic communication and interpersonal skills through staged interactions with mannequins. Collaboration is instilled when students work in groups to deliver patient care through participation in simulation. Faculty-developed case studies used in the lab should be structured with a communication component to include telephoning the physician to clarify an order or suggesting strategies to interact with a distressed family member.

Learning situations can be enhanced by the contained setting of the skills laboratory. With close supervision and responsive interactions between students and faculty, the students learn in an environment of collaboration and inquiry. Questions about new procedures or concepts can be answered and discussed promptly without the constraints of a fast-paced patient care area. Faculty members act as facilitators and have opportunities to present information regarding advances in evidence-based practice. Students feel confident to try new skills in a low risk situation without fear of harming patients. Mistakes are excellent sources of learning and do not have to possess penalizing consequences. However, if the skills laboratory is used for mastery performance evaluation of student abilities, the results can be recorded as a component of a course grade or used for remedial identification. Students who have weaknesses in psychomotor or critical thinking skills can use the environment of the skills laboratory for tutoring assistance from faculty. Through one-on-one interaction, the weak student can practice and receive immediate feedback from a qualified evaluator to gain knowledge and confidence.

TYPES OF LEARNERS

Undergraduate nursing students possess various learning styles. The skills laboratory can provide a rich learning experience for all types of learners. Whether the student learner is self-directed or takes a more dependent approach, the faculty can individualize instruction based on each student's abilities and learning style. (See Chapter 1 for an overview of cognitive styles, learning styles, and learning preferences.) Kolb's theory of experiential learning proposes cycles of learning along a continuum from concrete experience to abstract conceptualization of knowledge (Dobbin, 2001). Nursing students possess a more concrete, active pattern learning style characterized by the need for dynamic involvement when learning new concepts and skills (Schroeder, 2004). According to Dobbin (2001), "learners also can have a preference for reflective observation (watching to learn) or active experimentation (learning by doing)" (p. 5). For example, tactile exploration by touching and manipulating syringes and needles is essential for the concrete learner. Lecturing has only limited ability to educate in regards to psychomotor skill acquisition. As the student learns new skills in the lab, questions arise and "what ifs" are posed to enhance the learning experience. The use of return demonstration strengthens mastery and confidence.

Faculty must ensure that instruction in the skills laboratory is directed to students with a wide range of learning styles. Students may possess any one or a combination of the following learning styles: visual (spatial), aural (auditory-musical), verbal (linguistic), physical (kinesthetic), logical (mathematical), social (interpersonal), or solitary (intrapersonal) (Schroeder, 2004). Through the use of simulators, audiovisual software, graphs and diagrams, charts, pictures, demonstrations, practice, discussion, or even music, the skills laboratory can address the needs of all students when acquiring new nursing knowledge. The key to effective teaching in the lab is dependent on the faculty use of a varied and innovative approach to education.

Generational differences among students are addressed by the variety of teaching strategies that are offered by faculty in the skills lab. Whether a Generation X, Millennial, or Baby Boomer, each student approaches the learning environment with different characteristics and learning needs (Billings & Halstead, 2005). The skills lab offers an array of options to capture the attention of students in today's society. For example, the Millennial student prefers to work with a team and be socially involved. According to Godson, Wilson, and Goodman (2007), third year students working with first year students in a nursing program proved very effective. The third year students were asked to teach a psychomotor skill related to patient care to the first year students. The first year students then practiced the skill that they had learned from their fellow nursing students. The mentors' support helped to comfort and ease the anxiety of learning a new skill experienced by the beginning nursing students. Each group described benefits of working together as a team. (See Chapter 5 for an in depth exploration in the generations of learners).

CONDITIONS FOR LEARNING AND RESOURCES

Opportunities for learning skills in the clinical environment continue to dwindle due to fewer clinical placements available in healthcare institutions. With often fierce competition among educational programs for optimal student assignments in hospital and community resources, the skills lab takes on an increased importance for all clinical courses in the curriculum. Skills, which were once discussed and practiced briefly in the lab and then performed on clients, may no longer be practiced in the clinical area due to patient availability and legal ramifications. Practice in the skills lab may be the only opportunity for learning many basic as well as complex skills needed after graduation. Therefore, skills taught in each course must be identified and additional time and supplies allotted for practice in the lab. Skills will not only be taught in isolation with low-fidelity simulators such as static mannequins, but can also become a part of scenarios with high-fidelity human patient simulators. These scenarios offer the students opportunities to interact with simulators with specific problems, and the skills learned are carried out as interventions become necessary, rather than in isolation. Thus, scenarios based on learning objectives for each course throughout the curriculum and imbedded with increasingly complex skills become an important avenue for assisting the student in progressing from novice to higher levels of ability. Skills performed within scenarios also allow for the adult learner to apply knowledge and psychomotor ability to immediate learning goals.

Skills labs must take on a new look that parallels the hospital environment as simulators become patients and assist the student is the suspension of disbelief while practicing necessary skills. This environment includes not only sights, but also the sounds that are inherent in a busy clinical area. Labs must include the equipment, technology, and resources that are currently found in the clinical environment. The skills laboratory includes not only typical equipment, such as intravenous pumps, but also computers and personal digital assistants (PDAs) with evidenced-based resources that will be needed to assist students with problem solving and critical thinking as they work through scenarios. Informatics should be accessible as students must learn to work with databases and documentation software. Labs will need to be designed to provide rooms/bays that are essentially self-contained hospital units for scenarios to be carried out. Although the rooms may be used for a variety of scenarios, different rooms may need to be designed and equipped for areas such as obstetrics, emergency care, acute care, home care, pediatrics, and intensive care units in addition to ancillary units. As the hospital environment changes and innovations, such as telenursing and eICUs become commonplace, skill labs require design elements that provide multiple screen workstations connected to multiple simulators.

USING THE METHOD

Teaching within the new skills lab combines the best of the traditional methods of instructions with the new technological advances. Regardless of the complexity of the skill, acquisition begins with didactic instruction and practice in the lab on low-fidelity mannequins. Additionally, students may be provided with kits of equipment and supplies to continue practicing skills at home. These include such things as mock wounds for dressing changes and styrofoam wig heads with tracheostomy tubes for practicing tracheostomy care. As mentioned previously, performance of skills at this time is rule-governed and inflexible. These skills can then be imbedded within a scenario accompanied by the complexity of care based on the course objectives. Three to five students can work through the scenario on a high-fidelity human patient simulator, identifying indicators for various skills, perhaps obtaining orders for the skill, collecting supplies needed, performing the skills, observing the effects, and documenting and reporting the procedure and effects. Although only one student actually performs any one skill, other students actively participate in the skill through discussion and support. The importance of the skill takes on a new meaning as it becomes a part of patient care for an illness and a patient with specific needs and responses. Communication and professionalism is fostered with other team members, such as healthcare providers, and among other members of the student's peer group. Debriefing following the completion of the scenario should be considered integral to the process. Discussions with the faculty as facilitators can assist the student in applying theory to practice, correcting mistakes, answering questions, identifying learning needs, and making connections to the real world.

The use of appropriate scenarios and all levels of human patient simulators and mannequins are invaluable for teaching skills in a safe environment where patient cooperation is not needed, where repetition is essential, and especially where skills could potentially cause harm to the patient. Critical thinking and problem solving, obtaining appropriate supplies, manipulating equipment, looking up resources, performing procedures accurately and safely, and communicating verbally and in writing are all activities that require considerable amounts of practice by the novice learner. In the fast-paced clinical environment, time is of the essence and students are often expected to perform beyond the level of novice learner. Students can move beyond the novice level with the use of credible scenarios and simulated patients in the realistic, transferable environment of the skills lab.

Skill labs may include evaluation of specific skills as a part of outcome measurements at the end of the semester. Students are often evaluated performing a specific skill or skills as the faculty observe and record their performance. Return demonstration to determine mastery of specified skills is an effective method to determine the safety of transition to patient care in the clinical setting. If students demonstrate a poor performance when evaluated, immediate remedial action can be taken to correct deficiencies before exposure to patients. Patient safety must be the overriding consideration when documenting student abilities. For example, if during a lab check-off, a student draws up 10 ml of a medication instead of the required 3 ml dose, the faculty can reeducate the student immediately, validate that accurate knowledge is mastered, and avert a potential patient injury in subsequent clinical encounters.

Simulated patients also are used in effectively evaluating skills. The required skills are developed in a short scenario. Three to five students care for the patient and perform the skills as the intervention becomes necessary in the scenario. Students should be aware of the criteria and expected behaviors, having practiced all the skills to be evaluated previously. At the beginning of the scenario, students can draw for the skills they are to perform during the scenario. As the scenario progresses, students care for the patient together, except when a specific skill is needed. Peers then become observers as the student who was assigned a skill performs according to the criteria outlined, and is evaluated by the instructor. Peer observers become active learners as they mentally rehearse and evaluate the skills as they are being performed. Once the skill has been completed, the scenario resumes until another skill is needed. The process is repeated throughout the scenario until all students have demonstrated their selected skills. Verbal and/or written feedback can be given to the students individually by the instructor following the scenario. Students may also give their peers feedback about their performance.

Video recording may be used as an adjunct to learning or evaluation of skills. This method of assessment offers findings that are very objective when used for grading purposes. Students can learn by video recording and critiquing their own performance or viewing the video and discussing their performance with a faculty member. They can also video record and submit their video for evaluation and feedback by a faculty member. In a study by Brimble (2008), skills assessment using video analysis in a simulated environment was an effective evaluation tool. The nursing students completed a questionnaire before, during, and after video taping a simulation in the skills lab. The most common, positive theme that students expressed was the ability to learn from their mistakes by watching the reenactment of their performance on video. Subjects indicated that the visual feedback that they received from viewing their actual performance complemented the verbal critique offered by their faculty member. Negative themes included feelings for anxiety, being judged by others, and being embarrassed.

However, Miller, Nichols, and Beeken (2000) found that students prefer faculty member presence during skill demonstrations and immediate feedback rather than video recording and delayed feedback.

POTENTIAL PROBLEMS

Major problems inherent in the development of the modern skills laboratory are the cost to provide the needed technology, supplies, and the physical space to house them. In order for students to practice with the equipment used in the profession, it must be purchased from medical vendors. Supplies are very expensive, especially when they are the most recent equipment used by the clinical agencies. Needles with integral safety devices are often more costly than traditional needle systems. Students must see and practice with the tools that they will use in their clinical experiences, which requires frequent equipment revision in the laboratory. As enrollment in schools of nursing increases due to shortage mandates, the skills lab provides space that is available from early morning to late in the evening for student use.

Skills labs have typically been large rooms with multiple beds and static mannequins. Large numbers of students often practice the same skill at the same time. Although this type of space and instruction are a beginning, additional smaller simulation rooms are needed for the more costly high-fidelity human patient simulators with all of the equipment, technology, and added supplies needed for implementing simulations. In addition, some labs have a small control room with a one-way mirror attached to each simulation room.

Other problems include lack of faculty willingness to embrace new technology and other services offered by the skills lab. Implementation of high-fidelity simulation, evidence-based case scenarios, and the additional time it takes to have students, three to five at a time, complete the skills within the case scenarios requires dedicated faculty participation. Learning new simulation teaching strategies and management of the simulators requires additional faculty time and energy. Writing evidence-based scenarios that contain the necessary skills is another time-intensive faculty activity, unless these are purchased. According to Childs (2002), faculty and students must be interested and motivated to use the skills lab for the multiple teaching opportunities that are possible. Often, a core group of faculty members use the services of the skills lab on a routine basis, but all instructors should be informed about the applicability of skills lab services to augment the delivery of the curriculum content. In return, the skills lab must be responsive to the faculty and their needs to maximize the use of available technology.

Communication with faculty and students about the skills lab services is a critical element of an effectively functioning lab. This challenge is often addressed through the use of Web-based software. Currently, most colleges and universities support a Web-based framework such as Blackboard or WebCT. The skills lab should offer a Web site directed to students and faculty where policies and procedures, calendar events, and contact information for lab personnel are posted. A schedule of open lab times and remedial sessions should be easily accessible for students who need those services. Communication is an essential key to allow users to take full advantage of all the services offered by a well-equipped skills lab.

Every skills laboratory must be a safe environment for faculty, students, and staff. Skills labs are required to follow strict safety procedures to protect personnel and students in the lab from injury or spills. Needles, sutures, and performance of certain procedures pose daily threats. The expense to adhere to federal and local government regulations may prove costly but are a necessary component of a safe and effective skills lab.

CONCLUSION

The skills laboratory provides an enriched teaching and learning atmosphere that encourages active and involved exploration and mastery of new knowledge and skills to develop competent graduate nurses. Theory is applied to practice and validated in the skills lab through teaching and technology. The faculty member can use unlimited strategies to educate students who have a spectrum of learning needs in order to foster critical thinking. In the protected environment of the skills lab, students learn, make mistakes, question conceptual ideas, practice psychomotor skills, and expand knowledge to a new level of understanding. Students learn by doing through experimentation that would be impossible and dangerous in direct patient care situations. Faculty members have direct observation and supervision of all student activities which is often difficult in a busy clinical agency. Transition to the role of graduate nurse is enhanced by effective and innovative use of the new skills laboratory.

APPLIED EXAMPLES

Comprehensive Nursing Skills Experiences

In a fundamental skills course offered by various disciplines, skills are a primary focus requiring didactic instruction and demonstrations first given in lecture and then reinforced in the skills lab. Skills that are appropriate for beginning nursing students include the complex task of medication administration: obtaining or understanding healthcare provider orders, learning the appropriate dosages and where to research information about the drug, calculating dosages from the correct amount of drug available, safely and competently handling the syringe during drawing up of medication, administration, disposal of the syringe, recognizing appropriate sites for administration

(subcutaneous or intramuscular), performing the five rights prior to administration, and recording the medication in the permanent patient record. All these basic skills must be understood and practiced repeatedly by the student. To meet the wide range of learning styles, instruction should include verbal and written material as well as audio-visual demonstrations and one-on-one interactions and demonstrations with the students. Kinesthetic learning is provided by the use of different types of syringes, vials, and pills; and solitary practice is combined with discussion, reflective observation, and active experimentation.

Administering insulin and digoxin can be used as examples for student practice. Sliding scale insulin orders could be written in a mock chart, and students could be given various blood glucose results so that different amounts of insulin would need to be drawn up. In the lab, students practice drawing up insulin, selecting an appropriate site, administering the medication on a manikin, discarding the syringe, and documenting on the mock chart. They should also practice giving oral medications such as digoxin correctly, which would include auscultation of the apical pulse. Not only must they be able to perform the skill of giving the medication correctly, but they would also need to recognize that an apical pulse rate must be taken before administration, under which circumstances the medication should be withheld based on current literature, and when the healthcare provider must be notified for future actions.

Once the skills have been practiced, three or four students are introduced to the high-fidelity simulator. They are presented with the history and physical findings of a patient who is hospitalized with selected clinical problems. A mock chart is available with healthcare provider orders, which include treatment and medication orders. Medications are noted on the medication administration record, including insulin sliding scale, oral medication, and prn medication orders. The students are made aware of the time of day and results of lab studies such as blood glucose readings. Students at this point are assigned selected skills to perform, such as wound dressing change, urinary catheterization, administration of pain medication via the intramuscular route, application of bandages, or performance of a basic head-to-toe assessment. The skills are embedded in the scenario and must be performed according to patient need and healthcare provider orders. The students must prioritize their actions based on the dynamic events unfolding in the patient scenario. This complex situation fosters critical thinking and problem solving to meet patient demands. The faculty member acts as facilitator to encourage competent participation by individual students and provides immediate feedback to correct problems in cognition and performance of skills. As the student progresses in level of learning ability across the curriculum, the faculty member offers less prompting to increase the independence exhibited by the student. By applying adult learning principles, the student is allowed to demonstrate more creativity in a learning environment that supports personal knowledge and meets immediate learning goals.

Evaluation of required skills is an important function of the skills lab. The lab provides unlimited opportunities for faculty to observe and test acquisition of psychomotor skills as well as cognitive processing. For example, the evaluation process in the form of a formalized checkoff can be implemented at the end of a semester to determine mastery of required skills. Before the checkoff is completed, students receive detailed procedural (step-by-step) information or criteria regarding the skills that they must master. By knowing the exact expectation before the evaluation, the anxiety level experienced by the students is decreased, and the faculty member can more easily determine the skill level of an individual student unclouded by psychological barriers. Practice opportunities are provided to reinforce skills the week before checkoff. The lab is arranged to represent the hospital setting with a patient in bed, a medication room, and a supply area. The student receives an assigned skill, reviews

the patient's mock chart, assembles the necessary equipment to perform the skill, and prepares the patient for the procedure. The interaction with the manikin should appear as authentic as possible. This situation can be achieved by encouraging the student to communicate with the patient in a normal manner. The faculty member observes the performance of the skill based on the criteria previously provided to the student. A checkoff form is used to document and evaluate the student's actions in relation to the criteria. The faculty member does not interact with or prompt the student in any manner. If the student fails to follow the criteria, points are deducted, affecting the final score. The criteria contains selected critical behaviors that must be accomplished successfully to pass the evaluation. Examples of critical behaviors are contamination of a sterile field or recapping a used needle. If the student fails to acquire sufficient points or neglects to perform critical behaviors, the student fails the checkoff and is provided the opportunity for remediation and a repeated attempt. Failure of the course is possible if the student is unable to successfully master the performance of the skill. The skills lab is an excellent venue to assess competency and determine learning needs. By utilizing theory combined with innovative teaching approaches and technological advances in the skills laboratory, faculty members optimize learning opportunities.

REFERENCES

Benner, P. (2001). *From novice to expert: Excellence and power in clinical nursing practice*. Upper Saddle River, NJ: Prentice-Hall.

Billings, D. M., & Halstead, J. A. (2005). *Teaching in nursing: A guide for faculty*. St. Louis, MO: Elsevier Saunders.

Brimble, M. (2008). Skills assessment using video analysis in a simulated environment: An evaluation. *Pediatric Nursing, 20*(7), 26–31.

Childs, J. C. (2002). Clinical resource centers in nursing programs. *Nurse Educator, 27*(5), 232–235.

Clarke, D., Davies, J., & McNee, P. (2002). The case for a children's nursing skills laboratory. *Pediatric Nursing, 14*(7), 36–39.

Dobbin, K. R. (2001). Applying learning theories to develop teaching strategies for the critical care nurse: Don't limit yourself to the formal classroom lecture. *Critical Care Nursing Clinics of North America, 13*(1), 1–11.

Duffin, C. (2004). Simulated 'skills labs' to ease pressure on training. *Nursing Standard, 18*(39), 7.

Godson, N. R., Wilson, A., & Goodman, M. (2007). Evaluating student nurse learning in the clinical skills laboratory. *British Journal of Nursing, 16*(15), 942–945.

Infante, M. S. (1985). *The clinical laboratory*. New York: John Wiley.

Knowles, M. (1989). *The making of an adult education: An autobiographical journey*. San Francisco: Jossey-Bass.

Miller, H., Nichols, E., & Beeken, J. (2000). Comparing video-taped and faculty-present return demonstrations of clinical skills. *Journal of Nursing Education, 39*, 237–239.

Pravikoff, D. S., Tanner., A. B., & Pierce, S.T. (2005). Readiness for US nurses for evidence-based practice. *American Journal of Nursing, 105*(9), 40–52.

Schroeder, C. C. (2004). *New students – New learning styles*. Retrieved March 19, 2006, from http://www.virtualschool.edu/mon/Academia/KierseyLearningStyles.html

CHAPTER 16

Innovations in Facilitating Learning Using Simulation

Kimberly Leighton and Judy Johnson-Russell

INTRODUCTION

A new world of teaching opportunities has opened up to faculty in the healthcare industry in the last few years, and continues to grow in sophistication. These opportunities come at a time when educators are struggling with the realization that they are unable to prepare students adequately to assume the role of the healthcare provider. The vast amount of content, technical and interpersonal skills, and professional role expectations coupled with the increased number of incoming students and decreased availability of clinical placements (Nehring, 2010) have created a frustrating and sometimes dangerous situation. Clinical sites, which once were the primary place of learning, now restrict student activities leading to suboptimal experiences for content integration and mastery. Observational experiences and mentor–apprenticeship are not always beneficial as preceptors are frequently preoccupied with pressing patient problems and are not as invested in student learning.

The use of high-fidelity simulators creates a learning environment that closely resembles the clinical setting and can present learners with almost any situation they might find in a patient care setting. Although the technology still intimidates many, the techniques of facilitating learning are at the essence of this pedagogy. For those who embrace this pedagogy, teaching with high-fidelity simulators using realistic scenarios is exciting and rewarding. This methodology provides a safe environment for educating students without risk to human life and helps learners transfer knowledge and skills into actual clinical practice (Morgan, Cleave-Hogg, Desousa, & Lam-McCulloch, 2006). This chapter is intended to present innovative ways of utilizing simulation.

DEFINITIONS AND PURPOSES

Simulation and patient simulators are commonly referred to as low, medium, and high fidelity; however, there is no accepted classification that differentiates each from the other (Gaba, 2004). Fidelity of simulation follows a continuum beginning with low-fidelity simulation experiences, such as use of role play, or may incorporate a static mannequin that does not respond to intervention. Medium-fidelity simulations build on the degree of realism presented and may involve task trainers or moderate-fidelity simulators that provide a degree of feedback to the participant. At the upper range of the continuum lie high-fidelity simulations that provide for more immersive simulated clinical experiences (SCEs), using realistic and sophisticated computer technology to enhance the abilities of the patient simulator to provide feedback to learners (Decker, Sportsman, Puetz, & Billings, 2008; Hovancsek, 2007; Jeffries & Rogers, 2007a; Nehring, 2010). For an overview on background and use of the high-fidelity patient simulator, please see Chapter 14.

The purpose of integrating simulation into any curriculum is to provide students with beneficial learning experiences that will assist in meeting course and program objectives, while promoting safe patient care. The focus of the simulated patient experience is on the needs of the learner, rather than being on the needs of the patient, as it must be in the hospital or other clinical environment. Carefully chosen SCE provide the opportunity for multiple objectives to be met by multiple learners at the same time.

Task trainers or low-fidelity trainers and mannequins provide for repeated skill practice, such as catheter insertion. The catheter is inserted and removed according to a defined order of skill demonstration. Higher-fidelity simulators, sometimes referred to as human patient simulators, challenge students to reach higher level objectives by prioritizing care and promoting critical thinking. Students must critically think about why the catheter is important to the patient's care, its correlation to the illness or disease process, expected outcomes, and plan for additional care and safety needs of the patient as the scenario proceeds. The communication component is added as the patient simulator or the patient's family may question the student, asking for explanation of the procedure. Although the skill of catheterization is the same, it has not occurred in isolation, but in context as a part of the total care of the patient. As the simulation continues, students see the results of their interventions and the impact on the patient's condition (Leigh & Hurst, 2008).

An advantage to simulation is that an SCE can cover any desired time span to demonstrate the changes in the patient's condition. Students may take care of the patient upon admission to the emergency department, continue several hours later during admission to the patient care unit, as the patient's condition improves with intervention over time, and culminate with discharge planning and teaching. The time span of an SCE may cover anywhere from a few hours to days. Students experience the physiologic changes in the patient's condition over time, an advantage that is rarely available in the traditional clinical environment.

Faculty control the progression of the SCE by moving from state to state as objectives are met or appropriate student behaviors are demonstrated. Students benefit from being able to experience and participate in the whole process of managing the patient's illness or condition.

When sufficient time is provided for simulation, students in nursing have the opportunity to work through the process of completing assessments, analyzing data, planning appropriate care, prioritizing care, providing interventions, and evaluating the responses to their interventions. Rarely is there time in clinical to proceed purposefully at this slower pace.

Another purpose of simulation is to enhance communication. Communication in the simulation laboratory can occur face-to-face, via the phone, or via written documentation, which will be discussed later in this chapter. Students can be provided opportunities to communicate face-to-face with the off-going nurse (role played by faculty) during shift report, while being encouraged to ask questions or seek out additional patient information. Students communicate with each other as they determine priorities for care and problem solve situations that arise.

Communication with the patient and any present family members provides for experiences that may not occur in the traditional clinical environment and can be tailored by faculty to present specific concepts. For example, while receiving discharge instructions, the simulated patient may state that they do not have money to purchase their prescriptions. Perhaps as a simulated patient deteriorates, the student decides to call and notify the patient's family. It is at that point that the student learns that the phone has been disconnected because the bill has not been paid.

The simulation laboratory is also a safe place to practice communication with other healthcare providers, including physicians. Many, if not most, new nursing graduates have never been allowed to place a phone call to a healthcare provider while on the traditional clinical unit. Therefore, it is vital that this opportunity be included in simulated experiences. This communication may occur face-to-face with a faculty person role playing the provider or via phone. If the students place a call about early findings and the faculty wish to encourage further critical thinking, the caller can be told that the provider is not available because their cell phone is out of service range, they are busy in the operating room, or in a patient room at their office. Students should also practice communication with other healthcare providers by calling the laboratory, radiology, or other ancillary departments for test results.

It is important to make these exchanges as realistic as possible; however, it is equally important to not perpetuate stereotypes. For students who are novice at this type of communication, provide guidance and ask questions to promote critical thinking and organization. Using organizational tools, such as situation-background-assessment-recommendation (SBAR), will help to arrange thoughts prior to initiating communication. As students progress through the program and become more proficient, the realism of the verbal exchange should increase accordingly.

SCEs provide numerous opportunities for faculty to observe intrapersonal, interpersonal, and communication among small groups of students, as well as other professionals. It is often difficult to observe communication in the traditional clinical environment as clinical faculty attempt to meet the needs of all students. In the simulation laboratory, faculty can observe communication skills and provide immediate feedback (Pagano & Greiner, 2009).

The five core competencies for integrating safety and quality into nursing education developed by the Institute of Medicine (IOM) can be addressed in the simulation laboratory. The competencies are: (1) provide patient-centered care, (2) work in interdisciplinary teams, (3) employ evidence-based practice, (4) apply quality improvement, and (5) utilize information (IOM, 2003). Patient-centered care could include patient education and support interventions as patients learn to manage their health problems. Interdisciplinary teams can be formed with students working together to meet the scenario objectives. Nursing schools often collaborate with respiratory, pharmacy, social work, seminary, and medical students and together plan and carry out patient care. Evidence-based guidelines should be utilized to develop the SCE and to define interventions to be completed during the SCE. All SCEs can contain a safety issue so that students are able to identify hazards and take steps to prevent errors and accidents. Computers and personal digital assistants (PDAs) can be utilized in the simulation laboratory so that students experience working with computerized documentation systems and clinical decision support systems.

Policies and procedures from the traditional clinical environments should be available during the SCE, along with additional resources for students to reference prior to and during care provision. Students need to become expert seekers and processors of information in this ever expanding healthcare environment. Having appropriate resources and references, as well as the time to utilize them, during the SCE will assist graduates to know where and how to find needed information.

A real advantage to simulation is that it assists students in learning their role in emergency situations. When an emergency occurs in the hospital, generally students are not allowed to participate. However, in the simulation laboratory they can practice their role repeatedly without fear of harm to a patient. In addition, when incorrect decisions or interventions are completed in the simulation laboratory and the patient has a poor outcome, the opportunity exists to redo the SCE after debriefing occurs and correct patient management has been discussed. This allows the learner to see a better outcome and add experience.

Faculty often comment that participating with their clinical students in simulation provides them with knowledge of each student's strengths and limitations. This assists in individualizing clinical experiences and provides focus for remediation and assignments. It is particularly helpful if an SCE is in the beginning weeks of the rotation. It is also possible to see growth and changes in behavior when an SCE is conducted some weeks later.

DESIGNING THE SIMULATED CLINICAL EXPERIENCE

Deciding How to Integrate SCEs into the Curriculum

Deciding on appropriate SCEs to include into any curriculum takes careful thought and planning. All clinical courses and some didactic classes, such as pathophysiology, pharmacology, and cultural issues, can incorporate simulation. A review of the program's specific strengths and limitations will assist in choosing SCEs that will best meet student needs. Concepts that seem hard for students to grasp or that are difficult to teach are excellent choices for SCEs. Test scores such as from the National Council Licensure Examination-Registered Nurse or Practical Nurse (NCLEX-RN; NCLEX-PN), Assessment Technologies Institute (ATI), Health Education Systems, Inc. (HESI), or faculty developed tests for specific courses give indications of content and concepts that students are not comprehending. SCEs that address these areas should be chosen to facilitate learning in weak areas.

When choosing SCEs, patients with conditions or illnesses that are not readily available in the clinical agencies are beneficial, as all students then have the opportunity to care for that type of patient. SCEs that prepare students for specific clinical experiences, for high-risk situations, or for complex patients are also excellent choices. The timing of the simulation is another important consideration. Some schools incorporate simulation at the beginning of each course to assist with preparation for entering a new clinical rotation and again at the end of the rotation as a capstone experience. Another factor to consider is participation in the SCE in correlation to the presentation of didactic content. Most faculty utilize simulation after the content has been assigned or presented. Test scores after simulation may reflect a deeper understanding of the content than before simulation. Each course within a program will have its own needs and objectives that can be addressed through carefully planned SCEs.

Scheduling Students in the Simulation Laboratory

Scheduling of SCEs is often a major hurdle for faculty to overcome. For most educational institutions, class scheduling is part of a complex process that includes many departments, faculty, resources, and buildings. Making one change can be very disruptive. Therefore, it is valuable to consider a variety of options when integrating simulation into the curriculum, beginning with a critical look at current teaching methods and clinical experiences.

Often, nursing schools have been challenged to increase enrollment but have limited clinical resources. As a result, clinical experiences may have been added to the curricula that do not provide the best opportunity to meet learning objectives for the student. The site's experiences may be too complex, or too easy, for a given level of learner. Available hours may not fit easily into the course schedule. Occasionally, professional behaviors of the clinical site do not mesh with those of the nursing program. Faculty are encouraged to critically review all clinical placement sites to determine if needs are being well met in that environment. If not, consideration should be made for moving the experience to the simulation lab.

The question is often raised about the number of hours that can be provided in the simulation lab. This is dependent on the state Board of Nursing regulations in each state and may be prescriptive as to the number of hours or percentage of hours. Other states leave discretion to the faculty as long as program outcomes continue to be met. A more difficult question is, "How many hours of simulation are needed to replace the same number of clinical hours?" This question is much more challenging to answer and the answer needs to be supported by research.

Scheduling simulation throughout the curriculum is best achieved by using a variety of scheduling methods. This allows for increased simulation use with less disruption to the course schedule. Several methods can be utilized: stations in a lab, set blocks of time, postconference, entire day, and class time. It is important to remember that the students will always take longer to make decisions and perform skills than faculty expect, as this is part of their learning process. To decrease frustration and "catching up" during the day, allow more time than thought necessary to schedule SCEs.

Stations

This method works well for integrating SCEs into assessment and fundamental skills courses. These courses are often designed so that students work in pairs and small groups to practice psychomotor skills, communication techniques, and critical thinking. Students often rotate through different learning activities during lab time. A short SCE can be added that allows students to apply what they have learned in context of a patient situation. Using this method may result in adding time to the existing lab, but more often, another learning station is deleted.

Blocks of Time

This method creates a set period of time for self-determined groups or faculty-assigned groups to participate in an SCE. All blocks of time might be together during a specific week of the course, or the blocks of time could be distributed throughout the semester until everyone has completed their time. Blocks of time must be long enough and filled with enough activity to make it worth the students' time to come to campus for the experience. For programs with set amounts of student contact hours, some faculty have decreased their clinical time by 10 minutes/week over a 15-week semester, resulting in the ability to reassign that time (150 minutes) to simulation.

Postconference

This scheduling method can be planned in advance or done impromptu based on activities of the clinical day. Typically, postconferences last approximately 1 hour and occur at the end of the clinical day. They are designed to serve as a time to reflect on the day's activities, but are often used for various other activities such as topical review of difficult theoretical concepts, review prior to exams, or even as time to remain on the clinical unit to observe an unusual activity. This time frame is included in the schedule of the clinical day and some faculty facilitators have found that SCEs designed to include concepts unique to their clinical unit, are a valuable use of this time. For example, a postoperative unit may have several patients with chest tubes but not every student has the opportunity to care for those patients. Managing a chest tube patient in the simulation laboratory provides an opportunity for every student to care for that type of patient.

Entire Day

In this scheduling method, a clinical group participates in various SCEs over an entire day. Rather than attending a hospital unit or clinical agency for clinical, the students report to the simulation laboratory. The simulation laboratory is placed on the clinical schedule rotation instead of an agency site. A typical day's schedule should begin and end at the usual clinical times. Students can provide care for a variety of patient types, depending on the length of the scenarios. It is helpful to assign rotating roles to keep students engaged. Expectations for preparation, care, resource use, and documentation should be the same as on the clinical unit.

During Class

Simulators can be used during class time by either moving a portable simulator to the classroom or using video to transmit from the simulation laboratory to the classroom. Portable simulators are designed for ease of movement and can be placed in the front of the classroom to demonstrate various concepts. Students can be chosen to participate in caring for the simulated patient either randomly, based on skill level, or based on identified learning needs. Students remaining in the audience can participate in directing the care, prioritizing care, or observing for various aspects of care, such as communication techniques. Using video, especially two-way interactive video, provides the same in-class learning advantage without moving the simulator. Another learning opportunity is provided when both an adult and pediatric simulator is moved into the classroom, setting the stage for comparing and contrasting between the care of an adult patient and pediatric patient with the same illness or disease process.

An additional in-class learning opportunity exists through use of the simulation software. The computer running the simulation software can be connected to the classroom projector, allowing all students to see the patient parameters. After orienting students to the various parameters, the faculty member can demonstrate the hemodynamic changes that occur with hypervolemia, hypovolemia, pneumothorax, pericardial tamponade, different cardiac rhythms, and numerous medications. The simulator does not have to be connected to this computer in order to demonstrate these features. Further discussion of classroom use of simulation is provided later in this chapter.

Fidelity of the Simulated Clinical Experience

Realism of the SCE is commonly referred to as fidelity. There is no consensus as to how much fidelity is necessary for learning to occur, but many believe that the closer to real a scenario is, the more engaged students become and the opportunities for learning to occur increase. Medley and Horne (2005) recommend that in a high-fidelity SCE, the real-life situation be recreated in as realistic manner as possible. Cantrell, Meakim, and Cash (2008) identified the theme "the more real the simulation, the better the learning" when analyzing the qualitative portion of their study of student evaluations of a simulation experience. In a small pilot study, researchers found no statistically significant difference in pretest/post-test scores of a group learning with low-fidelity simulation and a group learning with high-fidelity simulation (Kardong-Edgren, Anderson, & Michaels, 2007). It is important to match the level of fidelity to the desired learning outcomes, as some SCEs require higher levels of fidelity than others (Gaba, 2004).

The learning can be positive or negative and, while it is hoped that only positive learning is transferred to real patient care, the potential for negative transfer of learning also exists. Therefore, it is important that processes and procedures in the simulation laboratory as closely mimic reality as possible. Four major areas of fidelity should be considered when creating the SCE: the simulator, the physical patient, holistic aspects of the patient, and the environment. Simulator fidelity was addressed previously in this chapter.

Physical Patient

Fidelity of the simulated patient's physical condition should impact as many of the student's senses as possible: sight, smell, touch, and hearing. This involves significant creativity on the part of the faculty member but can often be accomplished at little cost. Creating this type of fidelity is often referred to as moulage, a word often associated with the military. Examples of low-cost solutions to create physical conditions are provided in Table 16-1. Always test new moulage in an inconspicuous area if there is a risk for staining to occur.

Table 16-1 Physical Fidelity of the Simulated Patient

Sense	Physical Condition or Disease	Moulage
Sight	Vomit	Egg white whisked with fork; streak yellow food coloring with toothpick tip
	Blood clots	Cherry pie filling; thick lumpy tapioca with red food coloring
Smell	Incontinence	Water with yellow food coloring and ammonia
	Vomit	Add grated parmesan cheese to vomit
Touch	Edema	Memory foam covered with ace wrap or antiembolism stockings
	Clammy skin	Spray with water bottle
Hearing	Hospital sounds	Loop a recording and play back
	Hospital pages	Announce random overhead pages via microphone

Holistic Aspects of the Patient

Nursing care of the patient involves not only physical care, but developmental, cultural, psychosocial, and spiritual care as well. These important aspects are often left out of the SCE. Undergraduate nursing students were asked their perceptions of how well their learning needs were met in the traditional clinical environment and in the simulated clinical environment (Leighton, 2007). Learning needs related to holistic patient care were better met in the traditional clinical environment ($P = .000$).

Positively impacting these learning needs is easy to do in the simulation lab and costs little or no money to do so. In most cases, adding more information to the patient's story or health history can add this dimension. Table 16-2 outlines several ways in which holistic patient care can be added to the SCE.

A variety of props can be added to the simulated patient's room to help prompt students to address holistic aspects of care. A picture frame with a family picture including several children might be placed at the bedside to see if students address the patient's role in the family. A Bible, Koran, or other religious book or icon can be placed at the bedside to shift the focus to spiritual aspects of care. It is helpful to have resources available to students to look up information about different cultural and religious beliefs while caring for the simulated patient.

Environment

Simulation centers or laboratories come in all shapes and sizes, from the corner of a skills lab to a large, free-standing space with individualized and very realistic patient rooms. No matter the space, it is important to make it appear as realistic as possible to the intended clinical environment. While this is typically a patient's hospital room, many SCEs can occur in a patient's home, an outpatient setting, or in the recovery room. Having the equipment and props characteristic of the desired environment will help learners to be engaged and learn use of appropriate equipment and supplies.

Obtaining supplies and equipment can be a costly endeavor. Consider discussing simulation needs with clinical nurse managers who may be able to divert opened sterile kits to the simulation laboratory if they cannot be used with human patients. Many hospitals have warehouses where unused or overstocked equipment is stored. Simulation laboratories are often able to purchase at discount or borrow equipment. Many pharmacies now return expired medications for account credit; however, simulation personnel may be able to obtain these medication vials or ampoules. Different regions of the

Table 16-2 Holistic Care of the Simulated Patient

Aspect	Patient	Concern
Developmental	45-year-old male with heart attack	He and wife have five children and he is unable to return to construction job
	14-year-old with abdominal pain	Sexually active and has contracted a sexually transmitted infection
Cultural	26-year-old female speaks only Vietnamese	Only available person who knows Vietnamese is the hospital's maintenance man
	88-year-old Native American patient who urgently needs medication	Prefers to wait for medicine elder
Psychosocial	8-year-old boy requires appendectomy	Parents recently moved to area and father's health insurance has not yet taken effect
	72-year old patient with chronic obstructive pulmonary disease requiring several medications	Unable to afford medications with current finances
Spiritual	52-year-old female requires abdominal surgery	Refuses to remove jewelry with religious icons
	66-year-old patient who was just diagnosed with cancer	Refuses treatment because believes the illness is a result of past sins

country have differing rules and regulations as to disposal of expired items. Some simulation laboratories have reported obtaining syringes and expired intravenous fluids from veterinarians and from patients who no longer require home care services. Be creative in seeking out solutions to supply and equipment needs.

Student Preparation/Professional Expectations

In the previously mentioned survey of undergraduate nursing students (Leighton, 2007), it was reported that students did not prepare to the same level for simulated experiences (0–1 hour) as they did for human patients (2–4 hours). Many reasons exist for this difference, such as the student may have already experienced caring for the type of simulated patient and therefore need less preparation time, personal or social obligations limit preparation, or the student may perceive the simulated experience as less stressful and without consequence if performance is poor.

It is recommended that students prepare for SCEs in the same manner and to the same degree as they do for traditional clinical experiences. Providing the student with focused preparation activities is also more efficient than the time spent seeking out information from the chart, the patient, the family, and other caregivers. Preparation activities contribute to learning and allow the simulation facilitator to answer questions, clarify misconceptions, enhance the knowledge base, and facilitate learning rather than teach. Time in the simulation lab is therefore more likely to be focused and intense.

Professional behavior and dress is important to the learning experience in the simulation laboratory. In fact, observations have been made that students behave more professionally when in uniform than when in street clothes (Ravert, 2010). While learning to manage a variety of patient types and conditions, nursing students are also learning professional behaviors and communication techniques. Providing an environment in which professional behaviors are modeled and practiced will likely enhance professionalism. At the same time, state boards of nursing are often being asked to consider patient simulation as a replacement for traditional clinical experiences. If this is to occur, then efforts should be made to ensure that the experiences in the simulation laboratory are as realistic as possible.

IMPLEMENTING THE SIMULATED CLINICAL EXPERIENCE

Faculty Roles

Faculty roles during simulation are primarily facilitative. Rather than the sage on the stage, faculty become the guide on the side (Kardong-Edgren, Starkweather, & Ward, 2008). Although the role varies somewhat depending on the level of the students, the faculty may provide the learner with prompts and cues. These are most often in the form of carefully asked questions that stimulate critical thinking and problem solving and assist the student in taking necessary actions with appropriate interventions. As students progress through the program, fewer prompts and cues are required or are given.

Critical thinking, problem solving, and planning care are aided in simulation when a large flip chart with removable paper is utilized. One person is assigned to be the documenter/recorder for the simulation. Beginning with report, the documenter writes down pertinent information and continues to record as assessments, new data, and interventions occur. The information can then be easily viewed by all participants and is referred to constantly. This documentation can be utilized as the student calls the healthcare provider, as the faculty asks questions about the meaning of newly acquired lab data, or as students plan care based on new orders. The paper can easily be removed and taken to debriefing for further evaluation and discussion of care. Alternatively, a whiteboard may be used for data gathering documentation.

The Dreyfus and Dreyfus' model of skill acquisition, adapted for use with nursing by Benner (1984), supports learning on a continuum beginning with novice and progressing through advanced beginner, competent, proficient, and expert stages. This model has implications for faculty who facilitate in the simulation laboratory. Learning the skill of facilitation is a new challenge for most faculty and they begin at a novice level. It is important for faculty to recognize this and to not attempt a SCE that is overly complex and detailed for their first effort. Begin with simple scenarios as they can often have as much impact as those that are complex. As the level of comfort with facilitation grows, so will creativity and willingness to attempt more complex scenarios. Trying to do too much at the beginning will only frustrate the facilitator and the students, making the next attempt at simulation more of a challenge.

The novice-to-expert approach has also been used to help determine the role of facilitators when interacting with students in the simulation laboratory. Novice students may experience increased stress or anxiety when placed in an unfamiliar environment and given new expectations to care for a simulated patient. They have little to no experience to draw from and it may be of value for the faculty to be present at the bedside, assist in proper assessment techniques, and respond to questions immediately.

As the students progress to advanced beginner, the facilitator can play the role of a family member. Continued presence in the room provides a level of comfort and reportedly decreases anxiety among students. The facilitator asks questions of students while in the family member role and is able to determine if students understand the care they are providing and can provide appropriate education and responses to the patient and family.

When learners reach the proficient stage, facilitators become further removed, although depending on the laboratory set up, they might remain in the room with the students. However, at this point, they only observe unless it is essential to intervene and redirect the students. At the expert stage, the facilitator is completely removed from the simulated patient room and observes through a one-way window or via technology such as Skype.

Student Roles

One of the biggest challenges facing faculty in the simulation laboratory is that of group size. Defining roles for each individual student brings focus to the experience and decreases confusion. A variety of roles can be utilized, depending on the SCE. Roles can be assigned or chosen at random, or purposefully assigned based on identified student weaknesses. Suggestions of roles and responsibilities utilized by many simulation laboratories are provided in Table 16-3.

Facilitators are encouraged to utilize roles that are nurse specific as outlined in Table 16-3. Assigning roles of other healthcare providers, such as laboratory technician, respiratory therapist, or physician, are often troublesome, as the students do not have the background to know the roles of those providers. It is also challenging to have students play the role of the family member, again because most lack that

Table 16-3 Roles for Students in the Simulation Laboratory

Role	Responsibilities
Primary nurse	Assessment; final decision Consider two primary nurses so one student is not responsible alone if a poor outcome is experienced
Secondary nurse	Backs up primary nurse if two primary system not used Assists the primary nurse in assessment and decision making
Medication nurse	Administers medications safely according to orders
Documentation nurse	Documents on paper or electronically to maintain a patient record Documents on flip chart or whiteboard to keep all informed of assessment findings and care provided
Healthcare communicator	Provides information to healthcare provider in person or via phone calls; contacts ancillary departments for test results
Observer	Provides focused role for observer such as observing for communication between nurse and patient; identification of cultural care; patient education provided by nurse; recognition of psychosocial care; overall management of care

type of experience, but also because they have to perform in front of their peers. Those who are shy or introverted tend to struggle in these types of roles.

There is often concern expressed by facilitators that the students in the observation role will not learn as much as those actively caring for the simulated patient. In Phase III of the NLN/Laerdal project, *Designing and Implementing Models for the Innovative Use of Simulation to Teach Nursing Care of Ill Adults and Children: A National, Multi-Site, Multi-Method Study*, researchers reported that there were no significant differences in knowledge gain, satisfaction, or self confidence based on the role of the student (Jeffries & Rizzolo, 2006).

Use of Resources in the Simulation Lab

PDAs are beginning to be incorporated into simulation experiences. During the SCE, students can immediately access textbook information and can look up diseases, care plans, drug and laboratory guides, medical dictionaries, procedural guidelines, and literature databases. It is important in today's constantly changing healthcare environment that students learn where to access needed information rather than expecting to always rely on memory. Nurses need to be able to rely on the latest evidence-based information to make decisions and to have it available when needed at the point of care. PDAs are invaluable as students move from performing skills to making decisions about care based on the latest knowledge available. Clinical calculators are also utilized in simulation laboratories to more safely determine drug dosing, intravenous drip rates, and for other physiological calculations.

The Joint Commission (TJC) identified the leading root cause of sentinel events in the United States between 1995 and 2006 as a breakdown in hand-off communication (WHO, 2007). These sentinel events resulted in unintended harm to patients and prompted TJC to recommend that hospitals standardize hand-off communications. SBAR is being used by hospitals across the country to improve communication. During the SCE, students can have valuable practice in communication skills by giving hand-off reports, by calling healthcare providers, and by interacting with the interdisciplinary team utilizing the SBAR format. Use of the format assists students to become more organized and confident in their thinking and reporting.

Charting

Charts and forms, if not on the lab's computer, should be constructed for each SCE. Documentation forms should be as similar as possible to those the students utilize in their clinical areas. Additional forms that might be appropriate for the SCE, such as emergency department records, blood transfusion and blood bank forms, and incident reports, for example, should also be available

Various methods are utilized in simulation laboratories to create documentation opportunities for students. It is helpful to utilize a system as close to what students see on the traditional clinical unit as possible; however, many simulation laboratories do not have the resources to do this. There are several existing commercial products available, but many simulation facilitators create their own system.

Types of documentation can range from paper charting, using blank forms obtained from a local facility or creating one's own, to electronic charting similar to an electronic health record. The level of complexity in the design of these documentation systems is up to the faculty. Some faculty created realistic systems using Microsoft office products such as Word and Excel. There is no known research pointing to whether one method is better than another. The underlying principles and concepts of documentation are the important focus.

Multidisciplinary/Interdisciplinary Team Simulations

As nursing faculty become more comfortable with simulation, they are beginning to incorporate SCEs that foster an interdisciplinary team approach with other healthcare students. The IOM has said that "all health professionals should be educated to deliver patient-centered care as member of an interdisciplinary team, emphasizing evidence-based practice, quality improvement approaches, and informatics" (IOM, 2003, p. 3). As the population ages and lives with multiple comorbidities and chronic health needs, their care requires the collaboration of multiple healthcare professionals. Therefore, simulation provides the perfect opportunity for students to work together on complex patient care problems. Pharmacy, respiratory therapy, social work, seminary, and medical practitioners or students have all collaborated with nursing students during SCEs. Students learn the knowledge, roles, responsibilities, and frame of reference each brings to the patient situation. They learn to work together as a team, to share the information they have about the patient, and to communicate and resolve differences related to care.

Many hospitals and schools of nursing are utilizing the TeamSTEPPS program developed by the Department of Defense's Patient Safety Program in collaboration with the Agency for Healthcare Research and Quality. This program provides materials and a training curriculum for an evidence-based teamwork system to improve communication and teamwork skills. Information about this program may be obtained by going to http://teamstepps.ahrq.gov/. The goal of TeamSTEPPS, and all intradisciplinary training, is to assist in providing higher quality, safer patient care through more effective communication among health professionals.

Classroom Use of Simulation

Most faculty think of a laboratory space when envisioning the use of patient simulation in their courses; however, simulation can be added to the classroom experience as well. Three common methods of integrating simulation into classroom teaching follow.

Simulator in Classroom

Many patient simulators are portable and can be moved easily into a classroom. While this may seem overwhelming the first one or two times, it is not difficult to learn with repetition and can be accomplished in only a few minutes. Once in the classroom, place it at the front of the class and invite two or three students to care for the patient, who should be designed to facilitate learning of concepts currently being taught. Students often hesitate to volunteer for this role and may have to be assigned.

The simulated patient's condition or illness may be cared for to resolution during one time frame of the class or the care can be divided into sections corresponding to the didactic material as it is presented. Another option is to simulate two different but similar conditions, such as heart failure and chronic obstructive pulmonary disease. Selected students care for each patient and the subsequent patient management is subjected to contrast and comparison analysis.

Simulation via Two-Way Interactive Video

Some simulators and their environs are not designed for easy transport and cannot be removed from the laboratory. The simulated patient remains in the laboratory and the designated number of students leave the classroom to care for the patient there. This interaction is broadcast to the classroom using existing interactive video capabilities. Many schools do not have the resources for this type of equipment but there are now many free or low-cost options, such as Skype, now available via the Internet.

Simulation Software

The laptops that run the simulation software can be connected to an overhead projector in the classroom in the same manner that a computer is connected to project PowerPoint presentations. Once connected, the students are oriented to the instructor view and instructed on which visible parameters to monitor. Simple to complex material can be visually presented using the following examples:

- Administer the same medication and dose to a young healthy simulated patient and to a simulated patient with cardiovascular disease. Observe changes in blood pressure and heart rate (novice students) or mean arterial pressure and central venous pressure (advanced students).
- Provoke a pneumothorax through the software and have learners monitor the respiratory rate and oxygen saturation levels for changes.
- Create a pericardial tamponade through the software and have learners monitor hemodynamic changes with various amounts of fluid.
- Remove 2 to 3 liters of blood through the software and have students monitor hemodynamic changes. Conversely, administer 2 to 3 liters of crystalloids and monitor the same hemodynamics.

POSTSIMULATED CLINICAL EXPERIENCE

Debriefing

Debriefing is essential to the simulation experience. It is during this time when students have the opportunity to reflect on the experience that much of the learning occurs. Faculty function as facilitators in the debriefing by stimulating students to consider what they were thinking during the simulation, how they were feeling, what they did, what occurred as a result, and how they can apply what they have learned to their care with real patients. It is important for students to be able to follow the fast-paced simulation with a quiet time away from the simulator where they can cognitively process and reflect on what occurred. Video clips may also aid in the understanding of what transpired (Fanning & Gaba, 2007).

There are four parts to the verbal debriefing: the introduction, sharing of personal reactions, discussion of events, and the wrap-up (Johnson-Russell & Bailey, 2010). Although the first three are sometimes discussed simultaneously, all should be covered at some point in the debriefing.

The introduction sets the stage for the debriefing by letting students know that this is a safe place to discuss what went on and that what they share about their feelings and behavior will not be discussed outside the room. Many faculty have students sign a confidentiality statement at this time. Students appreciate when faculty also sign this statement so that they know that what went on in the SCE will not affect their future in school. At this time, the faculty inform students about their expectations for the debriefing. They remind them that the expectation is that all students will contribute to the discussions by analyzing the simulation and what transpired in depth. Students are also expected to look at not just what went on with the patient, but also at their own behavior as well as how they functioned as a team.

In the immediate postsimulation period, there is often excitement and/or anxiety from the tension built up during the simulation. Expressing these feelings or sharing of personal reactions is often necessary before students can cognitively process other aspects of the SCE. Assisting students to delve deeper into the events that led to these feelings may provide a new awareness of their functioning and thought processes.

The discussion of events focuses more on the patient, the condition, the interventions, and the outcomes. The facilitator can segue into this part of the discussion using comments the students have previously just expressed, or ask specific questions about their knowledge of the patient and their condition, what they anticipated the outcome would be, how the SCE unfolded, how they prioritized and instituted a plan to manage care, and what they might have done differently. Asking about what resources were utilized and others that were available but not used may be appropriate. Additionally, it is important to have students look at safety needs of the patient and if any of these were overlooked and the possible problems as a result of the oversight. Questions about their individual functioning, difficulties in performing care, and what each student needs to do to remedy their deficiencies should be asked.

Team functioning is important to discuss, especially in relation to communication with team members. Communication with family members and the patient may also need to be addressed. Debriefing is an excellent time to have students role play and practice more effective communication. Students frequently have difficulty relating the events of the SCE to the real world because their experience is limited. It is often valuable, therefore, to spend time discussing how the SCE applies to the clinical setting and to patients they may encounter in the future.

Video clips may provide additional stimulation for discussions. They should be used as an adjunct in the debriefing to assist students in understanding those things that they might have missed or when there have been procedural problems, missed cues, or poor decision making. Viewing the videotape is an excellent way of helping learners understand the events that transpired in the SCE and their participation in them. Viewing segments where they performed well is also important in reinforcing appropriate behaviors and instilling confidence.

The summary or wrap-up can be accomplished by the faculty using statements the students have verbalized about what they felt went well and what did not. Faculty can also remind students of areas that need improvement. Some faculty prefer to have the students summarize the session by verbalizing what they learned from the SCE. Students appreciate hearing positive comments from the faculty about their performance or the improvements in their functioning that were observed.

Additionally, some faculty post questions on their intranet, have the student reflect on the experience, and answer the questions within 24 hours of the SCE.

Students should complete an evaluation at the end of the debriefing. These can give the faculty valuable information about what was most helpful to the students and what might be changed to make the SCE an even better learning experience.

Faculty may want to utilize the debriefing assessment for simulation in healthcare (DASH) from the Center for Medical Simulation to evaluate and develop their debriefing skills. Information about the rating forms can be found at the DASH Web site (http://harvardmedsim.org/cms/dash.html).

Postsimulated Patient Death

Many simulation facilitators are fearful that simulated death experiences will cause the student to believe they killed the simulated patient or are responsible for its death, leading to feelings of guilt. There is also concern that buried feelings may rise to the surface leading to psychological trauma. There is no literature to support these assumptions; however, the facilitator is charged with recognizing and managing psychological stress of participants (Leighton, 2009a).

The debriefing process is vital to managing this psychological stress as students are given the opportunity to talk about their feelings and explore the events that occurred during the SCE in a safe, nonjudgmental environment. The facilitator may consider involving a chaplain or mental health practitioner in the scenario or during the debriefing. In some cases, the facilitator may need to refer the student for further psychological assistance (Leighton, 2009a).

Evaluation/Testing/Assessment

Considerable discussion occurs at simulation conferences and informal meetings about evaluating students in the simulation laboratory. Several schools have developed rubrics to use for this process, while formal research protocols have created other methods to evaluate learning, critical thinking, or components of critical judgment (Lasater, 2007). At this time, more nursing schools use simulation as a teaching strategy than do those who use simulation as an evaluation tool (Hovancsek, 2007).

It is imperative that nursing programs identify their philosophy related to evaluation or assessment in the simulation laboratory. To begin, definitions must be determined. During meeting discussions, participants use a variety of different terminology to describe evaluation, assessment, and testing. It is clear that many of these conversations are attempting the compare apples to oranges.

Questions that should be considered during discussions about evaluation, testing, and assessment could include:

- Is the simulation lab better suited for facilitating learning or for evaluating students? Is it possible to do both?
- Is it fair to test students if they have not had significant exposure to simulated clinical experiences?
- Are faculty all competent in their roles? How is this variable controlled for evaluation purposes?
- How do we account for the variety of student responses and interventions that are inherent in simulations?
- Are we sending mixed messages when we tell students that simulation is a safe environment to learn in and then use that same environment for evaluation?
- Do we test students in the traditional clinical environment? Is it then fair to test in the simulation lab?
- If the focus is on testing, will the experience become an experience about performing rather than about learning?
- What can you learn about your students in the simulation environment without formal evaluation or testing?
- If we say that most of the learning occurs in debriefing, can we fairly evaluate students before that debriefing occurs? (Leighton, 2009b, p. e57).

If the decision is made to evaluate simulations, the faculty must determine the purpose of the evaluation, decide when to evaluate, create an evaluation plan, utilize instruments to collect the data, and interpret the data (Jeffries & Rogers, 2007b). Various instruments can be found in the education and simulation literature; however, the facilitator must consider the reliability and validity of the tool to be used.

No matter what decision is made regarding evaluation or assessment of learning in the simulation laboratory, the SCE itself must be evaluated. Obtaining information about the design of the simulation, availability of resources, effectiveness of the facilitator, perception of learning outcomes, and suggestions for future SCEs provides valuable insight to the facilitator (Horn & Carter, 2007). This information should be trended and adjustments to the scenario made as necessary.

Research Opportunities

It should be clear to the reader of this chapter that a wide variety of research opportunities exist for the users of simulation. While simulation has been used in healthcare education for years, the use of high-fidelity patient simulation is still in its infancy in nursing education. While it is often bemoaned that there is little research pointing to the efficacy of this teaching strategy, the research base is growing as facilitators become more comfortable in their role.

Conducting research in the simulation laboratory has several advantages over research in the traditional clinical environment; namely, that there is no risk to patients. Facilitators are also able to control the scenario, patient responses, communication with healthcare providers, and what equipment is available. However, those same faculty are also as difficult to control as a variable. Faculty have different levels of education regarding the role of facilitator, respond variably to students' efforts to communicate, and often need to step outside of the planned script to respond to unpredictable student actions (Alinier, 2008).

There have been many obstacles to using research data to support increased use of patient simulation or to justify the expense and time required to learn. A systematic research review, over a 34-year period of time ending in 2003, revealed wide variety in research design, methods of measuring outcomes, journal report structure, as well as use of small sample sizes (McGahie, Pugh, & Wayne, 2008).

It is a responsibility of each of us as simulation facilitators and proponents to help move the field forward through well-designed research studies and documentation of best practice and standards of excellence. It is no longer enough to document that students like simulation or that they prefer this method to another. The time has come to document that learning occurs and that it is equal to or better than our traditional teaching methods. As the competition for clinical sites continues to build, simulation will take a vital role in the future of nursing education.

CONCLUSION

This chapter has provided information intended to help those who take on the challenge of facilitating learning in the simulation laboratory. While many nursing programs have managed to obtain funding for simulation equipment, there has often been little forethought into how faculty will manage to learn this type of teaching strategy and where the time will come from for that purpose (Kardong-Edgren & Oermann, 2009). This chapter was intended to help aide the process of faculty development by providing realistic ideas that can be easily implemented by facilitators of learning in simulation laboratories. The simulator and its features have little value if the faculty does not know how to effectively teach with the technology.

APPLIED EXAMPLE

STRATEGY

Incorporation of fidelity, role of faculty, and holistic aspects of patient care for a beginning assessment course SCE. Participants in the simulation laboratory include the course faculty member and up to eight students.

Expectations

The students are expected to obtain subjective and objective assessment data and inform the healthcare provider of their findings. Prerequisite knowledge should include anatomy and physiology of the cardiovascular system and corresponding assessment techniques. This is a young morbidly obese female patient whose symptoms are precipitated by a systolic heart murmur.

Setting

The simulator is lying on a bed or stretcher and has not been seen by a healthcare provider. Place two individual breast models (often used to teach palpation for lumps) on the chest of the simulator. The patient's obesity can be simulated by placing a pillow over the abdomen and securing it with an ace wrap or gauze roll. Put female clothes appropriate for the weather on the simulator (it is easiest to cut the shirt up the back leaving the collar intact; cut the pants along the back to the inseam to allow ease of application). Apply a female wig. Makeup can be applied to the simulator after it is tested in a nonvisible place for staining. Personal effects such as magazine, cell phone, and purse can be placed on the bedside table next to a bottle of sugared carbonated beverage.

Simulator Settings

Set systolic murmur (or other preferred abnormal heart sound). All other settings are normal.

Faculty Role

This is the first SCE for students and, therefore, they are at a novice level and will need faculty assistance. It is preferable to orient students to the simulator and its features prior to starting the scenario. Only tell students what they need to know to care for this patient, as providing information on intravenous (IV) sites, defibrillation, or monitoring is above their knowledge level and will be extraneous information.

Begin outside of the simulator's room and brief students on the patient who has just arrived to the healthcare provider's office. Report is as follows:

> "This is a 38-year-old female with complaints of fatigue, orthopnea, and palpitations. She is 5'2" tall and weighs 100 kg."

Student Expectations

- Knock on the door and announce entry
- Introduce self and role to patient
- Wash hands
- Ask subjective questions to obtain more information from the patient, such as:
    - How long ago did you symptoms start? (6 months ago; gradually worsening)
    - Any associated symptoms? (no dyspnea or chest pain)
    - What makes the symptoms worse? (walking and exercise)

- What makes the symptoms go away? (rest)
- How many pillows do you use at night? (three)
- Do you have any history of medical problems? (no)
- Do you have any family history of medical problems? (no cardiac disease)
- Do you smoke, drink alcohol, or use drugs not prescribed for you? (no)
- How much do you exercise in a week? (none)
- Has there been any change in your weight recently? (gained 40 pounds past 4 months)
- What is you typical diet? (fast food, soda)
- Do you take any medications? (ibuprofen as needed for back pain)
- When was the last time you saw a healthcare provider?

Questioning may continue until the facilitator believes that enough data has been collected. The facilitator then prompts the beginning of the physical assessment.

Student Expectations

- Wash hands
- Explain what will be done to patient
- Conduct general survey
- Provide for privacy
- Head-to-toe physical assessment with emphasis on cardiovascular system
- Wash hands
- Make sure personal items are in reach
- Ensure safe environment

During the physical assessment, the students will discover an abnormality in the heart sounds. Although it may be beyond their scope to recognize and define a heart murmur, they should be able to identify that an abnormality exists. All other findings, including vital signs are normal.

Holistic Aspects (one or more may be included):

- Psychosocial: Patient does not have health insurance and voices concern about how to pay for office visit, follow-up tests, or prescriptions.
- Spiritual: Patient may be anxious and ask student to pray with her.
- Cultural: Patient may be from a culture other than that of most of the students.
- Developmental: Patient may blame weight gain on a recent life experience, such as a divorce.

ANTICIPATED AND UNANTICIPATED EVENTS AND CONSEQUENCES

Nervousness

As this is often the first SCE for the students, they are prone to nervousness and have trouble getting started. The facilitator may need to go around the bed, student by student, and ask them to pose a subjective question to the patient. The person responding as the patient should be patient and allow time for questions to be formulated, not rushing the students.

Scattered Thought Processes

Novice students tend to randomly ask subjective questions without organization. Following subjective questioning, the facilitator can help them to prioritize their completed assessment questions and findings.

Incorrect Assessment Techniques

The facilitator is at the bedside with this novice group and can correct technique as problems occur. Unless the SCE is recorded, this level of learner may not recall what they did right or wrong by the time debriefing occurs.

Failure to Recognize Abnormality

This may occur in the novice student due to lack of experience. If this is the case, the facilitator should point it out and have all students listen to the heart sounds. The respiratory rate may be lowered on the simulator and the heart sound volume increased to facilitate hearing of abnormal heart sounds.

EVALUATION OF LEARNER ATTAINMENT

The intent of this SCE is to provide an introductory level experience for the student who has not yet interacted with a real patient and is just beginning to learn physical assessment techniques and concepts. The facilitator will often be surprised by the learner's inability to formulate subjective questions and conduct a basic physical assessment. Remembering that novice learners have no experiences to draw on will keep expectations in perspective. Learners should be able to demonstrate physical assessment techniques learned in class; however, they often need help finessing their technique and need reassurance that they are doing the assessment correctly.

REFERENCES

Alinier, G. (2008). Pitfalls to avoid in designing and executing research with clinical simulation. In R. R. Kyle Jr. & W. B. Murray (Eds.), *Clinical simulation: Operations, engineering and management*. New York: Elsevier, Inc.

Benner, P. (1984). *From novice to expert: Excellence and power in clinical nursing practice*. Menlo Park, CA: Addison-Wesley.

Cantrell, M. A., Meakim, C., & Cash, K. (2008). Development and evaluation of three pediatric-based clinical simulations. *Clinical Simulation in Nursing Education, 4*(1), e1.

Decker, S., Sportsman, S., Puetz, L., & Billings, L. (2008). The evolution of simulation and its contribution to competency. *The Journal of Continuing Education in Nursing, 39*(2), 74–80.

Fanning, R. M., & Gaba, D. M. (2007). The role of debriefing in simulation-based learning. *Simulation in Healthcare, 2*, 115–125.

Gaba, D. (2004). A brief history of mannequin-based simulation & application. In W. F. Dunn (Ed.), *Simulators in critical care education and beyond*. Des Plaines, IL: The Society of Critical Care Medicine.

Horn, M., & Carter, N. (2007). Practical suggestions for implementing simulations. In P. R. Jeffries (Ed.), *Simulation in nursing education*. New York: National League for Nursing.

Hovancsek, M. T. (2007). Using simulations in nursing education. In P. R. Jeffries (Ed.), *Simulation in nursing education*. New York: National League for Nursing.

Institute of Medicine. (2003). *Health professions education: A bridge to quality*. Washington, DC: National Academies Press.

Jeffries, P. R., & Rizzolo, M. A. (2006). Final report of the NLN/Laerdal simulation study. In P. R. Jeffries (Ed.), *Simulation in nursing education*. New York: National League for Nursing.

Jeffries, P. R., & Rogers, K. J. (2007a). Theoretical framework for simulation design. In P. R. Jeffries (Ed.), *Simulation in nursing education*. New York: National League for Nursing.

Jeffries, P. R., & Rogers, K. J. (2007b). Evaluating simulations. In P. R. Jeffries (Ed.), *Simulation in nursing education*. New York: National League for Nursing.

Johnson-Russell, J., & Bailey, C. (2010). Facilitated debriefing. In W. M. Nehring & F. R. Lashley (Eds.), *High-fidelity patient simulation in nursing education*. Sudbury, MA: Jones and Bartlett Publishers.

Kardong-Edgren, S., Anderson, M., & Michaels, J. (2007). Does simulation fidelity improve student test scores? *Clinical Simulation in Nursing Education, 3*(1), feature 4.

Kardong-Edgren, S., & Oermann, M. H. (2009). A letter to nursing program administrators. *Clinical Simulation in Nursing, 5*(5), e161–e162.

Kardong-Edgren, S., Starkweather, A., & Ward, L. (2008). The integration of simulation into a clinical foundations of nursing course: Student and faculty perspectives. *International Journal of Nursing Education Scholarship, 5*(1), Article 26.

Lasater, K. (2007). Clinical judgment development using simulation to create an assessment rubric. *The Journal of Nursing Education, 46*(11), 496–503.

Leigh, G., & Hurst, H. (2008). We have a high-fidelity simulator, now what? Making the most of simulators. *International Journal of Nursing Education Scholarship, 5*(1), Art 33.

Leighton, K. (2007). Learning needs in the simulated clinical environment and the traditional clinical environment: A survey of undergraduate nursing students. Dissertation completed August 2007. *ETD collection for University of Nebraska – Lincoln*, Paper AAI3271929.

Leighton, K. (2009a). Death of a simulator. *Clinical Simulation in Nursing, 5*(2), e59–e62.

Leighton, K. (2009b). What can we learn from a listserv? *Clinical Simulation in Nursing, 5*(2), e57–e58.

McGahie, W. C., Pugh, C. M., & Wane, D. B. (2008). Fundamentals of educational research using clinical simulation. In R. R. Kyle Jr. & W. B. Murray (Eds.), *Clinical simulation: Operations, engineering and management*. New York: Elsevier, Inc.

Medley, C. F., & Horne, C. (2005). Using simulation technology for undergraduate nursing education. *Journal of Nursing Education, 44*(1), 31–34.

Morgan, P. J., Cleave-Hogg, D., Desousa, S., & Lam-McCulloch, J. (2006). Applying theory to practice in undergraduate education using high fidelity simulation. *Medical Teacher, 28*(1), e10–14.

Nehring, W. M. (2010). History of simulation in nursing. In W. M. Nehring & F. R. Lashley (Eds.), *High-fidelity patient simulation in nursing education*. Sudbury, MA: Jones and Bartlett.

Pagano, M. P., & Greiner, P. A. (2009). Enhancing communication skills through simulations. In S. H. Campbell & K. M. Daley (Eds.), *Simulation scenarios for nurse educators: Making it real*. New York: Springer Publishing Company.

Ravert, P. (2010). Developing and implementing a simulation program: Baccalaureate nursing education. In W. M. Nehring, & F. R. Lashley (Eds.), *High-fidelity patient simulation in nursing education*. Sudbury, MA: Jones and Bartlett.

WHO Collaboration Centre for Patient Safety Solutions. (2007). *Communication during patient hand-overs*. (Volume 1, Solution 3). Retrieved January 25, 2010, from www.who.int/patientsafety/solutions/patientsafety/PS-Solution3.pdf

CHAPTER 17

Interprofessional Education

Jennine Salfi and Patricia Solomon

As the call for enhanced collaboration among healthcare professionals continues to rise, there is a need for practitioners to learn the knowledge and skills necessary for collaborative practicum in their preregistration education. Evidence has indicated that collaboration skills are not intuitive or always learned on the job (Rosenstein, 2002), and most health professional education currently involves students learning skills and content without interaction with their peers in other health professions programs. It has been argued that if individuals from different professions learn together in interprofessional education (IPE), they will work better together, enhancing patient care and the delivery of healthcare services (Hammick, Freeth, Koppel, Reeves, & Barr, 2007).

DEFINITION AND PURPOSE

IPE occurs when students of two or more professions learn with, from, and about one another to improve collaboration and the quality of care (Centre for the Advancement of Interprofessional Education [CAIPE], 1997). CAIPE (2008) uses the term "interprofessional education" to include learning in both academic and clinical settings, before and after qualification.

Effective Interprofessional Education

1. Works to improve the quality of care, because no one profession working in isolation has the expertise to respond adequately and effectively to the complexity of many clients' needs.
2. Encourages professions to learn with, from, and about each other because it provides an opportunity to introduce skills, languages, and perspectives associated with each profession. It is comparative, collaborative, and interactive (as is interprofessional practice) and takes

into account respective roles and responsibilities, knowledge and skills, powers and duties, codes of conduct, value systems, opportunities, and constraints. This cultivates mutual trust and respect, acknowledging differences, and confronts misconceptions and stereotypes, dispelling prejudice and rivalry.

3. Grounded in mutual respect, and honors the distinctive experiences and expertise that each participant brings from their respective professional field.
4. Enhances practice within professions as each profession gains a deeper understanding of its own practice, and how it can complement and reinforce that of others. It demonstrates and reinforces the importance of teamwork and collaborative practice as it helps ease occupational stress either by setting limits on the demands made by any one profession, or by ensuring that cross-professional support and guidance are provided if and when added responsibilities are upheld (CAIPE, 2008).

THEORETICAL FOUNDATION

Even though skills and content may be similar across professional programs in health sciences, there is generally minimal interaction between the students in each professional program, and few opportunities for faculty development in the area of IPE. This lack of attention to IPE could lead to undervaluing or misinterpreting each profession's contributions, with the potential of impairing communication, collaboration, and teamwork in the clinical work setting postgraduation. Thus, in order to address the calling for enhanced collaboration among healthcare professionals, IPE can be used as a mechanism to enhance professional practice and improve the delivery of healthcare services (Hammick et al., 2007).

IPE introduces a pedagogy with its own classification that aims to recontextualize traditional and distinct bodies of professional knowledge into the knowledge of collaborative practice. Through this influence on the constructs of traditional knowledge, IPE attempts to sensitize students to the role of other healthcare disciplines and teach the delivery of interprofessional care (Schmitt, 1994). This new form of teaching can overcome the traditional ways of knowing about how to be a professional practitioner, and has the potential to result in more effective relations within the healthcare team. The most predominant philosophical argument for IPE is that when IPE is offered at the prelicensure level, improvements will be made in interprofessional communication and collaboration in practice and, ultimately, will result in improved delivery of care and health outcomes for patients (Salvatori & Solomon, 2005).

TYPES OF LEARNERS

Some prelicensure programs are at the undergraduate level (e.g., nursing.) The introduction of IPE at the undergraduate level remains controversial. One of the arguments against the introduction of IPE at the undergraduate level is that most students at this level have not acquired a sense of their own professional characteristics, or sufficient practical experience to be able to experience the full benefits of IPE (Fraser, Symonds, Cullen, & Symonds, 2000). Some believe that premature introduction of IPE could have negative repercussions on undergraduate students because it might interfere with the establishment of a distinct professional identity (Miller, Ross, & Freeman, 1999). Conversely, students at the postgraduate level are able to take full advantage of the learning opportunities available through IPE because they possess considerable practical experience to base their insight and discussions (Barr, Freeth, Hammick, Koppel, & Reeves, 2000; Miller et al., 1999).

Currently, there are no studies demonstrating that early exposure to IPE hinders the ability to acquire or develop one's professional identity. Some advantages associated with integrating IPE within undergraduate curricula include the opportunity to overturn negative stereotypes at an early stage in an individual's professional socialization (Barr et al., 2000) and to improve the student's confidence and ability to communicate with other members of the healthcare team. It also introduces the concept of teamwork in the healthcare setting, and the importance of collaboration among a variety of professionals to enhance patient care.

One approach that considers both the advantages and potential disadvantages of introducing IPE into the undergraduate curriculum is to designate specific interprofessional competencies per level of the professional program. For example, in the nursing program, it would not be unrealistic to expect that by the end of their second year, students should be able to describe their own professional roles and responsibilities, as well as the general scope of practice of other health professionals. This would allow for the development of a distinct professional identity, as well as an awareness of the healthcare context in which the professional role is situated. As the level of practical experiences increases within the program, more sophisticated interprofessional competencies and opportunities can be integrated into the curriculum.

CONDITIONS

Interprofessional activities and opportunities should be offered to health professional students so that they will be able to expand their level of understanding and appreciation of other professional roles and will learn to respect and value the input of other disciplines in the team decision-making process. IPE competencies can provide the basis for interprofessional opportunities and activities. To cite an example, a university in Ontario, Canada, has established the following four core competencies as the basis for their interprofessional activities:

1. Describe their own professional roles and responsibilities, and the general scope of practice of other health professionals to colleagues and patients/clients
2. Know how to involve other professions in patient care appropriate to their roles, responsibilities, and competence
3. Collaborate with other professions to establish common goals, provide care for individuals and caregivers, and facilitate shared decision making, problem solving, and conflict resolution
4. Contribute to team effectiveness by sharing information, listening attentively, respecting others' opinions, demonstrating flexibility, using a common language, providing feedback to others, and responding to feedback from others (Barr, 2001).

These four competencies are embedded in three types of IPE activities: exposure, immersion, and mastery (Charles, Bainbridge, & Gilbert, 2008).

Exposure Activities

These activities are primarily knowledge based relating to the first two competencies, and focus on describing roles and responsibilities and demonstrating awareness of the scope of practice of other health professions. These activities are generally of short-term duration and examples include shadowing experiences, multidisciplinary panel discussions, a written reflection on an interprofessional interaction experienced in a clinical setting, and Interprofessional Student Council–approved activities (Program for Interprofessional Practice, Education and Research [PIPER], 2007).

Immersion Activities

These activities are typically of longer duration than exposure activities, and require higher levels of interaction between the health professional students. All four competencies may be addressed through these activities. Students will be required to collaborate with other health professional students, make decisions, and solve problems together. Some examples of immersion activities include tutorial courses, e-based learning activities, special events days (e.g., day in aboriginal health), and communication skills labs (which will be described in greater detail) (PIPER, 2007).

Mastery Activities

This is the most complex and integrative group of activities. Students will integrate their interprofessional knowledge and skills in a team environment. Typically this will be of longer duration, and students will build relationships in a team environment and be actively engaged in team decision making around client care. Although mastery activities are primarily clinical practices experiences, some extended courses or student projects may also be considered mastery activities (PIPER, 2007).

For some programs, participation in these activities is already mandatory. It is hoped that eventually all students in health science programs will be expected to demonstrate interprofessional competencies prior to graduation, with each student participating in at least one exposure, one immersion, and one mastery activity.

RESOURCES AND METHODS: COMMUNICATION SKILLS LABS

One example of an immersion activity is the communication skills labs, which were developed in 2004, and designed to address all four IPE competencies (Salvatori, Mahoney, & Delottinville, 2006). Communication skills must be effective to ensure connectedness between members of a team and the environment of the skills labs allow for an awareness of equal power and fosters shared decision making, responsibility, and authority (Selle, Salamon, Boarman, & Sauer, 2008). It has been suggested that students need to be challenged with complex, realistic healthcare problems using cooperative learning as part of the learning process, such as using a paper-based healthcare scenario or, better yet, a simulated patient with students from three to five disciplines (D'Eon, 2004).

Communication skills labs involve a small group of interprofessional students, gathered together to conduct an assessment of a standardized patient(s), formulate learning questions and prioritize health-related issues, and collaborate on a hypothetical plan of care for the standardized patient. The interprofessional nature of the group provides an opportunity to learn about each other's roles and skills set, and the students learn to respect the distinctive experiences and expertise that each participant brings from their individual professional fields (CAIPE, 2008). Mutual respect is fundamental in collaborative working, and may also promote the level of confidence in working with other healthcare professionals. Finally, the experiential learning associated with the communication skills labs reinforces the importance of communication and teamwork in providing quality care in the healthcare setting (Barnsteiner et al., 2007).

Developing the Scenario

The scenario provides the starting point for learning in a communication skills lab. Well-constructed patient scenarios provide a focus for learning, stimulate interest in the content, and provide a meaningful context within which prior learning is activated and new knowledge is gained (Drummond-Young & Mohide, 2001).

The design and development of a patient scenario is comprised of several steps. Using a design similar to that of Drummond-Young and Mohide (2001), the following framework was constructed to illustrate the steps of development used to create a scenario for an interprofessional communication skills lab.

Figure 17-1 Development of an interprofessional scenario. There are multiple steps involved in creating a scenario for an interprofessional communication skills lab.

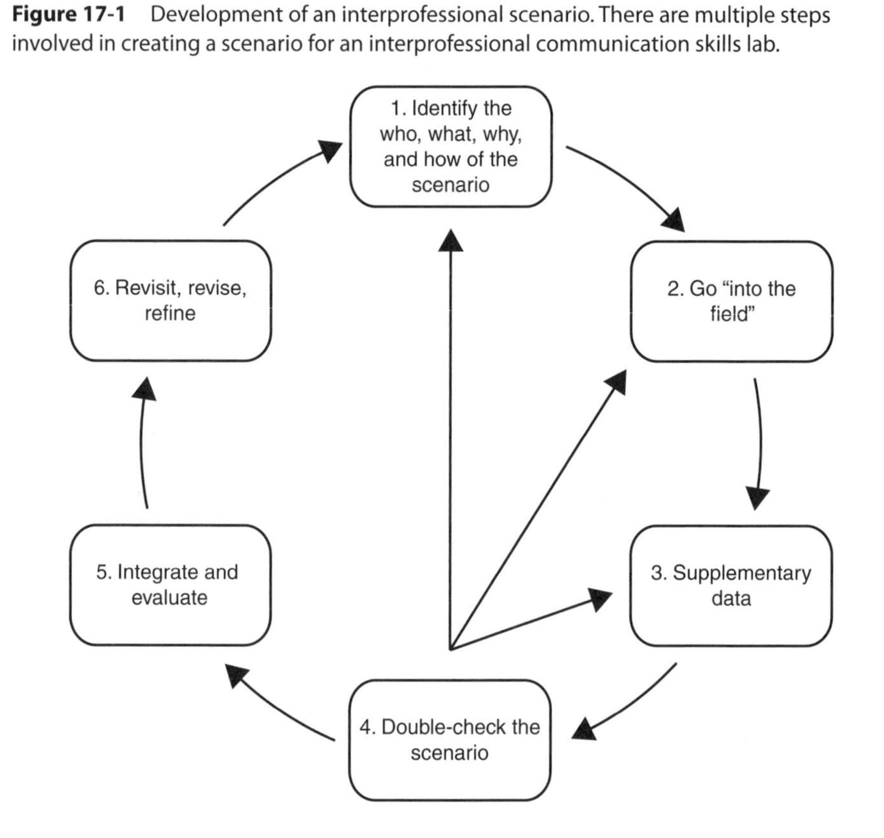

1. *Identify the Who, What, Why, and How of the Scenario*
   a. *Who will be the audience experiencing the scenario? Make sure the scenario has something to offer each profession.*

      In creating the scenario referred to in this chapter, the author had to first identify who the audience was going to be, so that the scenario could be designed to offer each profession opportunities for learning in terms of knowledge, skills, and dispositions (Drummond-Young & Mohide, 2001). With the current aging population and shift in focus from acute to chronic health care, a scenario involving an older adult in the community setting was chosen for its complexity, and for its requirement of a number of health and social care professionals to be involved in the delivery of care.
   b. *Why is this scenario being developed? What is the purpose?*

      The scenario was being developed for an interprofessional communication skills lab. The main purpose for this scenario was to provide an opportunity for collaboration with other professions to establish common goals and facilitate shared decision making, problem solving, and conflict resolution (Barr, 2001). Communication skills (sharing information, listening attentively, respecting others' opinions, demonstrating flexibility, using a common language, providing feedback to others, and responding to feedback from others) among professions is crucial in the healthcare environment, and are the main focus of these interprofessional labs.
   c. *What are the main concepts/issues of the scenario?*

      A scenario about an elderly person in a community setting could present several issues for exploration, but being cognisant of the target audience and the purpose of the communication skills lab, the author chose to focus the scenario on two main issues: caregiver burden and long-term care placement. The need for effective communication and efficient collaboration and decision making among a variety of healthcare professionals must be present, in order to develop a well-rounded plan of care that would resolve these complicated issues.
   d. *How will it play out? What is your vision for execution?*

      The author wanted to develop a scenario that would mimic a common situation in the community setting: determining when to have an elderly person assessed for long-term care placement. The vision for the scenario included a currently widowed elderly woman and a very tired and worried daughter, whose relationship had become very tense since the daughter suggested assessment for long-term care placement. It was at this point that it was decided the scenario would include two standardized patients—a mother and daughter dyad—so that the students could gain practice assessing and communicating to both individuals, as well as observe the dynamics of the relationship and communication patterns between an elderly women with impaired cognitive function and her daughter.

2. *Go "Into the Field"*

   Once the focus of the scenario has been determined, "go into the field." If possible, develop or adjust the scenario based on an actual clinical case(s). To further enhance the authenticity of the scenario, have a professional who has had experience with a similar case provide detail and feedback. Authenticity and customization of an interprofessional event so that it reflects relevant healthcare delivery and settings is important for a positive experience for the participants (Hammick et al., 2007).

   Once the backbone of a scenario is determined, it is time to dress it up. In this example, data were primarily gathered from a real clinical case. Additional description and feedback for the new scenario was provided by a case manager in the field who had had experience with a similar case. The case manager was also able to confirm and check details such as medications and medical history, so that all information was intelligible.

3. *Supplementary Data*

   The scenario itself should be brief, with enough detail to offer some focus for discussion, but open enough to stimulate critical thinking and encourage hypothesis generation. Previous research dictates that students prefer and appreciate a more complex scenario (Salvatori et al., 2006). Create supplementary resource material, for example chart data, to offer additional details of the scenario.

Scenario: The Case Manager's Home Visit

Mrs. Cooke is a 74-year-old woman who lives with her small dog in a one-bedroom apartment. Recently widowed, her community case manager came to reassess her ability to function on her own. Prior to this visit, Mrs. Cooke was receiving one hour of personal care per week to assist with her bath. Upon the case manager's arrival, the door to the apartment was wide open, Mrs. Cooke was wandering around without stockings, and her blouse was half open. Bruises were visible on her legs. Her wallet sat open on the kitchen table, next to an empty medication dosette.

A community case manager was selected as the lead professional in this case, as they are the individuals who primarily assess and coordinate home care services, and potentially initiate the process for long-term care assessment. They also tend to be one of a variety of healthcare professions (i.e., nurse, physical therapist or occupational therapist, social worker, dietician, speech language pathologist).

The previous scenario was created with enough information to steer the interprofessional group of students toward the author's intended focus for the scenario: an elderly woman with a decreased ability to function safely at home with a daughter experiencing caregiver burden—candidate for long-term care placement? However, the scenario also included a few added details to augment discussion, for example, other topics that could be explored from this scenario:

- What is the cause of her current state?
    - Polypharmacy?
    - Alzheimer disease?
    - Other sources of confusion: Diabetes? Urinary tract infection? Brain tumor?
- Depression? Grief and bereavement?
- Was there an intruder?
- Falls? Other safety concerns?
- Social isolation? Social supports?
- Able to stay in own home with increased home care service?
- Support for daughter

After the group has had a chance to brainstorm and generate hypotheses, they can access the chart data for additional details, before they proceed with collaborating on a hypothetical plan of care for the elderly woman (and her daughter) in the scenario (Please see Appendix 17-1 on the Web site that accompanies this book). Supplementary data could also include lab tests and procedure results, medical-related letters, etc.

4. *Double Check the Scenario*

After the scenario has been created, seek evaluative feedback, preferably from other healthcare professionals with similar experiences. Once feedback has been received and adjustments made as necessary, recruit and train standardized patients for the scenario. Standardized patients are individuals who "are specially trained, by a specific yet not complex method similar to 'method acting' to simulate an actual patient in every detail" (Barrows & Tamblyn, 1980, p. 63). In the example provided previously, there were two standardized patients trained: an elderly mother and daughter. In training this dyad, the author of the scenario simply narrated her vision of the situation describing in detail the personalities of each individual, the relationship between the mother and daughter, the communication (verbal and nonverbal) techniques to be employed by each individual, and any other details that were included in her vision for the scenario. One example of an additional detail might include the appearance of the standardized patient; in this case, the elderly woman was to appear a bit dishevelled, indicating probable difficulty in completing activities of self care.

Once details and plausibility of the scenario has been checked out and the standardized patients have been trained, pilot the scenario to observe how it unfolds. Does it unravel as you had envisioned it? Did it meet the objectives of the skills lab, and have something to offer each discipline in the group? Did the scenario promote communication, teamwork, and collaboration? Make adjustments and add information to the scenario as necessary.

5. *Integrate and Evaluate*

   Integrate into the program, and continue to evaluate the content and process associated with the scenario. Gather feedback on a regular basis from multiple sources: faculty, students, and standardized patients. Students, faculty, and standardized patients each bring a unique perspective to the scenario, which can elicit valuable comments and suggestions for change.

6. *Revisit, Revise, and Refine on a Regular Basis*

   Scenarios grow old and outdated, so to remain current in the field of health care and to continue to offer exciting new challenges for the students, scenarios must be revisited on a regular basis. Review the scenario and determine whether it needs to be refined, revised, or re-created.

Small Group, Problem-Based Learning Approach

The communication skills lab unfolds similar to a small group, problem-based learning class. Small group learning allows students to develop a sense of responsibility for their learning progress. Small group learning in an interprofessional environment further enhances learning as students develop a sense of responsibility for accurately representing the knowledge and skills base of their profession. Furthermore, students in a group environment learn about human interaction, develop interpersonal skills, and may become more aware of their own emotional reactions and moral standing. Learning how to listen, and provide and receive evaluative feedback are also skills that small group learning helps to cultivate (Neufeld & Barrows, 1974), which are all essential in a healthcare environment.

The composition of a small group in a communication skills lab may vary from week to week (depending on the availability of students), but generally consists of a variety of students from different programs. A minimum of three professions in the health sciences should be represented in each small group (Salvatori et al., 2006). The purpose of the meeting is to collaborate and work through a client healthcare scenario. Sessions typically run for approximately 3 hours in length, with a 15- to 20-minute break midway.

The lab begins with introductions, and a general orientation to the purpose and process of the group session. A clinical scenario is introduced as the focal point for learning, which might be read aloud or quietly, played out by a standardized patient(s), or be presented in an audiovisual format. After being introduced to the scenario, obvious health-related issues are identified, and hypotheses of other potential issues are generated. Once this has been completed, an initial interview with a standardized patient(s) takes place, so that additional information can be collected, and hypotheses verified or rejected.

Once the group has had a chance to discuss the findings and agree on the issues that are of priority in the healthcare scenario, they collaborate on a treatment or discharge plan. The standardized patient(s) returns to the group, and a follow-up interview is conducted to discuss the plan of care. The final hour of the skills lab allows for time to debrief about the scenario, and provides an opportunity to exchange feedback between students, and receive feedback from the standardized patients and faculty present (Salvatori et al., 2006).

Role of Faculty

The main roles of faculty are to observe the interprofessional group of students from behind a one way mirror, intervene (if necessary), and provide feedback using a standard observational guide (Salvatori et al., 2006). Ideally, tutors are familiar with the small group, problem-based approach to learning so that they are able to quickly distinguish the group's dynamics, and identify individual roles within the group. The faculty should also be efficient in providing evaluative comments, specifically constructive feedback, so that the students can grow from the experience.

Role of Students

The role of the students is very similar to that of the role of a student in a small group, problem-based learning class. Students need to demonstrate behaviors in critical thinking, effective group participation, and professional conduct. They need to be well aware of their role and scope of practice because they will need to represent their profession in this multidiscipline environment.

Students may also assume one of two functional roles, as described by Sampson and Marthas (1990): task roles and maintenance roles. Task roles are actions such as initiating, clarifying, informing, sharing information, and evaluating whether or not group goals are being achieved. Setting up an agenda at the beginning of a group session is a common example of a task role (Uys & Gwele, 1999). Maintenance roles are behaviors that act to strengthen the group and maintain harmony, for example, offering encouragement and support, open and effective communication strategies, and compromising (Sampson & Marthas, 1990).

The role of the student in a communication skills lab is comparable to that of a health professional involved in a multidiscipline team meeting about a client in a healthcare setting. Working in student "teams" establishes mutual respect and enhances collaboration, and the relatively equal status of students contributes to a sense of safety, allowing them to take more risks that they normally would not be ready to take in clinical practice (O'Neill & Wyness, 2004).

One key finding from a systematic review of IPE was that interprofessional activities are generally well received by participants, especially when the context for learning reflected the students' current or future practice (Hammick et al., 2007). Research from another study revealed that students enjoyed their experience in the communication skills lab, in particular, interacting with students from the other health science programs. Students reported an increased awareness of other professional roles, and agreed that the feedback provided on their individual communication skills and overall group performance was informative (Salvatori et al., 2006).

POTENTIAL PROBLEMS

There are many barriers to interprofessional activities, despite the many benefits associated with this style of learning. IPE is "complex and time consuming to arrange and sustain" (Kilminster et al., 2004, p. 719). It can be very challenging to identify available time for IPE initiatives within preregistration professional courses (Hammick et al., 2007). Incompatible clinical shifts and timetables, as well as rigid curriculum were identified as the most significant barriers in establishing IPE (Morison, Boohan, Jenkins, & Moutray, 2003).

Another barrier to the delivery of IPE in health science programs includes faculty interest and expertise in IPE. As identified by Hammick and colleagues (2007), a key mechanism for effective IPE involves faculty development. Faculty need to be knowledgeable, competent, and confident if they are to be effective in implementing interprofessional core competencies into the health sciences curricula. Faculty also need to be proficient in applying principles of adult learning, as this has also been cited as a key mechanism for well-received IPE (Hammick *et al.*, 2007).

In some institutions, the number of students varies across professional programs, and this is a barrier to effective coordination of IPE activities into the health sciences programs. For example, one professional program might be three times the size of the others, making it difficult to create groups that have a balance and variety of professions. Or some health science faculties may only have a few professions to choose from, again affecting the ability to create balanced groups of at least three different professions.

Regardless of the challenges, awareness of the importance of IPE on safe clinical practice and strong professional partnerships continues to build, so too does the drive to establish mandatory IP activities into the health sciences curricula.

CONCLUSION

Students in health professional programs do not learn interprofessional concepts from sitting side by side in lecture halls, and they do not develop skills in communication, collaboration, and teamwork by simply observing or shadowing a different health professional. The communication skills labs provide the opportunity to collaborate with students from a variety of health professions and participate in experiential learning, which has been shown to promote role understanding, and the importance of working together as a team. Only when an awareness and appreciation of others' professions has been established, and skills such as communication and collaboration have been acquired, can solid healthcare partnerships be built, and high-quality healthcare services be delivered.

REFERENCES

Barnsteiner, J., Disch, J., Hall, L., Mayer, D. & Moore, S. M. (2007). Promoting interprofessional education. *Nursing Outlook, 55* (3), 144–150.

Barr, H. (2001). *Interprofessional education: Today, yesterday, and tomorrow*. London: Westminster University, Learning and Teaching Support Network Centre of Health Sciences and Practices.

Barr, H., Freeth, D., Hammick, M., Koppel, I., & Reeves, S. (2000). *Evaluations of interprofessional education: A United Kingdom review for health and social care*. Retrieved August 2008 from http://www.caipe.org.uk/publications.html

Barrows, H., & Tamblyn, R. (1980). *Problem-based learning*. New York: Springer.

Centre for the Advancement of Interprofessional Education. (1997). *Interprofessional education—a definition*. London: CAIPE.

Centre for the Advancement of Interprofessional Education. (2008). *Interprofessional education—a definition*. London: CAIPE.

Charles, G., Bainbridge, L., & Gilbert, J. (2008). *The College of health disciples and the UBC model of interprofessional education*. British Columbia, Canada: UBC.

D'Eon, M . (2004). A blueprint for interprofessional learning. *Journal of Interprofessional Care, 19,* 49–59.

Drummond-Young, M., & Mohide, E. A. (2001). Developing problems for use in problem-based learning. In E. Rideout (Ed.), *Transforming nursing education through problem-based learning*. Sudbury, MA: Jones and Bartlett Publishers.

Fraser, D., Symonds, M., Cullen, L., & Symonds, I. (2000). A university department merger of midwifery and obstetrics: A step on the journey to enhancing interprofessional learning. *Medical Teacher, 22*(2), 179–183.

Hammick, M., Freeth, D., Koppel, I., Reeves, S., & Barr, H. (2007). A best evidence systematic review of interprofessional education: BEME guide no.9. *Medical Teacher, 29*(8), 735–751.

Kilminster, S., Hale, C., Lascelles, M., Morris, P., Roberts, T., Stark, P., et al. (2004). Learning for real life: Patient-focused interprofessional workshops offer added value. *Medical Education, 38,* 717–726.

Miller, C., Ross, N., & Freeman, M. (1999). *Shared learning and clinical teamwork: New direction in education for multiprofessional practice*. London: The English National Board of Nursing Midwifery and Health Visiting.

Morison, S., Boohan, M., Jenkins, J., & Moutray, M. (2003). Facilitating undergraduate interprofessional learning in healthcare: Comparing classroom and clinical learning for nursing and medical students. *Learning in Health and Social Care, 2*(2), 92–104.

Neufeld, V., & Barrows, H. (1974). The "McMaster philosophy": An approach to medical education. *Journal of Medical Education, 49*(11), 1040–1051.

O'Neill, B., & Wyness, M. (2004). Learning about interprofessional education: Student voices. *Journal of Interprofessional Care, 18*(2), 198–200.

Program for Interprofessional Practice, Education and Research. (2007). *Description of IPE activities and competencies*. Retrieved September 2008 from http://fhs.mcmaster.ca/ipe/competency_intro.htm.

Rosenstein, A. (2002). Nurse-physician relationships: Impact on nurse satisfaction and retention. *American Journal of Nursing, 102,* 26–34.

Salvatori, P., Mahoney, P., & Delottinville, C. (2006). An interprofessional communication skills lab: A pilot project. *Education for Health, 19*(3), 380–384.

Salvatori, P., & Solomon, P. (2005). Interprofessional education. In P. Solomon, & S. Baptiste (Eds.), *Innovations in rehabilitation sciences education*. Germany: Springer.

Sampson, E., & Marthas, M. (1990). *Group process for the health professions*. Albany, NY: Delmar.

Schmitt, M. (1994). USA: Focus on interprofessional practice, education, and research. *Journal of Interprofessional Care, 8,* 9–18.

Selle, K. M., Salamon, K., Boarman, R., & Sauer, J. (2008). Providing interprofessional learning through interdisciplinary collaboration: The role of modelling. *Journal of Interprofessional Care, 22*(1), 85–92.

Uys, L., & Gwele, N. (1999). A descriptive analysis of the process of problem-based teaching/learning. In J. Conway & A. Williams (Eds.), *Themes and variations in PBL*. Callaghan, Australia: PROBLARC.

SECTION IV

EDUCATIONAL USE OF TECHNOLOGY

Educational technology continues to grow by leaps and bounds and has vastly changed the world of education. The technology can be as simple as communicating by e-mail, or as complex as presenting full degree-granting programs by distance learning. Classroom teaching is utilizing more and more technology, from PowerPoint documents and student- and faculty-made videos, to blended learning, a combination of in-class and asynchronous discussions. Libraries have become accessible to distance learners by use of technology, and full-text articles are now available online. The Internet has opened a new and extensive world of information that was not previously available, and both faculty and students need to learn how to take advantage of what is out there, but also how to use it with caution. Students are increasingly involved in social technology where they communicate with wide audiences. Teaching in a technological world requires faculty collaboration with academic information technology specialists, a specialty field in itself, to learn how to use the ever changing systems, but also to keep abreast of new resources as they become available and provide technological support for students.

The discussion in these chapters provides a look at different ways of utilizing available technologies and discusses strengths of the system and problems that may occur. As technology has grown in the past few years, the technology discussion in this edition has increased as well. Social networking is now being included in teaching strategies as discussed in the chapter Web 2.0 and Beyond. Distance learning techniques are now moving into the classroom in blended or hybrid classes and faculty need to learn to incorporate these strategies as a way to better achieve their learning objectives. Technology may be used to assist learning, but it does not replace the instructor. Teaching methods require adaptation to be effective in this new environment and should be evaluated for that effectiveness. The amount of Internet information may be overwhelming, and it is critical that faculty and students begin to cull the material to a reasonable amount, and validate accuracy. The use of educational technologies may require extra time and effort from faculty, but can be very effective in enhancing learning and rewarding for students and faculty alike.

CHAPTER 18

The Use of Video in Health Profession Education

Clive Grainger and Alex Griswold

INTRODUCTION

Video is the strongest medium we can use to reveal interpersonal relationships. It is nearly impossible to fully communicate through the use of words alone what may be revealed in a person's eyes, face, and gestures. Video production can be a collaborative or solitary venture but in either case it should be fun.

In this chapter, we aim to provide the reader with ideas about how video might be used in the education of the health professional. Our aim is to offer advice to both faculty and students so that they acquire greater confidence through the use of simple techniques to improve their technical knowledge. We will review some of the uses of video in education, as well as the process of "production" in layman's terms. We will highlight some simple tips, learned from many years of video production in both the classroom and in the broader field of education. When we use the term *video*, which is technically the visual part of a recording, we are using it in a colloquial form meaning sound and picture together.

In addition to improving technical knowledge, we aim to increase the effectiveness of communicating a message without the need to involve technologist specialists in the process. This is not an exhaustive "how-to" and our aim is not to swamp the reader with technical language. There are many excellent reference books and Web sites to consult about the process of video production and we suggest you refer to some of these for more in-depth study.

USES FOR VIDEO IN EFFECTIVE TEACHING

As a tool for learning, video is useful for documenting events for later study and/or for communicating with large numbers of people. For example, a lecture can be recorded and made available on the Web to people who could not attend

Table 18-1 Video Use in the Classroom

Creating clinical records A video camera can make more useful and comprehensive records of patient progress than a written chart or even a still photograph.
Documenting presentations/training sessions These can be reviewed later in the classroom so that instructors can fill in gaps, or offer interpretations. Time can also be shortened—points can be illustrated by fast-forwarding or with judicious editing.
Recording interactions between students and patients Instructors may show videos as examples of what went well and what might be improved. Students can use these materials for study outside the classroom.
Communicating case studies for individual or group study Video case studies enhance traditional print case studies by revealing body language and other subtle clues. As a teaching tool, video can serve to provoke thought and encourage students to express their opinions.
Recording clinical or informal interviews Interviews may be logged and transcribed for later study. Some patients may find it easier to reveal thoughts and feelings to a camera with no operator, than to talk to a medical professional behind that camera.
Revealing patient understanding and misconceptions Many clinicians are aware of the most commonly held misconceptions about various ailments. Both hearing and seeing patients present their incorrect ideas is far more effective than reading about them. New misconceptions might also be revealed.
Comparing and contrasting examples of both "good" and "bad" professional interaction Videotaped interviews may be especially helpful in conveying the interaction between health professional and patient. A little humor might be used to illustrate the "wrong" way!
Demonstrating clinical procedures Videotaping procedures that are not easily demonstrated to groups of students can be very effective—saving the instructor from becoming a "sage on the stage."
Communicating specific medical information Video is an excellent tool for the elderly, for those who face mobility challenges, or who are unable to read. It is possible to use alternative audio tracks or subtitles for ESL patients. Such material may also be used for review by the caregivers of such patients.

Continuing education
In-service training is naturally an important part of every medical professional's career. The presentation of development materials via video on the Web can be the most convenient way for busy professionals to choose where and when they might study.

Evaluating student progress
Students may be encouraged to produce their own video projects. These may be used to measure how well a sequence of concepts has been understood. Presentation for classroom peer review may also be simplified.

in person. Video allows events to be studied in multiple dimensions: A recording of a patient–caregiver interview can be used as a record of the interview. It can also be used for diagnosis, treatment, or in an educational setting.

There are a number of uses for video in the classroom that may be considered by both educator and student. Table 18-1 is by no means an exhaustive list—you may come up with ideas of your own.

NEW TECHNOLOGY/ACCESS

Video has become a ubiquitous medium. The use of video materials is integrated into most health professional education college courses. It is particularly effective when used for distance learning. During recent years, there has been a revolution in access to affordable video equipment. Many families now own and use relatively sophisticated video cameras. To most students, this technology is not as unfamiliar or expensive as it once was.

One can readily access modestly priced camera equipment along with relatively sophisticated editing software, often bundled with computers. Examples of bundled editing and recording software are Apple's *iMovie* and *iDVD*. The reader will find similar Windows-based editing programs such as *Windows Movie Maker*. Cheap hardware and software have also enabled the creation of DVDs for the dissemination of materials.

New uses for video are being rapidly developed for the Web, on cell phones, and on the ever-popular iPod. We are witnessing a merging of technologies where a little bit of video goes a long way. Use of innovative multimedia continually increases the effectiveness of educational communication.

With successful use of new technologies come challenges for both the educator and student. Learning to effectively use yet another technology may be daunting. It is possible to lessen any anxiety by researching and leveraging resources that may be available locally, consulting with your technology specialist and discussing concerns with fellow faculty. Many of your colleagues may have, or have had, similar concerns to your own. It may be possible to sponsor professional development sessions related to the use of emerging technologies.

The term "video tape" may soon be as obsolete as "record"—how many of today's students would know what a 33 or a 45 looked like, let alone a 78? Technological development is always in a rapid state of flux, but we are heading into an exciting future with unpredictable possibilities.

WHY USE VIDEO? ADVANTAGES AND DISADVANTAGES

The old adage that "a picture is worth a thousand words" may be true, but the moving image can be worth even more! Try to describe each shot of a short film, or even a television ad, and see how many words it takes.

Video production at the highest levels may appear to be challenging but many of the techniques used by professionals are within the grasp of those with even the simplest of tools. Classroom viewing of the moving image allows the audience to witness inaccessible events with a sense of immediacy that other media cannot convey. Video may be coupled with other forms of interactive media to produce powerful learning tools.

If there is a choice about presentation method, the first question you may want to ask is whether video is really the correct medium for the task. Watching video in its simplest form can be a very linear, passive experience—there is a beginning, a middle, and an end. Is this the most effective way for you or your students to tell a story or to present material? We have already highlighted many of the ways that video might be used—we recommend that you view various excellent and innovative examples that may be found on the Web.

Perhaps you may want to consider breaking your material into smaller sections, or perhaps an audio-only "radio" treatment may be a more appropriate (and less time consuming) choice? Sometimes, just listening will help participants fill in their own visuals allowing for more active or thoughtful participation. Video has an "authority" and many of us are visual learners. Production can be time consuming—do you really have enough time?

There are many advantages to using video for the right project; perhaps you have an assignment that must be videotaped for presentation. Some learners "see" a lot better than they write; use of a visual and audio medium can help these students overcome potential written communication problems.

Video professionals use many terms that may be unfamiliar to the new user but most can be easily deciphered, for example, "streaming video." Streaming video consists of a sequence of moving images sent in compressed form over the Internet. It is displayed on the viewer's computer as it arrives rather than as a large file that must be fully downloaded in order for it to be viewed. You will find many excellent books and Web sites that may be used to decipher such terms.

THE PRODUCTION PROCESS

In order to produce videotaped material the minimum equipment required is:

- A camera with plenty of tape (or other recording medium) and batteries, and/or a wall adapter. There is nothing worse than your tape or batteries running out at an inopportune moment—we have all experienced it and, yes, even the most seasoned of producers too (but you only do it once!)
- Preferably a tripod for taping interviews, or at least a pair of steady hands.
- A microphone separate from the camera.
- A friend. Though you certainly can tape single-handedly, not having to concentrate on every aspect of your "shoot" will relieve much stress. It is nice to have someone help to carry your equipment, write notes to help you edit later, and to commiserate with you should anything just happen to go wrong!

ADAPTING TO THE NEEDS OF YOUR PRODUCTION

We previously listed some of the many uses for video in teaching and learning. We will revisit some of those examples and offer a few tips for each one. The most straightforward shooting is usually preferable. The background should not be distracting and, if necessary for close analysis, it is often useful to incorporate a measured grid or distance scale as part of the backdrop.

Presentations

When there is one speaker at a podium, it is usually quite easy to obtain a clear video image of his or her presentation. Use a tripod, if available. The audio may be more problematic. If there is a public address (PA) microphone, there may be a way to tap into the audio directly from the PA amplifier. If not, try to place a microphone on the podium, but test it ahead of time and, by all means, try to find out if the speaker wants to walk away from the podium. In that case, a wireless lapel microphone may be your best choice. PowerPoint presentations or other graphics can be either captured with a second dedicated camera, or imported directly into the editing system as digital files.

Interviews

There are many types of interviews. One of the most common is the "clinical interview," where a researcher and interviewee sit opposite each other across a table. The camera should be set up at the side, not directly in the interview subjects' line of sight. The height of the lens on the tripod is very important. The inexperienced videographer will often set the camera too high, so it "looms" down on the subject. This creates an impersonal feel to the interview. It is better to adjust the tripod so that the camera lens is level with the top of the interviewer and interviewee's heads. Adjust the shot so that whatever is of interest is included in the frame, zooming in on the subject of interest and panning to adjust so that it is clearly visible. Audio can be captured with a microphone placed unobtrusively on the table, aimed at the interviewee, but if you need to hear the interviewer clearly you may need a second microphone for the interviewer.

Demonstrating Clinical Procedures

The key (perhaps obviously) is to make sure that the area of interest is clearly visible. The use of a tripod is optional; sometimes it is better to have the mobility of a handheld camera. This will help you to avoid the area of interest being blocked by the person demonstrating the procedure.

In-service Training

Video used to illustrate a point or trigger discussion can be very useful in training sessions. These do not have to be too elaborate; often they can be shot with available lighting and in real settings. Here is where the "reality TV" approach could actually make a presentation more believable.

PLAN YOUR VIDEO

Planning is the most important part of video production—it requires much preparatory work before any material is shot. This may seem tedious but will more than pay for itself in the long run. What goes right or wrong during production is often related to the time spent in purposeful planning. Careful planning will also help you to consider other issues that you may not have thought about.

SOME DIFFERENCES: PROFESSIONAL VS AMATEUR VIDEO

We realize that our readers will have varying degrees of expertise but please stick with us as we describe a few key differences between video produced by the experienced and inexperienced cameraperson.

Audio

Audio is critically important—the recording of quality audio is one of the most overlooked elements in successful video production. You may not realize this until you listen to the difference between clear and noisily recorded speech in an interview. After all, is it not the point to hear what the interviewee is saying? Your pictures may be very pretty but are of little use if your audience cannot hear what is being discussed!

A built-in camera microphone is convenient, but unless you are very close to and pointing directly at your subject, it will record noise around the area as well as your subject. If you choose to be distant, or a fly-on-the-wall, the problem is compounded. Use of an external microphone on an extension cable will allow you to record an interview clearly and to cover many situations. Look at TV reporters—they handhold a microphone, moving it between interviewer and interviewees. You can try that technique too, if your interviewee is not seated.

Composition

Take a look at holiday "snaps" or home video. Compare them to material taken by a "professional." What differences do you observe? Quite often the framing of the experienced shooter will be more pleasing; heads are not in the middle of the frame, nor is there an excess of space above the subject. Also, the camera will often be closer to the subject, creating a more intimate interview. Unless the action dictates that you do so, avoid shooting too wide.

Always be aware of what is happening in the background of your shot; it is very distracting to see plants growing out of people's heads. Avoid shooting into crowds of people—they can be distracting and have been known to steal the scene by waving at the camera.

The "Wobbles"

It is helpful to steady your camera when taping to avoid a seasick viewer. The use of a tripod will also help you to step out from behind the camera to consider matters that you may not be able to attend to otherwise. "Scenic" shots will be easier to record with use of a tripod.

Lighting

In most clinical situations, it is impossible to set up additional lighting. Ambient lighting is all that can be used. Modern video equipment will record at very low light levels, but the images look best if illuminated at least to the level of a typical office. To avoid silhouetting your subject, do not show the light source (i.e., an exterior window) in the field of view, unless there are other light sources that illuminate the subject. Most video cameras have automatic exposure control. Experienced users will often set the exposure on their camera to manual to avoid the overall changes in light levels as the camera pans around the scene.

Transcripts

Although typing an unabridged copy of any spoken word on your tape might seem tedious, there are a number of benefits. A transcript will save you time when you edit interviews; the process will force you to review all of your material, making you aware of what was actually said. You may think you know what was recorded but it may be different from the reality—this is sometimes good and sometimes bad. It is possible that you only need, or have time to present, a taste of the full interview in the version shown to an audience. With a transcript you will be able to distribute a verbatim copy of all, or part, of the interview at a later time.

Editing

It is not always necessary to edit taped material, but without judicious editing you may very quickly bore your audience.

Less is more! Pull out the most important, salient material and place the rest onto "the cutting room floor." Your material should follow a logical progression. Do not show only the talking head(s) but put it into context, that is, what is the environment that your material is being recorded in? Is there any accompanying action? Try to reveal the relationship between people in the room. It is possible to help explain some of what is happening through the judicious use of voiceover or graphics. There are no hard and fast rules—be creative.

Etiquette

The relationship between videographer and interviewee is often the key to success. Being aware of a "fly on the wall" can be very disconcerting for a subject. Put them at ease first. Just as the microphone is the surrogate for the viewers' ears, the camera lens takes the place of their eyes. In effect, the camera is a stand-in for the audience, one that can be oppressive and overbearing, or if handled well, a kind friend or confidant.

Most television documentaries do not ask interview subjects to speak directly to the lens. This journalistic style allows the interview subjects to make eye contact with the interviewer and forget about the machine that is actually in the room. More experienced television personalities can be trained to peer naturally into a lens, ignoring the people around it. This is a skill that takes training and practice. Often, the greatest challenge for many nonactors is speaking directly to the camera. Remembering lines while speaking into the lens can be especially frustrating. If you are creating this kind of segment, leave lots of extra time for retakes. While sometimes having the presenter's script on poster boards can help, it is easier to use a teleprompter that projects the script on the front surface of a half-silvered mirror mounted directly in front of the camera. This kind of equipment may be available from your media department. Another solution is to plan to shoot only a few sentences while the host is on camera, then read the rest from a script. In editing, the sections that are read from the script can be covered with other pictures.

If you are able to incorporate comedy into your video, it can help to produce more effective, attention-grabbing materials—but use a little bit of humor. A small amount of light relief goes a long way in the right place, BUT what is humorous to you may not be to someone else.

GENTLE WARNINGS

Receipt of written consent should be sought from subjects recorded outside the classroom setting. We will assume that your classmates do not mind. It is best not to attempt covert recording unless you want to invite trouble.

Many medical professionals are used to obtaining informed written consent; various institutions have their own formalities for acquiring this consent. We would strongly urge you to consider obtaining written consent, most especially if your material may be viewed by a number of people, or in a number of different settings. It is *very* important to receive (and file!) WRITTEN, informed consent from the parents or guardians of minors. When dealing with this legal paperwork it can be daunting for the signer.

Words of caution also apply to copyright. Please be aware that the majority of music, video, and photographic material found on the Web, in libraries, or on disk that may seem to be "free" is copyrighted. This means that legal protection has been assigned to authors protecting them against unauthorized copying of their work. The good news is that you can find noncopyright "public domain" media in many places, but it is your responsibility to confirm this.

In Exhibit 18-1, you will find an example of what we call a "release form." You can base your own release on this. The wording can be adapted for adults only. Please be aware that this is a legal document and as such should be approved by your institution before use.

EXHIBIT 18-1

Acknowledgment, Consent, and Assignment

I, [***Parent/Guardian's Name***] ______________________ acknowledge as the parent/guardian of my child [***Child's Name***] ______________________ that [***Institution's Name***] is producing videotaped materials.

I acknowledge that this videotaped material is being produced for the purpose of furthering the educational goals of [***Institution's Name***]. Any profits from the sale or commercial use of this material will be applied to the educational work of [***Institution's Name***].

I hereby grant and release to [***Institution's Name***] the right to film, tape, and photograph my child and record his/her voice in connection with the materials and hereby assign all of his/her right, title, and interest in the materials, and their footage, including his/her copyright interests therein, to [***Institution's Name***].

I acknowledge that [***Dept. of Institution's Name***] will be the sole owner throughout the world of the copyright and all other rights in this material, as well as in any photographic materials, written works, bibliographies, syllabi, or other materials based upon the Programs ("Related Works").

The [***Dept. of Institution***] and its respective licensees and others acting with their permission have my consent to use my child's name, likeness, picture, and appearance in the materials and associated projects. I also grant my consent to use the above, as well as any biographical materials I have provided or may in the future provide, to advertise and publicize the material and related works.

The rights and releases granted herein apply to all formats in which the material may be marketed or presented, including, but not limited to television, the Web, cable casting, written works, educational and home video use.

This acknowledgement, consent, and assignment has been signed as a contract under seal on this:

__________ Day of __________________ 200X

Name: ______________________________

Signed: ______________________________

Home Address: ______________________________

____

____

Home Tel: ______________________________

Email: ______________________________

Example 1

Thomas Allardi

Physical Therapist, Massachusetts General Hospital, Boston

We frequently videotape our patients for a number of reasons. A common one is to complete a basic gait analysis. In order to accomplish this, a patient's step must be broken into its component elements. Video helps us to observe each component many times over.

Videotaping helps us work with children with cerebral palsy who are often diagnosed with muscular imbalance. In order to offer treatment we carefully analyze interrelated movement between knees, hips, and toes. A recording allows us to efficiently evaluate this and to communicate to both colleagues and our patient's parents alike the specific nature of the case.

Videotaping is an important tool used after an examination in order to consult with colleagues without need to use the physical therapist's unique language. As you can imagine, as with most medical specialties, when a puzzling case comes to our attention it is far more effective for us to consult our colleagues with a review of video.

Parents are often reluctant to see their child wearing an assistive device but we have been able to show before and after examples of recommended appliances, whose use is in best interest of their child. Video evidence often reassures these parents.

A bonus of using video recording is that because most of our child patients do not stand still long enough to repeat their movement, we can use video for immediate review!

Example 2

Amanda Pike

Nursing Student, Northeastern University School of Nursing, Boston

The students I study with have a wide range of learning styles but we are all very comfortable using technology. I think all of us use social networking sites like Facebook, watch videos on YouTube, and nearly every laptop computer we have has a built in Web cam.

Some of our textbooks are actually packages of textbooks with accompanying DVDs and links to video on the Web. I find watching the videos really helpful, especially when studying for tests.

We use video in a number of our course components. I found it very useful to record myself before my internship interviews. It helped my self confidence and although I wasn't required to, I showed the video to some of my friends and my tutor to get their feedback.

I learn a lot through my experience observing and working in clinical settings but I sometimes watch videos about techniques that I have seen during my time in the hospital. I have also watched videos that show correct procedures for use of technical equipment—some of this cannot be easily demonstrated in the class, for example, how to correctly use a patient lift without hurting either the patient or the caregiver. Some of the video we see illustrates rarely experienced situations in our internships and so watching video might be the only way to learn about them.

One of my friends recently recorded and edited a short video for a kinesiology class that she then put into a PowerPoint presentation. It illustrated the range of motion of her father's arm after his rotator cuff surgery showing his motion from different angles. All of her classmates were asked to make simple presentations using video recorded on their compact cameras, cell phones, or on normal video cameras.

CONCLUSION

We live in an environment ripe with moving images. Visual and aural media can be powerful tools for education. As we have seen, video materials can be simple or complex and may be used on their own or in tandem with other technologies and may also be used to supplement more traditional materials.

It may be challenging to stretch your technical abilities but any serious amateur can make a video worth watching. The onus to understand, or to interpret a piece of video, should not be left to the viewer. Your work may make complete sense to you but the audience does not know, or usually care about how you made it. Stand back, put yourself in the shoes of someone viewing it cold, and try it out on your friends or colleagues. Is it really accomplishing what you intended it to?

We hope that the process of making a video will open up new avenues of creativity and imagination for you. Good luck!

ADDITIONAL RESOURCES

American Medical Association. (2009). Patient physician relationship topics: informed consent. Retrieved November 24, 2009, from http://www.ama-assn.org/ama/pub/physician-resources/legal-topics/patient-physician-relationship-topics/informed-consent.shtml

Annenberg Media (2009).. [Live streaming video]. Retrieved November 24, 2009, from http://www.learner.org

Brigham and Women's Hospital. (2009). [Surgery webcasts]. Retrieved November 24, 2009, from http://www.or-live.com/BrighamandWomens/

Cleese, J. (2009). [Learning through humor video series]. Retrieved November 24, 2009, from http://www.rctm.com/Products/celebritiesgurus/johncleese.htm

Curran, V., Kirby, F., Allen, M., & Sargeant, J. (2003). A mixed learning technology approach for continuing medical education. *Medical Education Online, 8,* 5. Retrieved November 24, 2009, from http://www.med-ed-online.org/t0000036.htm

The George Lucas Educational Foundation. (2009). [Technology integration in the classroom]. Retrieved November 24, 2009, from http://www.edutopia.org/tech-integration

Makoul, G. (2001). Essential elements of communication in medical encounters: The Kalamazoo consensus statement. *Academic Medicine, 76*(4), 390–393.

McCombs, R. (2005). Shooting Web video: How to put your readers at the scene. *Online Journalism Review*. Retrieved November 24, 2009, from http://www.ojr.org/ojr/stories/050303mccombs/

Rose, J. (2008). *Producing great sound for film and video*. St. Louis, MO: Elsevier.

Schneps, M. H., & Sadler, P. (2005). *A private universe*. Retrieved November 24, 2009, from http://www.learner.org/resources/series28.html

Science Media Group. (2009). Factors influencing college success in science (FICSS). Retrieved November 24, 2009, from http://www.ficss.org/

Utz, P. (2006). *Today's video* (4th ed.). Jefferson, NC: McFarland Publishing.

Utz, P. (2009). Learn video equipment, setup, operation, and production. Retrieved November 24, 2009, from http://videoexpert.home.att.net/

CHAPTER 19

Multimedia in the Classroom: Creating Learning Experiences with Technology

Karen H. Teeley

INTRODUCTION

Health professions educators have new roles to fill in an era of increasing technology. "Multimedia" has grown from simple A-V (audio-visual) to a never-ending, ever-growing list of technological opportunities. The challenge for the instructor is not just to master new complicated technology but instead to find more meaningful ways to engage the students. Expectations are higher with each succeeding generation as students are exposed to technology at earlier ages. Today's students have grown up with technology; they have been raised on the Internet, they "Google" for information, and have thrived in the online communities of MySpace, Facebook, instant messages, chat rooms, and email. Students expect educators to be adept with the current technology and its applications (Prensky, 2001).

With increasing student enrollments in the health professions, the additional challenge is to be able to reach more students, with more content, yet maintain that all-important student–teacher relationship so vital in educating health professionals.

Aside from technological sophistication, today's students are skilled in the art of multitasking or parallel processing (Prensky, 2001) and lose interest quickly if the learning environment is not dynamic or interesting or both.

How can instructors use technology to reach and engage students and create opportunities for students to apply what they learn? This chapter will look at multimedia and multidelivery formats including Web-based course tools, the Internet, and other learning activities designed to create meaningful learning experiences.

DEFINITION AND PURPOSE

There are numerous definitions of multimedia, but for purposes of this chapter, multimedia simply means using more than one type of media and integrating the use of text, graphics, audio, and/or video. Barr and Tagg (1995) describe paradigm shifts taking place in higher education from teacher centered to learner centered education.

Educators are no longer the "experts," teachers have become "persons with expertise" (Wilson, 2004). Since students have access to volumes of information via the Internet, the instructor can no longer possibly keep ahead of the abundance of information but instead must guide the student into making the information meaningful. Students struggle with prioritizing information and organizing it in meaningful ways. The instructor's role changes from the traditional "sage on the stage" to the role of the "guide on the side" (Collison, Elbaum, Haavind, & Tinker, 2000).

Educators must be knowledgeable in new and emerging multimedia technology to be able to reach and engage students in ways the students are willing to learn.

With increased competition for students, institutions must reach more students more effectively. Multimedia technology and a variety of delivery methods provides the flexibility for faculty and institutions to engage both in the classroom and online.

THEORETICAL FOUNDATIONS

Creating learning environments through multimedia technology has roots in our knowledge of adult learning. Components of adult learning are described by Malcolm Knowles (1990) and emphasizes that adults are self-directed, are interested in topics that are relevant to their lives, like to be actively involved in the learning process, and have control over where and how they learn so they can learn at their own pace. Knowles' theory of andragogy makes the following assumptions about the design of learning: (1) adults need to know why they need to learn something, (2) adults need to learn experientially, (3) adults approach learning as problem solving, and (4) adults learn best when the topic is of immediate value (Knowles, 1990).

It is important that the instructor knows the learner's needs and design learning activities that are relevant to those needs. The student should be actively involved in learning, with the instructor acting as a facilitator or guide. The instructor that recognizes that adults have different learning needs can tailor their instruction design to the characteristic ways adults prefer to learn.

Adult learning theory is important in multimedia instructional design for several reasons. First, it is important to tailor the content specifically to the learner's level or it will not be effective (Lee & Owens, 2000). Second, learner goals and objectives must utilize a variety of learning activities if adults are to be engaged in the learning (Fink, 2003), and, lastly, by engaging in meaningful activity students feel like they are making significant, sustainable contributions (Teeley, Lowe, Beal, & Knapp, 2006).

Educators are familiar with Benjamin Bloom's taxonomy of educational objectives, as they have been a standard framework since the 1950s (Bloom, 1956).

Educators generally refer to the cognitive domain most frequently. They include, from the lowest to the highest:

- Knowledge
- Comprehension
- Application
- Analysis
- Synthesis
- Evaluation

Fink (2003) responds to the changing needs of students and educators by introducing a new taxonomy, called a *taxonomy of significant learning,* in his 2003 publication, *Creating Significant Learning Experiences* (Fig. 19-1). He addresses needs that are not easily met by Bloom's taxonomy such as learning how to learn, leadership and interpersonal skills, ethics, communication skills, character, tolerance, and the

Figure 19-1 The taxonomy of significant learning.

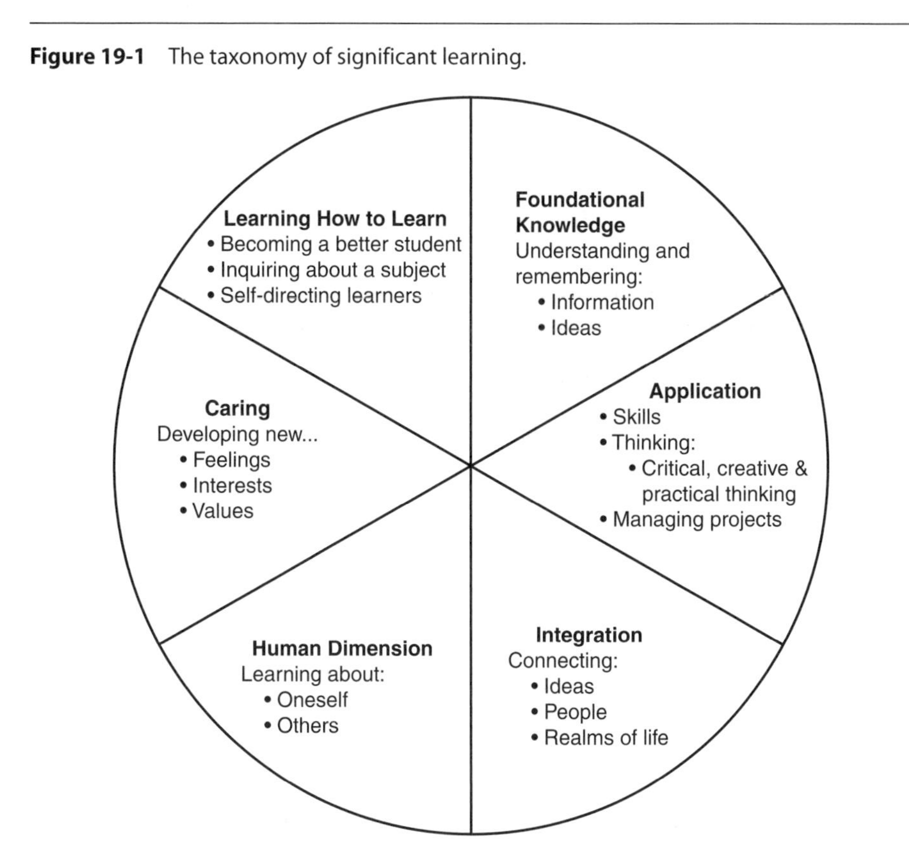

Source: From Fink, L. D. (Ed.). (2003). *Creating significant learning experiences*. San Francisco: Jossey-Bass, pp. 31. Used with permission.

Table 19-1 Fink's Major Categories in the Taxonomy of Significant Learning

Foundational Knowledge. At the base of most other kinds of learning is the need for students to "know" something. Knowing, as used here, refers to students' ability to understand and remember specific information and ideas. It is important for people today to have some valid basic knowledge, for example, about science, history, literature, geography, etc. They also need to understand major ideas or perspectives, for example, what evolution is (and what it is not), what capitalism is (and is not), and so forth. **Special Value:** Foundational knowledge provides the basic understanding that is necessary for other kinds of learning.

Application. This familiar kind of learning occurs when students learn how to engage in some new kind of action, which may be intellectual, physical, social, etc. Learning how to engage in various kinds of thinking (critical, creative, practical) is an important form of application learning. But this category of significant learning also includes developing certain skills (e.g., communication, playing the piano) or learning how to manage complex projects. **Special Value:** Application learning allows other kinds of learning to become useful.

Integration. When students are able to see and understand the connections between different things, an important kind of learning has occurred. Sometimes they make connections between specific ideas, between whole realms of ideas, between people, and/or between different realms of life (e.g., between school and work or between school and leisure life). **Special Value:** The act of making new connections gives learners a new form of power, especially intellectual power.

Human Dimension. When students learn something important about their own self and/or about others, it enables them to interact more effectively with themselves or with others. They discover the personal and/or social implications of what they have learned. What they learn or the way in which they learn sometimes gives students a new understanding of themselves (self image) or a new vision of what they want to become (self ideal). At other times, they acquire a better understanding of others: how and why others act the way they do, or how the learner can interact more effectively with others. **Special Value:** This kind of learning informs students about the human significance of what they are learning.

Caring. Sometimes a learning experience changes the degree to which students care about something. This may be reflected in the form of new feelings, interests, and/or values. Any of these changes means students now care about something to a greater degree or in a way than they did before. **Special Value:** When students care about something, they then have the energy they need for learning more about it and making it a part of their lives. Without the energy for learning, nothing significant happens.

Learning How to Learn. This occurs when students learn something about the process of learning itself. They may be learning how to be a better student, how to engage in a particular kind of inquiry (e.g., the scientific method), or how to become self directing learners. All of these constitute important forms of learning how to learn. **Special Value:** This kind of learning enables students to continue learning in the future and to do so with greater effectiveness.

Source: Fink, L. D. (Ed.). (2003). *Creating significant learning experiences*. San Francisco: Jossey-Bass Used with permission.

ability to adapt to change (Fink, 2003). Fink defines learning in terms of change, stating that, "For learning to occur, there has to be some kind of change in the learner. No change, no learner. And significant learning requires that there be some kind of lasting change in the learner" (Fink, 2003), (Table 19-1).

TYPES OF LEARNERS

Students enter the health professions in different stages in their lives. While some are traditional college students, most students have very busy lives with jobs and children and other additional family obligations. With the added expense of college tuition, it is a rare student who does not have to work in addition to attending school and fulfilling clinical placements. This changing profile of the learner suggests that most students fulfill the pedagogical requirements of the adult learner (Jairath & Stair, 2004). The more flexible and self paced the course delivery is, the more likely the students will be able to fit it in to their schedule, and be successful.

Web-based courses using a learning management system such as Blackboard require a comprehensive orientation to the format. Students must become quickly proficient in navigating the tools and how to troubleshoot common problems such as disabling pop-up blockers and mastery of email and attachment functions. Most importantly, students need to know how to access help.

Students in higher education in the first decade of the 21st century fall into the generation called "Millennials" (Howe & Strauss, 2000). These are students born between the years of 1982 and 2002. They are global, connected, and interactive. Although they grew up in a media age, they will undoubtedly have varying levels of proficiency that will require access to support functions.

Prensky (2001) differentiates *digital natives* from *digital immigrants*. He describes digital natives as the students today who are *native speakers* to the digital language of computers, video games, and the Internet, while those who are not native to the digital language (most instructors) are said to be *immigrants*. Immigrants have to learn a new language and adapt to a new environment. "Digital natives are used to receiving information really fast, they like to parallel process and multi-task and they function best when networked" (Prensky, 2001). He suggests that it is unlikely that digital natives are going to learn the immigrant's language, so in order to reach these students, immigrant instructors must learn to communicate in the language style of the student.

CONDITIONS FOR LEARNING: BLENDED LEARNING

A Web-based, or blended design, course requires that the students are self directed and are accustomed to working independently. Although beginning college students may do well with the technology, the discipline and organization required means that the more mature student will be better prepared and ultimately more successful.

The course must be well planned out in advance because the students will have access to the entire course once they are registered and enrolled. Clear instructions and troubleshooting guides should be readily available and included in a course orientation or overview.

Blended design is the best of both worlds; it allows for the development of independent study style and self discovery in the online portion, yet the classroom component provides the intimacy found in the face-to-face classroom environments. The design promotes community building both online and in the classroom, once the students have been assigned to their "groups."

Multimedia delivery formats have the potential to better engage the students by creating self-directed, lifelong learners.

Goals for multimedia–multidelivery format include:

- Create a positive learning environment
- Greater interactivity and increased engagement in course
- Address different learning styles
- Retain information after the course
- Develop and ability to transfer knowledge
- Make information meaningful
- Develop self directed learners
- Develop a love of knowledge and lifelong learners
- Create collaborative learners
- Promote community building

RESOURCES

Personnel

The most essential resource for a blended or Web-based design is the availability of experienced faculty facilitators to manage the smaller discussion groups of 6 to 12. A group that is too small does not have the diversity of input and opinions to make it interesting but a group that is too large becomes unwieldy for both the students and the facilitator especially if there are multiple posting and responses required within a small time.

Technology

Students and faculty need access to home computers with access to high-speed Internet and email accounts. Classrooms must also have computer and

Internet access plus projection equipment for CDs, tapes, videos, and PowerPoint. Faculty must be proficient in the use of the classroom technology. If the educational setting offers training for faculty, it is advised to take advantage new and emerging technology. Nothing seems to diminish the important role of the faculty quicker than stumbling through technological set up in front of a class.

FACULTY DEVELOPMENT

Faculty development for online course development is essential in addition to ongoing design support and technology support.

USING THE METHOD

There are numerous *how to* texts available for Web design courses and many of these resources are listed in the Additional Resources section at the end of this chapter. This section will look specifically at developing a blended course and incorporating within the course design multiple media types aimed at engaging the student in the learning experience.

The key to successful implementation of a blended course is allowing sufficient time for planning the course itself as well as allowing time to train faculty facilitators (see Table 19-2).

PLANNING

Taking an existing course and adapting it for use online requires *reconceptualizing* the learning material (O'Neil, Fisher, & Newbold, 2004). Each module or learning section needs to be reassessed in light of new available options. How are the module's objectives best met given the skill level of the faculty and the available technology? Can the content be packaged and available online for viewing at the student's own pace? Does the content lend itself to small group discussions that can be facilitated on a discussion board? If the students read the material online in preparation for the next face-to-face class, then can class time be better spent in classroom activities and discussions instead of simply imparting content? What activities, case studies, and discussions are better suited for an online discussion or a face-to-face class?

For integrated planning, use a course design worksheet based on goals and learning objectives. See Table 19-2 which is based on Fink's taxonomies (Fink, 2003).

Table 19-2 Taxonomy Design Worksheet

Goals	Fink's Taxonomy	Learning Activities, In Class	Learning Activities, Outside Class	Types of Media/ Delivery	Feedback and Assessment
1. Describe basic elements of the financing of healthcare delivery including Medicaid, Medicare, and managed care options	Foundational knowledge	Lecture Textbook CD interactive game	Online vignettes Self-paced PowerPoint Clinical setting	Instructor-led lecture CD interactive game PowerPoint Web-CT	Preclass online quiz Midterm or final exam 1-minute papers
2. Evaluate opportunities for disparities in present day system	Application Integration Caring Human dimension	Discussion Debate Case studies	Clinical setting Online discussion question Online reflection Literature/stories	Web-CT Text-based case studies Discussion board Internet audio Internet video	Discussion grade Weekly reflection Project presentations
3. Investigate resources for eliminating disparities	Integration Caring Learning how to learn	Discussion Debate	Clinical setting Links to Web sites	Self directed Internet exploration	Project presentations

FEEDBACK AND ASSESSMENT

How will the students receive feedback? And how will they be assessed and graded? Discussion questions need to be carefully constructed to elicit thoughtfully researched responses. Clearly defined rubrics are helpful for the students as well as the faculty facilitators to assure uniform grading criteria.

EXPECTATIONS

In addition to the traditional course content with objectives and outcomes, the online and blended faculty need to clearly set the tone and the expectations. The students will most likely have access to the online component of the course before they meet face-to-face (of course this is optional). What the students see on their first "visit" will most likely determine their first impressions of the class. Will it be visually appealing and friendly or chaotic and hard to navigate? A friendly "Welcome from the Professor" with the blended course expectations clearly explained will ally fears and set the tone for a positive learning experience.

Dispel the myth that less class time means less work. Clearly define the student's expectations for workload plus the expectations of the new role for the faculty facilitators. When can the students expect responses from the faculty and how will their grades be communicated? Develop a list of course frequently asked questions and add to it as the course evolves.

TRAINING AND ORIENTATION

New roles and expectations for faculty facilitators must be clearly defined, as this is most likely a brand new role. Time involved should not be underestimated and should be agreed on at the start of the course to prevent any unwelcome surprises. Rubrics for grading are helpful for new faculty as well as timelines and sample responses to the student's discussion postings. *How to* resources for moderating online discussions will help support the faculty as they grow in this new role.

Group faculty training with hands-on Internet and Web course access is ideal for introducing the faculty facilitators to the course design and to hear concerns and questions before the class begins. Practice discussion questions help the faculty work together to anticipate student issues. Once the training period is over, it is helpful to establish a private discussion area on the course's Web site just for faculty to communicate with each other, they will undoubtedly have common questions from students and it will be helpful to have a *community* as a resource.

Student orientation to the blended design needs to be just as thorough as the faculty orientation, especially if this is a new way of learning. In addition to online resources, the first face-to-face class should be spent going over required computer skills, course

Table 19-3 Course Development Workflow Checklist

1. Outline the course into teaching modules.
2. Identify online and face-to-face segments.
3. Define learning objectives for each module.
4. Outline module content.
5. Define feedback and assessment strategies.
6. Identify integration link each week between online and classroom.
7. Identify resources for content support.
   a. Web sites, books, articles
8. Determine teaching/learning activities to address course content and objectives.
9. Determine assessment tasks.
   a. Quizzes/tests
      i. Develop test questions based on objectives.
      ii. Provide rationale for answers.
   b. Discussion board questions/case studies
      ii. Develop questions based on module objectives.
      ii. Clearly define instructions for posting and responding including length and deadlines (visual chart).
      iii. Provide rubric for correct answers.
      iv. Communicate rubric to other course faculty.
      v. Design method for weekly faculty communication with course coordinator.
   c. Other written assignments
10. Develop grade plan based on assessment tasks.
11. Communicate all the above in the course syllabus.
    a. Include time management expectation for students (3 hours prep per hour class)
    b. Include help desk resources and academic technology support
12. Communicate all of the above to clinical faculty in a faculty orientation/training session.
    a. Develop clinical faculty training materials.

layout and navigation tips, expectations for timely assignment submissions, organization tips, appropriate communication strategies (netiquette), and, most importantly, how much time will be expected to complete the assignments (Table 19-3).

POTENTIAL PROBLEMS

For Students

The most challenging problem is for the students to embrace a new way of learning. Although the students may be accustomed to the technological features, this blended course requires a lot of independence and self direction, and the student who is not ready for this different way of learning can feel lost and resentful. Poor organizational skills and impaired time management can also derail a student if they get behind. Students who are not Web savvy need to get up to speed quickly. Varying computer skills and access to high-speed Internet can also be problematic in this course style. Online quizzes are a particular challenge for varying Internet speeds, and students can experience a high degree of frustration on top of the quiz anxiety when the Internet is inaccessible.

For Faculty

Course development takes a considerable time commitment just in the planning stages. Once the course is implemented, the first few "editions" need continued tweaking and modifying to work out unforeseen bugs. Because of the nature of technology, plus the addition of new areas of content, the course will never be finished, but will always be evolving.

Applied Example

Community Health Nursing–A blended course

The decision to use a blended model emerged from growing class sizes and increased need to deliver more content in less time. A creative way was needed to better engage the students in learning and increase the connectivity between the students and the faculty in light of the larger class sizes.

The course coordinator/designer, met with instructional designers and Web course experts from the college's academic technology department. Goals and timelines were established with an 8-month planning time frame. In addition, the first blended model was scheduled to run as a pilot project with only three modules online. Once some of the bugs were worked out of the pilot, the full blended course had five modules online with seven face-to-face classes.

The community health nursing class content was already organized in modules and posted online in a Web-enhanced format; most of the documents, such as the syllabus, handouts, and forms, were already online as well as the test question database.

This reduced some of the redesign time.

The course modules were reevaluated taking into consideration the best way to engage the students with the material. Online and Web-based activities were selected with multiple learning styles in mind. The class was scheduled to meet every other week online, alternating with face-to-face classes.

One of the major hurdles in the online course management is the increased faculty time required for the reading and responding to multiple discussion posts. With a class size of 70+ students and 2 to 3 posts per week, it quickly becomes unmanageable to respond to more than 200 posts each week.

Because the course already employed clinical faculty for a student/faculty ratio of 6 to 7 students per faculty, it seemed logical to include the clinical faculty in the course design as *faculty facilitators*. As the students were assigned to their clinical groups, the same groups were carried over into the classroom, and the clinical /faculty facilitator was responsible for managing the discussion posts for their group. This worked out especially well by engaging the clinical faculty in the classroom portion and provided much needed continuity for the students, connecting the classroom and the clinical settings.

For the online component, the students had assigned readings and activities followed by a Part I and Part 2 discussion questions and responses due on specific dates. The responses were important as they were designed to engage the students in an online community and promote a back and forth discussion as opposed to just posts. Faculty facilitators were guided in their role as *facilitators* and were encouraged to not jump into the discussion but rather let the discussion flow among the students. The facilitators graded the student's posting individually but responded to the groups' postings as a whole once all the postings were complete. Once the faculty facilitators posted their response to the student group, they were encouraged to share their response with other faculty members on a private (faculty only) "Faculty Forum" discussion board. The faculty forum was also available to faculty to share ideas and concerns throughout the class.

In order to keep the classroom times interesting by leaving time for activities and discussions, the students were required to read the assignments *before* class and complete an online quiz based on the material. Because this was structured as a learning experience rather than a test, the students could take the test up to two times and only their highest score was recorded. This worked well because the students came to class with questions and were already engaged in the material. The students also liked this because they received immediate feedback from the online test.

Academic misconduct was minimized as much as possible by stating up front that the quizzes and tests were *open book*. The questions were designed to be higher level, that is, *application* and *integration* rather than simply *knowledge based* (Fink, 2003) and required fuller comprehension of the material. Midterms and final exams, while also online, were built on a Blackboard feature of a computerized random selection of questions so that no two tests were alike. Misconduct is always a concern with online tests but by enabling the students to take the quizzes more than once and enabling the random selection feature, the opportunities were minimized.

One of the most successful features of the course was the student's presentation project based on reading current literature about a selected vulnerable population group (Leffers & Martin, 2004). The learning goal was to evoke a caring response by immersing the reader into the personal struggles of the population. This goal is consistent with Fink's *Taxonomies of Significant Learning* (Fink, 2003) of both the caring and human dimension taxonomy.

The students presented their project as a group to the class utilizing creative multimedia methodologies. A selection of their presentations included formats such as video production, radio show simulation, a Jeopardy game, and others that engaged the rest of the class and communicated the message of heartfelt vulnerability.

The best way to keep up with new and meaningful delivery methods is to take notes from the students, they will let instructors know how they like to learn.

Feedback for the blended delivery method was elicited from both students and the clinical faculty facilitators. The responses were organized into four themes: time management, participation, learning opportunities, and technology. The results were favorable for the blended style in general as most students like the flexibility and opportunities to participate. Some students still would prefer to sit in class and *be passive learners*, but for the most part, the students enjoyed the learning experience and students and faculty alike benefited from the increased engagement in the discussions. See survey results in Table 19-4.

Table 19-4 Feedback for Blended Learning

	Student: Advantages of Hybrid Model	Student: Disadvantages of Hybrid Model	Faculty Facilitator: Advantages of Hybrid Model	Faculty Facilitator: Disadvantages of Hybrid Model
Time/ Schedule	"Fits schedule better" "More flexible—less stressful" "Quizzes can be taken in a relaxed environment" "More time for readings" "Less commuting time" "Lets me organize my time better"	"Writing out the discussions is time consuming" "Seems to be more work involved, too much time researching answers to discussions" "Hard to keep organized, the time management is difficult" "Very time consuming, makes you prefer classroom lectures"	"The students seem to manage their time better"	
Participation	"More engaged with material" "Really enjoy learning other's opinions" "More communication with classmates" "Students who don't speak easily in class, speak up online" "More time for a better prepared response" "More feedback from peers" "Smaller groups, more attention" "Good for someone like myself who does not speak up in class yet has a lot to say"	"Don't like sharing with other students" "Feel disconnected from the classroom professor" "Miss the classroom interaction with other students" "Online discussions feel like busy work" "Online doesn't feel 'real,' hard to take it seriously" "I would rather sit in class for 2 hours and listen to the professor than to read on my own and share my thoughts on the Internet" "Too much computer screen time, would rather more face-to-face time" "Other's discussions are too long to read"	"Very interesting discussions, I love reading them!" "Allows the students to clearly express their thoughts" "I learn a lot about the students from their postings, I would never get that otherwise" "Would love to see more of the course online!"	"The students don't like reading all the discussions and responses" "I worry that the students view the online sessions as an 'off' week"

(continues)

Table 19-4 Feedback for Blended Learning (Continued)

Learning Opportunities	"Forces you to look things up and learn more" "Like the independent learning—I learn more on my own" "Enables students to learn in different ways" "Need to really read to participate in class" "I am learning more through the discussions and quizzes than I am in the classroom" "The discussions allow us to think about what we read" "The Internet connectivity leads us to different Web sites with a lot of new information" "The discussions make you really think about the readings instead of just memorizing" "Ties in the clinical practice with class" "The discussions revealed whole new areas of interest for me"	"Feel different instructors grade discussions differently, it's not fair" "Find the different assignments confusing" "We have to learn quite a bit on our own"	"The students did great research in preparation of the discussion questions" "The discussion questions seem to cover a great deal of material" "The students seem to learn more from the assignments" "The students seem to be able to organize their thoughts better by putting them in writing" "The students seem better at tying together the classroom and the clinical"	"Hard to give feedback—at this level students still need feedback on basic grammar and APA format, I find that hard to use this format to make comments"
Technology	"Improves my technology skills by forcing me to use the WebCT features"	"If the Internet is down, participation is difficult" "The technology is confusion" "Frustrating to work on an old PC" "Culture shock compared to other nursing classes"		"I don't like correcting online, I would rather have a word document I can print out and make comments on"

CONCLUSION

Students entering the health professions in the 21st century are different learners than their instructors. Internet access to new information and the convergence of technology is a way of life and must be an integral part of the classroom if the goal is to be meaningful engagement and lifelong learning. Instructors need to learn to reach students in ways they will use the material and foster a love of learning. A successful student is one who knows that learning will not end with graduation but will graduate with the necessary tools and skills to make lifelong contributions to their profession.

REFERENCES

Barr, R. B., & Tagg, J. (1995). From teaching to learning—a new paradigm for undergraduate education. *Change, 27*(6), 12.

Bloom, B. S. (Ed.). (1956). *Taxonomy of educational objectives. the classification of educational goals handbook I: Cognitive domain*. New York: McKay.

Collison, G., Elbaum, B., Haavind, S., & Tinker, R. (2000). *Facilitating online learning: Effective strategies for moderators*. Madison, WI: Atwood Publishing.

Fink, L. D. (Ed.). (2003). *Creating significant learning experiences*. San Francisco: Jossey-Bass.

Howe, N., & Strauss, W. (2000). *Millennials rising: The next greatest generation*. New York: Vintage Press.

Jairath, N., & Stair, N. (2004). A development and implementation framework for web-based nursing courses. *Nursing Education Perspectives, 25*(2), 67.

Knowles, M. (1990). *The adult learner: A neglected species* (4th ed.). Houston: Gulf Pub Co.

Lee, W. W., & Owens, D. L. (2000). *Multimedia-based instructional design*. San Francisco: Jossey-Bass.

Leffers, J., & Martin, D. C. (2004). Journey to compassion: Meeting vulnerable populations in community health nursing through literature. *International Journal of Human Caring, 8*(1), 20.

O'Neil, C. A., Fisher, C. A., & Newbold, S. K. (Eds.). (2004). *Developing an online course: Best practices for nurse educators*. New York: Springer Publishing Company.

Prensky, M. (2001). Digital natives, digital immigrants. *On the Horizon, 9*(No.5).

Teeley, K., Lowe, J., Beal, J., & Knapp, M. (2006). Incorporating quality improvement concepts and practice into a community health nursing course. *Journal of Nursing Education, 45*(2), 65–71.

Wilson, L. O. (2004). *Teaching millennial students*. Retrieved August 6, 2005, from http://www.uwsp.edu/education/facets/links_resources/millennials.pdf

ADDITIONAL RESOURCES

Bonk, C. J., & Zhang, K. (2008). *Empowering on-line learners*. San Francisco: Jossey-Bass.

Brookfield, S. (2005). *Adult cognition as a dimension of lifelong learning*. Retrieved June 22, 2009, from http://www.open.ac.uk/lifelong-learning/papers/393CD0DF-000B-67DB-0000015700000157_StephenBrookfieldpaper.doc

Brookfield, S. (1986). *Understanding and facilitating adult learning*. San Francisco: Jossey-Bass.

Clark, R. C., & Mayer, R. E. (2003). *e-Learning and the science of instruction*. San Francisco: Pfeiffer.

Conrad, R., & Donaldson, J. (2004). *Engaging the online learner*. San Francisco: Jossey-Bass.

Fink, L. D. (2005). *A self directed guide to designing courses for significant learning*. Retrieved June 22, 2009, from http://www.ou.edu/idp/significant/Self-DirectedGuidetoCourseDesignAug%2005.doc.

Garrison, D. R., Vaughn N. D., (2008) *Blended Learning in Higher Education*. San Francisco: Josey-Bass.

Horton, W. (2006). *e-Learning by design*. San Francisco: Pfeiffer

Howe, N., & Strauss, W. (2000). *Millennials rising: The next greatest generation*. New York: Vintage Press.

Krug, S. (2006). *Don't make me think: A common sense approach to web usability* (2nd ed.). Berkeley: New Riders.

Matthews-Denatale, G., & Cotler, D. (2005). *Faculty as authors of online courses: Support and mentoring*. Retrieved June 22, 2009, from http://www.academiccommons.org/commons/essay/matthews-denatale-and-cotler

Novotny, J. M., & Davis, R. (Eds.). (2006). *Distance education in nursing*. New York: Springer Publishing Company.

Palloff, R. M., & Pratt, K. (2005). *Collaborating online: Learning together in community*. San Francisco: Jossey-Bass.

Palloff, R. M., & Pratt, K. (2003). *The virtual student*. San Francisco: Jossey-Bass.

Palloff, R. M., & Pratt, K. (2001). *Lessons from the cyberspace classroom*. San Francisco: Jossey-Bass.

Pink, D. H. (2006). *A whole new mind*. New York: Riverhead Books.

Wiske, M. S. (2005) *Teaching for Understanding with Technology* San Francisco: Jossey-Bass.

ELECTRONIC RESOURCES

Blended Learning at Simmons College. Retrieved from http://at.simmons.edu/blendedlearning/

Faculty Resources for Hybrid Learning. Retrieved from http://www4.uwm.edu/ltc/hybrid/faculty_resources/index.cfm

Illinois Online. Retrieved from http://www.ion.uillinois.edu/resources/tutorials/id/index.asp

University of Calgary: Teaching and Learning Centre Resource Library. Retrieved from http://tlc.ucalgary.ca/resources/library/

University of Michigan: Center for Research on Learning and Teaching. Retrieved from http://www.crlt.umich.edu/tstrategies/tsot.php

CHAPTER 20

Electronic Communication Strategies

Gail Matthews-DeNatale and Arlene J. Lowenstein

DEFINITION AND PURPOSES

Educational institutions are increasingly becoming computer-enriched environments in which technology is integral to all aspects of academic life and work (Green, Brown, & Robinson, 2008; Mitra & Steffensmeier, 2000). Electronic communication has grown significantly in educational settings and has brought about dramatic changes in communication between students, faculty, and staff. The use of computers for electronic communication takes many forms. In addition to well-established technologies such as email, learning management systems (e.g., Blackboard, Angel, Moodle, Sakai) provide educators with a bundled set of tools for communication, including instant messaging, threaded discussions, chat rooms, and Web-based live classrooms. Personal response systems (PRSs; clickers) allow students to pool communication, immediately registering a vote or collectively answering a survey question in the classroom. Podcasts can be recorded so that students can listen to, or review, lectures at a time and place of their convenience. Online, there are a host of free, easy-to-use tools that are sometimes referred to as "Web 2.0" or the "social web," including blogs, wikis (Web pages that can be modified by anyone visiting the site), VoiceThread, Google Apps, LinkedIn, and Facebook.

With all of these options readily at hand, it is understandable if some educators feel overwhelmed by myriad possibilities. As 21st-century educators, we are challenged to explore the possibilities associated with new technology and to reinvent ourselves as teachers. Recent research conducted at Memorial University in Newfoundland indicates that "the [online] medium itself changed the dynamics of class interactions, not only those between students and professor, but also the interaction between students themselves" (Reid, 2009). This chapter provides a pedagogical analysis of options for electronic communication, along with a recommended process for selecting an electronic communication option that best suits a given situation or learning scenario.

Effective use of this technology depends on a clear understanding of the desired learning outcomes and the type of communication that will best further goals for learning in a given situation. For example, online journaling may be most appropriate for learning that is individualized and reflective, whereas threaded discussions or wikis may be more appropriate for learning that improves collaboration and group analysis.

Likewise, the needs of the learners are also a factor in deciding which tools to use. Electronic communication makes it possible for a wider range of students to become actively involved in the teaching–learning process. Presented with a range of easy-to-use tools, students can become active and self-directed participants in the teaching–learning process. Online communication can be asynchronous, which does not require that both parties communicate at the same time. Introverted students have time to reflect before composing a message to a threaded discussion, contributing thoughts that might go unspoken in a face-to-face (or ideas that might only become lucid after class lets out). Online communication can also be synchronous, with all participants taking part at the same time. Tools like chat and Web-based live classrooms can provide students with a place to meet and make in-the-moment decisions about their group projects. These options are particularly helpful for students who live off campus and therefore have difficulty finding a mutually agreeable time to meet with their peers.

Electronic communication is not just a back and forth between one student and the instructor. Communication can be between the instructor and groups of students, or communication between group members, with the instructor acting as a "guide on the side," rather than as the "sage on the stage" (Collision, Elbaum, Haavind, & Tinker, 2000). People who are unfamiliar with this "constructivist" approach to teaching sometimes wrongly assume that it is completely spontaneous and unplanned.

According to Reid (2009), "online courses are a disruptive technology in the sense that it requires different pedagogical methods which may not yet be fully understood. In many ways it is a break with the past and requires professors to rethink their teaching practices."

Successful integration of electronic communication into the course plan requires a thoughtful process of instructional design that sets the stage and provides appropriate resources for learning. The instructor is able to transition into a facilitative role because the plan for learning is well thought out, articulated clearly, engaging, resource rich, and so generative that students are equipped to take responsibility for their own learning. Sarah Haavind describes this as "front loading" learning (Haavind, 2007).

The instructor is also responsible for introducing students to the resources available, providing guidelines for use, and troubleshooting with the student when technical problems occur or referring student to appropriate technology support for assistance. It is a good idea for the instructor to build in time to experiment with electronic tools and strategies under consideration, developing personal mastery and ensuring that the technology functions as anticipated. The course design process may begin months or even semesters before the course is launched, and instructors may find themselves collaborating with one or more instructional designers or instructional technologists on the development of a course. In writing about ePortfolios (a Webspace where students or faculty can store and reflect on their accomplishments among other uses), as a tool for enhanced meta cognition, Trent Batson states that "if we in higher education wish to learn the most and leverage the most during this knowledge revolution, we have to recognize the active agent in the revolution. The active agent is humanity." In the same way that faculty should read and understand a book before assigning it to their students, instructors should also spend time using technology in their own lives as learners to "discover in themselves what talents and abilities come forward" (Batson, 2008). Likewise, Ruth Reynard also extols the virtues of "getting your hands dirty," piloting ideas to solicit student input, and making sure that the technical implementation strategy is explicitly aligned with learning goals (Reynard, 2008).

THEORETICAL RATIONALE

In the face-to-face classroom setting, decisions about verbal communication are relatively straightforward, and there is also a commonly held understanding among students about the forms and strategies for communication. For example, issues that are of general importance are raised during class, whereas communication with individuals takes place during office hours, before class, or after class. Seasoned educators develop an intuitive sense for appropriate formats: when to lecture, convene small group discussions among students, or host a question and answer session.

The advent of electronic communication greatly increases options for communication, offering the opportunity for enhanced interactions between teachers and learners. Communication can be text-based, include images or video, and even take place through an avatar (an online character). Likewise, interactions can take place in real time (e.g., chat, text messaging) or asynchronously (online discussion forums, email). With this opportunity comes a new set of responsibilities:

- to reflect on the goal and desired effect of each act of communication;
- to select a communicative strategy and tool that is appropriate to the goal;
- to understand the range of options available, as well as the affordances and constraints of each tool; and
- to consider issues of access, including the needs of students with disabilities.

To make pedagogically sound decisions about how to communicate with students, it is helpful to first take a step back and consider how communication happens among people. Although communication is fundamental to everyday life, communications experts will tell you that it is deceptively complex. From Aristotle to the present day, academics grapple with the challenge of developing a theoretical model for communication that captures nuances of the process. Early models described a linear process that involved the transmission of information from a sender (e.g., speaker, writer) to a receiver (e.g., listener, reader) (Shannon & Weaver, 1949).

But communication, particularly electronic communication, is anything but linear. Contemporary theorists describe communication as a multidimensional process that can take place over extended periods of time, for distinct purposes (persuasion, inquiry, etc.), and within complex systems in which the specific context can dramatically alter perceived meaning (Littlejohn, 2002).

For example, a single instructor (sender) can podcast a presentation to hundreds or even thousands of people, yet each person (receiver) will probably listen to the podcast in a different context (e.g., in the car, at the gym, while cooking supper), stopping and starting to complete the process of listening in different increments of time. At first glance, this might appear to be problematic, but listener control over the time, place, and increment of playback is central to the dramatic rise in podcasting use and popularity. Anxieties that podcasting might contribute to increased absenteeism proved to be irrelevant in a recent study conducted by the University of Washington (UW). Eighty-four percent of student respondents in UW's podcasting pilot initiative reported the same or increased levels of attendance, and faculty reported that even if attendance did decline, in podcast-enhanced courses "those who were there were truly present" (Lane, 2006). This is yet another example of the ways in which electronic communication challenges educators to rethink assumptions about teaching.

Questions to Consider in Devising an Electronic Communication Strategy

The following questions are designed to guide readers through a pedagogically grounded process for integrating electronic communication into teaching and learning

1. What are the overarching goals for student learning? First, it is important to consider goals for the course as a whole, because that helps inform the suite of tools to be used during the semester. Unless your course has technology as its focus (e.g., an informatics course), it is advisable to be judicious in your selection of technology. It is better to use a few tools extremely well than to overwhelm students with different technologies

each session. If your learning management system allows you to hide tools that are not in use, doing so will make your course easier to navigate and less overwhelming.

2. What are the session- or unit-specific goals for student learning? Some tools lend themselves particularly well to specific tasks. For example, PRS clickers are particularly good for polling large classes to get a snapshot of student learning in the aggregate (persistent misconceptions, concepts that have been mastered), and then involving students in personalized with neighbors or with the group as a whole.
3. What evidence (artifacts of student work) will be needed so that the instructor and the students can assess and improve progress toward learning goals?
4. To what extent should a given act of communication be public (e.g., discussion and debate) or private (e.g., reflection and self-assessment)?
5. What is the desired level of interactivity (give and take) associated with the act of communication? Is it a one-way broadcast (content delivery) or is it an open-ended question that is best understood by hearing from a range of perspectives?
6. How complex is the act of communication? Text messages and chat rooms are great for simple questions (e.g., "Did you mean for us to read Chapter Three AND Four?"), but they are inadequate for following a nuanced thread of extended discussion among multiple participants.
7. How collaborative is the assignment? Do you want students to work as a team to produce a product, report, or analysis? If so, then choose a tool that can provide each group with their own work space (e.g., wikis, live classroom breakout rooms).
8. What are the learners' time constraints? If class members live in different time zones, it could be disastrous if students are required to login at a given time for synchronous interaction.

After you have considered these questions, Table 20-1 will help you identify electronic communication strategies that meet your needs.

CONDITIONS

If possible, gather information about the conditions under which students will access the course. For example, if many students will be accessing the course through a dial-up connection, bandwidth-intensive strategies such as video are not advisable. Likewise, some institutions place storage and upload limits. It is better to know the institutional policies beforehand to ensure that course materials are within file size limits.

Table 20-1 Electronic Communication Styles

Use	Texting	Chat	Email	Online Journal (Private)	ePortfolio	Blog (Public)	Wiki	Threaded Discussion	Podcast	PRS Clickers	Live Classroom
One to self				×	×						
One to one	×	×	×		×						
One to many		×	× (list, carbon copy)		×	×		×	×		×
Many to one							×			×	
Many to many			× (list)				×	×		×	×
Presentation and content delivery					×	×	×		×		×
Quick questions and clarification	×	×	×					×		×	×
Reflection and individualized interaction			×	×	×						
Collaboration and group work							×	×			×
Synchronous		×								×	×
Asynchronous	×		×	×	×	×	×	×	×		

Wherever possible, build technology orientation into the learning experience well in advance of the time that it will be needed. For example, in the first week of class require that students complete an online scavenger hunt that uses key technologies. In addition to the scavenger hunt, provide self-based tutorials, quickstart guides, and practice areas so that students can experiment, troubleshoot, problem solve, and self teach. Include information on where to go for technical support in the syllabus and in the support materials. In this way, technical glitches can be resolved before they have a chance to compromise the learning and the instructor is less likely to be inundated with technical questions.

Internet users are increasingly concerned about the loss of privacy that can result from uninformed interaction online. In particular, parents wonder about the safety of their underage children, and adolescents learn too late that youthful indiscretions have considerable staying power online. As an instructor, it is your responsibility to keep apprised of privacy laws and to take steps to provide a safe learning environment whose privacy is appropriate to the learning scenario. Instructors also are responsible for ensuring that course materials and assignments do not result in copyright infringement.

Some projects may be appropriate for public consumption (e.g., a vetted online poster presentation that presents original student research), but the vast majority of coursework should be password protected. If a password-protected learning management system is used, many privacy concerns become moot. However, security measures in cutting edge, free technologies will vary, and the stability of these platforms should be carefully considered as well. If a company goes out of business midcourse and shuts down its servers, student work may be at risk if there is no offline copy of the files. Familiarize yourself with FERPA and TEACH Act regulations so that you can be mindful about how privacy laws relate to electronic communication in the classroom. For more information, see privacy and copyright links listed in the resource section of this chapter.

TYPES OF LEARNERS

When thoughtfully designed and judiciously implemented, electronic communication improves an instructor's ability to meet the needs of heterogeneous learners. PRS clickers engage kinesic learners, podcasts address the needs of auditory learners and those for whom English is a second language, and threaded discussions are great for introverts who like time to reflect before contributing to a discussion. However, a strategy that opens doors for one type of learner may also be a strategy that presents a barrier to entry for another. For example, podcasts may not be accessible for students who are hearing impaired. Ideally, coursework is offered in a range of formats using a range of strategies, embodying the principles of "universal design" (Burgstahler & Cory, 2008). If assistance is needed to convert course content into an accessible format, contact the institution's Academic Support Center or Instructional/Academic Technology to request help. Mention Section 508 ADA compliance—things need to be accessible for people with disabilities (e.g., low vision, deaf).

RESOURCES

Although most faculty members and students have been exposed to and use computers, there are still those who are uncomfortable with new or different programs and few have high-level expertise. Regardless of expertise level, training with technical support follow-up must be made available (Bates & Poole, 2003). Knowledgeable and friendly technical support is very important for both faculty and students. Working with computers and other electronic means of communication can be extremely frustrating and stressful for novices unless an adequate support system to troubleshoot problems and encourage the uses is in place. Technical support personnel can alert faculty members to new programs that are available. Learning to work with computers and new programs takes practice and persistence, but the process can be well worth the time and energy. For example, in our setting, technical support personnel work with faculty to learn to use the technology needed to develop blended or hybrid learning models, using wikis and voiceover PowerPoints, and developing podcasts. Coordination between the information systems department and faculty is needed to avoid problems caused by underestimating the use and need for assistance. Specific resources are noted here:

Emerging Technologies (Technologies on the Horizon)

New Media Consortium Horizon Project, http://www.nmc.org/horizon/

Instructional Design and Curricular Innovation with Technology

Educause Learning Initiative, http://www.educause.edu/eli/16086

Innovate, an online journal dedicated to the creative use of technology in education http://innovateonline.info/?view=about

Privacy and Copyright

http://www.ed.gov/policy/gen/guid/fpco/ferpa

http://www.etown.edu/Registration.aspx?topic=Downloadable+Forms:+FERPA+Explained

http://www2.nea.org/he/abouthe/teachact.html

Universal Design

CAST (Center for Applied Special Technology), http://www.cast.org/publications/UDLguidelines/version1.html

USING THE METHOD

The choice of which technology to be used depends on the learning objectives, the need for synchronous or asynchronous processes, and the resources available. The use column in Table 20-1 demonstrates the various uses of some of the electronic communication programs, and the questions to consider outlined previously provide a guide to decision making in the use of available technology. While students may be asked to use the Internet for finding references and in-depth research, they must be taught to understand the need to validate the data found. Many Web pages are not peer reviewed, and the accuracy of the material cannot be guaranteed unless it is an electronic version of a journal article.

An online course might use both a chat room and threaded discussions. Mobile technology including handheld personal digital assistants (PDAs), cell phones, and laptop computers can be used in the clinical area to maintain contact with the faculty member and provide a way to explore additional information onsite (Effink et al., 2000). MP3 players can be used for more than music, and students can store and transmit data (Read, 2005). Choice of communication also depends on the need for group interaction, peer-to-peer-interaction, or student-to-instructor interaction. For example, a wiki might be used for group projects because it allows group members to edit documents directly, without the need for emailing changes to group members. Clickers may work well in large classrooms to allow students' anonymous responses to the instructor's questions be viewed by the total audience. This has been shown to increase student involvement, can keep students involved in the lecture, and allow the instructor to assess student learning and provide immediate guidance or additional information (Weerts, Miller, & Altice, 2009). Passwords may be necessary to gain access for some venues.

Technology changes and evolves rapidly. Cell phones take pictures and videos; MP3 players collect data. It is important for faculty to be aware of new methodologies as they develop. Faculty should also be aware of potential financial issues involved for students interested in purchasing or required to purchase their own equipment, and may need to provide rationale for equipment purchases.

Instructions for use must be clear. It is important to assess students' comfort level with computers, programs, and equipment and to provide resources to assist them. The process for finding help for technological problems should be developed and communicated to students. Email messages can be more informal than student papers or written journals. Typos, spelling, and grammar may not need correction in email messages, as long as students understand that good grammar, spelling, and proofreading are required for paper assignments. Many schools have ethical policies for computer usage and email. Students should be informed of those policies and be expected to adhere to them.

POTENTIAL PROBLEMS

Faculty and student comfort with the systems is the first major problem that needs to be considered. Although younger students are growing up with computer technology today, health professions often have older students in classes who have not had that advantage and younger student knowledge cannot be taken for granted. Many individuals are technologically challenged and avoid using computers, especially if they have had bad or frustrating experiences in beginning attempts. Technological problems often occur, from full computer crashes to loss of messages that have not been saved or were overwritten. Knowing where to go for help becomes very important to minimize frustration in these instances. Remembering passwords when they have not been used frequently can be difficult, and a system needs to be available to retrieve a password without compromising security. Misspelled addresses can be frustrating and time consuming when a minor error, such as an extra dot, causes the message to go astray. Finding the error in an address or message can be difficult because of the tendency to read the word as the reader thinks it should be, thereby reading over the error. Computers are famous for carrying out commands literally. What the user wrote in the command may not have been what the user intended, but computers do not recognize intentions. Small errors can cause major problems and are often difficult to discover. At the same time, however, with the proper support computers can enhance learning and be fun and enjoyable to use.

Privacy and avoiding embarrassment can be important issues. Email messages are not private, even though they feel as if they are. Both students and faculty need to be made aware of that fact. In chat rooms and other group venues, it is possible for students to use an alias or pseudonym, as Parklyn (1999) had students do in the discourse communities he developed. He found that students expressed more opinions when they were free of personal harassment or disparaging remarks directed at their true self.

Time for email and discussion boards is an important issue for the instructor, especially if the selected method involves one-to-one student–instructor conversations. Class size is an important parameter in deciding if the instructor has the time to respond effectively to students. There are other methods to work with larger classes. Oosterhof's (2000) method of individualizing email allowed for consolidating messages and providing some automatic answering options when working with large classes. Replies to students can be brief, but need to be meaningful. Both large and small classes can benefit from the use of electronic communication when the technology is geared to meet specific teaching–learning objectives.

FUTURE DIRECTIONS

The present context offers a wealth of options—sometimes it can even feel like there are *too* many possibilities. But it is also important to stay abreast of new developments, as well as to anticipate technologies that are fading from use. The New Media Consortium's Horizon Project, an annual report, is a relatively easy way to keep current. Looking toward 2010 and beyond, as smart phones make it possible for people to access the Web, podcasts, email, and text messages from a pocket-sized device, expect that electronic communication with become increasingly ubiquitous, as well as infinitesimally smaller. At first glance, as with the time shifting and incremental listening associated with podcasts, these tiny devices may seem to raise as many problems as they solve. But as educators open themselves up to considering the possibilities, to rethinking assumptions about teaching and learning, the opportunities could be vast even though the mechanism for communication is small.

EXAMPLE

Electronic Journaling

The history of nursing ideas course was developed to enable graduate students to view nursing theory in the context of nursing history and growth of the profession. The course description and objectives are shown in Exhibit 20-1. A major mission of the nursing program and the school is to prepare students for leadership within the profession. Understanding dynamics of change and recognizing decision makers is important to the development of leadership skills necessary to carry out that mission. The critical thinking objective is used to prepare students to recognize decision makers and those dynamics of change within the nursing profession and in the provision of health care.

EXHIBIT 20-1

History of Nursing Ideas Course Syllabus

Course Description

This course focuses on the contributions of nursing history, nursing theory, and contemporary issues in the social evolution of nursing as a profession. The nature of nursing theory and the relationship between philosophy, theory, and science are explored. The evolution of nursing knowledge within the social context of history is emphasized.

Objectives

Upon completion of the course, the student should be able to:

1. Identify major issues associated with the development of nursing as a profession.
2. Examine the influences of hospitals and the rise of medicine in the development of nursing.
3. Utilize critical thinking to analyze the components of theories and the history of development in nursing.
4. Examine the relationship between historical development in nursing, nursing theory, and nursing science.
5. Apply theory in domains of practice. Analyze contemporary nursing within the framework of its historical development.

The nursing program offers a generic master's program for students who have no nursing background but hold a baccalaureate in another field. This course is taught to those students in the first semester of their first year in the program. This course is also required for all registered nurses (RNs) who enter the graduate program, although they have the option to take the course at any point in their program plan of study. For entry-level students, the course attempts to establish an understanding of the profession in which the students will be entering, and specifically the importance of theory-based practice. This course also emphasizes the use of theory-based practice for the RN student. For both groups, the course sets the groundwork for the development of leadership skills and understanding the expectations of scholarly work in graduate study. Other courses in the curriculum build on the leadership and theory framework of this course, and a scholarly project that requires self-directed scholarly work is the culmination of the program.

These students bring a variety of backgrounds to the course. Entry-level students have included students with a previous master's degree in public health or another field, a heavy science background, or a doctorate in another field; professional musicians; emergency medical technicians; peace corps volunteers; or, at the other extreme, students fresh out of college with a liberal arts or science degree. Some have had experiences with the healthcare system or cared for an ill friend or relative, and that experience influenced the decision to enter nursing, whereas others have different reasons for their decision. The RNs also have varied backgrounds and enter the program with clinical expertise that they can share with the entry-level students. All of these students have something special to offer their fellow students and the instructor. They range in age from 21 to well older than 50, all bringing life experiences with them. It is a wonderful group to work with, but it is challenging because of the students' expertise and status as adult learners. Principles of adult learning must be considered in the design of teaching strategies for this course.

The course is presented along a timeline, looking at past to present to future. Influences on the development of the profession are explored over that timeline. Students look at such issues as the impact over time of sociocultural influences and changes, war, religion, economics, immigration, new diseases, new technologies, the development of medicine and health care, nursing practice, and nursing education. The era of the late 1960s and 1970s brings in the impact of the civil rights, women's rights, and consumer rights movements and the reaction of nurse leaders in recognizing the need for a stronger professional view of nursing and the development of nursing science. The development of a nursing body of knowledge becomes a major focus of the course for many weeks. Students conduct group presentations for their colleagues, explaining a specific nursing theory, including appropriate research, critiques, and applicability to practice.

No single reference book can be used for the content of this course. In order to effectively contribute to class discussions, students must read various articles and book chapters and become familiar with other sources, which may include the Internet. Students must be actively involved in the learning process to benefit from this course. Students must carry out a certain amount of discovery on their own, with instructor assistance in finding appropriate resources.

In designing the course for my first time teaching, I followed the format that other instructors had used—the development of weekly topics with reading assignments for each. A book of readings, developed for purchase and adhering to copyright laws, was made available to provide students with easy access to the articles. Special attention was given to the reading selections to be sure they would provide different perspectives for discussion and new information applicable to course objectives. In addition, students formed groups in which they were responsible for a nursing theory presentation. They were expected to conduct a literature review for the particular theory and present a bibliography to the class. A term paper was also required, which presented another aspect of the students' theories or discussed the historical issues that were presented in class.

The group presentation and paper assignments required students to seek out literature and be able to discuss it orally or in their term paper. Preparing for class discussions was problematic, however. Some students took advantage of the reading collection and contributed well to the class discussion, whereas others were quiet or contributed general knowledge that did not relate to readings. These students were missing out on the richness that the readings provided. Another problem was finding ways for the instructor to assist students in preparing their presentations and papers. Although regular office hours were available, many students used the time just before or after class to talk with me. The time was rushed, and, although I was aware of some resources that could help, I did not have time to explore additional resources that would have been helpful to them.

All students in the school had access to an email account that could be used within the learning resources center, but it was a new experience for many of them. I had become quite comfortable in using email and found it to be a valuable form of communication. The next time the course was offered, I decided to require an electronic journal that would allow students to discuss readings with me prior to class and to turn in their term paper outlines and/or project for feedback and assistance (see Exhibit 20-2). My objectives were to encourage students to read before class, to encourage students who found it difficult to speak in class to discuss what they had read, and to be available for questions about assignments. In addition, papers from the previous class had shown that students were not comfortable with the format for citing references and needed feedback prior to turning in the final paper. I added an annotated bibliography to the assignment to help them understand citation formats and to gain skill in abstracting information from a journal article.

This was only one of four courses that the entry-level students took as part of their program. They were beginning basic nursing, with clinical experience that took time and was their primary interest. It was important to keep the assignments at a manageable level and to keep their interest in the topic. The basic nursing course was designed so students would begin to recognize and use a theory base in their practice. For that class, they were able to use the information they worked with in history of nursing ideas class, which helped them to see the relevance of what we were doing.

EXHIBIT 20-2

Email Journal Examples

Student No. 1

In Carper's article, "Fundamental Patterns of Knowing in Nursing," the author states the importance of wholeness and incorporating all of the patterns of knowing in nursing. The American Nurses Association (ANA) policy statement states that, "Nursing is a scientific discipline as well as a profession" (ANA Policy Statement, p. 7). I concur that all of the components stated [earlier in this email] explain the profession of nursing well; however, I do not believe the theorists have put enough emphasis on the synergistic effect of the different components that constitute the profession of nursing. Although placing the branches of nursing together is great, one needs to look beyond that and see what happens when they work together and create this new dimension of nursing. The sum of these components truly makes the nursing profession unique. I believe it is important for nurses to be aware of the synergistic effect of the wholeness of nursing.

Student No. 2

Hello, Dr. Lowenstein, this is [name omitted] from your Nursing History class. I'm e-mailing this from my house, but if you need to reply to anything, I use my [email address omitted] email address more.

Well, I'm not sure if anyone had picked this one either, but I read "The Seeing Self: Photography and Storytelling as a Health Promotion Methodology," by Mary Koithan. I enjoyed how this article addressed the issue of our world being too fast paced and impersonal these days because I believe this is very true. It also cited that more and more diseases today are related to stress, which is obviously detrimental to our well-being.

The author stresses the importance of finding other ways to block out the confusion and busyness of everyday life and to center ourselves and concentrate on our wellness. She referred to these methods as aesthetic modalities that would promote health, empower the person, and make them aware of the connection between mind, body, and spirit. Such aesthetic modalities must work wonders for some people who are skeptical about modern medicine. It is good that we have these additional ways of healing because it is very individual and self-promoting. I found this article very interesting and hope to read more on similar subjects. I will see you in class on the 18th!

Student No. 3

The article I found dealt with the use of drawing to gain information about children and their experiences and feelings. The article "Children's Drawings: A Different Window," by Judy Malkiewicz and Marilyn L. Stember discussed that children will offer more of their feelings and experiences through drawings than through conversation with a healthcare provider. It is thus very useful for nurses to use this artistic technique to help them understand their younger patients and know how to address their needs, especially since younger children cannot express themselves well through verbal communication. The only obstacles that the authors presented were those involved with the interpretations of such artwork. Many times healthcare providers overanalyze these pieces, as well as underestimate their significance.

The article also discussed several different types of drawing exercises that can be used. Draw-a-Person, Kinetic Family Drawing, House-Person-Tree, Draw-a-Situation, and others provide the means to enter the child's world in various situations and roles that the child encounters. Each specific type of drawing serves a unique and specific purpose.

On a personal note, I worked at [employer omitted] for 3 years as a Child Life Assistant. In this position, I worked with the kids to keep them occupied with arts and crafts, tutor them on schoolwork, help them understand procedures using medical play, and educate them and their families on the things that were happening during their hospital stays. Most of the children on the unit were experiencing chronic illnesses such as cystic fibrosis, cancer, AIDS, spina bifida, and others. Thus we saw the children repeatedly and for long durations of time. Among our many activities and tools was the use of drawing. It provided a great release for the kids, and it told us a lot about how they were feeling about their care. It tuned us in to their fears, how we could reduce them, and how we could prevent them. I thought it was a wonderful thing. Also, the drawings were a source of pride for the kids. We displayed them all over the units and entered them into national competitions with the hospitals of the Children's Miracle Network. That was why my interest was struck by this particular article, but I can attest to the fact that these drawing exercises are valuable for both caregiver and patient. The article was from the book *Art & Aesthetics in Nursing*.

The use of theory-based practice was not as clear for the RN group, which was a factor that I needed to acknowledge in my responses to their emails. The RNs were encouraged to read articles relating theory to practice and to comment on how they viewed using the theory in their own nursing practice.

Instruction to students included the following:

A journal and annotated bibliography are responsible for 20% of the course grade. A **weekly journal** discussing your reactions to the readings and class discussion should be submitted by email. For the weekly journal, pick out the major points within the reading and comment on them. This can be somewhat informal, I do not need the whole citation for that reading, and try to keep your comments to two or three paragraphs in length. Of course, if you feel that a reading deserves more depth, I will gladly look forward to reading your comments. I will respond to each message, to acknowledge receipt or to discuss some of your points. I may also ask you to bring up the point you are making in the class discussion, so the rest of the class can benefit from your thoughts. I understand that you may not be able to read every article every week in advance of class, but that should be the exception, not the rule. If that happens, please read the article after class and comment on your reactions to the article in light of the class discussion.

An **annotated bibliography**, consisting of a minimum of four articles over the course of the semester, should also be submitted by email, in addition to the weekly journals. The annotated bibliography should follow the following guidelines:

- The content of the article should be relevant to the course objectives; include one article from the journal *Advances in Nursing Science*; and include the article citation in APA format, an abstract of the article including major issues and findings, and a brief critique and reaction to the article. The selection of articles is in addition to the assigned readings but may include articles to be used in the presentation or final paper.
- You are also encouraged to use email to correspond with me regarding any questions you may have about your presentation, paper, or any other issue you feel the need to discuss. I will be pleased to give you feedback in these areas. Of course you may schedule an appointment if you wish further assistance with these projects.

I have been very pleased with the response from the journals and annotated bibliographies. Students who were not familiar with email found it to be very helpful by the end of the semester and were often proud of their new skill. They usually became comfortable after a few tries, although it may have been stressful at first. Although technical problems did arise periodically, most students were successful in using the system. Technical problems included difficulty getting an email address and being unable to open attachments, especially when different operating systems were being used. To address that problem, I suggested that students not use the attachment feature, but rather paste the text directly into the email message, which was usually successful. Computer crashes and lost messages occurred sporadically, but most students were able to cope. To avoid complaints about needing to be on campus to use email, I accepted emails from school or home addresses.

The responses added much to the class discussions. Students did contribute experiences or ideas that they had expressed in the emails and that I felt would benefit the class discussion. Students demonstrated a deeper understanding of issues and content. I did not penalize students for missing a week or two, but instead worked with them to be sure they had met the course objectives.

An added advantage to using email was the ability to discuss email and other computer applications during the technology topic discussion. Class discussion included looking at the present and future, identifying the technology issues and how they have and potentially will influence both nursing practice and nursing education.

The amount of emails can be difficult to manage for the instructor. With a class of 35, I needed to set aside time to read and respond to emails in a timely fashion. In some cases, no long response was necessary; I was able to acknowledge the e-mail with few words. For others, a longer conversation was in order. I have learned to pay attention to each email as soon as I receive it and to respond immediately and not allow them to pile up. I was able to move the emails into a permanent file, sorted by student, with a separate permanent file for my responses. This allowed me to return to the messages if questions arose and to be sure students had met course objectives.

Although some students do read early, most of them wait until it is close to class. There were times when I was unable to read all of the messages before the class discussion, but these instances were usually spread out enough to allow me to at least acknowledge and possibly bring something up in the class discussion that I was not able to reply to in the message. Overall course and professor evaluations have improved with use of the email journals (see Exhibit 20-3). Students have felt a closer relationship with me, and I have been able to assist students with problems or issues that would not have surfaced in other formats. Students have demonstrated improved skills and benefits from the course content. I will continue to use journals to achieve those learning objectives.

EXHIBIT 20-3

Evaluation Comments

1. "I liked the structure of the course in regards to the group project on theorists rather than doing a lot of heavy reading. I also liked the seminar/discussion style of the course. The reading was intensive, though, but the email system was *great!*"
2. "I really enjoyed the readings and found the journal keeping and emailing very rewarding. I felt I definitely learned a lot about nursing that I didn't know about. Acceptance of my comments and experiences made the work very unthreatening."
3. "Enjoyed use of email, very effective, allow for better student/teacher interaction. Thank you."

REFERENCES

Bates, A. W., & Poole, G. (2003). *Effective teaching with technology in higher education*. San Francisco: Jossey-Bass.

Batson, T. (2008). Machines are dumb. *Campus Technology*. Retrieved November 24, 2009, from http://campustechnology.com/Articles/2008/11/Machines-are-Dumb.aspx

Burgstahler, S., & Cory, R. (Eds.) (2008). *Universal design in higher education*. Cambridge, MA: Harvard University Publishing Group.

Collision, G., Elbaum, B., Haavind, S., & Tinker, R. (2000). *Facilitating online learning: Effective strategies for moderators*. Madison, WI: Atwood.

Effink, V. L., Davis, L. S., Fitzwater, E., Castleman, J., Burley, J., Gorney-Moreno, M. J., et al. (2000). The Nightingale Tracker Clinical Field Test Nurse Team: A comparison of teaching strategies for integrating information technology into clinical nursing education. *Nurse Educator, 25*(3), 136–144.

Green, T. D., Brown A., & Robinson, L. (2008). *Making the most of the WEB in your classroom: A teacher's guide to blogs, podcasts, wikis, pages, and sites*. Thousand Oakes: Corwin Press.

Haavind, S. (2007). Designing questions for dialogue. Retrieved November 24, 2009, from http://eduspaces.net/sarahh/weblog/178061.html

Lane, C. (2006). UW podcasting: Evaluation of year one. *Catalyst Papers*. Seattle, WA: University of Washington Office of Learning Technologies. Retrieved November 24, 2009, from http://catalyst.washington.edu/research_development/papers/2006/podcasting_year1.pdf

Littlejohn, S. (2002). *Theories of human communication*. Belmont, CA: Wadsworth.

Mitra, A., & Steffensmeier, T. (2000). Changes in student attitudes and students computer use in a computer-enriched environment. *Journal of Research on Computing in Education, 32*(3), 417–432.

Oosterhof, A. (2000). Efficiently creating individualized e-mail to students. *Journal of Computing in Higher Education, 11*(2), 75–90.

Parklyn, D. L. (1999). Learning in the company of others: Fostering a discourse community with a collaborative electronic journal. *College Teaching, 47*(3), 88–90.

Read, B. (2005). Duke U. assess iPod experiment and finds it worked—in some courses. *Chronicle of Higher Education, 51*(43), A26.

Reid, S. (2009). Online courses and how they change the nature of class. *First Monday, 14*(3).

Reynard, R. (2008). 6 ways not to become rote using instructional technology. *Campus Technology*. Retrieved November 24, 2009, from http://campustechnology.com/Articles/2008/11/6-Ways-Not-To-Become-Rote-Using-Instructional-Technology.aspx

Shannon, C. E., & Weaver, W. (1949). *A mathematical model of communication*. Urbana, IL: University of Illinois Press.

Weerts, S. E., Miller, D., & Altice, A. (2009). "Clicker" technology promotes interactivity in an undergraduate nutrition course. *Journal of Nutrition Education & Behavior, 41*(3), 227–228.

CHAPTER 21

Web 2.0 and Beyond: Emerging Technologies that Enhance Teaching and Learning

Gail Matthews-DeNatale

INTRODUCTION

In looking forward to the future of Web-enhanced and online learning, it is helpful to begin with a retrospective of the past. Because past is prologue, revisiting the history of technology in higher education can provide insight into motivating factors for current and future developments.

Those of us who have used technology in their teaching for more than a decade will remember the early days when email and listservs were considered to be cutting-edge technology. Email was useful for one-on-one communication, whereas listservs supported one-to-many messaging and discussions. The first iterations of these tools were clunky and unforgiving; command-based interfaces made it difficult to correct even simple typos without having to start over. But over time, these tools improved and, over time, they have become central to the endeavor of higher education (Online degree, n.d.).

In the early 1990s, the increasing popularity of the World Wide Web gave rise to learning management systems (LMSs). "Web Course in a Box," one of the first LMSs to be used widely in higher education, provided faculty and students with a suite of password-protected tools especially designed for learning contexts: a syllabus-builder, threaded discussions, Web-based quizzes, and a class roster that could include student-written biographies and their photos. The invention of the LMS is important because it signaled a shift to perceiving technology as an online *place* where learning could happen, a virtual classroom that could accommodate many modes of learning, including many-to-many discussions, group work, and the development of coherent learning communities over extended periods of time. These first learning management systems were inexpensive or free to use, but commercial products such as WebCT and Blackboard soon followed, along with a series of mergers and acquisitions. Today, only a few commercial LMS products dominate the field.

We have come a long way from the early days of blinking cursors, glowing iridescent green on tiny black screens, yet our expectations have become increasingly sophisticated as well. Even though faculty and students assume that their institutions will provide some form of LMS for coursework, many wish that these educational resources were more visually appealing and easier to use. In addition, LMS costs have skyrocketed since Blackboard acquired most of its competitors and captured the market, leading many institutions to explore "open source" alternatives such as Moodle. But open source products require a level of technical expertise not available in many small institutions. We find ourselves longing, simultaneously, for more and less: more flexibility to accommodate a wider range of learning styles and teaching scenarios, less complexity to shorten the learning curve and lower barriers to entry.

This is the context in which Web 2.0 arrived on the scene in 2004 to 2005, bringing with it an explosion of Web-based free resources that are multimedia rich, elegantly designed, and easy to use. Web 2.0, sometimes referred to as "emerging technologies," felt like a breath of fresh air given the increasingly stodgy context of technology in higher education. These resources opened up a host of possibilities for creative, pedagogically effective assignments that could engage all types of students in active and collaborative work.

What educational possibilities are afforded by Web 2.0? By way of example, each semester students in Michael Wesch's Cultural Anthropology at Kansas State University (KSU) conduct primary research, translate results into polished 3- to 5-minute videos, and post the videos for public viewing on YouTube. This is not necessarily a novel teaching scenario. What is striking is that, as of September 2009, one student-produced piece entitled "A Vision of Students Today" has been viewed more than 3,340,000 times and viewers have posted more than 8,500 comments about the piece (http://www.youtube.com/watch?v=dGCJ46vyR9o). The work of these students extends beyond the KSU campus, serves as a catalyst for intellectual discussion that spans continents, and is a topic of conversation in both formal and informal learning contexts. Imagine the sense of accomplishment that these students feel; no LMS-based assignment could claim that level of impact on society as a whole.

Yet, over time, educators have also found that Web 2.0 can be confusing and somewhat intimidating. Even the associated terminology sounds like something penned by Lewis Carroll (e.g., blog, wiki, and mash-up). Unlike LMSs, emerging technologies come unbundled; each tool is selected "à la carte" and therefore it is up to the educator to weave technologies together into a coherent learning environment.

The accelerated pace of change is also dizzying—each week dozens of new resources arrive on the scene while others are either acquired or go out of business altogether. Just as the public is becoming accustomed to the term Web 2.0, pundits are starting to speak about Web 3.0, resources that are mobile and therefore always available (e.g., accessed through smart phones such as a Blackberry or iPhone), context sensitive (e.g., using global positioning systems [GPSs] to only return search results that are relevant to the user's geographical location), and community tailored (e.g., capable of identifying the recurring needs and interests of a person or group to offer only relevant resources and information).

THEORETICAL FOUNDATIONS

Given that technological options grow exponentially on a daily basis, how can educators avail themselves of emerging technologies without sacrificing precious time for teaching and research? All too often, teachers who want to experiment with technology begin by selecting the tool and then determine its educational use. This strategy is both *inefficient*, because it forces educators to learn about all technologies regardless of their relevance to a particular course, and pedagogically *ineffective*, because it takes the focus off of the most important drivers for course planning and development: learning goals, desired outcomes, and evidence of learning.

Lee Shulman, President Emeritus of the Carnegie Foundation for the Advancement of Teaching, describes five dimensions that are central to effective teaching: vision, design, interactions, outcomes, and analysis (1998). A good course functions as a coherent whole; discrete assignments are engaging and often creative in design, yet the pieces are interconnected, adding up to a synergistic learning experience. Likewise, good courses are responsive to learner needs, some of which are unique to the specific population enrolled in the course. Georgetown University's Randy Bass (1999), describes this process as identifying "the problem":

> I realized I didn't know really if the better students in a course who demonstrated a real understanding of the material by the end of the semester were actually acquiring that understanding in my course, or were merely the percentage of students who entered the course with a high level of background and aptitude. Similarly, I realized I didn't really know if the students who I watched 'improve' from their early work to later work were really understanding the material and the paradigm from which I was operating, or merely learning to perform their knowledge in ways that had adapted to my expectations.

In response to these uncertainties, Bass and other proponents of the "scholarship of teaching and learning" advocate focusing on "the relationship between student prior understanding and their capacity to acquire new understanding" to investigate how students' "self-awareness of learning might help them develop a deeper understanding of certain disciplinary principles more quickly and meaningfully" (1999). With this approach, courses and assignments are developed in response to, and as an investigation of, student learning needs.

This problem-based approach is the process by which faculty can select emerging technologies that are appropriate to desired learning outcomes, and this is the context in which emerging technologies may realize their full potential for transforming higher education. To use emerging technologies effectively, faculty must begin with a vision for learning that

- is responsive to learner needs, both intellectual and social;
- fosters connections between the course at hand and students' life experiences (e.g., friends, family, regional, ethnic, and cultural affinity groups);
- creates a bridge between the course and students' larger learning contexts (e.g., other courses, internships, service learning);
- taps into a diverse range of learning "styles" so that all students can play to their strengths as they grapple with course concepts and endeavor to communicate what they have learned; and
- helps students achieve deeper conceptual understanding and develop core capabilities in relationship to the course topic or discipline.

TYPES OF LEARNERS

Historically, higher education has best served students who learn best through reading, listening to lectures, note taking, and sequential problem solving, such as mathematical calculation. In 1983, with the publication of his seminal work on multiple intelligences, Gardner challenged the very notion of intelligence itself, and since then the concept of multiple intelligences has crossed over from academic educational circles into popular thought and understanding (1983). This new taxonomy of intelligence has far reaching pedagogical implications. Logic dictates that if there is more than one way to be "smart," there should also be more than one way to learn and be taught. In the intervening years, educational theorists have developed a host of learning styles models and inventories in an effort to represent the types of learners found in a heterogeneous classroom (Butler, 1986; Felder & Soloman, 2009; Kolb, 1984). The four part model put forth by Felder and Soloman is particularly useful in exploring the relevance of emerging technologies to higher education:

- *Reflective and Active*
  - Reflective involves learning by thinking
  - Active involves learning by doing
- *Sensing and Intuitive*
  - Sensing involves learning by facts and verifiable experience
  - Intuitive involves learning through innovation and possibility thinking
- *Verbal and Visual*
  - Verbal involves learning through the written and spoken word
  - Visual involves learning through images, diagrams, and timelines

- *Sequential and Global*
  - Sequential involves drawing on details and facts to construct larger understanding
  - Global involves starting with the "big picture" and then analyzing the whole to understand the sum of its parts

Note that these pairs are continuums of style, not dichotomies. All learners exhibit these eight styles in greater or lesser degrees. Yet emerging technologies are particularly good at addressing students' needs to experience active, intuitive, visual, and global learning. By way of example, the blog *100 Essential Web 2.0 Tools for Teachers* categorizes tools according to their capacity for fostering interactivity, engagement, motivation, empowerment, and differentiated learning. Some of these 100 tools are mapped to Felder and Soloman's learning styles framework in Table 21-1.

Table 21-1 Learning Styles and Emerging Technologies

Style	Emerging Technology Example
Active (learning by doing)	Students pool labwork or field-gathered data into a wiki, authoring a collaborative analysis of their primary data
Intuitive (innovation and possibility thinking)	Students browse the TED Talks video site identify thought leaders who can provide a "big picture" analysis of a given topic (for epidemiology students, access a talk on pandemics given by Larry Brilliant)
Visual (images, diagrams, timelines)	Students identify stories of previous experiences that relate to a given topic, then create and share "digital stories" using Voicethread (3- to 5-minute videos that combine images and words); classmates use Voicethread's annotation tool to comment on each other's stories
Global (big picture thinking)	Students use Gliffy to create mind maps that provide a holistic picture of a topic or concept, then use a blog or Twitter aggregator to compile an overview of all recent posts written about that topic

USING THE METHOD

When technology developers set out to create a new product, they begin by surveying the needs of their users. The next step is to develop a "spec," a specification document that describes all the things that the product will need to be able to do. In integrating emerging technologies into teaching, a similar process is useful. Begin with the following questions:

1. What should my students know and understand by the end of the course (or assignment or module)?
2. What skills or capabilities, academic or disciplinary, are essential to achieving the goals for learning?
3. What is the "problem" (à la Randy Bass) that I am trying to solve—which of the goals for learning have been difficult to accomplish when I taught this course in the past?
4. What do I want for myself and for my students? For example, the teacher may want to obtain a clearer picture of students' thought processes, or she may want her students to connect course concepts to everyday life.
5. By the end of the learning sequence, what evidence will you and your students need to be confident that learning goals have been achieved? Along the way, what evidence would help you and your students identify trouble spots to address areas of concern and make adjustments as necessary?
6. What modes of learning are particularly relevant to the topic or leaning goals? For example, epidemiology may lend itself to mapping, clinical decision making to visual and other data analysis, and cultural competence or medical ethics to multimedia storytelling.

The answer to these questions provides a "spec" that can be used to seek out an emerging technology that best meets learning scenario goals. This preliminary work, often called "instructional design," also saves time because the faculty member only needs to investigate technologies that will accomplish these specific criteria for learning.

In evaluating emerging technologies, faculty need not be alone. Educause, the national organization dedicated to technology in higher education, publishes a series entitled *7 Things You Should Know About . . . .* Each brief focuses on a single technology or practice, describing: what it is, how it works, and why it matters to teaching and learning. At the time of publication, there were 52 briefs in the series, with approximately 12 publications added to the collection each year. The Educause Learning Initiative (2009) in collaboration with the New Media Consortium (2009), also produces the *Horizon Report,* an annual digest of technologies that are likely to have a significant impact on teaching and learning in the near future, along with examples of those technologies at use in higher education. The *23 Things* online self-paced workshop developed by the Public Library of Charlotte and Mecklenberg County (2009).

In addition, most colleges and universities have centers dedicated to academic or educational technology. These centers employ instructional designers and instructional technologists who are expected to keep current with recent developments in technology, and they are eager to share their knowledge. Whether consulting with academic technologists or browsing *7 Things* briefs, the result will be more satisfactory and efficient if the faculty member first articulates their desired learning goals, processes, and outcomes.

POTENTIAL PROBLEMS

Web 2.0, 3.0, and other emerging technologies are a grand adventure that can add a new dimension to learning, but there is a price to pay for teaching "outside the box" of institution-supported LMSs. Educational institutions take care to make regular backups of courses in their LMSs—they cannot risk losing credit-bearing discussion posts or test results. In contrast, emerging technologies exist outside the context of higher education, with no guarantee of backups, security, or ongoing existence of the tool. An assignment that previously worked well using a given technology may need to be adapted in response to new versions, acquisition by another company, or even the disappearance of a much loved tool.

Students also can become frustrated when a course uses too many different types of technology. When using an LMS, the student experiences it as *one* software application even though the learning system can do many things. When using emerging technologies, students experience each one as a different tool: a different "place" to go to do coursework, a different interface to learn, and a unique application that has its own technology troubleshooting challenges. One strategy is to use the LMS as a portal or door through which students can access all other tools used in the class. This is can be accomplished by inserting a links to all technologies on the course home page or as needed in course modules. Another strategy is to integrate emerging technologies thoughtfully and sparingly: no more than 2 to 3 tools unless the course is about technology itself.

When taking the leap into emerging technologies, it is important to realize that this is uncharted territory. These technologies require a pioneering spirit, so plan accordingly and encourage your students to take an adventurous approach as well.

CONCLUSION

Emerging technologies provide educators with a rich palette of opportunities for enhancing student learning. These technologies are particularly well suited to active, visual, intuitive, and global learning and therefore accommodate the needs of learners who have been underserved historically by higher education. Those who want to incorporate emerging technologies into their teaching are cautioned to focus on pedagogy first and select tools that best meet learning needs, instead of selecting a tool and then deciding what to do with it in an assignment. Even though emerging technologies can breathe new life into coursework, enrich discussion, and increase student engagement, these technologies often transition and, therefore, it is wise to have a contingency plan in place.

APPLIED EXAMPLE

Digital Storytelling

While taking a capstone course in clinical decision making at Simmons College, students were also involved in clinical preceptorships in various settings and specialties. Assistant Professor Priscilla Gazarian wanted her students to make intellectual connections between their course concepts and their firsthand clinical experiences.

The instructional design for this assignment was informed by narrative pedagogy theory, which posits that phenomenological and interpretive thinking is improved when "students and teachers can have conversations based on common everyday experiences that arise from nursing practice" (Gazarian, in press). Digital storytelling was one part in a three part, semester-long project:

Part 1: Each student identified a recent clinical experience to explore in detail. The experience needed to be relevant to at least three course concepts.

Part 2: Student use technology to produce 3- to 5-minute audiovisual presentations, "digital stories" about the clinical situations told using a first-person voice (Matthews-DeNatale, 2008). Stories are "told" through an oral narrative approximately 250 words in length that is accompanied by images that illustrate or are relevant to the topic. Technologies recommended include VoiceThread, iMovie, and voiceover PowerPoint (Figure 21.1).

To accommodate verbal learners less attracted to visual imagery and those who with limited access to computers, students are given the option to complete the assignment without the use of technology (note: all students choose to use some form of technology in telling their stories). In the event that a given week's topic is particularly relevant to a given story, students are asked to screen their story in class. In addition, several "movie days" (including popcorn) provide an optional opportunity for other students to voluntarily show their pieces to the class.

Part 3: Students each submit a final paper that synthesizes what they have learned about the three identified concepts in relation to the clinical experience.

Figure 21-1

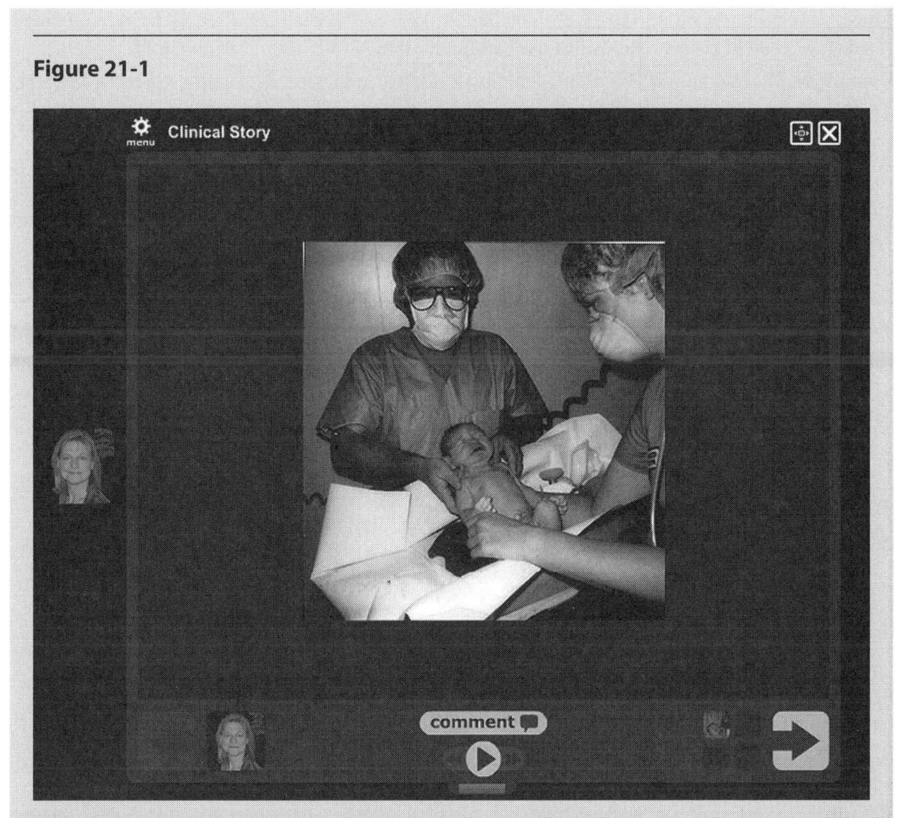

Source: From http:www.flickr.com/photo/jynmeyer

Of the technologies used in this assignment, only VoiceThread is considered to be an emerging technology. It is a Web 2.0 application because it is free, allows users to upload images and record audio easily without sophisticated multimedia expertise, provides an option for viewers to write or record comments that are posted on the same page as a story, and includes a "tagging" feature so that potential viewers can search for a piece using key words.

Planning was key to the success of this assignment. Gazarian contacted Academic Technology staff in advance to identify format options and to arrange for technical support in the event that students needed help creating their digital stories. Despite preliminary concerns that some students might be reluctant, Gazarian reported that "willingness to use technology to tell their stories was overwhelming" and the assignment was a "rich learning experience for all involved."

REFERENCES

Bass, R. (1999). The scholarship of teaching: What's the problem? In *Inventio: Creative thinking about teaching and learning*. Retrieved November 28, 2009, from http://www.doit.gmu.edu/Archives/feb98/randybass.htm

Butler, K. (1986). *Learning and teaching style: In theory and practice*. Columbia, CT: Learners' Dimension.

Educause Learning Initiative. (2009). 7 things series. Retrieved September 7, 2009, from http://www.educause.edu/ELI/ELIResources/7ThingsYouShouldKnowAbout/7495

Felder, R. M., & Soloman, B. A. (2009). Learning styles and strategies. Retrieved September 7, 2009, from http://www4.ncsu.edu/unity/lockers/users/f/felder/public/ILSdir/styles.htm

Gardner, H. (1983). *Frames of mind: The theory of multiple intelligences.* New York: Basic Books.

Gazarian, P. [in press]. Digital stories: Incorporating narrative pedagogy. *Journal of Nursing Education.*

Kolb, D. A. (1984). *Experiential learning: Experience as the source of learning and development.* Englewood Cliffs, NJ: Prentice-Hall, Inc.

Matthews-DeNatale, G. (2008). Digital story-making: Understanding the learner's perspective. Educause Learning Initiative Annual Conference, San Antonio, TX. Retrieved September 7, 2009, from http://www.educause.edu/Resources/DigitalStoryMakingUnderstandin/162538

The New Media Consortium. (2009). The horizon project. Retrieved September 7, 2009, from http://www.nmc.org/horizon

Online Degree. (2009). *100 essential Web 2.0 tools for teachers.* Retrieved September 7, 2009, from http://www.onlinedegree.net/100-essential-2-0-tools-for-teachers

Public Library of Charlotte and Mecklenberg County. (2009). *23 things.* Retrieved September 7, 2009, from http://plcmcl2-things.blogspot.com

Shulman, L. S. (1998). Course anatomy: The dissection and analysis of knowledge through teaching. In P. Hutchings (Ed.), *The course portfolio: How faculty can improve their teaching to advance practice and improve student learning.* Washington, DC: American Association of Higher Education.

ELECTRONIC RESOURCES

50 Ways to Use Twitter in the Classroom. Retrieved September 7, 2009, from https://tle.wisc.edu/solutions/engagement/50-ways-use-twitter-classroom

50 Web 2.0 Ways to Tell a Story. Retrieved September 7, 2009, from http://cogdogroo.wikispaces.com/50+Ways

Twitter in Higher Education Report. Retrieved September 7, 2009, from http://4tm-services.com/wp-content/uploads/2009/08/twittersurvey_facultyfocus.pdf

Web 2.0 in Plain English. Retrieved September 7, 2009, from http://www.pueblo.gsa.gov/cfocus/cfweb2009/focus.htm

Web 3.0 Concepts Explained in Plain English. Retrieved September 7, 2009, from http://www.labnol.org/internet/web-3-concepts-explained/8908/

CHAPTER 22

Blended Learning

Arlene J. Lowenstein

To an experienced educator, who was also a digital immigrant,
the first entry into online teaching was a challenge,
but has now become a love affair.
—*Arlene*

DEFINITION AND PURPOSES

Garrison and Vaughan (2008) define blended learning as "a coherent design approach that openly assesses and integrates the strengths of face-to-face and online learning to address worthwhile educational goals" (p. x). They note that it is a *thoughtful* fusion of classroom teaching and online learning experiences. Thoughtful is the key word here, because the learning opportunities and experiences are crucial, and the course needs to be specifically designed to allow students to discover and work with those opportunities. Blended learning requires a restructuring of class contact hours with the goals of engagement of the student in the learning process and extending access to learning opportunities that may be found on the Internet (Garrison & Vaughan, 2008).

Online teaching can be *synchronous*, where students will be online (OL) at the same time (e.g., chat rooms and teleconferences), or *asynchronous*, where students can access the course and post responses at any time, day or night, in different time zones. Blended learning, also known as *hybrid or mixed mode*, is a combination of online plus face-to-face (f2f) classroom sessions. Blended learning may utilize less class time but adds asynchronous learning time. A blended course may be designed 50% onsite classroom and 50% asynchronous online time, or 70% and and 30%, or other percentages. The ratio will vary depending on the course and needed content. Synchronous class time may also be used, but that is not required. The method chosen and class design depends on the learning objectives.

Understanding the Blended Course Environment

An online platform is used to allow students to access course information by logging in with the user name and password anytime, beginning a few days before the first day of class and ending when the course ends, after final exams. The course syllabus and other posted classroom materials, including PowerPoint presentations, videos, or other lecture materials, allow students to review materials and refresh their memory if they so choose to do so. Announcements and communication methods, such as emailing the students and group discussion boards, may also be available. The instructor can post materials anytime during the course, so that lecture materials may be posted before the class during which the lecture is given, to encourage preparation, or after the lecture has taken place, to allow the students to review for exams or assignments.

Discussion Posts

Discussion posts may be assigned at varying times during the course, or weekly, again depending on class design. Each student is expected to post a 200- to 300-word statement to each assigned discussion, commenting on the readings and addressing the instructor's discussion questions, thereby beginning what is known as a threaded discussion. Students then respond to two or more of their classmates' threaded discussion postings. Faculty may encourage additional replies in order to set up a learning community dialogue, where discussions provide a conduit for learning for both students and the instructor. A scheduled due date for original posts and responses assists students in organizing their work. Discussion posts may be graded or not, but students should receive feedback on their posts from the instructor and other students.

Assignments

Papers and group and individual projects can be assigned along with specific assignments, such as searching for additional resources and Web sites to share through the postings. Assignments may be posted and graded online or turned in on class days, depending on teacher preference.

THEORETICAL RATIONALE

In the 1990s, Badrul H. Kahn (2005, 2007) was concerned with what it takes "to provide the best and most meaningful flexible learning environments for learners worldwide." His answer to this question was developed into a framework for online learning, and this model is used internationally. He understood that e-learning did not include just teaching, but required a combination of factors to be effective. His framework consisted of eight elements, the first being *institutional*, which discusses administrative elements and the need for administration understanding and support. *Pedagogical* refers to the learning goals and design, and the need for adaptation to the expansion of opportunities available through online learning. The *technological* section refers to the infrastructure available to produce effective online teaching, avoiding the frustration that can occur with poor technology, and this goes along with the *interface*, which discusses how the user interfaces through the technology with those learning opportunities. *Evaluation* is critical for both learners and content to understand the problems and seek solutions to improve the learning. The *management* section is the management of the learning environment, who is responsible, and how is it done, and the *resource support* refers to required resources other than the nontutorial components. The *ethical* portion is related to diversity issues, and ethical concerns in the learning (Fig. 21-1).

Harvey Singh (2003) adapted Kahn's framework to blended learning programs to serve as a guide to planning, developing, delivering, managing, and evaluating blended learning programs. He noted that blended learning includes several forms of learning tools and mixes various event-based activities, including face-to-face and e-learning that can include both synchronous and asynchronous learning activities along with self-paced learning.

Figure 22-1 A framework for e-learning.

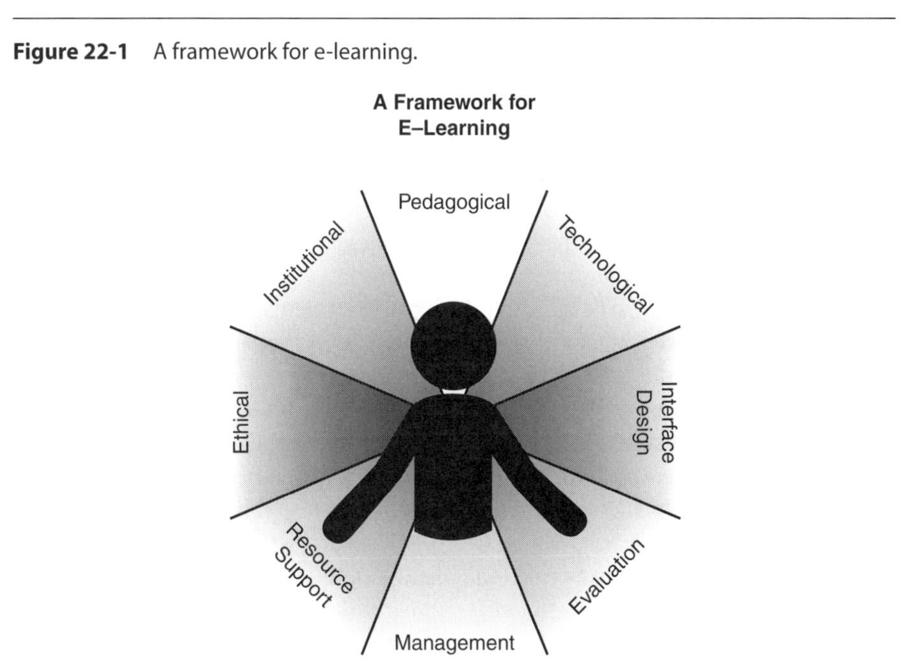

Source: Badrul, H. (2009). E-learning framework. Available at: *http:badrulkhan.com*. Accessed January 21, 2010.

Singh's (2003) studies have found that blending provides various benefits over using any single learning delivery medium alone. He recognizes that learning is not a one-time event, but it is a continuous process. The concepts in the Kahn framework demonstrate the need for a broad base of support, as well as the instructional or pedagogical issues to implement and carry out blended learning offerings. Singh has looked at each piece of Kahn's framework in relation to how it can be developed to establish effective blended learning.

Ausbum (2004) explored instructional features most important to adult learners in blended classes. She found that most adults in her study valued course designs that contained options, personalization, self-direction, variety, and a learning community. They enjoyed and highly valued two-way communication with their classmates and instructor, and felt that they benefited from frequent announcements and reminders from their instructors. However, she also found that in online instruction, as in more traditional environments, learners with different learning styles and characteristics do prefer and benefit from various instructional features and goals, depending on their previous experiences or learning style. Their preferences were not all the same. Active and self-paced learning established in blended learning can relate effectively to different learning styles and student preferences.

CONDITIONS

Developing the Learning Community

Discussions can be set up for specific weeks during a course or used every week, depending on the course objectives. It is important to develop a discussion learning community where students feel safe to talk to each other with little interference, except for guidance and nurturing from the instructor. Trust takes time to build, and the instructor needs to support students in this, so they do not keep quiet or hold back in the discussion because of fear of criticism. Students need to be given guidelines for discussion posts. Students need to be instructed about *netiquette*, for example, derogatory personal comments or attacks must be avoided. Instructor responses must demonstrate that mistakes are expected in a learning environment, and students do not need to be embarrassed, punished, or ashamed of those mistakes because they will learn from them. Instructors can provide constructive critiques via email to ensure privacy and avoid embarrassment for individual students as needed. Discussion boards can be more informal than required papers; however, students using traditional Internet speak may need to define those abbreviations for new computer uses, and our smiling face can be used to provide emotion :-).

Encouraging students to ask questions when unsure of the lecture or e-learning environment is valuable, and be sure they know not to hold back because they may feel the question was a "silly" one. There are no silly questions! One student's question may also be in the mind of other students who were afraid to ask because they may feel it was "dumb," or "they should have known" and did not want to receive criticism from the instructor and/or classmates or be embarrassed. It can be helpful to have a separate discussion board where students can ask the instructor questions, and the instructor's response is then available to all students. Depending on the technology available, it may be possible to allow a student to post a question anonymously. Personal questions or comments can be handled by email.

Discussions should promote evidenced-based practice, and encourage students to apply the research they are reading to their clinical environments. Asking students to apply the readings to case studies, to their clinical practice, and personal experiences promotes critical thinking and spurs interest by making the material come alive and relevant, thereby enhancing the lecture material. While classroom discussions are limited in the numbers of students that can be active, online discussions involve everyone. In large classes, small discussion groups can be established, and it can be exciting to see the different impressions and experiences that students talk about among themselves.

Instructors need to stay in the background during the discussions, allowing the students to create a dialog among themselves—the "guide on the side," rather than the "sage on the stage" (Collison, Elbaum, Haavind, & Tinker, 2000). Instructors can correct or add information to the discussions when specific points need attention, but the discussion needs to be student centered. Avoid a constant student-to-instructor and back again conversation, but encourage students to discuss with each other instead. The student who provides a main post should be instructed to return to that thread and answer classmates' response posts, challenges, and questions. Students should also be instructed to avoid "cheerleading," a one-line post that says nothing more than "that was a good post" or "great post," but to say why it was a great post, but also to constructively challenge and ask questions, and to express their own experiences that relate to the thread under discussions. As you monitor the discussions, you will get to know your students well and learn from them as they learn from you.

Planning and Modifying

Planning is very important to develop a coherent course that stays within the expectations for a student workload that is necessary, but not excessive for the topic. It is very important not to overload students with work for the course and that students

Table 22-1 Ten Questions to Think About for Blended Course Design

1. What do you want students to know when they have finished taking your blended course?
2. As you think about learning objectives, which would be better achieved online and which would be best achieved face-to-face?
3. Blended teaching is not just a matter of transferring a portion of your traditional course to the Web. Instead it involves developing challenging and engaging online learning activities that complement your face-to-face activities. What types of learning activities do you think you will be using for the online portion of your course?
4. Online asynchronous discussion is often an important part of blended courses. What new learning opportunities will arise as a result of using asynchronous discussion? What challenges do you anticipate in using online discussions? How would you address these?
5. How will the face-to-face and time out of class components be integrated into a single course? In other words, how will the work done in each component feed back into and support the other?
6. When working online, students frequently have problems scheduling their work and managing their time, and understanding the implications of the blended course module as related to learning. What do you plan to do to help your students address these issues?
7. How will you divide the percent of time between the face-to-face portion and the online portion of your course? How will you schedule the percent of time between the face-to-face and online portion of your course (e.g., one 2-hour face-to-face followed by one 2-hour online session each week)?
8. How will you divide the course-grading scheme between face-to-face and online activities? What means will you use to assess student work in each of these two components?
9. Students sometimes have difficulty acclimating to the course Web site and to other instructional technologies you may be using for face-to-face and online activities. What specific technologies will you use for the online and face-to-face portions of your course? What proactive steps can you take to assist students to become familiar with your course's e-learning and those instructional technologies? If students need help with technology later in the course, how will you provide support?
10. There is a tendency for faculty to require students to do more work in a blended course than they normally would complete in a purely traditional course. What are you going to do to ensure that you have not created a course and one half? How will you evaluate the student workload as compared to a traditional class?

Source: Blended Learning Institute: School for Health Studies. (2008). Academic Technology, Simmons College, Boston, MA.

feel that the work is doable, which can encourage student motivation in self directed learning (Keller, 2008). The Simmons College Academic Technology Department presented a workshop for instructors interested in establishing a blended learning course, and participants were asked 10 specific questions to think about as they worked on their course plans (see Table 22-1). Planning takes time and needs to be carried out well before the classes begin. The online portion must be completely developed and posted prior to the beginning of the course. Last minute preparation that may occur with traditional classroom lectures must be avoided, although modifications, such as adding additional information and resources or correcting information, can be made during the course with appropriate notification to students.

Working with Technology

Success in online teaching requires close collaboration with the school's instructional technologists. Make them your best friend, and try to have a specific person to work with. Encourage students to attend technology orientations and to contact them with computer issues. Orientation to a course may include a scavenger hunt for students within the e-learning environment, which may allow students to download certain files, take practice quizzes, send an email, etc., and enter the results, information from the documents, or a special word from mail message to guarantee that they can access all e-learning tools and successfully access the tools required for the course.

Faculty need to work with instructional technology to learn to work with the online platform and keep up-to-date with changing technology. Technologies such as wikis (excellent for group projects because students can access and edit a group paper, rather than using email), blogs, voiceover PowerPoints, podcasts, and other technologies can be incorporated within the course, but too many different technologies can be overwhelming to students. It is critical to meet technology deadlines in preparing your classes, so the course template can be set up on time.

TYPES OF LEARNERS

Blended learning can be used with graduate and undergraduate students. Digital natives are usually younger students who grew up with and are familiar with computers and facile in using them, but there still may be younger students that require assistance. Digital immigrants are those of us who did not grow up with computers (Prensky, 2001). Some of the student "immigrants" have been able to adapt well, while others take longer, and may require assistance. It takes time for some students to understand this format and how to work with it, especially when they have not previously worked in online course work. A blended learning course requires students to be self directed and take responsibility for their learning. It is active learning, and it may take time for them to learn that their behavior needs to be different from attending a totally in class lecture course, and changing behaviors is not easy. Faculty need to assist students with learning new organizational ways to manage their course responsibilities and reduce confusion. All students need to know where to go for help with technical problems. Technical glitches cause frustration for both students and instructors.

USING THE METHOD

Begin planning a blended course by defining course objectives (see Table 22-2).

Meeting objectives is a prime responsibility in designing a course lesson plan. The next step is to carry out a literature review of articles and Web sites that will be used for course readings, and can be assigned to students to supplement the textbook and used for discussion post assignments. During the course, asking students to research and post appropriate articles and Web sites expands their learning opportunities.

Develop a detailed lesson plan for each class, which includes each area of the f2f and online course environments, and noting quizzes, exams, and other learning assessment strategies as appropriate (see Box 22-1). This is the "thoughtful" portion of the class, designing the course around the objectives and determining appropriate learning activities. Objectives and learning activities should be determined for each week of the course. It is important to develop a grading

Table 22-2 Blended Learning Preparation

- Define course objectives.
- Carry out a literature review of articles and Web sites
- Develop a detailed lesson plan for each class that includes each area of the f2f and online course environments, and noting quizzes, exams, and other learning assessment strategies as appropriate.
- Write discussion questions, and assignments for each week of the course.
- Prepare quizzes and exams.
- Develop grading rubric and clear expectations for discussions and other assignments.
- Prepare the course syllabus to be posted on the Internet platform
- Prepare a welcoming letter.
- Materials for student access should be posted prior to the first day of class, although access dates may be controlled.

rubric and clear expectations for discussions and other assignments (see Box 22-2). Writing discussion questions and assignments for each week of the course comes next. Discussion questions should relate to the weekly class objectives, and the overall course objectives. Students can also be asked to research articles or other materials and present them in the discussion board for that week, so that the other students can see and develop a conversation about them. The next step is to prepare quizzes, exams, and guidelines for assignments. Exams may be offered in class or online. The instructional technologist should be able to help faculty with learning how to utilize and post online quizzes.

Once the instructor has compiled the information and learning activities that will go into the course, it is time to prepare the course syllabus that puts the lesson plan information into a document explaining what will be expected from students for the course, includes the grading rubric and contains a schedule of the dates and time students are expected to be in class or posting on the discussion board, with deadlines for the posting process. Instructors can provide individual feedback by email to students when needed instead of using the discussion board, but students need to know that, and when they should, or should not, utilize email rather than the discussion board. Email is usually used for personal or grading issues that allow for student privacy. It is helpful to prepare a welcoming letter that clearly explains your teaching methodology, expectations for student participation, and who students should contact for technical issues and help. Materials for student access should be posted prior to the first day of class, although access dates may be controlled.

Course evaluations may be carried out in class on the last day of class, or online if the last class is a scheduled online class. As with quizzes and exams, evaluations can also be developed in an online format. Online capabilities also allow for keeping statistics, such as how often students access the course online, to assist in course evaluation (Ginns & Ellis, 2009). A caution to be considered is that steps need to be taken to see that course instructors does not have access to the evaluation posted online that includes identifying information from the student. Students need to be sure that their online posting is anonymous from their instructor, and this may be a technical issue to be resolved.

POTENTIAL PROBLEMS

Student Self Direction

Successful students are self disciplined in completing assignments and discussion posts on time. Patterns of late or missed discussions need to be recognized and challenged using a positive and nonpunishment-oriented approach, especially early in the course as students are getting used to the process. Avoid criticizing students on the discussion board for everyone to see, but use email or conferences to discuss the problems individually with students. There will be some students who are exceptional in their postings, and others who will barely meet the minimum requirement. It is helpful to provide feedback to both types of students. It is important to remember that life can interfere with a student's ability to participate at times. Illness, family celebrations, or a death of someone close needs to be recognized and students supported as much as possible. Students need to understand that they need to notify the instructor of such occurrences as soon as possible and make arrangements for missed work if possible.

Plagiarism

Plagiarism policies need to be clearly spelled out. Many online platforms use or provide programs to examine papers for evidence of plagiarism. Instructors need to emphasize the importance of citing references.

CONCLUSION

Overall, I have found that students in my online and blended courses learned better, faster, and retained more information that they were able to apply, than students in my f2f classes.

Comparison of Blended and F2F Courses

Blended Course Advantages

- Blended courses encourage active learning and student responsibility for their own learning. Increased student participation can increase retention of learning.
- Students learn from each other as well as the instructor, as experiences and resources are shared among them.
- Required onsite classroom time may be reduced, and students can work on their own time and able to avoid conflicts with family and work schedules.
- The online and in-class interactions allows faculty to get to know their students well, if not better than in the straight classroom, through constant individual communications via the discussion board.

Blended Course Disadvantages

- Students require knowledge of working with computers. This can be more difficult for digital immigrants, usually older students, than for digital natives, younger students who have grown up with computers, although both groups may need to be strong support.
- Technical glitches can be frustrating and time consuming
- Some students have difficulty with being self directed and taking responsibility for their learning. This approach may be new to them, and they have been used to lectures where all they had to do is sit in class. Change can be difficult. Patience, encouragement, and support may be needed until they become accustomed to the process.

I have also learned an inordinate amount of new information from those students, which is a great benefit to me, and has added to my reference and resource lists. I found that I was able to have students learn as much or more in a shorter period of time than the traditional 12- or 14-week semester. The example following this discussion demonstrated that idea to me, as this was a summer, 6-week session while the usual fall semester was 14 weeks in length. I found that I was able to include all the information from the longer semester, and students were able to retain the material. However, adjusting to a new format definitely takes some getting used to for both students and faculty. Faculty may need to experiment to see what teaching strategies work best at which time. All in all, I have found the rewards much greater than any problems that have surfaced, and so have my students.

Box 22-1 Lesson Plan Template

Course Title: NUR 390 Theory and Research, Integration and Synthesis for Professional Nursing Practice

Course Developer: Arlene Lowenstein

Course Objectives
Upon completion of the course the student will:

1. Address the historical influences in health care, nursing research, and in the nursing profession and their influences on the nursing profession today.
2. Explore the application of theories within the discipline of nursing and other disciplines and consider their use in practice and research.
3. Identify and explore the various research methods utilized to advance nursing science.
4. Recognize the responsibilities of the professional nurse to advance nursing through research critique and utilization.
5. Consider the role of nurse in formulating research questions and contributing to conduct and dissemination of research findings.
6. Apply principles of evidenced based practice and research utilization as related to clinical practice issues.

(Example 22-1 lesson plan continues here.)

Goals for Learning (what graduates will know, understand, be able to do)	**As Evidenced By** (products of student work that correlate with the goal)	**Experiences** (course experiences that will generate this evidence)	**Online** (experiences most suited to OL)	**Face-to-Face** (experiences most suited to f2f)	**Blend** (integration/synergy between OL and f2f)
Become aware of historical influences in the areas of health care, nursing research, and the nursing profession that have influenced the current day nursing profession	Discussion posts relate readings that discuss historical issues to their nursing practice	Viewing movie *Sentimental Nurses Need Not Apply* Lecture/discussion on historical issues—timeline		Week 1 Viewing movie Classroom lecture/discussion	
Explore the application of a theory from nursing and one other discipline and explain how they can be used in nursing practice and research	Following guidance from the instructor, select one nursing theorist and one theory from another discipline and search the literature for two to three articles and an appropriate Web site for each theory that include use in practice and research. Post the resources to the discussion with a short explanation of key points and how they have been used.	Theory and theorist lecture will introduce them to basic areas to explore		Part 2 of Week 1 Lecture introducing nursing theory and theories from other disciplines Classroom discussion	Week 2 Online assignment to find Web site from one nursing theorists and one additional theorist

Understand basic elements of quantitative and qualitative research design	Submit two 6- to 8-page papers, one critiquing a qualitative research and one critiquing a quantitative research article. Papers will follow guidelines that include analyzing the basic elements of the research design.	Textbook readings Research Examples	Discussion posts	Week 3 session 1 quantitative research concepts Week 3 session 2 qualitative research concepts Classroom discussion	Discussion posts
Recognize the responsibilities of the professional nurse to advance nursing through research critique and utilization	Critiques of quantitative and qualitative research studies. Select two articles and disseminate to the class	Textbook readings and lecture re: critiquing	Exploring Web and articles online	Week 3 concepts of critiquing Classroom discussion	Posting resources online Week 4 quantitative paper due Week 5 qualitative paper due
Consider the role of the nurse in formulating research questions and contributing to conduct and dissemination of research findings	Discussion posts show evidence of dissemination of research findings	Textbook readings Evidenced-based practice examples	Online literature search	Weeks 4 and 5 none	Discussion posts
Apply principles of evidence-based practice and research utilization as related to clinical practice issues.	Presentation identifying evidence-based practice with references and recommendations for practice	Textbook examples and literature review Course wrap up	Online literature search Develop PowerPoint presentation	Student presentations and discussion Course wrap up and evaluation	None

Note: This 6-week course was taught in the summer for 12 undergraduate RN to BSN students. Because of the accelerated nature of the course, a discussion board was used each week.

BOX 22-2 GRADING RUBRIC FOR DISCUSSIONS

A Grade	B Grade	C Grade
Utilizes knowledge of adult learning theory in discussions and responses—meets objectives most of the time with minimal guidance and/or shows growth in learning from guidance and other student responses. Usually keeps up to date in responses. Discussion submissions meet course objectives with minimal guidance and/or demonstrates growth in learning from guidance and other student responses. Usually keeps up to date in responses.	Utilizes knowledge of adult learning theory in discussions and responses most of the time with consistent guidance. Responds late some of the time. Discussion submissions meet course objectives in discussions and responses most of the time with consistent guidance. Responds late some of the time.	Content is usually satisfactory, but is late in responding much of the time. Content is usually minimally satisfactory but may lack thoroughness much of the time. Is often late in responding.

EXAMPLE

The following example is from a nursing research course I taught for RN to BSN students. The course was held in the hospital in which the students were working. This was a summer course for 13 students, taught in a 6-week time frame, rather than the traditional 12- to 14-week format used in the fall and spring courses. The traditional format for this four-credit summer course would have had two lecture sessions each week, but that would be difficult for the students, who were all working as RNs, and for the hospital in which they were employed. Although I had taught fully online courses prior to this course, I had no experience with a blended format, but knew about that possibility. I decided to try that for this semester. I spoke with our academic technology department for advice, and was invited to a blended learning workshop for other faculty members who were interested in blended learning, and I was welcome to attend to begin to develop and plan the course. That workshop was extremely valuable to me as I looked at the differences between a strictly online course, a strictly classroom course, and worked on the blended model of including both modalities. The course description and objectives were based on the traditional course description and objectives as follows.

COURSE DESCRIPTION

The course is an upper level course designed to assist the senior level student in the continued integration and application of research and theory in nursing practice. Theoretical and historical perspectives will be discussed as integrated within the research process. A spirit of inquiry will also be fostered as many clinical questions remain that require a nursing perspective for future study. Principles of nursing research, critique, and utilization in clinical practice will be highlighted and students will be given the opportunity to develop a research-based project. Independent learning, self-direction, and understanding of group interaction in the teaching–learning process are also stressed. Intellectual integrity, creativity, and open communication are fostered in an environment of cooperative learning.

COURSE OBJECTIVES

Upon completion of the course the student will:

1. Address the historical influences in health care, nursing research, and in the nursing profession and their influences on the nursing profession today.
2. Explore the application of theories within the discipline of nursing and other disciplines and consider their use in practice and research.
3. Identify and explore the various research methods utilized to advance nursing science.
4. Recognize the responsibilities of the professional nurse to advance nursing through research critique and utilization.
5. Consider the role of nurse in formulating research questions and contributing to conduct and dissemination of research findings.
6. Apply principles of evidenced-based practice and research utilization as related to clinical practice issues.

Based on the course objectives, developing the course lecture plan (see Box 22-1) was the first step, followed by the discussion board rubrics (see Box 22-2). The rubrics were developed on the basis of achieving the course objectives and each rubric dealt with one or more of those objectives. However, in some instances I found the rubric to be too subjective, and may need some revision in future classes, but it serves as an example of the process. The course was implemented very successfully. Here are some of the undergraduate RN to BSN student comments to their classmates about the research hybrid course:

"Thanks to all my classmates, I think the term 'learning community' really summed up the experience very well. I do like the format and flexibility of on-line discussion. I think it allows a more considered participation than that of just class room, often I will think about a discussion or response and have a question or comment later on. I think we did cover a really good amount of material in a relatively short time—and acquired some great skills to bring forward."

"First of all I want you all to know that I cannot believe how much I learned in this course. Although, I felt at times to be in an ocean without a life jacket, you were all there to help. Thank you for letting me whine. I really appreciate all of the support you ladies have given."

"I liked the idea of on line classes. this was my first one and i liked it,"

"Hi Susi, thanks for another great post. I enjoy reading other peoples interpretation of something I have read and getting their perception."

"Hi all, I just learned not to hit enter after the subject box or else it gets posted. And second thing I learned was if you save your thoughts as a draft, you have to remember to go back and actually post it. Thanks Arlene."

REFERENCES

Ausbum, L. J. (2004). Course design elements most valued by adult learners in blended online education environments: An American perspective. *Educational Media International, 42*(4), 327–337.

Collison, G., Elbaum, B., Haavind, S., & Tinker, R. (2000). *Facilitating online learning: Effective strategies for moderators*. Madison, WI: Atwood Publishing.

Garrison, D. R., & Vaughan, N. D. (2008). *Blended learning in higher education: Framework, principles, and guidelines*. San Francisco: Jossey-Bass.

Ginns, P., & Ellis, R. (2009). Evaluating the quality of e-learning at the degree level in the student experience of blended learning. *British Journal of Educational Technology, 40*(4), 652–663.

Kahn, B. H. (2007). *Flexible learning in an information society*. Englewood Cliffs, NJ: Idea Group.

Kahn, B. H. (2005). *Managing e-learning strategies: Design, delivery, implementation, and evaluation*. Hershey, PA: Information Science Publishing.

Keller, J. M. (2008). First principles of motivation to learn and e3-learning. *Distance Education 29*(2), 175–185.

Prensky, M. (2001). Digital natives, digital immigrants. *On the Horizon, 9*(5).

Singh, H. (2003). Building effective blended learning programs. *Educational Technology, 43*(6), 51–54.

CHAPTER 23

Distance Education: Successful Teaching–Learning Strategies

Kathy P. Bradley and Sharon M. Cosper

INTRODUCTION

Today, distance education is offered using a variety of media-based technology. The technology allows instructors to deliver content in live and delayed time formats. The use of technology allows teacher–learner interaction in two ways: synchronous and asynchronous. Synchronous interaction involves real-time, live conversation during the instructional delivery. Asynchronous is described as delayed, occurring either before or after the instructional setting (Miller & King-Webster, 1997). The purpose of this chapter is to describe the use of synchronous distance education learning methods used in teaching in the healthcare professions. Therefore, it is essential for new practitioners to understand the concept of distance education and its application (Zapantis & Maniscalco-Feichtl, 2008). The debate over the merits of distance education varies from blind adoration with assertions that teaching with technology can resolve weaknesses in traditional teaching methods, to opponents who insist distance teaching is not capable of producing the same learning outcomes associated with traditional teaching methods (National Education Association [NEA], 2000).

Synchronous videoconferencing allows for teaching professional students located at remote sites. Students enrolled in healthcare professional curriculums require the maximum level of interaction in order to facilitate the mastery needed for complex knowledge, skills, and behaviors required by the professions (Gallagher, Dobrosielski-Vergona, Wingard, & Williams, 2005). Healthcare professions are increasingly challenged to meet the needs of learners and provide care in remote areas. New technologically based instructional trends are available for providing needed health-related professional education. The educational trend for the 21st century continues to include the use of synchronous technologies to offer effective and innovative healthcare education. Examples of a planning process, benchmarks, identification of possible pitfalls, and strategies for success will be shared from the literature and from experiences (Jurczyk, Benson, & Savery, 2002; Tucker, 2001).

DEFINITIONS AND PURPOSE

The trended use of a variety of technologies and instructional systems has brought about a change in education and instructional delivery. Distance education is described as an instructional delivery method occurring when learners and educators are separated by time and/or distance during the teaching–learning process. Technology is integral to the learning experience for the new generations of learners (Bedord, 2007). The use of accelerated learning technologies has created dramatic changes in how health professions' students learn. Distance education represents the convergence of a host of opportunities and challenges (Keller, 2005). Greene and Meek (1998) described distance education as a quasi separation of the educator and learner requiring central involvement in the planning, development, and delivery of instruction. The use of distance education has provided alternative educational opportunities that may not otherwise be available because of learners' constraints such as family, work, or social commitments. Current technology is integral to the learning experiences for the new generations of professional learners (Bedord, 2007).

THEORETICAL FOUNDATIONS

Educational technological theories are also referred to as techno-systemic or systemic theories. They are generally focused on the improvement of the instructional message through the use of appropriate technologies. Historically, research efforts in distance education have focused primarily on the capacity of computers to process information and explore ways to improve the quality of interaction between the learner and the content. The technological upsurge in the last 20 years has had a significant influence on educational institutions in terms of the use of technological development and the evolving concept of curriculum development and instructional delivery methods (Anderson, Beavers, VanDeGrift, & Videon, 2003).

In the 1960s, technology was viewed as the pioneering methodology of education. In 1968, the United States established the Commission on Instructional Technology to analyze the benefits of technology for educational purposes. The commission's report identified the use of technology as a contributing force to an educational revolution. The report called for studies to examine methodologies that effectively improved the acceptance, and progression of the use of distance education (Bertrand, 1995). The report motivated future studies, resulting in the creation of the NEA and establishment of research-driven quality benchmarks for distance education in higher education. These benchmarks were formulated from practical strategies in use by leading US universities. The categories of quality measures included institutional support, course development, teaching–learning strategies, faculty support, student support, and evaluation and assessment methods (NEA, 2000). These benchmarks are used to establish standards for distance education courses.

The term *technology* is broadly used in the literature to describe all technology including computers, videoconferencing, Internet, and resources to provide instruction from the systematic application of scientific knowledge to solving practical problems. The main focus of a synchronous educational theory is to propose an organization for the use of instructional methods that could be used to effectively transmit learning content to individuals at another site. The use of learning or instructional technology is an approach that places emphasis on components of communication and the selected learning methodologies. Instructional technology is a method to systematize learning in a general applied method (Ely, 2000). Pregent (1994) described distance education as a meta approach to the relationship between theory and practice. Instructional technology is an interdisciplinary process and applicable in all fields of study. Instructional technology involves the process of organizing the learning environment with the selected instructional methods and means. It involves the systemic conception of instruction (Ely, 2000).

There are two main educational trends within the technological movement, system theory and hypermedia theory. The system theory offers numerous models that have been applied in secondary and postsecondary institutions. Von Bertalanffy (1998) expanded system theory's scientific roots to include an analysis of the parts and processes associated with a life form. Romiszowski (1986) outlined stages of the systems approach and instructional systems. The principal implementation methods included organizing the instructional process into a flowchart of performance objectives and then sorting the identified objectives into appropriate learning taxonomies for usage. Figure 23-1 highlights this process. The process then allows the instructor to select the necessary elements including groups, texts, audio-scripto-visual devices,

Figure 23-1 Outline of effective distance education learning process.

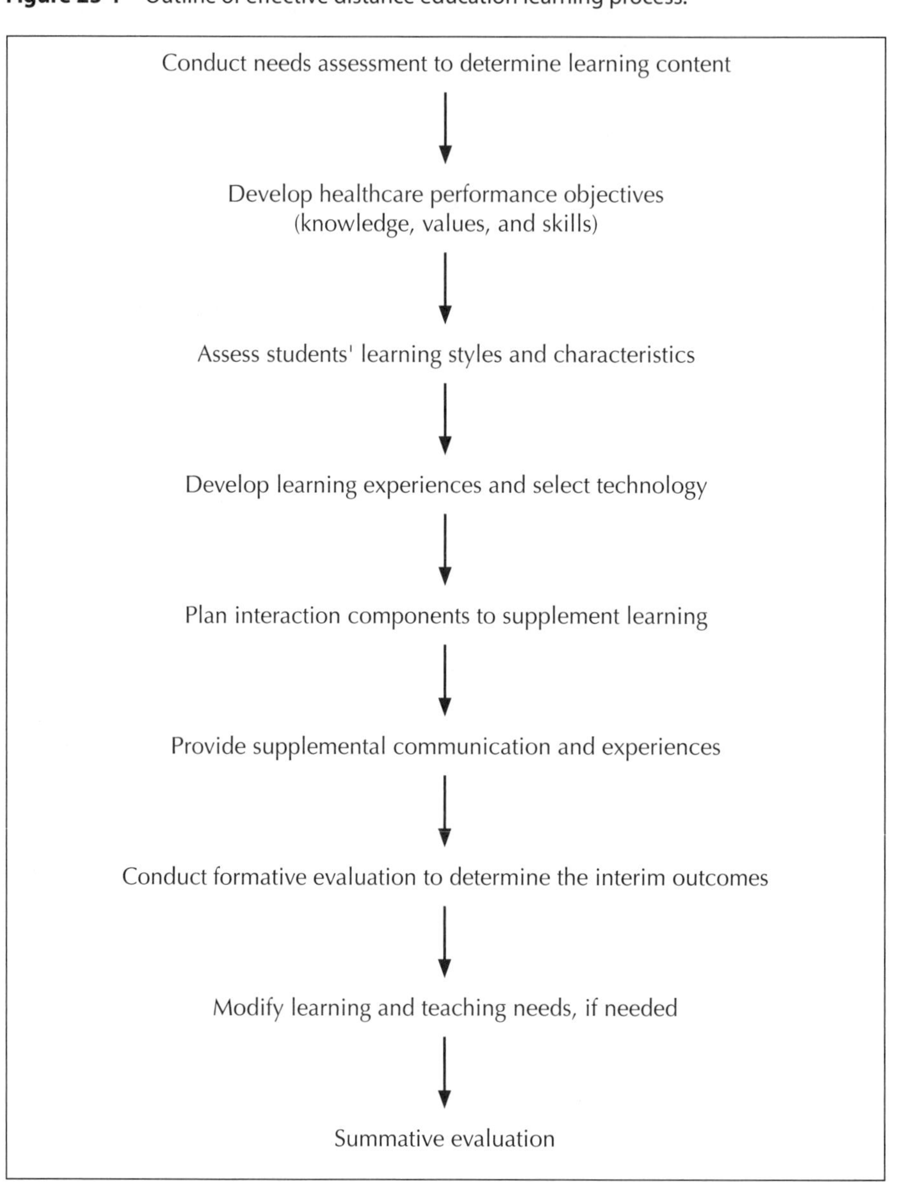

videoconferences, computers, etc. Information is gathered on the learners' characteristics and needs, and the learning objectives are modified accordingly. Operational plans for teaching and learning are developed. This method takes into account the learners, the performance needs, organization, use of systems theory, and the learning conditions.

Technology defines the external learning conditions, while internal learning conditions involve the cognitive processing required by the individual learner to master the performance or knowledge expectations (Anderson et al., 2003). Pregent (1994) described the applicability of the systems approach as appropriate for all disciplines. He described the instructor as the stage director, facilitator, coach, or informational engineer who determines what is to be learned. The instructor also develops the plan needed for learning to occur and assesses the activities and means necessary to promote accomplishment of the specific learning outcome. The instructor provides feedback and corrects any inadequate performance or learning. The instructor assumes the role of motivator (Bertrand, 1995).

Hypermedia educational theories originate with the selection of the use of the technology or cybernetics. Hypermedia theory is based on behavioral and communication learning approaches. The potential use of technology in healthcare education has become commonplace. Hypermedia theories originated with the use of media in education or cybernetics. This approach is based on behavioral and communication theories. The focus in the hypermedia approach is to model the informational processing by using the selected media. Early foundations of this approach were used in mathematical fields. Computers, discs, videoconferencing, and Internet-based instruction are examples of selected media. Five fundamental organizational principles of a hypermedia environment include a variety of interactions, open modeling, domain independence, cooperative instruction, and multimediatization of the presented information (Anderson et al., 2003). The use of multimediatization allows for learning using various forms of media in a variety of ways. The most important learning phenomenon is the evolution of the learning principles used in educational technology requiring experimentation of the content and interactivity. Interaction exploration and discovery of the needed content using technology allows greater student access to the learning process.

Learning theories related to distance education and the use of instructional technology research provides a foundational viewpoint for an interactive healthcare curriculum and the appropriate use of selected instructional technologies. The selected learning theories and technologies are used to enhance the learners' outcomes. Universities worldwide offer distance learning strategies. Implementation requires an acceptance of the learning technology, the use of innovative teaching methods, and interactive implementation methods as a required learning process (Keller, 2005). The primary instructional focus continues to be on the interactive process designed to obtain the targeted learning outcomes and performances, not the selected technology (Tucker, 2001).

TYPES OF LEARNERS

Distance education has become a routine aspect of higher education (Bedord, 2007). Most universities offer distance education courses. Universities that use distance education allow for a broader, more diverse student audience. Distance learning is appropriate for a variety of educational programs and learners. This chapter addresses the use of distance education in preparing healthcare professionals, who are generally upper division or graduate-level students. Rapid advances in the health professions and the related technology have fostered innovative teaching and learning methodologies. Healthcare students expect to be adequately prepared to practice as professional care providers. Consumers expect competent, knowledgeable practitioners. Studies involving a variety of health professionals have examined learning outcomes and the pros and cons of educating future health professions using distance education methodology. The literature regarding the effectiveness among healthcare professions continues to be limited in scope; however, numerous studies have described successful learning outcomes (Anderson et al., 2003).

Studies examining the success of distance education and student profiles indicate learner and instructor familiarity with technology was beneficial to the overall learning outcomes. Also, learner motivation and a sense of interactivity were highly predictable of learner success (Gallagher et al., 2005). Older adults tend to select distance education courses because of conflicting life priorities. Distance education programs allow these individuals more opportunities to pursue a healthcare career. The level of motivation to succeed among these learners is helpful for successful learning outcomes. Larger sample sizes and an examination of learning outcomes for the health professions are needed for more reliable and sophisticated statistical analysis. An important touchstone of distant education has been the ability to contribute to the development of individual learners regardless of life circumstances. Synchronous distance education is appropriate for all types of healthcare learners if attention is paid to the learners' access to education, adjustment to the new learning environment, individual development, knowledge and awareness of learners in context, and understanding the learners' perspectives of distance education (White, 2005).

CONDITIONS FOR LEARNING

The literature for distance education has provided various suggestions for implementation. Successful distance education methods allow for attention provided to the development of individual learners. This process requires an understanding of the learning needs of the distance learners and their individual learning contexts. Studies examining learning characteristics have identified a positive relationship between self-motivation and distance learning success.

Five central distance education themes have been described:

1. The learner's access to education is the first critical component of the teaching–learning process.
2. The learner should have easy access to the learning materials and an understanding of the technology.
3. Instructions should be given as to the best way to negotiate content mastery within the technological environment.
4. It should be expected that there will be an adjustment to the new learning environment.
5. It is recommended that the instructor spend time identifying the learners' needs and characteristics, individual development needs, have knowledge and awareness of learners in context, and understand the learners' perspectives of distance education (Sherry, 1996; Zapantis & Maniscalco-Feichtl, 2008).

Two crucial conditions for effective distance education are the quality of the instructional process and the technology. As an example, a telemedicine project was conducted to prepare a client education program for childbirth preparation classes. The instruction originated from a large regional hospital and was projected to a remote site at a small rural hospital. Over 6 months, three classes were administered. Formative learning outcomes were examined and the identified advantages included the availability of the learning programs, improved program attendance, and the convenience to the rural participants. The primary disadvantages of the project were technical problems that occurred, particularly audio quality. This study supported the importance of quality technology systems and support services to the learning process (Byers, Hilgenberg, & Rhodes, 2003).

The available studies examining distance education using videoconferencing or other synchronous teaching methods all indicated the quality of the instruction, the interaction of the learning, and attention to the learners' needs and characteristics are critical to the learning outcomes. These data are similar to traditional learning outcomes studies. When all of the aforementioned variables are controlled, the critical condition for success is the quality of the technology and immediate technology support (Hilgenberg & Tolone, 2000). With few exceptions, students learning in distance education programs have similar learning outcomes (McKissack, 1997). Studies have supported the need for student learning preferences to be honored, the provision of experiential educational experiences, and supportive learning conditions. It should be expected that technological problems must be immediately addressed in order to allow for learning to occur. University support for quality technology is critical for obtaining the required educational outcomes needed by healthcare professions.

Zapantis and Maniscalco-Feichtl (2008) also described the importance of the quality of the training and support of information technology staff. They described the importance of quality faculty preparation and early student communication for learner motivation and success. The methods included additional scheduling for technology downtime. Ground rules for students included reading the details offered in the course syllabi and the use of the syllabi as a critical source of information. Professionalism and participation expectations should be clearly explained. One major concern is whether the student is contributing to the class. The investment of preparation is essential for effectiveness in distance education.

One study in a clinical laboratory science program documented and disseminated possible difference in academic performance between distance students and on-campus students. The analysis revealed there was no significant difference in the mean final grade point averages and certification scores between the two groups. The findings documented the success of the clinical lab science distance program for educating entry level scientists (Russell et al., 2007). How do educators ensure their distance education efforts are successful? The NEA's (2000) published a multisite study establishing the following benchmarks as necessary for successful distance education strategic planning: (1) institutional support benchmarks; (2) course development benchmarks; (3) teaching–learning benchmarks; (4) course structure benchmarks; (5) student support benchmarks; (6) student support benchmarks; (7) faculty support benchmarks; and (8) evaluation and assessment benchmarks. Examples of a quality planning process, possible pitfalls, and strategies for success will be shared from the literature and from experiences of one allied health program with a distant education site.

RESOURCES

Identifying the needed resources for successful synchronous learning requires knowledge about how effective instruction is provided. Supportive learning aids need to be developed and the technology support must be seamless. Although the learners are participating in the learning process from an electronic classroom, the need for interaction with the content and the professor is critical to the learning process. Learners on the remote site may become codependent on written instructions. Educators need to be aware of the intended objective of written assignments and ensure the directions are clear. Learning outcomes are accomplished if the learning experiences are interactive. Also, handouts and readings supplement the presented content if the sound and video transmission are of a good quality. Poor learning outcomes have been noted with poor sound and video transmission (Mills, Bates, Pendleton, Lese, & Tatarko, 2001; Saba, 2005). When these resources are secured, distance education teaching and learning methods are appropriate for healthcare professionals.

Synchronous distance learning technology must support the learning ideas. New system technology includes Internet-based videoconferencing or the video over Internet protocol (VOIP). The distance learning course allows two or more sites to deliver and receive instruction. Communication is interactive between the sites. Each site is equipped with dedicated videoconferencing equipment, cameras, and microphones. Educators may need a personal wireless microphone. Televisions allow the instructors to view students on multiple campuses. The remote site views a video image of the instructor and other students at the transmission site. The instructor may use PowerPoint slides, SmartBoard, or transmission software such as Tegrity to supplement the projected learning content. A document camera may be used to project documents or demonstrations of practice techniques, such as the correct methods for management of a hand contracture. Various other technology, such as Webinars, for interactive classrooms also allow for interaction and demonstrations (Wimba, Inc., 2009). The process is effective with fostered faculty-to-student and student-to-student interactions with supportive experiential and flexible presentations (Anderson et al., 2003).

USING THE METHOD

A model has been developed by a southeastern graduate occupational therapy (OT) program located within a health sciences university to foster teaching–learning success. The literature describes the elements used in this model as supportive effective learning outcomes. A model for distance education is proposed to guide other healthcare programs considering the use of distance technology or the virtual classroom. The model may be applied to traditional classroom content as well as for practice application teaching–learning experiences. The model continues to advocate for the critical element of instructor–learner and learner-to-learner interaction using a variety of experiential teaching methods. The decision to consider the use of distance education centers on matching the appropriate technology to the appropriate learning need. The technology choice is always secondary to the learners' needs and the program's required knowledge, values, and skills competencies. The importance of the instructor–learner interaction is critical to the success of any professional educational program implementing instructional technology methods. The learner must also have experiential learning activities to support the retention of knowledge (Grimes, 2002).

Administrative (Institutional) and Financial Support

Within the proposed distance education model is the required prerequisite administrative commitment and support. Institutional support includes a documented technology plan with established security measures as well as established maintenance of the infrastructure. The administrative support will also require a financial commitment from the institution for staff and faculty training support as well as the hardware and software needed for success and upgraded technologies. University administration and the healthcare education program should create a financial pro forma to project the start-up costs of offering a synchronous educational program. The financial foundation should include: (1) the cost of selected instructional technology; (2) a determination of the number of enrolled students needed to justify the cost of financial expenditures; (3) the cost of faculty and staff development for learning how to appropriately use the technology with selected instructional design strategies; (4) the cost of the selected technology and technological support expenses; and (5) ongoing upgrades or operational expenses (NEA, 2000).

Faculty Support and Commitment

Faculty support and commitment, as well as student support and commitment, are collateral development areas needed to enhance the knowledge, skills, and buy-in for learning within a technological learning environment. In order for distance education to effectively meet the needs of the students, the level of commitment to success the educators have on developing and implementing instruction must be considered by the institution. Published literature examining motivators and inhibitors for faculty with regards to distance education have identified several motivators and inhibitors. With regards to motivators, most studies demonstrate that intrinsic motivators are more commonly the driving force behind faculty desire for involvement when compared to extrinsic motivators. Some of the top intrinsic motivators identified in the literature include the ability to reach new audiences, intellectual challenge, and personal motivation to use technology. The most prevalent trends in concerns related to inhibitors of faculty involvement included a concern with the lack of technical support available and increased time necessary to prepare for distance education curriculum. These areas of concern must be addressed by the institution in order for there to be a successful faculty commitment to distance education; otherwise, the success and quality of the program will be at risk (Cook, Ley, Crawford, & Warner, 2009).

Initial faculty skills in using the selected instructional technologies will be varied. Planning for faculty and student professional development skills will result in significantly improved skills within a short time period. Faculty will need technological assistance and the institution should plan to provide this support. Some faculty members may require support to successful transition from traditional teaching methods to using the technology. Peer mentoring may be helpful to faculty members that are new to distance education. Faculty should also plan to expose applicants and enrolled students to the distance videoconferencing by providing an orientation to guide the learners' acceptance of the technology. Faculty should be aware of their resources to assist the learners' acceptance with distance education as well as troubleshooting resources if access is problematic. Faculty should also caution students that their every move or comment may be broadcasted to more than one location at any given moment.

Development of Curriculum Design and Course Materials for Effective Outcomes

The selected curriculum design will remain constant for the required educational experiences for a curriculum taught by using technology or traditional curriculum design methods. Both areas require organized and planned educational experiences that are guided to promote lifelong learning, as well as individually motivational and experiential learning activities that involve a variety of experiential teaching methods.

The educational program should predetermine expected learning expectations and develop course benchmarks. Identification of programmatic outcomes and beliefs about learning and teaching effectiveness should be articulated. Curriculum design and learning themes should be formulated with instructional methods to ensure the instructional experience meets the curriculum's targeted learning goals and objectives. The curriculum components should be clearly communicated with the learners. The students' awareness of the learning objectives and expectations will enhance their efforts to successfully meet the program and course academic expectations.

The established teaching/learning benchmarks should include frequent faculty interactions and efforts to foster learner-to-learner interactions. Interaction is an essential distance education characteristic requiring prompt, thorough, and constructive feedback. The student enrolled in a distance education program will be dependent on faculty feedback for professional growth. Course structure should include benchmarks for professionalism, expected course participation, and learning outcomes. Faculty should clearly explain the learners' role with regard to self-motivation and the use of technology required by the distance education program design. Expectations regarding timely submission of student work should be established on the first day of class along with a course template with essential criteria for communication and expectations. Teaching–learning methods, grading rubrics, and targeted learning expectations should be explicitly explained in the course syllabus. Learning activities for the students enrolled in a distance education healthcare program should be designed to facilitate the learners' abilities to analyze, synthesize, and evaluate appropriate clinical reasoning decisions.

Selected Technology

The selected technology is identified to best meet the learners' needs. Too often instructors are pressured to use technology that is more cost-effective or available. It is inappropriate to select technology based on availability or the bells and whistles the selection offers. The technology selection should be guided by sound instructional designs choices that optimally facilitate the desired knowledge, skills, values, and interaction needed for competency and lifelong learning needs. Technology selection must have a faculty voice in the decision making. The model proposed in this chapter requires an interactive relationship between curriculum design, instructional design, technology selection, and the financial implications (Boettcher, 2000).

Student Support

Student support benchmarks should include access to student services, admissions procedures, communication regarding tuition and fees and related timelines, grading policies, and procedures regarding retention and progression criteria should also be shared with other policies in an electronic student manual. Students should be aware of procedures to obtain textbooks and other learning resources. Criteria for student advisement, academic support, and test proctoring requirements should be explained. Students should also be aware of procedures and contact information for technical assistance as well. Educational programs should be proactive in developing the resources for student support in a distance education program. Timely support enhances the students' satisfaction with the distance education experience.

Commitment

Many institutions embark on distance education without first analyzing the impact on the teaching, the faculty, and the learners. The financial impact on the administration and the control of intellectual property are also serious synchronous learning issues. The eagerness to join the technology marketplace has resulted in many distance education failures (Oblinger & Kidwell, 2000). The development of new higher learning administration strategic plans and policies that embrace distance education and change are needed. The process should create an organizational plan that anticipates consequences and develop troubleshooting resources. The level of administration, faculty, and student commitment is a good predictor of distance education success. Guidelines are available to assist the instructor in making the decision whether to enter into distance education arena. Educators need to respond to several issues before getting started in distance education, including the following:

1. ***How does one get started?*** For example, clarify the needed infrastructure of support and needed financial resources. Conduct a needs assessment to determine the number of potential learners. Determine what type of distance program is needed. Determine if the need is for entry level healthcare professions, postprofessional education, or client- and family-centered care. Determine the available technology and the learning needs of the faculty and learners. Critically analyze university support of the offered technology and other support systems. Determine if the faculty and adjunct healthcare providers would accept the distance learning concept and be prepared for technology mastery.
2. ***Identifying potential barriers to successful implementation.*** Assume the role of devil's advocate and self identify any barriers. For an example, technological errors or downtime interfere with the teaching–learning flow. Determine how faculty would assist learners to recapture the lost teaching–learning interaction for the needed learning competencies. Identify methods to report technology issues and record response and resolution times. Published opinions vary on the amount of extra time required for teaching using distance methods, but there is consistency in the literature in that distance teaching requires more instructor time. Recognize that

some faculty may experience degrees of technology discomfort. Discontentment with actual face-to-face student interaction also may be a concern. Many earlier publications revealed that educators feared the use of distance education as a potential job threat. Once the instructors engage in distance education, they are comforted that the role of the instructor is paramount to distance education success (Hilgenberg & Tolone, 2000). It is important to identify the potential barriers or threats to success and work with faculty to jointly pose effective strategies to resolve the potential barriers to success.

3. Preparation of successful distance education strategies requires the faculty and administration to jointly ***identify the strengths and weaknesses of initiating distance education.*** Action plans should be developed and planned, with targeted timelines. The faculty will need to develop a level of expertise in instructional technology and implementation strategies. Faculty will require more time to design these needed experiential learning materials and activities. Faculty will need to stay abreast of frequent technology advances (Martin, 2005).

Healthcare educators must carefully address the aforementioned identified needs and suggested strategies. Valuing the use of technology and synchronous distance education will be essential to successful applications. Faculty should identify the potential barriers and plan professional development and alternative solutions to resolve potential issues (Boaz, Foshee, Hardy, Jarmon, & Olcott, 1999; Dupin-Bryant, 2004).

POTENTIAL PROBLEMS

There are negative impacts on learning outcomes when the audio or video transmission is poor. The potential disruption needs to be anticipated with backup instructional plans to ensure student learning. Clear interaction and communication is required for effective professional learning. The literature clearly states technology problems directly contribute to poor learning outcomes (Hilgenberg & Tolone, 2000). Interruptions in audio and video have severe consequences for the learning environment for the transmission and remote learning sites (Anderson et al., 2003).

Experiential learning and interactivity are basic distance education requirements. If these events do not occur, the students at the remote site often disengage as they feel they are watching television. The lack of interaction results in poorer learning outcomes. The instructor must make assertive efforts to keep the students at the remote site engaged and promote active participation with meaningful learning activities. Initial assessment of the learning styles of the students is helpful in planning meaningful learning experiences.

The interaction between campuses should be positive, collaborative, and interactive. Faculty should role model the needed level of support and connection between the various learning sites. Students should be aware that casual conversations during class or break could be broadcasted. It is important that the faculty member present equal interaction time for all learning sites. Student expectations and faculty support should also be equal. It is important to avoid any tendency to respond to questions that are not open to all learners and all campuses. All learners should be included in course discussions, directions, communication of any changes, and all students need to feel valued.

Faculty need to be proficient with the technology and to be aware of projection expectations, such as the size of font used in PowerPoint presentations or the use of demonstrations that may be easily viewed by all students. Avoid the use of projected Web sites that are not easily viewed by all students.

New faculty will need to be coached in the most effective methods for distance teaching and for the most effective use of the technology. Knowledge of potential pitfalls assists new faculty members to minimize the negative impact of these issues.

CONCLUSION

A profusion of studies provide arguments both for and against distance education. The dichotomy of opinions is due to the complexity of variables that contribute to a successful distance education experience. Earlier studies focused on learner outcomes and satisfaction rates. Numerous studies indicated the overall outcomes were comparable to traditional educational methods if the instruction considers learning styles, interactivity, and the quality of communication and experiences. Student learning styles and motivation do have an effect on overall success. If learning preferences are effectively considered, the learning outcomes have been comparable to traditional education methods. Factors contributing to failures are the quality of the technology and the support personnel. Distance students prefer organization, experiential learning, and interaction with the instructor. Selection of the appropriate technology methods should consider the needed program competencies and learner characteristics. Technology should be suitable for the learning needs of health profession students. The quality of the technology support is critical to the students' learning and the overall success of the distance education program (Anderson et al., 2003; Zapantis & Maniscalco-Feichtl, 2008).

APPLIED EXAMPLE

The Medical College of Georgia's Department of Occupational Therapy offered a distance education program that included two campuses. The model of implementation for using VOIP included meetings with administration, academic leadership, technology services, and operational personnel from each campus to identify the needs for transitioning to this form for teaching and to develop an implementation plan. Key issues were identified from the onset of planning to ensure seamless teaching–learning outcomes prior to implementation of the new technology. The technology was used to project learning to 108 occupational therapy (OT) students. The institution and university system made the financial commitments to upgrade the technology prior to implementation of the program (thus meeting the administrative and financial support prerequisites discussed previously). Faculty attended a series of professional development seminars related to the new technology and brainstormed the development skills needed to use the technology in the most effective manner. The faculty team leader designed experiential teaching vignettes to illustrate how the technology could be used. The faculty then led a student orientation to demonstrate the use of the technology from the student perspective and provide guidelines for success. The VOIP was implemented gradually so that all glitches could be managed before the older technology as phased out, pending faculty and student support and commitment.

The Department of OT's academic affairs committee critically analyzed the implementation of the new technology and examined the program competencies to ensure the teaching–learning process remained the focal point. The OT profession's standards for educational effectiveness were reviewed, and the competencies and targeted outcomes were updated to ensure accreditation standards were fully realized. Benchmarks for technology, learning, and faculty and student outcomes were developed (curriculum design and program competencies were validated).

The curriculum design remained constant for the required teaching–learning experiences because the educational outcomes were the most important factor. Faculty mentors were assigned to faculty with less than optimal teaching effectiveness. It was noted that faculty who were organized, proficient with the technology, interactive, and provided experiential learning activities were the most successful. Student assignments and supportive efforts were developed to target analysis, synthesis, and evaluation level learning outcomes and critical reasoning skills. These methods included case-based learning, video analysis of real clients and their families, and client simulations. Resources for student support were also provided (Student Support).

Some faculty felt pressured to move to the new technology, so a team of participants from academia, administration, and the technological support departments met to troubleshoot any potential barriers or problems. A collaborative team effort was adopted by all groups in order to provide proactive communication, troubleshooting, and sound interaction between the curriculum design, instructional implementation, and the use of selected technology. The collaborative team interaction is a process, not an event, so communication needed to be ongoing (selected technology was identified).

As a part of the distance education process, all involved participants (students, faculty, administration, and technicians) needed to remain committed to the process. Benchmarks were established to critically analyze the impact on the teaching, the learners, and the faculty members. The financial impact and the control of intellectual property were examined each semester. Administrative decision making policies were established to critically examine the program's distance education success. Annually, the team conducted a strength, weakness, opportunities, and threats (SWOT) analysis to determine future distance education needs. Student satisfaction of the process was also analyzed. The team developed an annual strategic plan to ensure distance education success. The process requires the faculty and administration to jointly identify methods for enhancement of continued distance education success (faculty and others made a commitment).

REFERENCES

Anderson, R., Beavers, J., VanDeGrift, T., & Videon, F. (2003, November). Videoconferencing and presentations support for synchronous distance learning. 33rd ASEE/IEEE Frontiers in Education Conference, Boulder, CO, pp. 1–6.

Bedord, J. (2007). Distance education: Choices, choices, and more choices. *Distance Education, 15*(9), 18–22.

Bertrand, Y. (1995). *Contemporary theories and practice in education*. Madison, WI: Atwood Publishing.

Boaz, M., Foshee, B., Hardy, D, Jarmon, C., & Olcott, D. Jr. (1999). *Teaching at a distance: A handbook for instructors*. Monterey, CA: Archipelago Productions.

Boettcher, J.V. (2000). The state of distance education in the United States: Surprising realities. *Syllabus: New Directions in Educational Technology, 13*(7), 36–40.

Byers, D. L. Jr., Hilgenberg, C., & Rhodes, D. M. (2003). Telemedicine for patient education. *Distance Education in the Health Sciences, 8*, 135–147.

Cook, R. G., Ley, K., Crawford, C., & Warner, A. (2009). Motivators and inhibitors for university faculty in distance and e-learning. *British Journal of Education Technology*, *40*(1), 149–163.

Dupin-Bryant, P. A. (2004). Teaching styles of interactive television instructors: A descriptive study. *American Journal of Distance Education, 18*(1), 39–50.

Ely, D. (2000). Looking before we leap-Prior questions for distance education planners. *Syllabus: New Directions in Educational Technology, 13*(10), 26–28.

Gallagher, J. E., Dobrosielski-Vergona, K. A., Wingard, R. G., & Williams, T. M. (2005). Web-based vs. traditional classroom instruction in gerontology: A pilot study. *Journal of Dental Hygiene, 79*(3), 1–10.

Greene, B., & Meek, A. (1998). *Distance education in higher education institutions: Incidence, audiences, and plans to expand* (NCES-98-132). Washington, DC: National Center for Education.

Grimes, E. B. (2002). Use of distance education in dental hygiene. *Journal of Dental Education, 66*, 1136–1145.

Hilgenberg, C., & Tolone, W. (2000). Student perceptions of satisfaction and opportunities for critical thinking in distance education by interactive video. *American Journal of Distance Education, 14*(3), 59–73.

Jurczyk, J., Benson, S. N. K., & Savery, J. (2002) *Benchmarks of web based instruction: A comparative study of student and instructor expectations*. Columbus, OH: MERA.

Keller, C. (2005). Virtual learning environments: Three implementation perspectives. *Learning, Media, and Technology, 30*(3), 299–311.

Martin, M. (2005). Seeing is believing: The role of videoconferencing in distance learning. *British Journal of Education Technology, 30*(3), 39–50.

McKissack, C. E. (1997). *A comparative study of grade point average (GPA) between the students in traditional classroom setting and the distance learning classroom setting in selected colleges and universities*. Unpublished doctoral dissertation, Tennessee State University.

Miller, W., & King-Webster, J. (1997). *A comparison of interactive needs and performance of distance learners in synchronous and asynchronous classes*. Las Vegas, NV: American Vocational Association.

Mills, O. F., Bates, J. F., Pendleton, V., Lese, K., & Tatarko, M. (2001). Distance education by interactive videoconferencing in a family practice residency center. *Distance Education Online Symposium News, II*. Retrieved August 12, 2006, from http://www.ed/psy.edu/acsde/deros/deosnews/deosnews11_7.asp

National Education Association. (2000). Quality online: Maintaining standards in the distance education course. *Syllabus: New Directions in Educational Technology,* (10), 10.

Oblinger, D., & Kidwell, J. (2000). Distance learning: Are we being realistic? *Syllabus, 13*(7), 31–38.

Pregent, R. (1994). *Charting your course: How to prepare to teach more effectively*. Madison, WI: Magna Publications.

Romiszowski, A. J. (1986). *Developing auto-instructional materials: From programmed texts to CAL and interactive video*. London: Nickols Publishing.

Russell, B. L., Leibach, E. K., Pretlow, L., & Kraj, B. (2007). Evaluating distance education in clinical laboratory science. *Clinical Laboratory Science, 20*(3), 137–138.

Saba, F. (2005). Critical issues in distance education: A report from the United States. *Distance Education, 26*(2), 255–272.

Sherry, L. (1996). Issues in distance learning. *International Journal of Educational Telecommunications, I*(4), 337–365.

Tucker, S. (2001). Distance Education: Better, worse, or as good as traditional education? *Online Journal of Distance Education Administration, 4*(4), 1–13.

Von Bertalanffy, L. (1998). *General systems theory: Foundations, development, applications*. New York: Braziller.

White, C. (2005). Contribution of distance education to the development of individual learners. *Distance Education, 26*(2), 165–181.

Wimba, Inc. (2009). Retrieved May 24, 2009, from Distinguished Lecture Series: Simulations in Higher Education http://www.wimba.com/company/events/dls.fig

Zapantis, A., & Maniscalco-Feichtl, M. (2008). Teaching in a distance education program. *American Journal of Health-System Pharmacy, 65*, 912–920.

CHAPTER 24

Web-Based Instruction

Judith Schurr Salzer

INTRODUCTION

Rapidly evolving technology, in combination with the explosion in medical information and knowledge, has increased the use of Web-based teaching and learning during the past decade. Today's students in healthcare professions require fast access to the most current information on which to base their critical thinking and to apply evidence-based practice. Web-based instruction provides a variety of educational tools to broaden the scope of learning experiences and prepare students to function optimally in a technologically rich healthcare environment.

DEFINITION AND PURPOSE

As transition from the Industrial Age to the Information Age continues, the Internet offers educators an increasing range of teaching options. Courses may be developed that are totally Web-based asynchronous (no face-to-face or real time interaction), totally Web-based synchronous (no face-to-face interaction with class meetings online in real time), partially Web-based (hybrid/blended) with some face-to-face meetings either in a single classroom or multiple classrooms using distance technology (with asynchronous or synchronous online interaction), or traditional with supplemental Web-based components (email, forums, chat rooms, class content). A National Center for Education Statistics (NCES) survey found that 66% of degree-granting postsecondary institutions reported offering online, hybrid/blended online, or other distance education courses during the 2006 to 2007 academic year (Parsad & Lewis, 2008). Participating institutions estimated that 77% of the 12.2 million enrollments in college level credit-granting distance education courses were in online courses, 12% were in hybrid/blended online courses, and 10% were in other types of distance education (Parsad & Lewis, 2008). Although virtual colleges, which exist only in cyberspace, are increasing in number and gaining acceptance as a credible means of obtaining a degree, research indicates that employers continue to prefer applicants with traditional degrees (Adams & DeFleur, 2005). Online degrees from traditional colleges and universities are less controversial, perhaps because it is often difficult to ascertain whether a program was attended on campus or online.

Rather than being used as an all or none strategy, the Internet is often integrated into courses as one of many teaching strategies as educators transition pedagogy from face-to-face to online delivery. Research and documented experience are providing increasing evidence that Web-based instruction is applicable to a wide variety of students and subject matter including courses with clinical components or skill acquisition. As the rapid evolution of technological innovations continues, educators will be challenged to incorporate ever-new technologies into their instruction while developing pedagogically sound instructional strategies.

THEORETICAL FOUNDATIONS

Web-based instruction is the newest addition to a variety of distance education tools. Distance education began with correspondence courses and video tapes, then CD-ROM, and evolved to include two-way video with two-way audio and asynchronous or synchronous computer-based Internet instruction. Today, many courses and programs use multiple delivery systems such as combining asynchronous computer-based Internet instruction for delivery of didactic content with two-way video/audio for seminar discussions. Although technology has advanced to the point where personal computers support Web-based education to most individuals with computer and Internet access, the pace of technological advancement requires frequent updating of equipment, and individuals limited to dial up Internet access experience serious disadvantages.

As with any innovation, use of the Internet for educational instruction has had early adopters, late adopters, proponents, and detractors. Teaching online is different from traditional teaching and requires a paradigm shift. In online teaching, a shift occurs from instructor-focused to student-focused (Chaffin & Maddux, 2004), in which the authority figure instructor becomes instead a facilitator of student learning (Ryan, Hodson-Carlton, & Ali, 2005). This shift requires motivated instructors who are innovative, creative, and willing to learn and experiment with new teaching methods.

Published research provides insight into faculty and student perceptions of online learning and effectiveness of online teaching. Ali, Hodson-Carlton, and Ryan

(2004) investigated graduate students' perceptions of learning online. Students found online learning convenient and asynchronous discussions an effective means of communication. Timely faculty feedback has consistently been identified as a crucial Web-based course component for student success and satisfaction (Dennen, Darabi, & Smith, 2007; Menchaca & Bekele, 2008; Saritas, 2008). However, undergraduate and graduate students' perceptions may differ. Although undergraduate and graduate students were equally satisfied with online learning and equally willing to assume responsibility for their learning, undergraduate students felt more connected to instructors and classmates (Billings, Skiba, & Connors, 2005). Students' native language, gender, and prior computer experience do not appear to have an effect on their academic achievement or course satisfaction in an online setting (Barakzai & Fraser, 2005). Similarly, faculty find Web-based courses to be equal to or better than traditional courses in flexibility, student participation, and learning outcomes (Cragg, Dunning, & Ellis, 2008; Davis et al., 2007; Johnson, Posey, & Simmens, 2005). Anecdotal descriptions of successful Web-based courses range in content from critical care (Jeffries, 2005), health assessment (Lashley, 2005), and epidemiology (Suen, 2005) to methods of validating critical thinking skills (Ali, Bantz, & Siktberg, 2005).

Although the use of Web-based education will continue to expand in the future, a number of pragmatic issues have yet to be resolved. Online course development and teaching are more time consuming than traditional instruction. Many institutions fail to provide faculty with adequate time to learn the required technology and develop courses for online delivery, resulting in workloads that do not accurately reflect the time commitment required. As a result, significant disincentives currently exist for many faculty members to teach Web-based courses.

Some educators continue to be intimidated by rapid technologic advances in Web-based educational applications. However, the impact of the Internet on all courses and health professionals cannot be ignored. Students have quick and ready access to the most current information on the Internet and are increasingly expecting instructors and courses to be dynamic and interactive. In addition, computer literacy and Internet skills are now essential for survival in today's workplace and as a vehicle to lifelong learning. As a result, educators are recognizing that the traditional delivery system is only one of many varied ways of learning (Draves, 2000).

TYPES OF LEARNERS

Student age, gender, or computer skills should not be the deciding factors in determining whether Web-based courses are appropriate for an individual (Barakzai & Fraser, 2005). Instead, an individual's cognitive style is key to predicting successful academic achievement in an online environment. Individuals categorize and manage information in varying ways. Those with a field-dependent learning style who prefer a more social learning environment in which they are taught content are likely to do less well in a Web-based environment than those with a field-dependent learning style who enjoy conceptual challenges and are less dependent on face-to-face social interaction (see Chapter 1). Classes may also be composed of a mix of nontraditional adult and traditional young adult learners who have differing motivations, purposes, and intellectual skills (Neal, 1999). Successful Web-based learning requires students to be proficient in reading and writing skills, be self-directed, and self-motivated with at least basic computer skills (Kerr, Rynearson, & Kerr, 2006).

Before electing to pursue Web-based courses, students should assess whether their readiness and learning style are compatible with an online environment. Many self-assessment tools are now available through online organizations and schools offering Web-based educational options. After completing the questionnaire, students receive feedback with an assessment of their probability of success in a Web-based course. A sample of self-assessment tool Web sites is provided at the end of this chapter.

When students register for a Web-based or enhanced course, their technology skills and knowledge of Internet navigation should be assessed before class begins. A short preparatory class for those lacking required skills is needed, as well as a class for all students on navigating the institution's online library resources. The lack of adequate knowledge and skills in online navigation can prevent even the most motivated student from taking control of his or her own learning.

CONDITIONS FOR LEARNING

Variations of Web-based instruction integration into courses continue to evolve and gain in popularity. Although fundamental principles of good teaching and learning are applied in Web-based courses, a paradigm shift is required. Teaching online is simply not the same as teaching in person. The instructor is no longer the authority figure providing new information in a passive setting, but rather is a facilitator of learning in a dynamic, interactive environment (Chaffin & Maddux, 2004). This paradigm shift involves faculty learning new pedagogies and adjusting their roles to ones that require "high energy levels and creativity" (Ryan et al., 2005, p. 361). Further, faculty members often need to develop new skill sets, including the use of new technology and incorporating it into teaching.

Specific elements of Web-based instruction may be integrated into courses to enhance the learning process depending on the level of the course, course content, and instructor's experience with technology and Web-based instruction. Commonly, courses transition to a Web-based format over time as instructor comfort and experience increases. A traditional course may begin its transformation to becoming Web-based through the addition of an online syllabus, content outlines, and communication tools such as a bulletin board for posting announcements. Over time, content may be delivered online, replacing some face-to-face classes, and asynchronous and/or synchronous communication tools may transition courses to be completely Web-based. Alternatively faculty may find some combination that works best for them such as maintaining face-to-face interaction through monthly seminar discussions. Using multiple tools adds flexibility to the learning environment and appeals to varying learning styles (Menchaca & Bekele, 2008).

At the other end of the spectrum, entire programs and schools exist only on the Internet with faculty located all over the country or globe. Some schools are actually virtual, with no brick and mortar existence. Web-based degree-granting programs span the range from offering little interaction with faculty, a do-it-yourself type of program, to frequent faculty communication and specific, concentrated on-campus requirements.

It is impossible to say with certainty where the trend toward Web-based instruction will lead with the rapid development of new technology, but using the Internet to teach and learn is clearly here to stay. Although some may continue to prefer traditional teaching methods, it appears likely that this mode of instruction may soon become outdated. As instructors become increasingly creative in their online teaching, incorporating new technologies as they develop, there appear to be few limitations to the development of Web-based global education.

RESOURCES

Any instructor with a computer and Internet access is able to add several helpful online components to courses. Instructor Web pages with links to course-related material may be created by novice computer users with specialized software. Free software is available for download to provide chat rooms for synchronous student discussions, and new applications are under continuous development. More commonly, institutions provide a platform for online courses, which is often maintained on a server separate from the institution's main server. The platform provides course components that each instructor selects to include in a course template. Course content, links, communication tools, articles, videos, or other features may be loaded directly into the course template.

Courses that are developed and managed online require institutional support in the form of equipment (hardware and software), services, and faculty time and recognition. The infrastructure is expensive to establish and maintain. Faculty members require up-to-date computers, supporting software, and Internet access.

A server and educational platform must be purchased and regularly updated with security maintained. An expert staff specializing in using and maintaining the environment must be trained, updated, and available to students and faculty at all times. Faculty training on course development incorporating various teaching strategies in the online environment is essential. In addition, best practices and innovations in technology and the online environment must be communicated to faculty through periodic professional development.

Because not all faculty members adapt to the technical environment at the same pace, support and mentoring groups help those who may be overwhelmed or intimidated by the technology. Support groups also provide a forum for sharing implementation experiences and problem-solving strategies.

Institutional administrative support is required for faculty release time to develop online courses. Administrators must understand that an online course with faculty–student interaction requires a lower student-to-faculty ratio than a traditional course. Monitoring and guiding online communication among class members, in addition to direct faculty-to-student communication, requires a significant faculty time commitment. Institutions that commit resources to support online course delivery will likely require faculty to effectively use the resources provided. However, administrative policies for merit and tenure need to be adjusted to recognize the knowledge, skills, and time required to develop and teach courses in an online environment.

In addition to student course evaluations, a process for peer review of Web-based courses assists faculty to continuously improve their online courses. Excellent evaluation tools for Web-based courses are available online. Increasingly, institutions are developing their own evaluation criteria for online courses based on national criteria. A variety of free online newsletters is also available to inform instructors of best practices, new innovations, and methods of problem solving. Local, regional, and national conferences on Web-based teaching and learning enable faculty to network with others teaching online, share best practices, and evaluate new innovations.

USING THE METHOD

This discussion focuses on the practical integration of Web-based instruction into traditional courses, one of the most common applications of online instruction and often the first phase of transitioning courses to fully Web-based instruction. Regardless of the format, any course must be carefully planned, including identifying which online components will enhance the teaching and learning environment and considering students' varying learning styles. During course development, instructors must keep in mind that online tools themselves do not improve teaching or learning. The effective use of tools supports course objectives and learning outcomes and enhances communication between faculty and students and among classmates (Menchaca & Bekele, 2008).

Web-based tools generally impact communication through the transmission of information or by enabling two-way communication. Information may be transmitted to students by posting the syllabus, class outlines, or other resource information to be electronically accessed by the student at a convenient time. Chat rooms, email, electronic bulletin boards, forums, and quizzes provide means for two-way electronic "talking" between instructor and students and/or among classmates. Faculty members should become comfortable with using new tools prior to their implementation and should provide students with an orientation to the technology, new tools, and expectations for their use.

Although basic information transmission may be accomplished through instructors' personal Web pages created on the World Wide Web, tools available in commercial structured learning environments provide a standardized system for transmission of specific types of information. Information paths and pages enable instructors to provide the full syllabus, class content outlines, PowerPoint presentations with audio voiceover or video lectures, and link directly to online content, Web sites, or virtual demonstrations (e.g., heart sounds).

In courses delivering content online, course material should be divided by topic into 5 to 10 modules, with each module being a separate component of the course. Objectives, competencies, and outcomes are developed for each module (Draves, 2000). Module content is divided into lessons, which are chunks of information of less than 10 minutes in length (slide shows, videos, online lectures). Content outlines to guide study may be printed by students. Self quizzes and other learning exercises provide students with activities to reinforce learning and meet the needs of students with varying learning styles. Free, downloadable software is available to easily create crossword puzzles, matching, and multiple choice activities.

Pages created with faculty and student profiles help class members get to know each other and course faculty in courses that are completely Web-based or with limited face-to-face contact. Management tools enable instructors to track students' hits and identify students who may be falling behind. Students may track their grades and view statistics on each test or assignment, such as the class grade range, median, and mode. A calendar tool may be used by both instructors and students. Information about class schedules or content may be posted by instructors. Students may post clinical activities for instructor review or personal schedules that can be made visible only to the posting students. Posting and viewing slide shows and videos are generally supported by current technology except in areas with dial up–only Internet access. New user-friendly tools that are continuously under development are incorporated into frequent updates of commercial structured learning environments.

Online interactivity is essential for a Web-based course to promote student achievement and satisfaction. Two-way synchronous or asynchronous communication is facilitated by email, bulletin boards, forums, chat rooms, and quizzes. Because student access to the tools is available 24 hours a day, 7 days a week, faculty members must inform students of the limits established for faculty input. Some faculty members prefer to use the tools only during the traditional work-week, whereas others also check in during evenings and weekends. The more often faculty communicate with students, the more often students will take advantage of the communication tool. Fast response and feedback from instructors is commonly cited by students as an advantage of Web-based courses. Slow response and limited interaction from faculty results in low satisfaction and poor course evaluations. Some faculty hold office hours in chat rooms on a regular basis, enabling students to "drop in" to discuss content, ask questions, or "talk" about the course in a synchronous online environment. Although a high level of interaction is essential in an online environment, it requires a greater than usual faculty time commitment.

Email is familiar to most faculty and students. Either personal email accounts or email embedded in commercial structured learning environments may be used for asynchronous one-to-one communication. Email embedded in commercial structured learning environments may be used to communicate only with course faculty and those students who are registered in the course. Faculty members may send the same message to all class members or communicate with individual students. Students may provide information, clarify content, or ask questions directly of the instructor. Successful use of email requires an agreement among users on the frequency of checking for messages. More frequent checking results in greater interaction.

Electronic bulletin boards are used by instructors and students to post messages to the entire class. Similar to a bulletin board, a forum provides for asynchronous communication among members of a designated group. In large classes, forums provide for more productive conversation among students in smaller groups. Forums may be used by students to work through an assigned discussion question between scheduled classes. Forum discussions may be monitored by instructors for both content and student participation. Instructor comments provide positive feedback to the group, redirect the discussion, or suggest resources. Students have the opportunity to think about their answers or to do some reading prior to posting comments. Figures 24-1 and 24-2 demonstrate a student-initiated, faculty-monitored forum discussion. Again, expectations and rules must be communicated to students to avoid rambling pages that lack substance. The expected content and minimum number of postings per student need to be clearly stated and understood by students. Postings may be graded using a grading rubric, counted as class participation, or used as a critical thinking exercise.

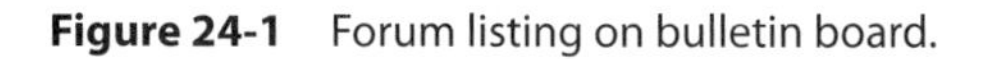

Figure 24-1 Forum listing on bulletin board.

Interesting case [Forum: Group 1]

- ☐ 144. Kathy Benton (Thu, Mar. 2, 2000, 16:40)
  - ☐ 145. Instructor (Thu, Mar. 2, 2000, 20:40)
  - ☐ 146. Annie Freund (Sat, Mar. 4, 2000, 15:24)
    - ☐ 147. Instructor (Sun, Mar. 5, 2000, 12:32)
      - ☐ 148. Donna Rider (Sun, Mar. 5, 2000, 13:38)
      - ☐ 149. Annie Freund (Sun, Mar. 5, 2000, 14:03)
  - ☐ 150. Kathy Benton (Sun, Mar. 5, 2000, 16:18)
    - ☐ 151. Instructor (Mon, Mar. 6, 2000, 08:45)

Figure 24-2 Forum dialogue under Figure 24-1 forum listing.

Subject: Interesting Case
[Prev Thread] [Next Thread]

[Prev Thread] [Next Thread]
Article No. 144: posted by Kathy Benton on Thu, Mar. 2, 2000, 16:40

I saw something this week that I haven't seen before and wanted to ask you guys about it. I saw a 3-year-old who we diagnosed with a right otitis media. She presented with serosanguineous drainage from the ear, but she did not have myringotomy tubes. She did have a perforated ear drum. We treated her with Floxin 6 drops twice a day and amoxicillin by mouth. I have not looked at the literature yet, but I wanted to know if you guys have seen this presentation of otitis media and how you treated it. Kathy
[Prev Thread] [Next Thread]
Article No. 145: [Branch from no. 144] posted by Instructor on Thu, Mar. 2, 2000, 20:40

What was the history on this child? Did she have upper respiratory infection symptoms, ear pain, fever? What dose of amoxicillin did you use? Prof. Sanders

---

[Prev Thread] [Next Thread]
Article No. 146: [Branch from no. 144] posted by Annie Freund on Sat, Mar. 4, 2000, 15:24

I saw a similar case this week. The child presented with bloody ear drainage and was diagnosed with acute otitis media with perforation. We treated the child with amoxicillin and Floxin. I haven't had a chance to look at the literature yet, but will let you know if I find anything. Annie

(continues)

Figure 24-2 Forum dialogue under Figure 24-1 forum listing *(continued).*

[Prev Thread] [Next Thread]
Article No. 147: [Branch from no. 146] posted by Instructor on Sun, Mar. 5, 2000, 12:32

It's interesting that each of you have seen this since it is not that common. Makes me wonder if there is an unusual underlying cause like a virus. What was the age of your patient, Annie? What other symptoms did she have? Prof. Sanders

---

[Prev Thread] [Next Thread]
Article No. 148: [Branch from no. 147] posted by Donna Rider on Sun, Mar. 5, 2000, 13:38

Dr. Patton saw a child this week whose mother reported seeing bloody drainage on the sheet when they got up in the morning. The mom described the drainage as a quarter-sized amount or slightly more, and she said she thought it came from his ear. On exam there was no evidence of ruptured ear drum. One tympanic membrane was slightly hazy, but the other was normal appearing. We did not find any evidence of bleeding from the nose, mouth, etc. We did not diagnose as a ruptured tympanic membrane. Kathy, what did the tympanic membranes look like on exam? Donna

---

[Prev Thread] [Next Thread]
Article No. 149: [Branch from no. 147] posted by Annie Freund on Sun, Mar. 5, 2000, 14:03

The child was 20 months and has had 2 previous episodes of otitis media this winter. She also attends daycare. She is the first case like this I have seen and I thought it was unusual. Annie

---

[Prev Thread] [Next Thread]
Article No. 150: [Branch from no. 144] posted by Kathy Benton on Sun, Mar. 5, 2000, 16:18
I found a good article online in Contemporary Pediatrics, May 1999. You can access it from www.contpeds.com and go to past issues. Kathy

---

[Prev Thread] [Next Thread]
Article No. 151: [Branch from no. 150] posted by Instructor on Mon, Mar. 6, 2000, 08:45

Good. Sounds like we need to discuss this further this week. Please see what else you can find in the current literature and bring the references to seminar. Also, make sure you have the relevant history and physical findings of children you have seen with ear drainage. See you Wednesday. Prof. Sanders

Real-time synchronous conversations can be conducted in chat rooms that are commercially available for free download or within a commercial structured learning environment. Use of a chat room requires setting a date and time to "meet" in a designated room. Student groups may use chat rooms to discuss projects or class content. Instructors may meet with small groups of students for topical discussions, to discuss problems, or to clarify content between scheduled class meetings. Some chat rooms permit the instructor or all participants to print conversations out at the completion of the chat session. A printed record of the discussion and action agreed upon is helpful to both instructors and students.

Online testing is widely available, often with immediate grading and student feedback. Although essay questions generally require hand grading at this time, programs for computer grading are under development. Quiz-type tools in commercial structured learning environments have several uses. Self-administered quizzes with immediate feedback aid students' study of online content. Graded tests assess students' knowledge throughout the course. In addition, a quiz tool may be used as another form of asynchronous communication. Open-ended questions provide a framework for students' clinical journal entries or notes and provide for timely instructor-to-student feedback. At the same time, students' clinical progress may be closely monitored to identify student problems and provide for early intervention (see Figs. 24-3 and 24-4).

Figure 24-3 Sample SOAP note using quiz tool construction.

Question 1: Enter complete, concise subjective information.

Student Response:

A 21-month-old female comes to clinic today for a sick visit accompanied by her mother. Child has had a fever, runny nose, and cough. The fever has been for 2 days up to 102 axillary. She has had a cough that sounds "hacky" for about 3 days, and she has had a runny nose for about 1 week. Her appetite has been decreased, but she is drinking okay. She has had 6 oz. of juice and 6 oz. of milk today. Her elimination pattern is normal. She has had 3 wet diapers already today. Her activity level has been decreased, and mom thinks that she is sleeping more than usual. Her cough is waking her up some at night, but then she goes right back to sleep. She has not had any vomiting or diarrhea. She is in a small daycare with 4 other kids, and mom does not think that she has had any illness exposures. She has not been to daycare in 2 days. The only medicine she has had is acetaminophen for the fever, and it has brought the temperature down, but after it wears off it goes back up. The last dose of acetaminophen was 3 hours ago. Dad smokes in the house.

(continues)

Figure 24-3 Sample SOAP note using quiz tool construction *(continued).*

Comments:

Allergies? Acetaminophen dose? The progression of this illness would be easier to follow if you begin at the beginning: Child was well until 1 week ago when she began having a runny nose. Hacky cough began 3 days ago and fever up to 102 axillary began 2 days ago. Add in when her decreased eating, decreased activity level, and increased sleeping began. Work on being more concise.

Question 2: Enter pertinent objective information.

Student Response:

Weight—29 lbs. Temperature—100.8 tympanic
General—ill appearing but in no acute distress; quiet and cooperative for exam
HEENT—normocephalic; sclera clear, conjunctiva pink, right tympanic membrane slightly injected with good light reflex, clear landmarks, good mobility; left tympanic membrane slightly injected with good light reflex, sharp landmarks, good mobility; nares patent, turbinates erythematous with purulent white drainage; pharynx clear, tonsils +2 with no erythema or edema; mucoid postnasal discharge
Mouth—mucous membranes pink and moist, lips dry
Cardiovascular—clear S1, S2, without murmur; capillary refill brisk, peripheral pulses strong and equal
Lungs—coarse breath sounds bilateral; crackles in lower lobes bilateral, posterior > anterior; no wheezing or retracting; respirations even, unlabored, rate 28; no grunting
Abdomen—soft, nontender, no masses or hepatosplenomegaly
Genital—normal external female genitalia without discharge or rash
Skin—warm, dry, without rash, good turgor
Lymphs—shotty, nontender, posterior cervical nodes bilateral

Comments:

Was the white nasal discharge really purulent? Was it thick or thin?

Question 3: Enter your assessment with rationale.

Student Response:

Pneumonia—bilateral, likely viral
Rationale: According to the articles by Schidlow & Callahan and Churgay, crackles and wheezes are sounds that indicate compromise of the lower respiratory tract. Churgay's article pointed out that most pediatric pneumonias are viral in origin, but a bacterial source should be considered because antibiotics would then be crucial to the treatment plan. The articles I reviewed all indicated that children with a bacterial pneumonia are usually sicker, in more respiratory distress, and with higher fevers than those with viral pneumonia. After my reading, I have a much better understanding of how to diagnose and differentiate pneumonia.

(continues)

Figure 24-3 Sample SOAP note using quiz tool construction *(continued).*

Comments:

Good job.

Question 4: Enter your plan with rationale.

Student Response:

My preceptor obtained a chest X-ray that showed patches of consolidation and admitted the child for treatment of pneumonia. After my reading, I would not have done this. Because the child was in no distress and appeared mildly ill, I'm not sure I would have obtained an X-ray. The articles indicated that pneumonia in young child is a clinical diagnosis because X-rays may be unreliable. In addition, obtaining an X-ray would not have changed my treatment for this child. My plan would have been:

1. Amoxicillin 400 mg/5 ml, 1 teaspoon by mouth twice a day (60 mg/kg/day)
2. Push oral fluids—juices, Gatorade
3. Cool air humidifier at night for the coughing—instruct mom on use and cleaning
4. Instruct mom on what signs to look for that would indicate the child was working hard to breathe—mom to call or go to emergency department if they occur
5. Discuss dangers of passive smoke exposure
6. Return in 48 hours if child is still running a fever > 101
7. Return in 3 days for follow-up

Rationale: Although 90% of childhood community-acquired pneumonias are viral, it is very difficult to distinguish them from the bacterial causes. Because of this, antibiotic therapy is usually given (James, 1999). Aside from viruses, *streptococcus pneumoniae, staphylococcus aureus*, H-flu, and group A strep are the main pathogens causing pneumonia. *Streptococcus pneumoniae* is by far the most common cause and can be treated with penicillin or erythromycin in those allergic to penicillin (James, 1999). I used amoxicillin because it can be given twice daily at 60–80 mg/kg/day, and it is generally well tolerated by children and is inexpensive.

Comments:

Good. Be specific when you ask parents to "push fluids." How much, how often? I would also have arranged to call the family the next day to see how the child has been doing since the visit. To implement your plan, you need to feel comfortable that the parents are capable of assessing the child accurately at home. In this case, it certainly sounds reasonable. I am not familiar with amoxicillin that comes 400 mg/5 ml. Please let me know what your reference is for this.

(continues)

Figure 24-3 Sample SOAP note using quiz tool construction *(continued).*

Question 5: What references did you use?

Student Response:

Churgay, C. (1996). The diagnosis and management of bacterial pneumonias in infants and children. *Primary Care: Clinics in Office Practices*, 23: 821–835.
Lassieur, S. M. & Jacobs, R. F. (1999). Pediatric pneumonia: Recognizing usual and unusual causes. *The Journal of Respiratory Diseases for Pediatricians*, 1: 42–50.
Latham-Sadler, B. & Morell, V. (1996). Pneumonia. *Pediatrics in Review*, 17: 300–310.

Comments:

You refer to an article by James (1999), but it is not listed in references. Please provide this reference. Nice job. I see much progress in your critical thinking on these cases.

Increasingly Web-based courses are being developed for interdisciplinary use. Interdisciplinary online discussions of clinical or ethical case studies and virtual patient scenarios enable students to view issues from the perspectives of different professions. Students gain a greater appreciation for varying approaches and teamwork in problem solving.

POTENTIAL PROBLEMS

Although innovative and state-of-the-art, Web-based instruction is not without problems and disadvantages for administrators, faculty, and students. Both faculty and students may be surprised by the increased time required in Web-based courses. Students may not understand the increased responsibility for their own learning that is required in online courses and may believe that expectations are the same as in a traditional classroom (Ryan et al., 2005). As students assume more responsibility for their learning, faculty must relinquish some control of the learning process that they had in traditional courses and instead become facilitators of student learning. Since online course development is time consuming, faculty may be unpleasantly surprised to find that online courses need frequent updating, not only of content, but also to incorporate new technology. Dynamic, ongoing interaction in an online environment is an advantage, but misunderstandings may easily occur when the written comments are interpreted differently than if the comments were spoken. Body language and voice inflections that contribute to interpretation are absent in the online environment.

Figure 24-4 Sample student weekly self-assessment using quiz tool construction.

Question 1: What are your strengths, weaknesses, and areas you need more experience in during your remaining clinical time?

Student Response:

I feel comfortable talking with parents and younger children. Parents seem to be responding to me by asking questions about their children and listening to what I have to say. I'm finally feeling like I know how to answer some of the questions. I'm not as comfortable with adolescents and have had limited experience dealing with them. Because we see few adolescents in this practice, is there somewhere I could get more experience with them?

Comments:

It is good when you start to feel like you know what you're doing! There is a teen clinic not far from you that we have used for students in the past. Let me see if they would be able to have you work with them for some of your clinical training. You can also ask around to see if there are other appropriate sites. Let me know if you find anything and I'll look into it.

Question 2: What problems have you encountered in the clinical setting that are obstacles to your learning? What can you do about them?

Student Response:

The only problem is that Dr. Towner is so busy at times that I don't get to ask him his rationale for a diagnosis or treatment. I don't feel that I can try to slow him down because there are so many patients to be seen. I'm not sure what to do.

Comments:

Have you thought about arranging for a routine, 15-minute meeting with Dr. Towner to ask your questions? Take a look at your day and see when 15 minutes might be convenient for him. Write your questions down and be very concise. Make sure you do not take more than the prearranged time. Keep me posted on what you decide to do.

The electronic environment poses several threats to courses dependent on Web-based instruction. Electrical outages eliminate the ability of individuals in affected areas to participate in Web-based courses, sometimes for extended periods. Users depend on Internet service providers (ISPs) for connection to the Internet, but ISPs vary in efficiency, reliability, and quality. As Internet users increase, access problems may increase as ISPs become overloaded. Users also depend on the efficient functioning of an institution's server for the commercial structured learning environment. When the server goes down or is undergoing maintenance, all coursework ceases. Security breaches through the invasion of courses by hackers could compromise student confidentiality or result in the modification or theft of course materials. Institutional firewalls must be continually updated and tested, and students should be advised to install a firewall on personal computers.

Administrators are faced with the expense of continuous maintenance and upgrading of servers, hardware, and software. Far from being a lucrative means of providing education, most institutions are finding that online courses are more expensive than traditional courses to develop and implement. Administrators initially anticipated that online instruction would enable faculty to teach larger classes and to positively impact the bottom line. The increased demand on faculty time arising from the ease of student–faculty online communication is beginning to be realized. Although Web-based instruction provides many advantages and is able to reach students who would not otherwise be able to continue their education, administrators no longer consider Web-based courses to be an extremely profitable venture in the short run.

Faculty members need to learn new technology skills and how to apply appropriate teaching strategies. High motivation and a willingness to invest time in the learning curve are required, but without the expectation of recognition or early reward. Developing online courses is teaching innovation that should be expected, respected, and rewarded, but in most institutions it is ignored as an important scholarly activity. Similarly, current intellectual policies for Web-based materials are inconsistent and often do not allow for faculty ownership of online courseware.

Courses with limited or no face-to-face meeting may lead some students to feel isolated and prevent them from developing the identity, cohesion, and rapport usually found in face-to-face classes (Funaro & Montell, 1999; Neal, 1999). Student isolation may also interfere with learning. Computer access is becoming less of a problem because many institutions now require students to have updated or new personal computers; however, high-speed DSL or cable Internet access might not be available to students in remote areas. Students limited to dial up access may be prevented from full participation in a Web-based course. The additional expense of a computer and Internet access may create an additional financial burden for students.

CONCLUSION

Adventurous educators are increasingly venturing into the realm of Web-based instruction. Although clearly a tread that will continue into the future, the parameters and limits of Web-based instruction are currently untested and unknown. Innovative educators must continue to document and share their experiences as they employ creative uses of the Internet in teaching and learning.

Applied Example

Hybrid Teaching and Learning: Combining the Best of Both Worlds

Elizabeth Friedlander

The educator's challenge to help learners develop problem-solving and critical-thinking skills has never been greater. Changing societal expectations for educational preparedness, the increased pace of knowledge development and the subsequent need to stay abreast of new information, and the dynamic technological culture pose tremendous challenges and opportunities for today's educators, learners, and educational institutions (Morton, 1999). Educators must remain focused on the task of designing and evaluating learning environments that support the development of skills for lifelong learning (Driscoll, 2000). This involves a reexamination of all components of the traditional pedagogy, including curricular design, the role of the instructor and learner, and content delivery methods (Knowles, Holton, & Swanson, 1998).

Asynchronous online learning environments have the potential to support learning that is collaborative, problem based, and facilitates the development of lifelong learning skills (Palloff & Pratt, 1999). However, many faculty and learners continue to prefer traditional classroom learning to online learning. The most frequently cited reason is a strong preference for face-to-face learning (Charles & Mamary, 2002). In a recent study, nurses expressed a strong need for personal interaction with faculty and other learners in a learning environment (Friedlander, 2006). One solution is to consider a hybrid approach that combines the online benefits of enhanced access, convenience, and innovative teaching and learning strategies with classroom opportunities for personal interaction, networking, and socializing.

Advanced Assessment and Diagnostic Reasoning of the Adult is a five-credit course designed to facilitate the development of comprehensive health history, physical examination, and diagnostic reasoning skills in nursing students enrolled in the acute care, adult, gerontology, women's health, and psychiatric nurse practitioner tracks of a graduate nursing program. The course description and objectives are shown in Figure 24-5. The course is taught in the fall semester of the second year of a 3-year curriculum for entry-level students. The course is also required for RN and post-master's students as it lays the foundation for the assessment and critical thinking skills required of nurse practitioners. The course consists of three credits of classroom theory and two credits of clinical practicum in the nursing laboratory and patient care setting. In response to a need for enhanced course access, improved class schedules, and classroom space, the theory component of the course was revised and placed online in the fall of 2005 using an online course platform designed by the institution. The courseware is user-friendly and hosts asynchronous course room discussions along with DL-101, an introductory course to online learning for new users, and access to electronic library resources, technical support, and email for course instructor(s) and peer learners.

The 14-week course is divided into 15 online learning units. The learning units are shown in Figure 24-6. Students progress through the units at a pace of one unit per week. With the exception of the introductory unit, the instructional design of each subsequent online unit is identical to minimize learner frustration, facilitate mastery of the technology, and keep the focus on the learning. The introductory unit contains a link to DL-101 and several Web sites offering information and tips on netiquette and a copy of the course syllabus. Students are asked to post a personal introduction along with individual learning goals for the semester. Each subsequent unit begins with a list of required

Figure 24-5 Course description and objectives.

Course Description: This course focuses on the performance of comprehensive wellness-oriented screening and symptom-driven exams with appreciation of normal adult life cycle variations. Emphasis is placed on mastery of interviewing and psychomotor assessment skills, diagnosis of common problems, and exploration of the health promotion and treatment plan.

Objectives: Upon completion of this course, the student will be able to:

1. Incorporate medical diagnoses and nursing diagnoses in the assessment and diagnostic reasoning of adult patient problems.
2. Perform a comprehensive and sensitive health history and physical assessment that reflects life-cycle variations and cultural diversity.
3. Utilize diagnostic reasoning skills in the assessment and differential diagnosis, of patient symptoms and physical examination findings.
4. Establish interpersonal skills during interviews with patients.
5. Communicate the health history, physical assessment, differential diagnosis, and health promotion plan verbally and in writing using appropriate format and terminology.

readings from the course textbooks, online articles, and Web sites. Course textbooks consist of a selection of health assessment, differential diagnosis, and health promotion texts. Articles are exclusively full-text downloads available electronically through the institution's library. Web sites are accessed through clicking active links on the reading list. Required reading materials are thereby readily available to students through remote access.

Following completion of required readings, students view a PowerPoint presentation outlining the essential learning for the unit. Students are encouraged to print a copy of the presentation to use as a guide during the laboratory practicum. Once the readings and PowerPoint presentation have been completed, students progress to the course room discussions. Each unit hosts one to four asynchronous discussions that surround the analysis of case studies designed to explore the differential diagnosis of common complaints pertinent to the unit's topic. For example, case studies for the unit on neurological assessment addressed the differential diagnoses of headache and confusion, while the musculoskeletal unit case studies assessed back pain and joint pain. Students are taken through the differential diagnosis process by a series of questions that prompt students to develop a list of potential differentials, elicit additional history, conduct a symptom-driven physical exam, order diagnostic tests, and consider health promotion education and screening. A sample case study is shown in Figure 24-7.

Students are required to post a response to each of the unit's case study discussions. For large case studies, students either work electronically in groups to produce a group posting to the case study, or students are assigned to analyze a specific portion of the case study. Postings must be well developed,

Figure 24-6 Online learning units.

Online Learning Units

Unit 1: Introduction

Unit 2: Health History and Differential Diagnosis

Unit 3: Assessment of the Skin

Unit 4: Head and Eye Assessment

Unit 5: ENT Assessment

Unit 6: Respiratory Assessment

Unit 7: Cardiovascular Assessment

Unit 8: Assessment of the Abdomen and Rectum

Unit 9: Musculoskeletal Assessment

Unit 10: Neurological Assessment

Unit 11: Health Promotion

Unit 12: Assessment of Elders

Unit 13: Women's Health Assessment

Unit 14: Men's Health Assessment

Unit 15: Adolescent Health Assessment

thoughtful, informative, and must demonstrate critical thinking. Students are also required to respond to at least one other student's posting each week. Postings must consist of more than an "I agree" type response. Questions, comments, and related learning that students would like to share with the group are posted to an asynchronous discussion thread titled "Questions/Comments." This helps to keep case study discussions on task and free of unrelated communication. Each unit ends with a 10-question online quiz designed to evaluate student learning of content presented in the unit.

Figure 24-7 Sample case study.

Unit 7 Case Study Discussion: Mrs. Brown is a 73-year-old female with a history of DM, HTN, dyslipidemia, atrial fibrillation, CHF, and is s/p an inferior wall MI 3 years ago. She presents for routine follow-up. This morning you received a phone call from her daughter who is her health proxy, stating that her mom has been more short of breath than usual, not sleeping well at night, and has developed swelling of her ankles and a weepy ulcer on the lateral aspect of her left ankle. The daughter is quite concerned about the possibility of an infection because that leg seems more red and swollen than the other leg. The daughter also asks you if you can refill her mother's acarbose, metformin, losartan, furosemide, verapamil, simvastatin, and warfarin. She also thinks her mother has run out of sublingual NTG tablets.

Please post a reply to one of the following questions:

Question 1:
What are the differentials for Mrs. Brown's symptoms, and what are your priorities as you approach the assessment of Mrs. Brown?

Question 2:
What else do you need to know for health history, and what information do you need to gather on physical examination?

Question 3:
What labs and diagnostic tests do you consider ordering, and what consults would you obtain?

Question 4:
You decide to assess how Mrs. Brown is managing her care at home. What data do you gather in order to make the assessment?

The practicum for each unit takes place the following week in the nursing laboratory. The session begins with a review of the online quiz and is followed by a question-and-answer period to clarify points of learning. Once students are clear on the concepts, an instructor-produced video of the physical examination pertaining to the system is shown. Instructor demonstration using student volunteers is discouraged to prevent embarrassment and protect student privacy. Following the video, students work with laboratory partners to practice a system-specific history and physical examination. The practicum is driven by a related chief complaint. Each student has an opportunity to role-play the nurse practitioner and elicit a symptom analysis and history of present illness and conduct an appropriate physical examination. The history and physical is written up, submitted, and critiqued. Students are encouraged to write up the "visit" on the spot to simulate an actual clinical encounter. Subsequently, student written communication skills improve dramatically over the course of the semester.

The nursing laboratory is equipped with state-of-the-art simulation technology and students gain experience in assessing abnormal lung and heart sounds through the use of clinical case-based scenarios. Synthetic models are available for demonstrating and practicing breast, rectal, and prostate examinations. Live, professional models are used for the gynecologic exam practicum. The capstone experience of the course occurs in the final 3 weeks, when students have the opportunity to perform complete histories and physical examinations on patients in a tertiary care setting. Students submit write-ups of their assessments, which include a complete history, physical exam, assessment (which often includes a discussion of differential diagnoses), and a problem list. Students consistently report the clinical experience helps to pull the learning from the semester together.

NS 760 Advanced Assessment and Diagnostic Reasoning ran for the first time as a hybrid course in the fall of 2005 with 19 students. Sixteen of the 19 students completed evaluations of the hybrid design. Fifteen of the 16 students had never taken a hybrid course before. All sixteen students felt the hybrid instructional design was better than an all-online or all-classroom design. One student commented,

> It was better than both the traditional and online courses. I learned much more from reading and writing posts related to case studies than I would have learned from a 3-hour lecture. The lab time gave us plenty of time to answer questions that were too difficult to ask online. (December 5, 2005, anonymous course evaluation.)

Another student commented, "It allowed for lab time and face to face interaction but also made you take responsibility for your own work" (December 5, 2005, anonymous course evaluation). Many students liked the convenience and independence and felt the course provided a greater opportunity for input and learning from every student. "I think online case discussion actually increased my class participation compared to other classes because it was less intimidating!" (December 5, 2005, anonymous course evaluation).

Students liked the online case studies and lab time best. They also liked the organization of the course and the freedom of doing work on their own time. They least liked the occasional problem with the technology and posting online late or last as the case studies seemed completely discussed and they felt they had nothing to add. All students felt the course met their individual learning goals and that they would take the course again and recommend the course to other students. Only one student felt she did not have enough contact with fellow students and the instructors. All students reported feeling satisfied with the course and the majority felt very satisfied. Several students commented that the course exceeded their expectations, including one who said, "The course was more beneficial than I had expected."

Another student commented, "I was really nervous as I had never taken an online course, but it worked out really well."

Yet another student noted, "The course exceeded my expectations. I am now an advocate of online learning!" (December 5, 2005, anonymous course evaluation).

Students identified organization, instructor presence in the course room, and instructor enthusiasm for and comfort with the method as the keys to successful online learning. As with all learning situations, understanding, patience, and a sense of humor go a long way toward supporting students and minimizing frustrating learning experiences. As one student noted, "The instructor made it both interesting and fun and was very understanding about time constraints and working out the 'kinks' of an online format" (December 5, 2005, anonymous course evaluation).

REFERENCES

Adams, J., & DeFleur, M. H. (2005). The acceptability of a doctoral degree earned online as a credential for obtaining a faculty position. *American Journal of Distance Education, 19*(2), 71–85.

Ali, N. S., Bantz, D., & Siktberg, L. (2005). Validation of critical thinking skills in online responses. *Journal of Nursing Education, 44*(2), 90–94.

Ali, N. S., Hodson-Carlton, K., & Ryan, M. (2004). Students' perceptions of online learning-implications for teaching. *Nurse Educator, 29*(3), 111–115.

Barakzai, M. D., & Fraser, D. (2005). The effect of demographic variables on achievement in and satisfaction with online coursework. *Journal of Nursing Education, 44*(8), 373–380.

Billings, D. M., Skiba, D. J., & Connors, H. R. (2005). Best practices in Web-based courses: Generational differences across undergraduate and graduate nursing students. *Journal of Professional Nursing, 21*(2), 126–133.

Chaffin, A. J., & Maddux, C. D. (2004). Internet teaching methods for use in baccalaureate nursing education. *CIN: Computers, Informatics, Nursing, 22*(3), 132–142.

Charles, P. A., & Mamary, E. M. (2002). New choices for continuing education: A statewide survey of the practice and preferences of nurse practitioners. *The Journal of Continuing Education in Nursing,* 33(2), 88–91.

Cragg, C. E., Dunning, J., & Ellis, J. (2008). Teacher and student behaviors in face-to-face and on-line courses: Dealing with complex concepts. *Journal of Distance Education, 22*(3), 115–128.

Davis, J., Chryssafidou, E., Zamora, J., Davies, D., Khan, K., & Coomarasamy, A. (2007). Computer-based teaching is as good as face to face lecture-based teaching of evidence based medicine: A randomised controlled trial. *BMC Medical Education, 7*(23). Retrieved November 29, 2009, from http://www.biomedcentral.com/1472–6920/7/23

Dennen, V. P., Darabi, A. A., & Smith, L. J. (2007). Instructor-learner interaction in online courses: The relative perceived importance of particular instructor actions on performance and satisfaction. *Distance Education, 28*(1), 65–79.

Draves, W. A. (2000). *Teaching online*. River Falls, WI: Learning Resources Network.

Driscoll, M. P. (2000). Constructivism. In *Psychology of learning for instruction* (2nd ed., pp. 373–396). Boston: Allyn and Bacon.

Friedlander, E. A. (2006). *Online continuing nursing education: A study of factors related to nurse practitioner participation.* Unpublished doctoral dissertation. Capella University, Minneapolis, MN.

Funaro, G. M., & Montell, F. (1999). Pedagogical roles and implementation guidelines for online communication tools. *Asynchronous Learning Networks Magazine, 3*(5). Retrieved May 4, 2009, from http://www.aln.org/publications/magazine/v3n2/funaro.asp

Jeffries, P. R. (2005). Development and testing of a hyperlearning model for design of an online critical care course. *Journal of Nursing Education, 44*(8), 366–372.

Johnson, J., Posey, L., & Simmens, S. J. (2005). Faculty and student perceptions of Web-based learning. *The American Journal for Nurse Practitioners, 9*(4), 9–18.

Kerr, M. S., Rynearson, K., & Kerr, M. C. (2006). Student characteristics for online learning success. *Internet and Higher Education, 9*, 91–105.

Knowles, M. S., Holton, E. F., & Swanson, R. A. (1998). *The adult learner* (5th ed.). Houston, TX: Gulf Publishing Company.

Lashley, M. (2005). Teaching health assessment in the virtual classroom. *Journal of Nursing Education, 44*(8), 487–491.

Menchaca, M. P., & Bekele, T. A. (2008). Learner and instructor identified success factors in distance education. *Distance Education, 29*(3), 231–252.

Morton, E. (1999). Transforming education: Don't reengineer the existing system. *Vital Speeches of the Day,* 65(16), 487–491.

Neal, E. (1999). Distance education. *National Forum, 79*(1), 40.

Palloff, R. M., & Pratt, K. (1999). *Building learning communities in cyberspace: Effective strategies for the online classroom.* San Francisco: Jossey-Bass Publishers.

Parsad, B., & Lewis, L. (2008). *Distance education at degree-granting postsecondary institutions: 2006–07* (NCES 2009–044). Washington, DC: National Center for Education Statistics.

Ryan, M., Hodson-Carlton, K., & Ali, N. S. (2005). A model for faculty teaching online: Confirmation of a dimensional matrix. *Journal of Nursing Education, 44*(8), 357–365.

Saritas, T. (2008). The construction of knowledge through social interaction via computer-mediated communication. *The Quarterly Review of Distance Education, 9*(1), 35–49.

Suen, L. (2005). Teaching epidemiology using WebCT: Application of the seven principles of good practice. *Journal of Nursing Education, 44*(3), 143–146.

ELECTRONIC RESOURCES

Recommended General Resource

Illinois Online Network. Available from http://www.ion.uillinois.edu/

Student Self-Assessment Tools

Center for Independent Learning. Available from http://www.cod.edu/dept/CIL/CIL_Surv.htm

Community College of Philadelphia. Available from http://faculty.ccp.edu/dept/ccpde/self_asmt.html

OnlineLearning.net. Available from http://www.onlinelearning.net/OLE/holwselfassess.html?s=425.k0404492r.016c302m60

Peterson's Distance Learning Assessment. Available from http://www.petersons.com/dlwizard/code/default.asp

The Test of Online Learning Success (TOOLS). Available from http://faculty.txwes.edu/mskerr/files/TOOLS.pdf

Educational Platforms-Commercial Structured Learning Environments

Blackboard. Available from http://www.blackboard.com

eCollege. Available from http://www.ecollege.com/index.learn

LogiCampus. Available from http://logicampus.sourceforge.net/index.php

Online Course Evaluation

Online Course Evaluation Rubric. Available from http://www.atlm.edu/irpa/ecollege/Publications/OnlineCourseEvaluationRubric.pdf

Quality on the Line-Benchmarks for Success in Internet-Based Distance Education. Available from http://www2.nea.org/he/abouthe/images/Quality.pdf

Rubric for Online Instruction. Available from http://www.csuchico.edu/celt/roi/

Virtual Clinical Sites

The Auscultation Assistant. Available from http://www.wilkes.med.ucla.edu/inex.htm

EKGs and Heart Sounds. Available from http://www.skillstat.com/ECGskills.htm

Epidemiologic Case Studies. Available from http://www2a.cdc.gov/epicasestudies/

Eye Simulator/Virtual Patient. Available from http://cim.ucdavis.edu/EyeRelease/Interface/TopFrame.htm

Lung Sounds. Available from http://www.rale.ca/Repository.htm

Virtual Hospital. Available from http://www.janela1.com/vh/docs/index.htm

Virtual Patient Reference Library. Available from http://research.caregroup.org/vptutorials/

Virtual Pediatric Hospital. Available from http://www.virtualpediatrichospital.org/

Open Courseware

MIT Open Courseware. Available from http://ocw.mit.edu/OcwWeb/web/home/home/index.htm

Multimedia Educational Resource for Learning and Online Teaching (MERLOT). Available from http://www.merlot.org/merlot/index.htm

Open Courseware Consortium. Available from http://www.ocwconsortium.org/

SECTION V

TEACHING IN UNSTRUCTURED SETTINGS

This section addresses teaching and learning in the most unstructured settings, such as that of the clinical care environment. Clinical teaching is one of the most significant features of a health professions education. Chapters in Section V are introduced by philosophical underpinnings that should guide each instructor when planning and carrying out clinical instruction. This edition presents a helpful how-to chapter for instructors who conduct a very structured clinical experience, such as in nursing. The clinical teaching chapters evolve from introductory skills lab to addressing complex situations, such as student preceptor issues and service-learning. Critical thinking and the development of higher-order thinking are key components of the chapter on concept mapping. To meet the challenges of finding diverse clinical experiences, chapters on faculty practice clinic and study abroad present creative ideas for enhancing clinical learning. With these opportunities, students can achieve a higher degree of independence, self-awareness of personal strengths and weaknesses, and enhanced critical thinking skills.

CHAPTER 25

Philosophical Approaches to Clinical Instruction

Martha J. Bradshaw

INTRODUCTION

The purpose of clinical instruction is to give the student opportunities to bridge didactic information with the realities of practice. Clinical learning within the realm of nursing education is best achieved when there is consistent and meaningful interaction between the student and the clinical instructor who is part of an educational institution. In guided situations, students blend theoretical knowledge with experiential learning in order to effect a synthesis and understanding of those endeavors known collectively as *nursing*. Clinical learning is directed by a nurse educator who operationalizes his or her practical knowledge about teaching. Through use of this practical knowledge, the instructor translates the didactic content into application for use in health care. Clinical instruction in all health professions has become more challenging because of changes in the healthcare environment and the need for health professionals to fulfill increasingly diverse roles. Instructors need to examine their personal philosophy (underlying beliefs) about teaching, especially considering the changes in traditional models of clinical learning. The need for clinical judgment, especially in complex patient settings, calls for dual competence: content-specific knowledge and an ability to use the information for clinical practice and decision making. However, constant changes in the practice settings make competence elusive and demanding (Little & Milliken, 2007).

ROLE OF THE CLINICAL INSTRUCTOR

The goal of the clinical learning experience is for the instructor to guide the novice in what constitutes safe practice and to develop clinical judgment. In the clinical setting, planning and selecting clinical learning activities tends to be instructor driven. Depending on the amount of experience and sense of self-efficacy held by the instructor, the nature of clinical learning may become more student centered. In either case, the teacher guides the students in applying theory to patient care. The faculty role in clinical instruction is as diverse and demanding as are the settings. The instructor is expected to be competent, experienced, knowledgeable, flexible, patient, and energetic. The instructor should be capable of balancing structure with spontaneity. Clinical learning is aimed at knowledge application, skill acquisition, and professional role development. The instructor must be aware of didactic information the students are studying, in order to provide parallel opportunities for application. Students are led in practicing and improving nursing care skills, and need guidance in valuing the skills (Clark, Owen, & Tholcken, 2004). By recognizing the importance of a skill and performing it safely and efficiently, students will increase confidence in their abilities to provide direct patient care. Clinical instructors also help students understand and respect the uniqueness of each client and family in order to individualize holistic nursing care (Northington, Wilkerson, Fisher, & Schenk, 2005). Nursing students have indicated that their most successful clinical experiences (over time, such as a semester or rotation) are ones in which the instructor uses strategies to improve self-confidence, foster learning of responsibility, and how to think critically (Etheridge, 2007). In summary, the role of the clinical instructor is to direct the student to think like a physical therapist, nurse, or dentist.

Paterson (1994) describes two approaches to clinical instruction: task mastery and professional identity mentoring. Task mastery instruction is based on the instructor's decisions about what behaviors and ways of thinking are important for nurses and, therefore, need to be reproduced in students. In essence, clinical instructors are gatekeepers, allowing students to enter the profession once they have demonstrated their ability. With the professional identity approach, the instructor serves as a mentor, guiding students in decision making and inculcation of hallmarks of professional practice. Task mastery may be suitable with novice students, but the professional identity approach has a far reaching effect on students as they progress in their nursing program.

The successful student clinical experience—measured in terms of learning outcomes and an internalized sense of fulfillment—is largely influenced by the planning and selection of learning activities available to the students. Selection of activities, as well as actual teaching, is value-laden and reflects the faculty member's philosophical approach to clinical learning and the role or roles the instructor chooses to fulfill. The roles in which individual instructors see themselves may include interaction with students, serving as a role model, or functioning as an expert reference. Roles that students see as important for clinical instructors to hold have been identified as knowledgeable and professionally competent, able to be encouraging and supportive, provider of helpful feedback, organizational skills, and respect for others, especially students (Cook, 2005; Hanson & Stenvig, 2008). Once this self image is determined, teachers consciously or subconsciously shape situations that enable them to enact their various roles. This action enhances teacher effectiveness because the instructor is most comfortable in fulfilling preselected roles.

There is some indication that background knowledge and preferences for orientation to practice strongly influence planning and decision making by teachers (Yaakobi and Sharan, 1985). Therefore, an instructor with a concrete, structured practice background (e.g., surgical nursing) may select or plan patient assignments that are more structured than those selected by an instructor from a less structured background (e.g., psychiatric nursing). The potential conflict exists between teacher and student regarding learning and practice preferences. Consequently, an effective clinical instructor is one who has the knowledge and practice experience while understanding students' learning preferences and educational needs. Furthermore, new graduates report that their best earning opportunities in clinical were when they had a variety of patient care experiences (Etheridge, 2007).

FOUNDATIONS FOR SELECTION OF CLINICAL ACTIVITIES

Another philosophical perspective that governs clinical learning is the instructor's view of the *purpose* of the clinical learning experience. The three most common purposes are for students to (1) apply theoretical concepts, (2) experience actual patient situations, and (3) see and implement professional roles. Based on the chosen perspective, the instructor selects the agency or unit and plans the type of clinical assignment that is best suited for the identified purpose. The realism of clinical activities brings added benefit to any of the three types of experiences.

The planning and supervising of clinical learning call for the instructor's own philosophical stance to be blended with the selected goal(s) of the clinical experience. Student assignments may have one of the following goals:

- Learn the **patient**: provide one-to-one total care
- Learn the **content area**: practice a variety of care activities in one setting
- Learn **role(s)**: function as a staff or team member, as a practitioner, administrator, or other selected roles

The instructor who selects a student focus for clinical assignments may value empowerment as part of his or her philosophical approach to teaching. The aims of this approach are the cultivation of responsibility, authority, and accountability in novice practitioners (Manthey, 1992). Selected clinical activities directed toward empowerment could include:

- **Analytic nursing**: use of actual experiences (instructor or student based) to define and solve problems
- **Change activities**: develop planned change and identify resources to effect this change
- **Collegiality**: professional interactions (instructor–student, student–student, student–staff) to solve problems and promote optimal care
- **Sponsorship**: collaboration and interaction with preceptors, administration; analysis of bureaucratic system (Carlson-Catalano, 1992)

Within the framework of the assignment, the instructor then makes decisions about which activities will enhance learning outcomes. This process again reflects the teacher's values, beliefs about how learning should take place, and how teacher role fulfillment will influence this learning. For example, the instructor who values participatory learning and role modeling will be actively involved in many aspects of the student's activities, and his or her presence will be felt by the student—at the bedside or interacting with staff members. Role modeling, an encouraging attitude, and serving as a resource person are attributes that decrease student anxiety about the clinical experience and strengthen the instructor–student relationship (Cook, 2005; Hanson & Stenvig, 2008). The instructor who wishes to foster independence in students may take on the role of resource person and become centrally available to students as needed. The instructor who places emphasis on organization and task accomplishment will oversee numerous student activities and facilitate completion of the assignments within a designated period. Many instructors value all of these activities as a part of student learning. Accomplishing all of these activities calls for a great deal of diversity and planning by the teacher. There are clear advantages for students to be engaged in more than one type of learning experience from one clinical day or week to the next. This broadens the possibilities for learning plus strengthens understanding of multiple roles and diversity of settings. Students who experienced multiple clinical placements described themselves as more adaptable in new environments (Adams, 2002).

Some philosophical approaches to teaching and role assumption by educators are more subtle, yet promote more complex, higher order learning. More specifically, the teacher who values empowerment and accountability in students will take on a less directive role and assume one that is more enabling for each student. The instructor who wishes to promote independence in students must be willing to release a certain amount of control, in order to give freedom for students to learn and grow.

Periodic, timely feedback is essential. Students can only recognize strengths and areas for improvement when they are given objective, constructive feedback. Feedback should be not only evaluative but also encouraging to bolster confidence and independence. Augustine (1992) investigated feedback by clinical instructors and discovered that, in addition to group feedback, such as in conferences or orientation, students felt the need for personal feedback from the instructor until they were certain what the instructor wanted from them. This need indicates not only the value of the instructor as a guide but also the emphasis students place on feedback for clinical success or failure. The topic of feedback and clinical evaluation is addressed in depth in Chapter 26.

CLINICAL ACTIVITIES AND PROBLEM SOLVING

The instructor who promotes problem-solving abilities in students fashions clinical activities to meet this goal. Discovery learning is one way in which student autonomy and problem solving can be enhanced. Students can have experiences where they can realize, or discover, patient responses to certain aspects of care, or how structuring an activity differently is more time saving. These discoveries boost self esteem when students see what they have learned on their own, or that they have the ability to resolve certain problematic situations. Discovery learning also has been found to increase student motivation, interest, and retention of learned material (DeYoung, 1990). The instructor then is rewarded by seeing growth take place in the students.

Another approach to promoting problem-solving abilities is by placing emphasis on the clinical, or patient, problem, rather than on the clinical setting. Student assignments that take place in familiar, repetitive settings enable students to deal with patients *in that setting*. In addition to learning how to deal with clinical problems, students in new or unexpected settings also experience professional socialization through role discontinuity. In making the transition from instructor-directed, structured, familiar assignments to empowering, unstructured, undefined patient problems, students experience new ways of defining their own roles and responsibilities as practitioners.

STUDENT-CENTERED LEARNING

The strategy of reciprocal learning not only meets clinical learning needs but promotes collegiality as well. Reciprocal learning usually takes the form of peer teaching, or student-to-student instruction. This learning informally occurs within most clinical groups and can become more purposeful and goal directed through instructor planning. By pairing students for specific learning activities, the student learner gains information, experience, and insight in new ways. Learners receive individualized, empathetic instruction and may feel more relaxed with a peer than with a faculty teacher. The student teacher also learns about instruction, helping, and working with others. Peer support is useful for building student self confidence, providing a mechanism for feedback from someone other than the clinical instructor, and as a means to initiate the students in to the collaborative role (Brooks & Morarity, 2009).

From the viewpoint of the instructor, student-centered learning increases student accountability and independence. This is especially beneficial for students who are closer to graduation and need to break ties to the instructor. As students increase independence, the instructor can receive satisfaction from this new level of student performance. Students appreciate the trust that the instructor conveys to them. In fact, the promotion of cooperative learning, active involvement, and the recognition of diverse ways of learning are attributes that students rank highly in effective teachers (Wolf, Bender, Beitz, Weiland, & Vito, 2004).

FACULTY DEVELOPMENT

The powerful influence of the instructor as a person should not be overlooked. Development of an effective clinical instructor and the evolution of a meaningful, positive clinical learning experience are based on insight, planning, and implementation by the faculty member. Therefore, individual teachers need to cultivate an appropriate self image as a teacher. In addition, the clinical instructor should indulge in periodic self reflection: Is my own clinical competence being maintained? Are my own views on nursing and the teaching–learning process congruent with student perspectives and needs? Should teaching strategies, types of assignments, or communication skills be revised? Just as encouraging self reflection in students guides them in viewing their clinical experience as a success (Hanson & Stenvig, 2008), self reflection by the instructor will also bring about synthesis of the experience and evaluation of successes and failures. The effective faculty member then may need to reshape his or her own teaching perspectives to better blend with those perspectives held by the clinical students.

CONCLUSION

The philosophical approach to teaching is the foundation by which the instructor operationalizes his or her own practical knowledge. The responsibilities for the instructor are great, calling for clinical expertise, role modeling, and understanding of teaching and learning principles for a variety of students, settings, and clinical experiences.

Carlson-Catalano (1992) pointed out that much of the instruction that takes place is related to how the instructor has internalized professional values and developed a self image as a practitioner and role model. The instructor who wishes to promote empowerment in students must see himself or herself as empowered to do so. Only then can needed socialization and empowerment take place. The empowered instructor is able to visualize the potential learning opportunities in the clinical environment (Chally, 1992). The nature of clinical practice has been redefined, as so must the nature of clinical learning experiences.

Effective clinical instruction emerges from conscious efforts by the instructor. These efforts should be based on background knowledge, strongly formed values, and a well-defined self image as a nurse–teacher. Applying these personal resources enables the teacher to bring about effective clinical instruction. Formal and personal learning outcomes then are achieved.

REFERENCES

Adams, V. (2002). Consistent clinical assignment for nursing students compared to multiple placements. *Journal of Nursing Education, 41*, 80–82.

Augustine, C. J. (1992). Dimensions of feedback in clinical nursing education. *Dissertation Abstracts International*, 54(2A), 433.

Brooks N., & Moriarty, A. (2009). Implementation of a peer-support system in the clinical setting. *Nursing Standard, 23*(27), 35–39.

Carlson-Catalano, J. (1992). Empowering nurses for professional practice. *Nursing Outlook, 40*, 139–142.

Chally, P. S. (1992). Empowerment through teaching. *Journal of Nursing Education, 31*, 117–120.

Clark, M. C., Owen, S. V., & Tholcken, M. A. (2004). Measuring student perceptions of clinical competence. *Journal of Nursing Education, 43*, 548–554.

Cook, L. J. (2005). Inviting teaching behaviors of clinical faculty and nursing students' anxiety. *Journal of Nursing Education, 44*, 156–161.

DeYoung, S. (1990). *Teaching Nursing*, (pp. 26–27). Redwood City, CA: Addison-Wesley.

Etheridge, S. A. (2007). Learning how to think like a nurse: Stories from new nursing graduates. *Journal of Continuing Education in Nursing, 38*(1), 24–30.

Hanson, K. J., & Stenvig, T. E. (2008). The good clinical nursing educator and the baccalaureate nursing clinical experience: Attributes and praxis. *Journal of Nursing Education, 47*, 38–42.

Little, M. A., & Miliken, P. J. (2007). Practicing what we preach: Balancing teaching and clinical practice competencies. *International Journal of Nursing Education Scholarship, 4*, 1–14.

Manthey, M. (1992). Empowerment for teachers and students. *Nurse Educator, 17*, 6–7.

Northington, L., Wilkerson, R., Fisher, W., & Schenk, L. (2005). Enhancing nursing students' clinical experience using aesthetics. *Journal of Professional Nursing, 21*, 66–71.

Paterson, B. (1994). The view from within: Perspectives of clinical teaching. *International Journal of Nursing Studies, 31*, 349–360.

Wolf, Z. R., Bender, P. J., Beitz, J. M., Wieland, D. M., & Vito, K. O. (2004). Strengths and weaknesses of faculty teaching performance reported by undergraduate and graduate nursing students: A descriptive study. *Journal of Professional Nursing, 20*, 118–128.

Yaakobi, D., & Sharan, S. (1985). Teacher beliefs and practices: The discipline carries the message. *Journal of Education for Teaching, 11*, 187–199.

CHAPTER 26

Crafting the Clinical Experience: A Toolbox for Healthcare Professionals

Stephanie S. Allen and Lyn S. Prater

Healthcare education historically has been based on the expert–novice or mentor–protégé model. Optimal learning outcomes are not achieved when the teacher is just an authority figure and content expert. Rather, optimal clinical learning is best achieved when the teacher is a true educator. In order for expert clinicians to become effective teachers in their professional programs, an additional knowledge base and skill set is required. The clinical experience is a time in which the student applies theory to practice. It is the role of the clinical instructor to facilitate this application and evaluate learner outcomes. Establishing and maintaining professional boundaries with students, remaining current in practice, teaching and implementing evidence-based practice is both an art and a science. It is the purpose of this chapter to provide a framework for how to implement and use best teaching practices in the areas of clinical teaching and evaluation.

ROLE PREPARATION

Role preparation for health professions faculty typically came from graduates completing educational preparation, clinical experience, and having an interest in teaching. So although the educator may be an expert clinician in his or her field, as a novice educator may not have the foundation necessary to be a successful clinical teacher (Bartels, 2007). It is thus incumbent on the educational institution to provide the necessary mentoring for new faculty so that not only the scholarship of discovery can be implemented, but the scholarship of integration, application, and teaching can be developed. These roles identified by Boyer (1990) provide a pathway for faculty to develop and flourish in the structure of higher education.

The scholarship of ***discovery***, as noted by Boyer (1990), is the need for scientific inquiry into the discipline of healthcare professions, and thus the faculty research role is imperative in higher education. "The degree to which faculty engage in the role of scholarly discovery, as well as the approach taken to actualize the role, will depend on the rewards and structure of the academic environment" (Bartels, 2007, p. 156). The scholarship of ***integration*** is that part of the faculty role where meaning, perspective, making connections across disciplines, and placing the specialties in a broader context can be explored and applied. Bartels (2007) reminds us that "nursing faculty must be prepared to assume this role of interdisciplinary integration, finding ways to connect not only with evidence discovered within the profession, but also with evidence generated across professions" (p. 156). The scholarship of ***teaching*** is the heart of health professions education, but is often not a part of the basic education for entry into practice. For example, Beitz and Wieland (2005), when analyzing teaching effectiveness of nursing faculty, determined that 70% said their educational program did not prepare them to teach clinically. This is unfortunate because formal preparation for the educator role has been best addressed in nursing and less so in other professional fields.

The scholarship of ***application*** is relevant in the healthcare professions because it calls for the educator to maintain competency in the clinical field. Remaining current in practice heightens the ability for the educator to blend academic and practice roles. The scholarship of application "requires that faculty come to their academic role with an advanced understanding and preparation in the profession and applies clinical experience in their area of practice expertise (Bartels, 2007, p. 156). Teaching will likely be the primary activity of most nursing faculty, and it is imperative that this role be articulated and developed in new faculty. Clinical teaching is especially challenging as the situation/clinical sites can vary greatly from institution to institution and faculty must help students assimilate into their role of caregiver in an increasingly more acute setting. Ongoing changes in technology along with a generation of students who must learn to conform to an intense and highly standardized system for healthcare delivery make the clinical teaching event both challenging and rewarding. Clear objectives, professional boundaries, and collegial relationships with healthcare staff are all important components for clinical faculty to realize a successful clinical experience for students. This area of scholarship is especially pertinent for nursing faculty because nursing is an applied practice. The scholarship of application is invaluable as faculty prepares and guides their students for the practice arena of the future.

In addition to incorporating Boyer's model into a personal teaching style, the clinical educator must be aware of and able to implement effective clinical teaching behaviors. Kelly's (2007) case report related to physical therapy education described five exemplary clinical instructor teaching strategies: (1) creating and maintaining an open, collegial relationship; (2) adapting the experience to the student; (3) facilitating clinical reasoning; (4) making time for the student; and (5) receiving environmental support. For instance, once the collegial relationship has been established, the ability to provide direct feedback, both positive and corrective, is achieved. The open collegial relationship is maintained by providing clear and consistent expectations. Adapting the experience to the student requires student participation in determining learning goals and needs. Kelly (2007) refers to this as "meeting them where they are" (p. 65). An important category of facilitating clinical reasoning is utilizing "thinking out loud" with the student. The benefit of receiving environmental support results in feeling valued. According to Beitz and Wieland (2005), interpersonal relationships between the instructor and the student that were respectful and caring resulted in supportive and approachable communication. Also, students viewed faculty as positive role models if they were currently working in their specialty.

In conclusion, role preparation is critical to the success of the healthcare professional as an educator. Utilizing resources available and garnering support from seasoned faculty will make the implementation of the educator role easier. Bartels (2007) reminds us "critically important to supporting and retaining faculty in their multiple roles is the creation of an environment that allows for flexibility, encourages creativity and sustains faculty energy" (p. 157).

IMPLEMENTING THE ROLE

Clinical Orientation: How to Get Off to a Good Start

It is the responsibility of the clinical instructor to complete all required agency orientation and be knowledgeable of agency policies and procedures. Good rapport will be maintained between the instructor and clinical site when students and faculty follow agency guidelines. This shows both respect for the agency and allows an opportunity for professional development in the students. Instructors cannot just "drop off" students on a unit or at a clinical agency and expect the staff to provide all of the teaching. Staff nurses appreciate an instructor who is present, acts as a team member, has experience, and is relaxed and organized. According to Matsumura, Callister, Palmer, Cox, and Larson (2004), instructors who dropped their students off and expected staff to do the teaching were resented by the staff nurses, which ultimately affected the quality of the student experience. A component of orientation will be identifying for the staff what their responsibilities will be. Frequently, the clinical staff as agency employees are called on to participate in the educational experience. Clinical staff are familiar with their role as a patient care provider and teaching patients and family members but may not have been provided any formal instruction on the teaching or precepting of students. Consequently, clinical instructors need to communicate clear expectations for each clinical experience. Unless the educational institution provides a structured orientation for this process, the clinical instructor will be responsible for this process as well. If this formal process does not take place, each student's clinical experience will differ due to the varying quality of instruction provided by the instructor/preceptor within each clinical setting. Establishing rapport with the clinical management and staff takes time and dedication. Refer to Appendix 26-1, which is a typical schedule for new faculty orientation. Please see Appendix 26-1 on the Web site that accompanies this book.

Crafting the Clinical Experience

Once faculty have oriented themselves and the students to the clinical site, it is critical to craft the clinical experience so that the assignments match the course objectives and are congruent with the theoretical concepts. For example, the instructor should make patient assignments that have fluid and electrolyte deficits during the time frame the students are learning about this concept in their theory course. Additional practice with calculating maintenance fluids and analyzing lab values will help the students make the connections between theory and practice. More background on the selection of clinical activities can be found in Chapter 21.

In clinical settings in which the patient care activity is very specific, the clinical instructor will want to use an assignment sheet. This communication tool provides an easy reference for the unit staff to know what students will be caring for which patients. Because this assignment sheet contains sensitive information, it must be posted away from public access. Outlining clearly on the assignment sheet which student is doing what/when helps the staff know what experiences to save for a student and which ones they themselves are responsible for. At the beginning of the clinical day, the instructor will review the student's preclinical preparation and determine whether there are any gaps or inconsistencies for care. The student will receive a report from the primary care giver assigned to his or her patient and assume care within the context of the agency guidelines and clinical assignment. In order for the clinical instructor to organize a number of students within a clinical setting, he or she must negotiate and communicate the student's responsibility. As an example, even if a student has read the procedure for lab blood draws, he or she will benefit from watching it done at least once before attempting it on the patient.

It is imperative to follow agency policies regarding the procedures in which students may and may not participate. Please refer to Appendix 26-2, which is an example of an agency schedule for student orientation. Please see Appendix 26-2 on the Web site that accompanies this book. Credibility as a clinical instructor may be initially tested by staff members as well as by students. This is not unusual and should not threaten the instructor's sense of clinical competence. Once trust is established, the clinical instructor will find that this testing dissipates. Purposeful assignments should, in addition, be congruent with the evaluation tool. By keeping detailed anecdotal notes and documenting the student's progress, or lack thereof, in meeting the course objectives makes the final evaluation process less subjective. Providing students with specific positive examples as well as examples of omission or errors helps guide them in reflective practice. An important question that is worth discussing is "what would you do differently next time?"

Clinical rounds provide an opportunity to observe students interacting with their patients and family members. Introductions by either the student or instructor are important to facilitate ongoing rapport. Rounds also provide the opportunity for spontaneous learning by using the teachable moment. An astute clinical instructor will use these teachable moments as she or he encounters the student engaged in the delivery of real-time care. Guidance and/or gentle prompting regarding additional resources for the teaching–learning event can be given and role modeling by the instructor can be provided at the bedside. According to Close and Castledine (2005), "it is felt that the rounds are particularly useful in developing clinical practice, evidence-based care, understanding patients and the conditions they experience, while linking theory and practice" (p. 982).

Ongoing care and teachable moments are excellent occasions for challenging students to grow by using directed questioning. An example of this type of questioning would be when the instructor asks the student to discuss the rationale for a medication's use as a treatment modality, which differs from the drug's primary action (e.g., nifedipine in the preterm labor patient). According to Hoffman (2008), clinical instructors should be utilizing higher level questions to facilitate critical thinking skills in the clinical setting. "These questions require the student to correlate clinical findings with textbook descriptions and apply this content to the care of their patients" (p. 234). It is important to avoid spoon feeding the answers. Make the students look up policies and procedures and medical terminology. This provides an opportunity to utilize resources and to become self directed in their pursuit of knowledge in the profession. One of the goals of the clinical teaching experience is to provide the students with an experience that keeps them engaged and places them in the role of a total patient care provider. By eliciting feedback from both the student and the staff members, the instructor will be able to determine whether the assignment is too challenging or is not keeping the student engaged and will be able to adjust accordingly. Developing self awareness in students is a professional priority. It is important to share observations made by the staff and instructor that are promoting a positive professional demeanor as well as those that detract from a student's professional demeanor. When a student is overly focused on programming an intravenous pump and not making eye contact with a family member when they are asking a serious question, the establishment of a therapeutic relationship is affected. Actions by students such as washing hands in the patient's room and then running those hands through their hair before putting on sterile gloves for a central line dressing change may diminish trust when observed by patients and family members. At these times the instructor must redirect the student to ensure safety using a professional approach.

In addition to clinical rounds, pre- and postclinical conferences provide a rich opportunity for clarification and teaching. There are advantages and disadvantages to planned conference activities. An instructor should have a planned conference activity, but should be able to be flexible and spontaneous when the need arises. Here are some examples to use in postconference:

Example 1: Taking action based on analysis of patient information

This exercise guides the students in cultivating analytical abilities and assuming accountability for their actions.

Step 1: Each student identifies abnormal assessment findings

Step 2: Each student analyzes what nursing implications those abnormals have for patient care

Step 3: Each student shares with the group how patient care was altered/revised and the team process for implementation

Example 2: Applying evidence-based research to practice

This activity prompts the student to examine current evidence regarding practices in which they have participated in during the clinical day. Exercises such as this will enable the practicing professional to remain current.

Examples of these activities include using current clinical situations from the day's experiences and pulling the current theory content threads out to interact with away from the bedside. This provides a nonthreatening atmosphere that is not time dependent and allows for exploration in greater detail. For example, the week that fluid and electrolyte content is covered in class the instructor could have students complete the following activities.

Step 1: Each student is assigned to look up abnormal lab values for every patient cared for

Step 2: The instructor prints the lab data and removes all patient identifiers

Step 3: The instructor lays the lab data out on the table and asks each student to identify which is their patient's labs

Step 4: Provide 10 minutes for research before asking the students to report back to the group the necessary implications the abnormals have for the care they provided

It will be instantly clear who included lab analysis into their preclinical preparation.

Another example for postconference learning and discussion would be incorporating evidence-based practice into their care for the day.

Step 1: The students are instructed to bring an evidence-based research article that is related to some aspect of their patient's care

Step 2: Students present the research findings along with an example of how they incorporated the findings into their patient care with the clinical group

Another example is peer-to-peer feedback. Guiding students through the process of critiquing each other's documentation emphasizes the significance of attention to detail and provides a model for future communication with professional peers. The ability to give and receive peer-to-peer feedback as students is a rehearsal for future practice as students pepare for peer interaction within their practice.

Lundberg (2008) states,

> Relating clinical experiences to others helps students develop realistic expectations of their clinical skills and allows for immediate feedback from others, thus reinforcing their perceived abilities to function as a nurse. Shared stories are another form of peer modeling where other students can witness how their peers work through difficult situations (p. 88).

Example 3: Peer-to-peer feedback

Step 1: Have students sit next to one another in pairs

Step 2: Provide each with a tool to analyze the written documentation they have completed during that clinical experience

Step 3: The students hand over their documentation to their peer, the peer evaluates it using the standardized tool

Step 4: Once the evaluation is complete, the peers share their findings and make suggestions for additions and corrections to the documentation

Closure at the end of the clinical experience is an important last step for both student and clinical instructor. One last question might be "what lessons did you learn that you would take up in your future practice?" (McAllister, Tower, & Walker, 2007, p. 311). This question prompts the students to reflect on their experiences and charges them to take a more autonomous role in their professional practice.

Constructive feedback regarding the student's performance is an important part of the clinical educator's role. Fink (2003) provides an acronym, FIDeLity, to guide educators in providing this much needed feedback: *f*requent, *i*mmediate, *d*iscriminating (based on criteria and standards), and done *l*ovingly (or supportively).

Frequent

Fink (2003) describes the widespread practice of giving feedback only in the form of midterm and a final grade as being insufficient. No matter how often feedback is provided, the students often request more. It is worth the instructor's time to elicit whether the feedback provided is meeting the students' needs or whether they require additional information.

Immediate

Utilizing a broad, open-ended question when exiting the patient's room such as "how do you think that went?" will allow the student the opportunity to self reflect on their clinical performance. If the instructor has observed a break in sterile technique and the student did not self correct, the instructor has to intervene at the bedside. If the student required excessive prompting during a procedure, the instructor needs to clearly articulate that the student is not performing up to speed. At this point, it is the instructor's responsibility to design remediation activities away from the clinical site to provide additional opportunities for instruction and practice.

The problem with delayed feedback is that students cease to care about why their answer or activity was good or not. When the feedback comes a week or more after the learning activity, they just want to know, "Wha'd I get?" (Fink, 2003, p. 96).

Discriminating

Discriminating and distinguishing features of good and poor performance in ways that are clear to students is imperative. One way to accomplish this is in postconference with the instructor asking the question of the group "What was the best part of your day and what was the worst part of your day?" This will give the students the opportunity to hear about their peer's issues and will provide a milieu for open sharing and debriefing. It is not uncommon for some experiences among students to be similar and this provides opportunity for peer-to-peer feedback and support. This situation may result in confidence building in the growing professional. Anderson and Kiger (2008) points out "[student] experiences of managing in different situations served to enhance their belief in themselves and their abilities" (p. 445). In addition, when giving feedback regarding written assignments, the instructor must provide detail as described by Fink (2003): "Knowing that their organization was good but their use of evidence and reasoning was poor provides more discriminating and useful feedback than either 'OK' or a 'B'" (p. 96).

Lovingly

Lovingly delivered feedback, with empathy and personal understanding, is an essential component. Providing feedback by acknowledging the students' feelings in their attempts to be successful communicates the instructor's personal empathy and understanding. There are times when the consequences of the student's unsafe actions will result in the removal from the clinical setting. This may be one of the most challenging aspects of the clinical instructor role. An example of this type of feedback provided by the instructor to the student is "I know you are trying, but you performed three unsafe actions in three hours and I am dismissing you from clinical for the day." As the instructor of record provides feedback to clinical students, they may wish to integrate the FIDeLity acronym as a communication tool.

Conducting the Clinical Day

Every instructor should develop a purposeful, organized method for conducting the clinical day. Typically, the structure is based on a plan for both instructor and students. Patient care assignments for each clinical experience must be tied to course objectives. The instructor will map his or her day by using a master jot sheet. This tool, which includes all aspects of patient care, helps the clinical instructor track and plan times for specific interventions such as medications and treatments. To ensure that interventions and medications are administered in a timely manner, restrictions will need to be placed on the number of students participating in direct patient care activities at one time. For instance, during a 12-hour shift, all eight students will have a medication administration experience; however, four students will give medications at the beginning of the shift while the remaining students will administer medications during the last 6 hours of the shift. During this process it is the responsibility of the student to keep the instructor and staff informed of the outcome of the interventions implemented. Documentation is an important aspect of the learning activity and may be regulated by the clinical institution. Regardless of whether the student or the staff actually document in the medical record, it is the responsibility of the student to provide accurate and timely patient status reports. An additional responsibility of the instructor is to keep accurate anecdotal notes during the clinical day for use in formative and summative evaluations.

Anecdotal notes are an important tool for the clinical educator because they can be used to evaluate the student's progress and are a critical component in the documentation process of formative and summative evaluation. A word of caution regarding written notes was described by Mintie Indar-Maraj (2007): "teachers must carefully examine their value systems, philosophies and beliefs and not allow these to influence their evaluation of students" (p. 8). Record keeping of clinical student behaviors over time are captured in the form of instructor generated anecdotal notes. Instructors may wish to develop a tool to be used during each clinical experience that is directly related to the institution's formal clinical evaluation tool. Please refer to Appendices 26-3 and 26-4, which are formats for anecdotal notes. Please see Appendices 26-3 and 26-4 on the Web site that accompanies this book.

STUDENT ISSUES

A hallmark of a good clinical educator is the knowledge of the student's background and learning needs (Hanson & Stenvig, 2008). Please refer to Chapter 5 for further information regarding emerging workforce generation characteristics. In addition, instructional strategies need to be tailored to the cognitive style of the student. This requires the educator to be flexible and adapt his or her teaching style to the needs of each student in the clinical setting (Noble, Miller, & Heckman, 2008). Please refer to Chapter 1 for more information regarding cognitive styles.

Hopkins (2008) found that early identification of at-risk nursing students is related to success and retention in their academic program. This early identification begins with the admissions process where academic and nonacademic predictors can be utilized for student selection. Early intervention is recommended with students who are not doing well in clinical to improve their performance (Stinson, 2009). It is prudent to have a clinical faculty member serve on the admissions committee as the admission criteria can make or break the clinical experience for students. "Admission policies can either promote success or facilitate failure in a baccalaureate nursing program" (Newton, Smith, & Moore, 2007, p. 440).

Once the program identifies which predictors of success are valid, the next step is to develop a model of student support. Academic institutions may have this additional support in the form of a success center or additional student services.

At times, the clinical instructor may be called on to manage a challenging student situation. The purpose of this section is to address some issues which may challenge the clinical instructor. For this reason, setting and enforcing boundaries is a key element in establishing the instructor–student relationship. By defining and maintaining clear boundaries, the instructor is role-modeling behavior that will be expected in future practice. Setting emotional boundaries with the student will facilitate the educator's role in managing the clinical experience. Maintaining this professional boundary prevents the clinical instructor from usurping his or her power and getting off track with the student. To maintain this balance will require focus, vigilance, and self awareness.

Unprofessional Behavior

Another challenging student situation involves unprofessional behavior on the part of the student. This may be something that the clinical instructor observes while it is occurring or it may be reported by someone else. These could range from a minor infraction such as nontherapeutic communication to a major issue, such as a HIPAA violation. "Students should be engaged early-on in the significance of professional accountability for security and confidentially related to information technology" (Day & Smith, 2007, p. 141). It is within the instructor's role to enforce compliance with professional issues such as tardiness, absence, and dress codes. Consistency among faculty related to enforcing policies such as these provides the student with a standardized approach and allows for integration of these professional behaviors over time. Infractions involving unprofessional behavior must be dealt with immediately and the student must be confronted with the issue and given the opportunity to problem solve future prevention strategies. This is an appropriate time to explore with the student the question of "what would you do differently next time?" Many evaluation tools include professional behavior as a grading criterion, and any infraction may cause the lowering of the final clinical grade.

Incivility

Incivility is another form of unprofessional behavior. Entry into professional practice requires individuals to conduct themselves with a professional demeanor. The instructor must role model these professional behaviors at all times. Defining clear guidelines and setting boundaries should begin on the first day of the clinical experience as this will set the tone for the entire instructor–student interaction. Regardless of the instructor's clear expectations for professional behavior, there may be a student who is unable to conform. Uncivil acts such as challenges to faculty knowledge or credibility, general taunts or disrespect to faculty or other students, inappropriate emails, telephone conversations, vulgarity, harassing comments, and threats of physical harm are issues that require addressing and reporting through appropriate institutional channels. If the clinical instructor's interventions with the student are unsatisfactory, seeking the guidance of a more seasoned faculty is a prudent strategy. One should never feel as though they are faced with decisions in isolation. According to Clark and Springer (2007), "evidence suggests that incivility on American college campuses, ranging from insulting remarks and verbal abuse to violence, is a serious and growing concern" (p. 7). The effect of uncivil behavior on faculty members may affect productivity, self esteem, loss of confidence in their teaching abilities, and overall job dissatisfaction, which may result in the instructor leaving the teaching profession (Luparell, 2007b). Uncivil encounters disrupt the teaching–learning environment; therefore, it is incumbent on clinical faculty members to help students learn to cope with conflict in healthy and constructive ways.

Academic Dishonesty and Unethical Behavior (Honor Code)

Most institutions have an honor code policy. It is the responsibility of the clinical instructor to be familiar and comply with the policy as well as to report violations in a timely manner. Baxter and Boblin (2007) found in their study that students may view unethical clinical behaviors differently from unethical classroom behaviors. Altering charts or failing to report a mistake may result in patients experiencing negative outcomes. At times these aberrant behaviors may be a symptom of a more serious problem, such as chemical dependence, that may contribute to unsafe patient care. Reporting guidelines and testing of students for chemical usage may be covered by both agency and educational institution policies. For healthcare professionals, it is crucial that this moral development be examined for entry-level practice. "As nurse educators, we have the responsibility to ensure that we are preparing competent, autonomous, ethical practitioners who can provide quality nursing care" (Baxter & Boblin, 2007, p. 26).

Safety

Safety in the clinical setting is imperative and receives unprecedented attention on several fronts. Because of the ethical imperative of first do no harm, the integration of quality and safety content into the clinical curriculum is paramount. Safety issues related to patient care center around near misses and adverse events and require healthcare professionals to comply with a code of ethics. Reporting, investigating causal systems failures, and revealing the primary error to the physician and possibly the patient is a primary role of the healthcare professional (Lachman, 2007). It is the instructor's responsibility to assess each student's preparation for delivering safe patient care prior to the beginning of the clinical experience. If the instructor determines that the student is inadequately prepared, he or she may choose to dismiss the student from the clinical setting in order to prevent a breach in patient safety. A breach in patient safety is commonly a critical point for failure in the clinical course. An example of this breach of safety is a student coming inadequately prepared for medication administration. As Harding and Petrick (2008) remind us, "the practice of purposefully incorporating medication safety knowledge throughout connected theory and practice courses . . ." is beneficial to student learning (p. 47). Medication administration is an opportunity for the student to incorporate theory into practice. It is incumbent on the clinical instructor to document and provide feedback to the student who has had a breach of patient safety. The clinical instructor must also follow agency guidelines for reporting such incidents. In conclusion, "educators should monitor student errors and incidents over time (i.e., quality assurance determinants) to identify how education structures and processes are contributing to potential and actual student error" (Gregory, Guse, Dick, & Russell, 2007, p. 81).

EVALUATION OF CLINICAL LEARNING

The purpose of evaluation is to help the student grow in his or her profession. Traditionally, evaluation is looked upon as a negative or punitive act and can be viewed as adversarial between the student and faculty member. This, however, is not the case because evaluation is an opportunity for growth. The evaluation of clinical performance should not be subjective because it is based on a standardized evaluation tool and the instructor must collect data sufficient to base the evaluation against the behavioral outcomes over time.

Although the instructor has given oral and written feedback during the clinical day, a formal midterm and final evaluation of the student's performance is necessary to provide formative feedback and serves as a mechanism for grade assignment. The purpose of formative evaluation is to provide specific and detailed feedback to the student and observe his/her ability or inability to integrate this feedback into his/her clinical practice. One of the goals of this formative evaluation is to allow the students the opportunity to internalize the process of self reflection and self discovery, in his/her personal practice. It is the hope that this ongoing communication between the student and instructor will promote insight into the strength and weaknesses of the student's professional practice. Susan Luparell (2007a) makes a good point when she encourages clinical instructors to "say what you mean and mean what you say" (p. 105).

Luparell states,

> I have come to realize that, although there is some good to be found in the sandwich approach to providing feedback, this may contribute to the meat of the message being lost. When the student does not hear the true message, he or she cannot make the necessary adjustments for success. It is not caring to inhibit student progression toward the goals. I now realize that sugar coating the message is not equivalent to caring for my students. Rather, caring is demonstrated when a respectful tone within the context of trust is used to deliver a sometimes tough message. (p. 105)

Sample formats for midterm evaluations as shown in Appendices 26-5 and 26-6 can be utilized as a means to provide specific formative feedback on clinical performance. Appendix 26-5 is a narrative response tool where the instructor provides areas of strengths and weaknesses to this point in the clinical experience. Please see Appendix 26-5 on the Web site that accompanies this book. Appendix 26-6 is an example of a tool that describes specific behavioral outcomes that the student must display in order to be a safe and effective care provider. Please see Appendix 26-2 on the Web site that accompanies this book. Often students ask, once they see a letter grade, "What can I do to improve my grade?" By providing a list of outcome behaviors the student has the opportunity to incorporate them into his or her practice. "Be specific" was a common phrase used by a colleague during midterm evaluations. She often wrote "increase specificity" on assignments and the students would question what that meant. By providing specific examples the instructor helped students understand what to do differently before repeating the assignment.

Anecdotal notes are an important means by which the clinical instructor can provide specific details regarding the student's performance that will require remediation as well as documenting areas of superior performance. Although the tools are standardized, it is important for the clinical instructor to individualize his or her evaluation comments.

The final clinical evaluation allows the instructor to analyze and deliver to the student the progress of clinical performance over time. This summative event prepares the student to move forward in their program with guided input regarding their current state of practice. Edgecombe and Bowden (2009) remind us that "learning outcomes were expressed as both intrinsic and extrinsic" (p. 97). The summary evaluation will examine the student's ability to meet the course objectives that were imposed by the program curriculum. The intrinsic objectives of each student's personal need to learn upon exposure to nursing practice in the clinical environment should also be documented and discussed. To prepare for final clinical evaluations, an appointment time frame should be scheduled that is agreed on by both faculty member and student. The meeting place should provide privacy because the evaluation content and conversation should remain confidential. When the student arrives for the evaluation, a copy of the completed tool is provided for the student to read and sign, following any discussion of reflective practice, clarification of evaluative comments, and an opportunity for self appraisal on the part of the student. When meeting with students to give midterm and final evaluations, it is a good practice to have two clinically based faculty members present. This could be two faculty members who have simultaneously taught the student during the evaluation period or two faculty members from the same content domain. This practice validates for the student the significance of the evaluation comments as well as providing for physical and emotional safety for the primary instructor in situations in which the evaluation becomes emotionally charged. Learning contracts or clinical warning forms are documents used by clinical instructors to delineate unsafe clinical practice or a breach in professional practice. These contracts become a part of the evaluation process and typically include a remediation plan. The purpose of these learning contracts is to provide additional structure and clear communication as to what the student must do to be successful in the clinical course. Orientation for clinical faculty assists in their providing effective clinical instruction. "For example, use of a clinical warning form to document inadequate, unsafe student performance may help with optimal formative and summative evaluation of a struggling student in that it creates a paper trail for legal purposes and an educational wake-up call for the student" (Beitz & Wieland, 2005, p. 44).

As Barrington and Street (2009) found in their research regarding learner contracts, these tools improved learner–faculty communication and reflection on learning. For a sample document regarding safety in the clinical setting, refer to Appendix 26-7. For an example of a breach in professional behavior, refer to Appendix 26-8. Please see Appendices 26-7 and 26-8 on the Web site that accompanies this book. Writing and delivering the learning contract to the student who is not performing at an acceptable level should not be a contentious process, but should be communicated in a clear and compassionate manner. The clinical instructor cannot ensure success solely through the use of the contract but is responsible for designing the plan for success. The learning contract outlines the roles both instructor and student play in any additional remediation sessions that may take place outside the clinical setting. Part of the process for implementing the learning contract is to provide the student with feedback during each clinical experience. This may be referred to as meeting or not meeting the terms of the contract. If safety issues are not remediated, the student may not be allowed to continue in the clinical setting, which may result in a course failure.

Nurse educators need to be fully present with students who are at risk of failing clinical courses in ways that foster personal and professional growth rather than distance themselves. This is not easy work. As educators we are inclined to disconnect from students to protect our own vulnerability, particular when performance issues arise (McGregor, 2007, p. 509).

Ultimately, the student must display the outcome behaviors necessary for success in the course that are directly related to the standardized final clinical evaluation tool. The learning contract is signed by both clinical instructor and student and a copy is placed in the student's academic file.

Clinical Failure

Clinical failure is the lack of clinical competence and the inability of the student to meet the course objectives. Issues such as unsafe clinical practice, unprofessional behaviors, poor attendance, inability to implement appropriate interventions, falsification of patient records, omissions in documentation, and nontherapeutic communication and errors in medication administration are all examples of critical elements of practice that may result in clinical failure. "Not all nursing students can be successful, yet when failure is the outcome, students' dignity, self-worth and future possibilities must be preserved" (McGregor, 2007, p. 504). Some clinical failures indicate that the student needs more exposure or time in the clinical setting to be successful.

There are implications for clinical instructors as well as their students when clinical failures occur. From the student's perspective, the clinical failure may result in a wake-up call resulting in a revised method of preparation for and implementation of clinical. A second outcome for the student may be the revelation that the health profession chosen is not for them, at which time they may choose to revise their degree plan. At other times, the student may become angry and blame his or her failure on the clinical instructor. This reaction of the student will have implications for the clinical instructor as he or she may become a part of an appeals process. Rutkowski (2007) reminds us that assessing nursing students' competence during practice placements may result in a clinical failure. Safeguarding the public is the goal of safe clinical practice. Each healthcare professional's code of conduct must be the standard against which competency is measured. McGregor (2007) summarizes the picture of clinical failure by stating:

> In the face of a clinical failure, what really matters is how the student and the teacher interact. When tensions about clinical performance arise, teachers need to become partners who stand with, rather than against, vulnerable students who are struggling to become competent nurses. (p. 510)

Light at the End of the Tunnel

The outcomes of our teaching experience directly advance our chosen health-care profession. It is continually rewarding to write letters of recommendation for students as they enter the clinical practice arena and prepare for graduate school. The ebb and flow of the academic calendar can provide a predictable schedule for those who like a beginning and ending point to their work. The clinical day may be unpredictable and the generation of learners may change but clinical teaching still provides a stimulating and rewarding practice field.

REFERENCES

Anderson, E., Kiger, A. M. (2008). 'I felt like a real nurse'-Student nurses out on their own. *Nurse Education Today, 28*, 443–449.

Barrington, K., & Street, K. (2009). Learner contracts in nurse education: Interaction within the practice context. *Nurse Education and Practice, 9*, 109–118.

Bartels, J., (2007). Preparing nursing faculty for baccalaureate-level and graduate-level nursing programs: Role preparation for the academy. *Journal of Nursing Education, 46*(4), 154–158.

Baxter, P. E. & Boblin, S. L. (2007). The moral development of Baccalaureate nursing students: Understanding unethical behavior in classroom and clinical settings. *Journal of Nursing Education, 46*(1), 20–27.

Beitz, J. M., & Wieland, D. (2005). Analyzing the teaching effectiveness of clinical nursing faculty of full- and part-time generic, BSN, LPN-BSN, and RN-BSN nursing students. *Journal of Professional Nursing, 21*(1), 32–45.

Boyer, E. L. (1990). *Scholarship reconsidered: Priorities of the professoriate*. New York: The Carnegie Foundation for the Advancement of Teaching.

Clark, C., & Springer, P. J. (2007). Incivility in nursing education: A descriptive study of definitions and prevalence. *Journal of Nursing Education, 46*(1), 7–14.

Close, A., & Casteldine, G. (2005). Clinical nursing rounds, part 4: Teaching rounds for nurses. *British Journal of Nursing, 14*(18), 982–983.

Day, L., & Smith, L. (2007). Integrating quality and safety content into clinical teaching in the acute care setting. *Nursing Outlook, 55*(3), 138–143.

Edgecombe, K., & Bowden, M. (2009). The ongoing search for best practice in clinical teaching and learning: A model of nursing students' evolution to proficient novice registered nurses. *Nurse Education and Practice, 9*, 91–101.

Fink, L. (2003). *Creating significant learning experiences*. San Francisco: Jossey-Bass.

Gregory, D. M., Guse, L. W., Davidson, D. & Russell, C. K. (2007). Patient safety: Where is nursing education? *Journal of Nursing Education, 46*(2), 79–82.

Hanson, K. J., & Stenvig, T. E. (2008). The good clinical nursing educator and the baccalaureate nursing clinical experience: Attributes and praxis. *Journal of Nursing Education, 47*(1), 38–42.

Harding, L., & Petrick, T. (2008). Nursing student medication errors: A retrospective review. *Journal of Nursing Education, 47*(1), 43–47.

Hoffman, J. (2008). Teaching strategies to facilitate nursing students' critical thinking. In M. Oermann (Ed.), *Annual review of nursing education, 6* (pp. 225–236). New York: Springer Publishing Company.

Hopkins, T. H. (2008). Early identification of at-risk nursing students: A student support model. *Journal of Nursing Education, 47*(6), 254–259.

Indar-Maraj, M. (2007). Clinical evaluation of nursing students: Challenges and solutions. *MedSurg Matters, 16*(4), 6–8.

Kelly, S. P. (2007). The exemplary clinical instructor: A qualitative case study. *Journal of Physical Therapy Education, 21*(1), 63–69.

Lachman, V. (2007). Patient safety: The ethical imperative. *MEDSURG Nursing, 16*(6), 401–403.

Luparell, S. (2007). Managing difficult student situations: Lessons learned. In Oermann, M & Heinrich, K. (Eds.), *Annual review of nursing education* (pp. 101–110). New York: Springer Publishing Company.

Luparell, S. (2007). The effects of student incivility on nursing faculty. *Journal of Nursing Education, 46*(1), 15–19.

Lundberg, K. (2008). Promoting self-confidence in clinical nursing students. *Nurse Educator, 33*(2), 86–89.

Matsumura, G., Callister, S., Cox, A., & Larson, L. (2004). Staff nurse perceptions of the contributions of students to clinical agencies. *Nursing Education Perspectives, 25*(6), 297–303.

McAllister, M., Tower, M., & Walker, R. (2007). Gentle interruptions: Transformative approaches to clinical teaching. *Journal of Nursing Education, 46*(7), 304–312.

McGregor, A. (2007). Academic success, clinical failure: Struggling practices of a failing student. *Journal of Nursing Education, 46*(11), 504–511.

Newton, S., Smith, L., & Moore, G. (2007). Baccalaureate nursing program admission policies: Promoting success or facilitating failure? *Journal of Nursing Education, 46*(10), 439–511.

Noble, K. A., Miller, S. M., & Heckman, J. (2008). The cognitive style of nursing students: Educational implications for teaching and learning. *Journal of Nursing Education, 47*(6), 245–253.

Rutkowski, K. (2007). Failure to fail: Assessing nursing students' competence during practice placements. *Nursing Standard, 22*(13), 35–40.

Stinson, S. (2009). Maximizing minority students' success in clinical. *Minority Nurse, Spring*, 1–5. Retrieved June 11, 2009, from CINAHL with Full Text database.

CHAPTER 27

Nursing Process Mapping

Suzanne Sutton and Charlotte J. Koehler

INTRODUCTION

There has been a great revolution in the concept of teaching over the last 20 years. The nature of students, as well as the vast quantity of information to be learned, has changed to the point that it is impossible for the learner to successfully assimilate knowledge without changing the manner in which it is presented and learned. Students must learn basic facts and concepts, but they must also be taught to see linkages and connections between them in order to understand the complex whole (De Simone, 2007).

Concept mapping, also known as mind mapping, is a tool in which information can be presented and processed and allows the learner to see relationships and link the ideas in ways that make sense to them. Concept mapping helps to develop critical thinking skills, as the students considers the basic facts and how they are linked or affect other concepts within a complex system (Novak & Cañas, 2008).

DEFINITION AND PURPOSES

According to Novak and Cañas (2008), concept maps are visual and spatial representations of knowledge arranged in a hierarchical manner with linkages identified between the concepts using action verbs. They consist of *nodes*, which are concepts or ideas, represented by words or pictures, arranged in a general to specific manner. Between the nodes are *linkages*, which describe the relationship between the nodes. A node and its linkages are a *domain*. *Cross-linkages* are relationships between nodes in different domains (Fig. 27-1).

In practice, concept maps are used to organize facts, visualize relationships, and understand knowledge. A student or instructor clusters data in meaningful ways and uses linkages to enhance the learning experience and knowledge acquisition.

Figure 27-1 Sample concept map showing nodes, linkages, and domains.

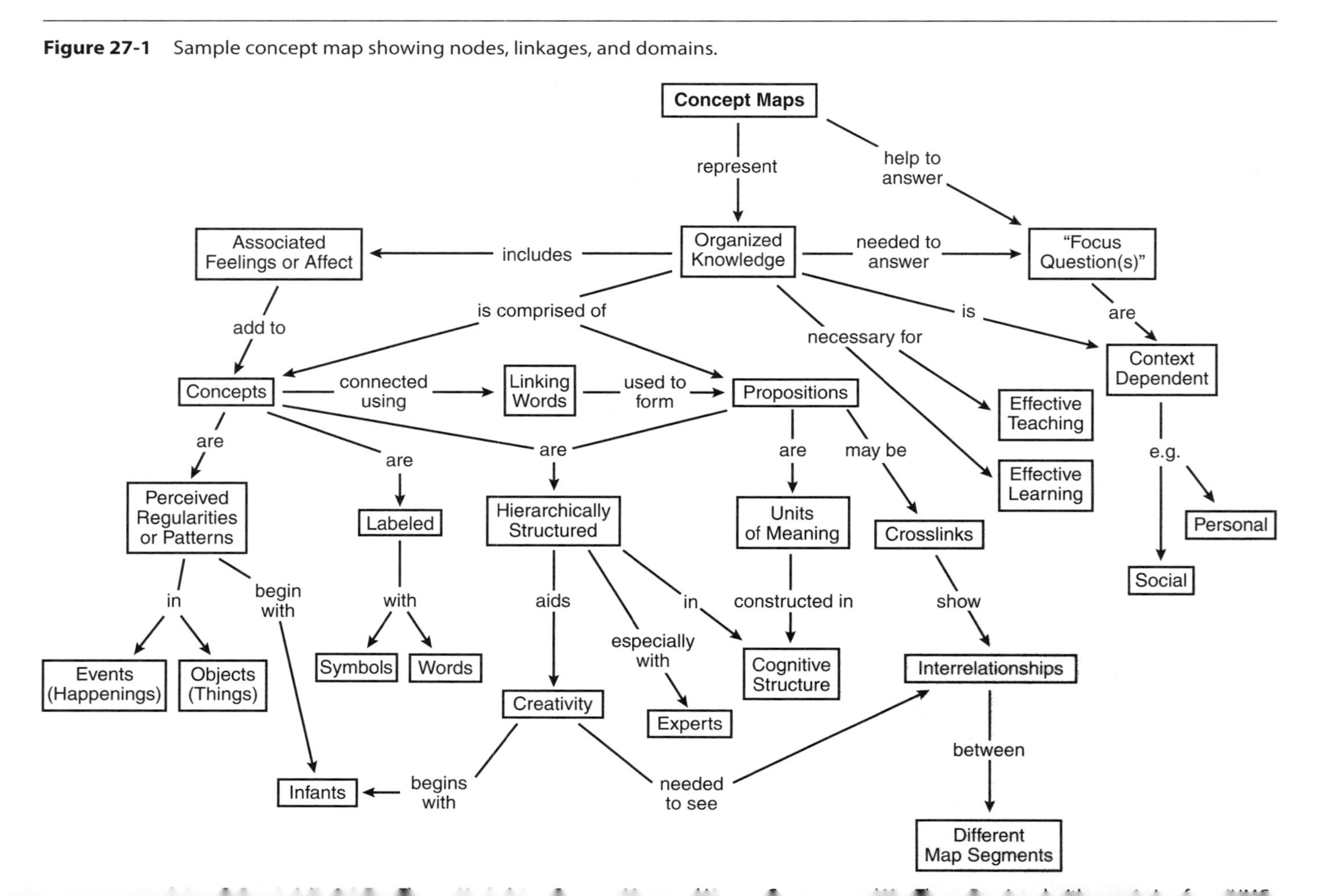

By drawing a picture of facts and the relationship, one can visually comprehend the whole. Rote or linear learning—arranging facts in text or outline format—tends to lead to disconnection of the concepts, rather than assimilation (Ausubel, 1963; Novak & Cañas, 2008).

THEORETICAL RATIONALE

Ausubel (1963), in his seminal work *The Psychology of Meaningful Verbal Learning,* states there is a great deal of difference between *rote learning* and *meaningful learning*. Rote learning is the memorization of facts or knowledge without context or perspective. This type of knowledge is quickly recalled, but not usable with other facts to draw conclusions or make inferences when considered in a different framework.

Rote learning is frequently accomplished by memorization and repeated recitation. For example, multiplication tables are learned by rote. Rote learning is a necessary technique when learning basic facts, such as anatomy and physiology, normal lab values, and basic assessment techniques and data. However, in order to be a successful healthcare provider, meaningful learning and critical thinking must also be employed (Ausubel, 1963; Ausubel, Novak, & Hanesian, 1978; Novak & Cañas, 2008).

Meaningful learning occurs when facts are learned in relationship to other facts. New knowledge is related to old knowledge and then assimilated. This results in an understanding of the knowledge, rather than knowledge of individual facts or ideas. In order for learning to be meaningful the information must be "conceptually clear and presented . . . relatable to the learner's prior knowledge" (Novak & Cañas, 2008, p. 3). Also, the learner must have a knowledge framework that supports the new knowledge and the learner must be actively engaged in the learning process (Ausubel, 1963; Novak & Cañas, 2008).

If we think of learning as constructing a building, the foundation will be the prior knowledge. In order to learn, the foundation, or prior knowledge, must be strong. The learner must have a good understanding and ability to recall the knowledge in order to build on it. New knowledge can be considered the bricks, wood, or other materials that are incorporated into the building to complete it. It becomes part of the building, a separate component, yet necessary to make the whole. In meaningful learning, new knowledge is integrated and leads to understanding of complex ideas; however, it remains a piece of separate fact, usable in assimilation of other knowledge.

Continuing this metaphor, we can use concept mapping as scaffolding or a hammer—a support or tool to complete the construction. Concept maps are about visualizing knowledge and relationships between facts and theory.

Visualization allows the student to incorporate knowledge and stimulates critical thinking.

CONDITIONS

Mapping is a versatile technique that can be used in a variety of situations. The process requires instructor flexibility and students whose anxiety level is low enough to be introduced to something new and different. Since mapping is a process, it can be used in a variety of ways and can be very simplistic or developed to a very complex format. Because the process is so adaptable, it can be used with a learner of almost any age and in a variety of situations. The application is limited only by the imagination of the user (Covey, 2005; De Simone, 2007; Vacek, 2009).

Planning and Modifying

Teachers who are new to this technique can become more familiar and comfortable with it by using it in a structured classroom setting. Mapping can be used in lecture to represent a concept or idea (Wagner, 1994), such as the relationships among information, psychomotor skills, cognitive skills, and attitude as they related to competence in giving care. It is used more informally to organize thoughts for classroom presentations. Devising interesting but familiar ideas for students to map as a classroom activity is one strategy for introducing the mapping process.

As learning assignments, concept maps help students organize their thoughts and reveal knowledge they may not know they possess. Students can use mapping techniques to categorize information from lecture and texts. They can then see connections and perceive relationships between concepts that improve their understanding and develop critical thinking.

Mapping can be a successful tool in leading and guiding discussions during post-conferences. This is especially appropriate with a complex patient with whom many students have been involved or as part of a simulation experience. The greater the number of student who can participate in the mapping process, the more meaningful the discussion will be. Students can assist each other to draw relationships among large amounts of data and to eliminate data that is irrelevant.

The mapping of clinical concepts also assists the beginning student to prioritize assessment data and develop meaningful and relevant information about the patient. Liling and Suh-Ing (2005) found students needed time to develop their mapping skills, but once the skills were mastered, the students were able to interpret problems systematically, identify priority problems, and find proper interventions.

Initially, students may have difficulty developing concept maps. Revisions are cumbersome using paper and pencil and can be very time consuming. There are several software packages, free or at a cost, available to assist in the development of concept maps. Revisions are easily made using software packages; however, they lack the flexibility and free-form capacity of pencil and paper maps (De Simone, 2007).

TYPES OF LEARNERS

Mapping is appropriate for undergraduate and graduate students. It is adaptable to independent learning, small group work, and very large classroom situations. Critical thinking, which is required for this process, helps students assimilate the interrelatedness of new information. Simple or complex, mapping varies widely to suit many learning situations. It is important to introduce this process in a way that students with a variety of experiences and knowledge relate to and in a way that allows them to see its usefulness.

Many theorists have described various learning styles and learning preferences that fit well with the use of concept mapping. Gardner and Hatch's (1990) discussion of visual/spatial form of intelligence emphasizes the ability to visualize and create mental images (see Chapter 1). Students who have strengths in this form of intelligence find mapping to be an easy and fulfilling method of relating their understanding of theoretical and clinical concepts. The ability to spatially describe the concepts helps them to better comprehend. Kelly and Young (1996) noted that a connection between experiences brings about meaningful learning.

Faculty need to enable the students to become more aware of their own personal learning styles and to offer varied experiences to facilitate different learning styles. Concept mapping is one avenue to learning that will assist with different types of learners as well as allow faculty and students to become more creative in teaching and learning (Covey, 2005).

USING THE METHOD

Concept mapping can be used to augment lecture, promote learning, or to organize patient care. It is best introduced in the classroom environment, as visual aids or handouts, to illustrate information. Then, in groups, students can develop concept maps to illustrate recently presented knowledge. This collaborative learning technique allows them to share knowledge and skill, enhancing the experience. Further, concept mapping, in a format known as *care mapping,* can be used to plan and document the care of patients.

While Novak and Cañas (2008) define the process of developing concept maps very specifically, instructors and students may adapt it to fit their particular teaching or learning styles. Using concept maps to organize ideas, consider relationships between ideas, and link new information to old knowledge is central to the use of this tool (Vacek, 2009).

Augmenting Lecture

Despite all the advances in education and the changes in students, lecture continues to be a standard technique in health education. It is an important and necessary method of presenting information. However, it can be overwhelming as the information being presented becomes more complex. Utilizing concept maps during lecture can greatly enhance the understanding of material being presented. Since most lectures are organized in an outline format, they lend themselves to mapping quite well.

For example, when teaching the pathophysiology of diabetes mellitus, the instructor will start with the fact that a lack of insulin triggers the symptoms of diabetes. Students must have the basic knowledge that insulin allows glucose to enter cells and provides energy. Rather than using bulleted lecture notes in a slide presentation, concept maps can be used as a framework for the information, supplementing the information presented via lecture (Fig. 27-2).

An additional benefit of using concept maps as the visual allows the lecturer more flexibility presenting material. Slide-based lectures (such as with PowerPoint) are linear in arrangement and can be restrictive. Slide presentations may limit deviation from what the instructor thinks is salient as opposed to what students actually have difficulty grasping or where gaps exist in knowledge. Slide presentations may direct the lecture more than the learners. On the other hand, lectures augmented by concept maps allow for visualization of concepts and their relationships and will stimulate the students to ask questions, reveal gaps in knowledge, and allow flexibility.

Learners, especially visual ones, enjoy concept map–based lectures, as it allows them to follow presented information more easily. One student states, "Seeing the connections between the symptoms helps me understand and remember better than just reading about it or hearing it in lecture." Another states, "It's easier to study the concept map and I can add to it and make notes on it that I understand."

Figure 27-2 Concept maps showing pathophysiology of diabetes mellitus. **(A)** Lack of insulin leads to two basic problems. **(B)** Cell starvation and hyperglycemia cause specific reactions in the body. **(C)** Further reactions and derangements occur. This represents a domain of the concept map. *(continues)*

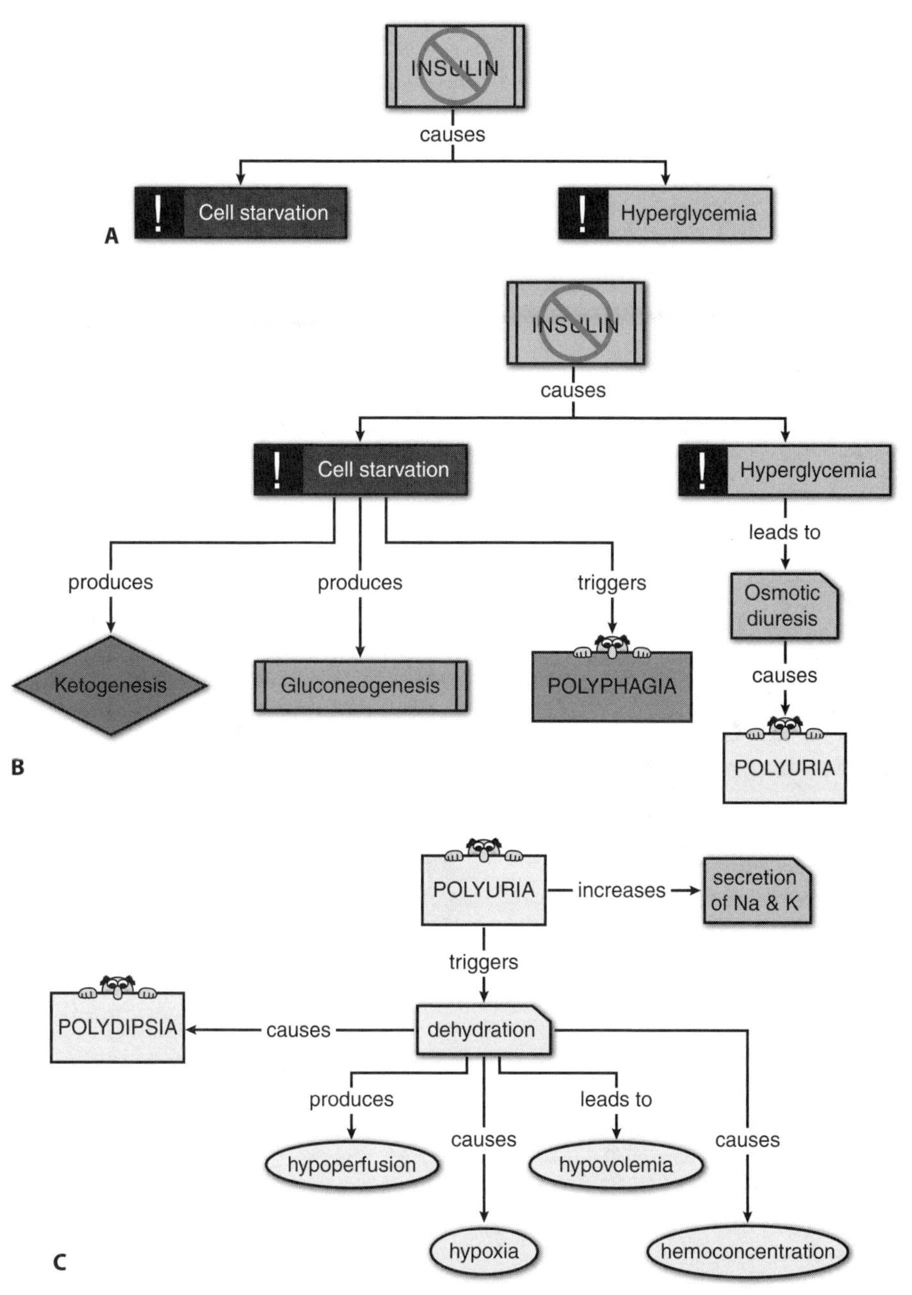

Figure 27-2 **(D)** Continuing pathophysiology leading to metabolic acidosis. *(continued)*

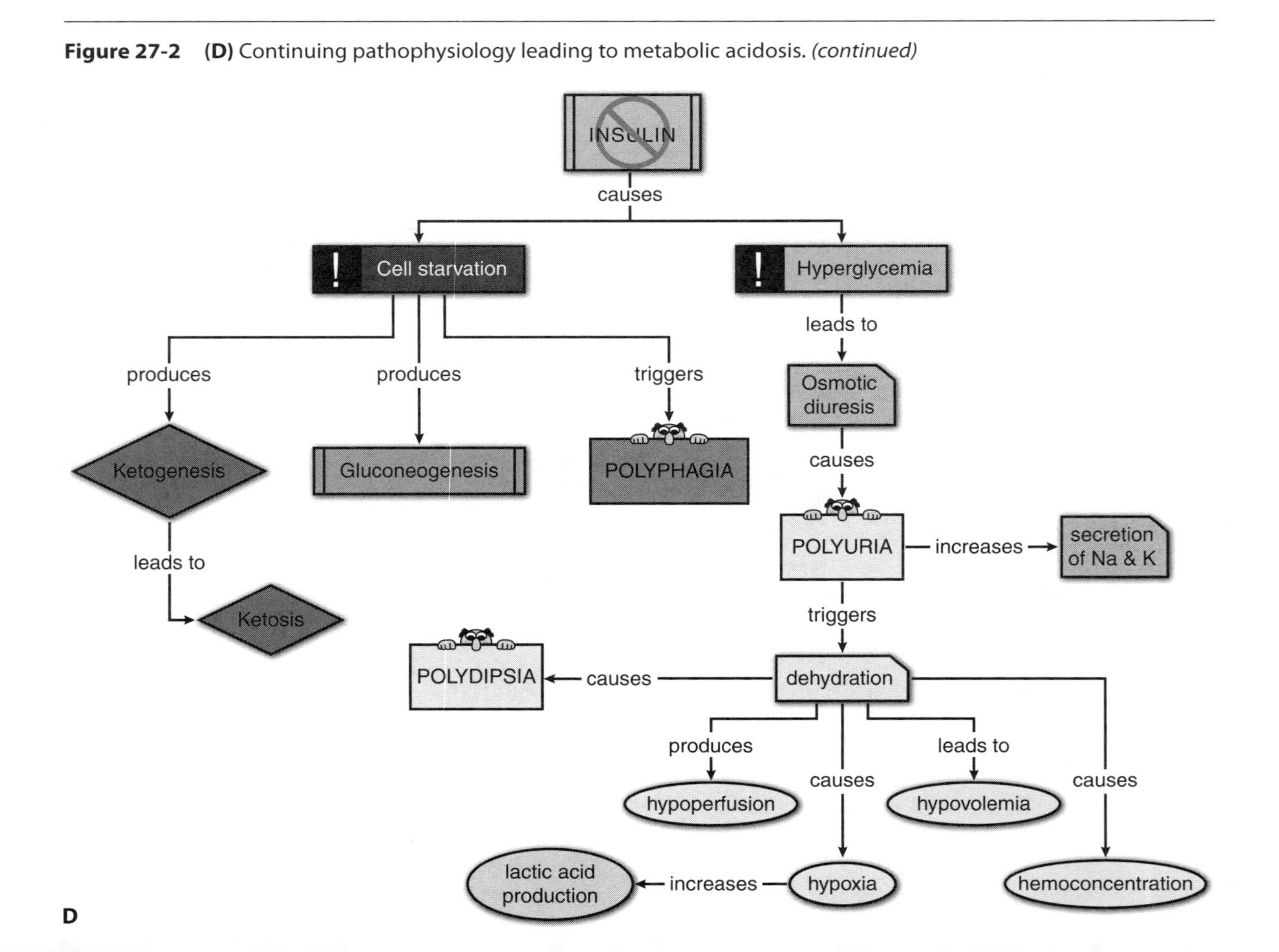

Figure 27-2 **(E)** The complete concept map, representing four of the manifestations of diabetes mellitus, polyuria, polydipsia, polyphagia and metabolic acidosis and their relationships.

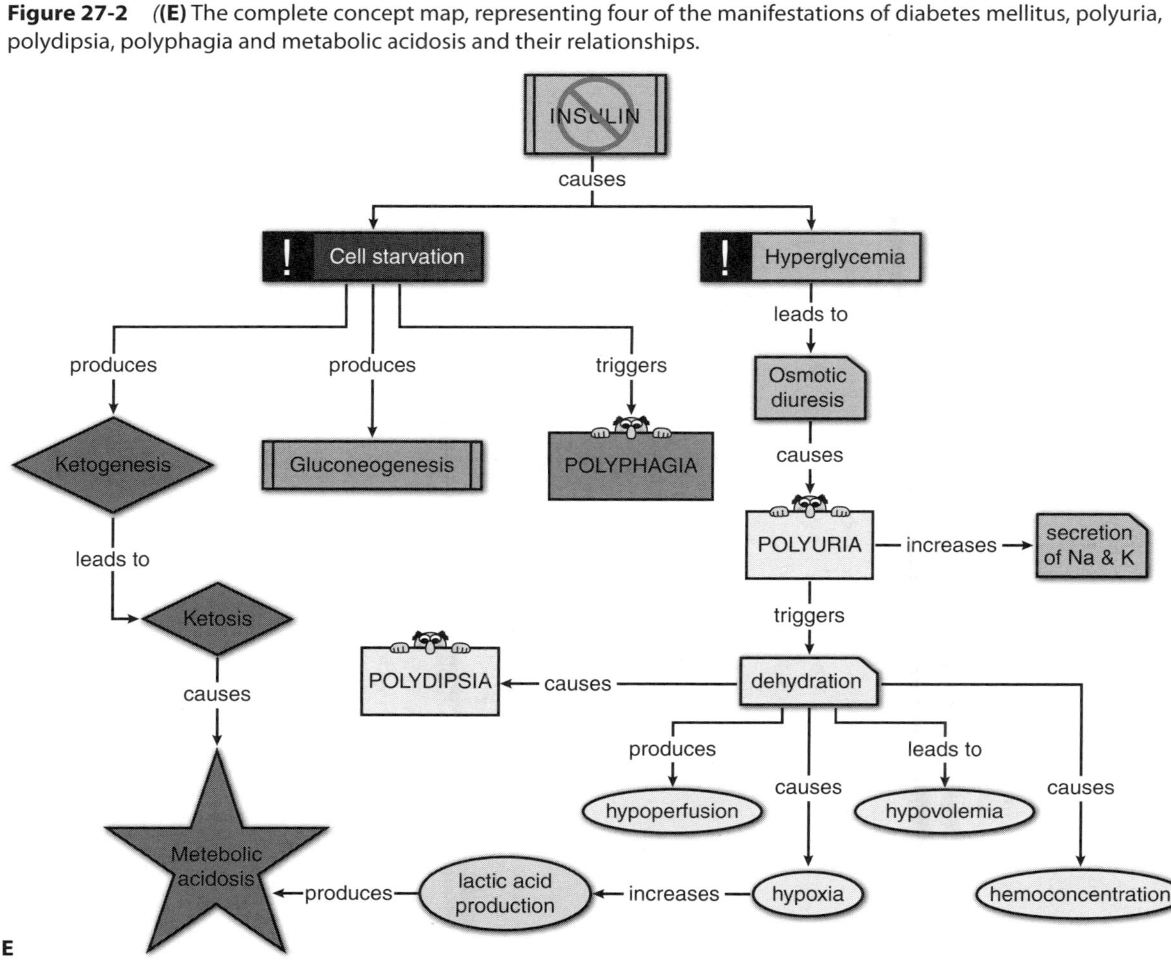

Teaching this way is adaptable to almost any pathophysiology and can also be used to teach anatomy and physiology, pharmacology, and treatment modalities. Inspiration 8, a concept mapping software, allows the user to input information in an outline format, a foundation of the lecture format. The outline is easily converted to the map format and the instructor can edit as needed. It is a great and simple way to utilize concept maps in lecture.

Enhancing Learning and Critical Thinking Skills

Traditional note taking and study techniques, such as flash cards and outlining chapters, tend to fracture knowledge. Concepts are not seen in relation to other knowledge using these techniques and are not assimilated (Vacek, 2009). According to De Simone (2007), concept mapping allows students to classify and arrange information on paper. Thus, they can see missing information, areas that need to be further explored and relationships between facts. Students who utilize concept maps in this way have a higher degree of involvement in learning and retain more knowledge (Covey, 2005; De Simone, 2007; Vacek, 2009).

Cmap tools, a free downloadable software package, allows users to work collaboratively to develop concept maps. Students work in groups to answer questions assigned in class. For example, one group may answer the question, "What causes hypertension?" while another works on "What are the macrovascular effects of hypertension?" Once completed, the concept maps are available, via the Web site, for all students in the class to use or modify. Working together, the students develop skills necessary for critical thinking, as well as interpersonal skills useful in their chosen profession (Fig. 27-3).

Introduction to concept mapping as a learning tool can be done in a nonthreatening way in the classroom. Case studies are a proven means of stimulating critical thinking in the classroom. This is an active learning technique that requires analysis of information, recall of facts, and reasoning to understand pathophysiology, patient problems, or other concepts (Sandstrom, 2006). After the case study is presented, students are divided into groups, provided with large sheets of paper (bulletin board paper works well) and markers. They may be given focus questions and key words to guide their map-making experience. During the first encounters with this process the instructor may need to provide significant guidance. However, students become adept at this process with a few experiences (De Simone, 2007).

Organizing Care

The traditional nursing care plan, linear and columnar in design, prevents visualization of the patient as a whole. Significantly, the patient is seen one problem at

Figure 27-3 Concept map showing causes of hypertension.

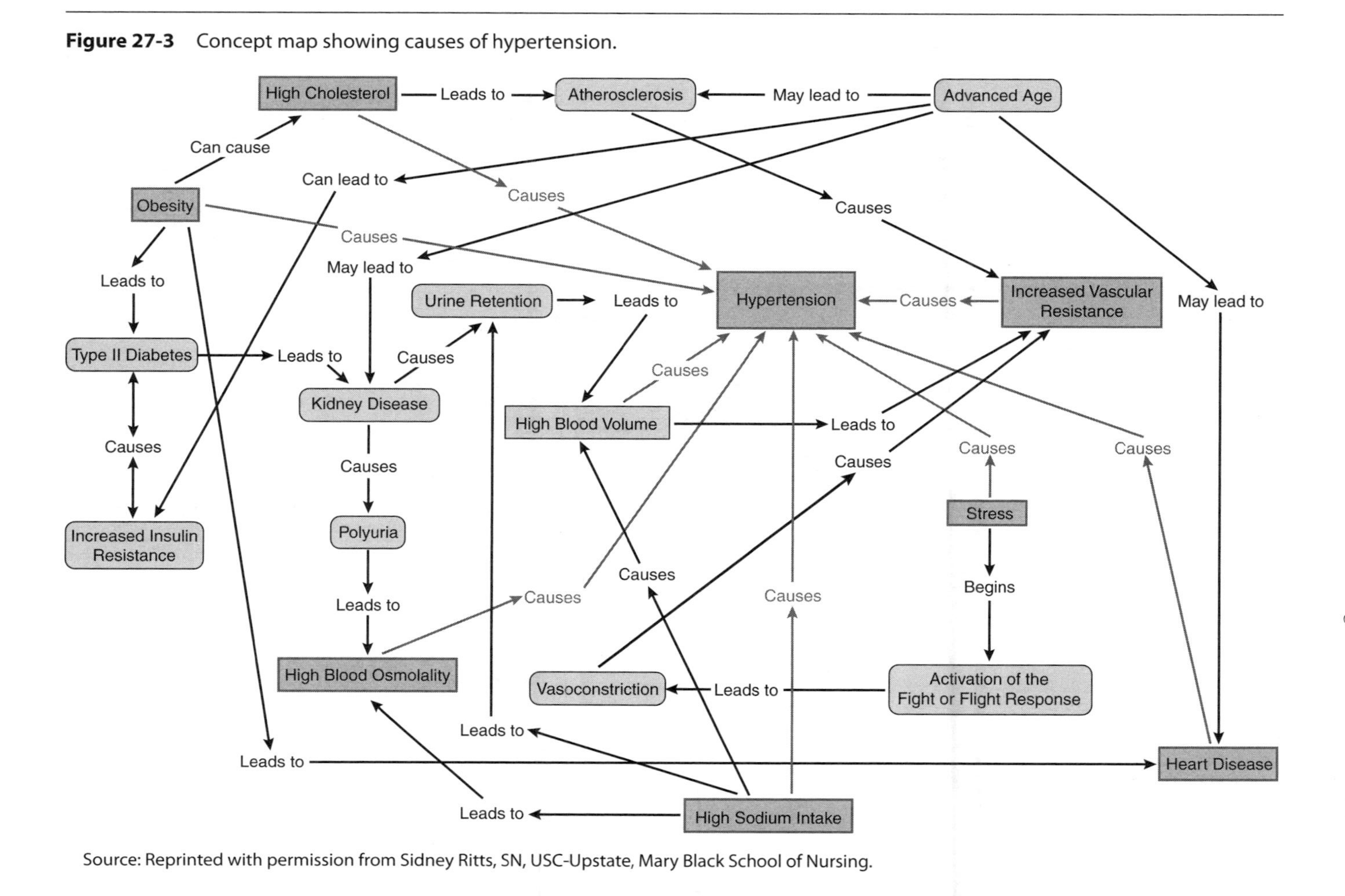

Source: Reprinted with permission from Sidney Ritts, SN, USC-Upstate, Mary Black School of Nursing.

Figure 27-4 A care map is an overview of what the student plans to do for their patient during the clinical day.

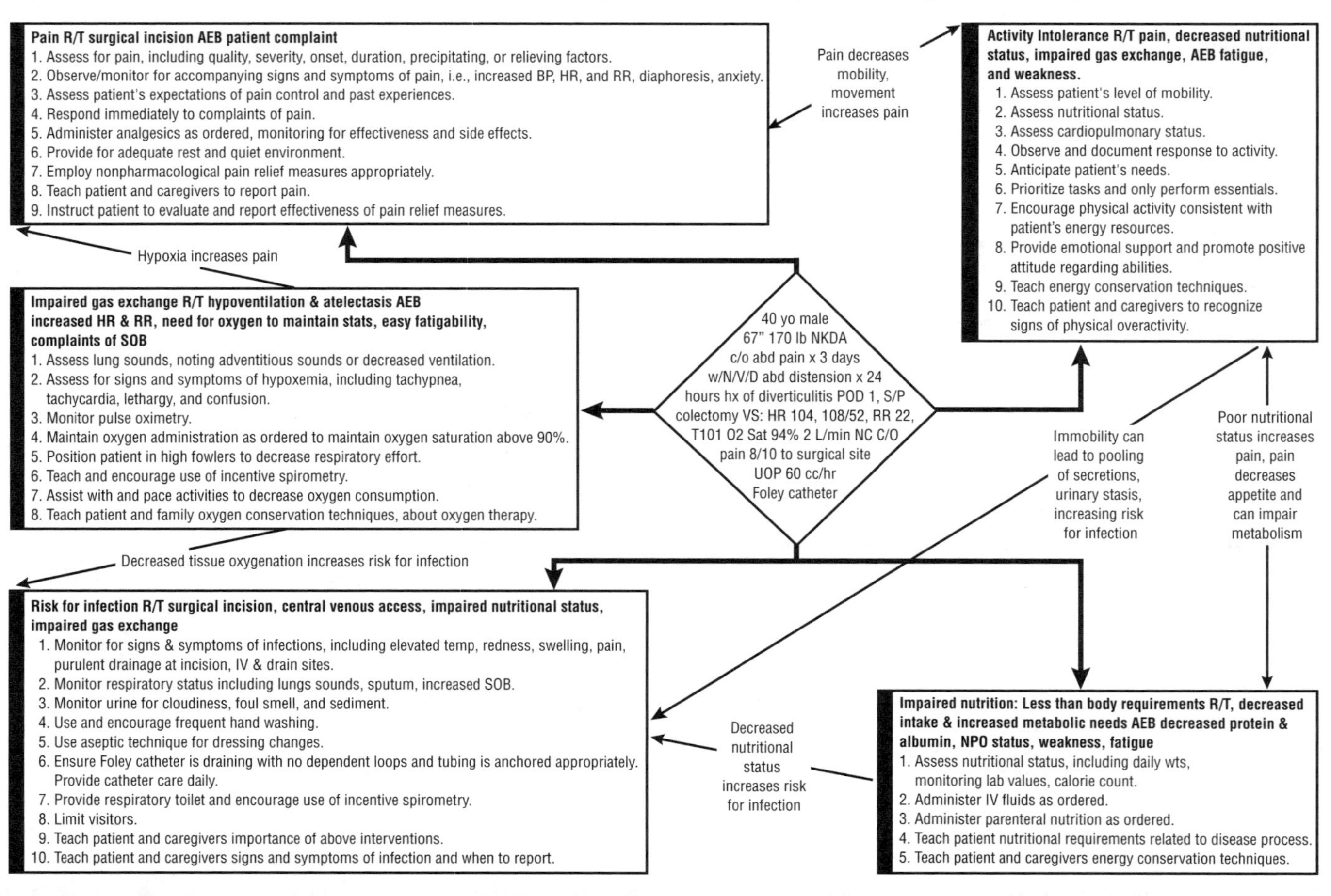

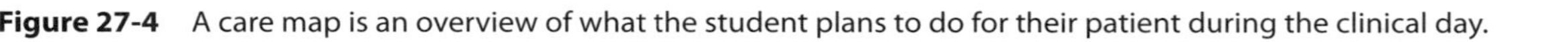

a time, with no connection indicated between the problems. Also, these care plans are not usually used for planning; rather they are used to summarize care provided or that *should have been* provided (Covey, 2005; Taylor & Wros, 2007).

Care mapping can be used as a component of a traditional care plan. It puts the patient's problems on one page and organizes problems in a way that makes sense to the student. A care map is not the *complete* care plan, but is an overview of what the student plans to do for their patient during the clinical day (Fig. 27-4). It is completed after the student has gathered information during preplanning. A complete nursing care plan includes the care map, attached forms that detail each nursing diagnosis (including rationales and outcomes), the client database, assessment, medication sheets, etc.

An attractive element of the care map is that important information, including problems, assessment data, and planned interventions, is on one page and can be easily carried and referenced throughout the clinical day. Notes regarding patient response and other relevant data can be jotted down on the care map.

Additionally, the care map allows the student to make connections between different nursing diagnoses and interventions. It is sometimes difficult for students to grasp that interventions for one nursing diagnosis can negatively impact another nursing diagnosis. For example, the common intervention of giving the patient an opioid for pain can impact that patient's gas exchange. When these nursing diagnoses are on separate pages they are easily compartmentalized and the student can overlook these connections. With a care map, connections are indicated using lines and arrows with words that indicate the connection. Students frequently state that care maps help them understand that patient problems have complex links to each other that need to be considered when planning care.

CONCLUSION

Nursing and health education are by no means unique in the requirement of their students to develop critical thinking skills. The development of these skills is imperative for the healthcare provider to successfully care for their patients. Critical thinking allows the user to take rotely learned concepts and connect or link them to understand the complex problems that affect their clients. Utilizing concept maps offers a method that is easily adaptable throughout the curriculum and is inherently individualized. It provides a visualization of knowledge guided by the particular student's learning style and understanding of material. While initial implementation may be difficult and seem unwieldy, the benefits of concept mapping as a teaching and learning tool are unquestionable. If we are to educate students to become the best nurses possible, we must continually adapt and modify our teaching methods to meet the demand of the constantly changing profession and student.

REFERENCES

Ausubel, D. P. (1963). *The psychology of meaningful verbal learning*. New York: Grune and Stratton.

Ausubel, D. P., Novak, J. D., & Hanesian, H. (1978). *Educational psychology: A cognitive view*. New York: Holt, Rinehart, and Winston.

Covey, D. (2005). Using concept maps to foster critical thinking. In L. Caputi, & L. Engelmann (Eds.), *Teaching nursing: The art and science* (pp. 634–651). Glen Ellyn, IL: College of DuPage Press.

De Simone, C. (2007). Applications of concept mapping. *College Teaching, 55*(1), 33–36.

Gardner, G., & Hatch, T. (1990). *Multiple intelligences go to school: Educational implications of the theory of multiple intelligences* (Tech. Rep. No. 4). New York: Center for Technology in Education.

Kelly, E., & Young, A. (1996). Models of nursing education for the 21st century. *Review of Nursing Research in Nursing Education, 7,* 1–39.

Liling, H., & Suh-Ing, H. (2005). Concept maps as an assessment tool in a nursing course. *The Journal of Professional Nursing, 3,* 141–149.

Novak, J. D., Cañas, A. J. (2008). The Theory Underlying Concept Maps and How to Construct and use them, Technical Report IHMC CmapTools 2006-01 Rev 01-2008. Florida Institute for Human and Machine Cognition. Retrieved January 8, 2010 from: http://cmap.ihmc.us/Publications/ResearchPapers/TheoryUnderlyingConceptMaps.pdf

Sandstrom, S. (2006). Use of case studies to teach diabetes and other chronic illnesses to nursing students. *Journal of Nursing Education, 45*(6), 229–232.

Taylor, J., & Wros, P. (2007). Concept mapping: A nursing model for care planning. *Journal of Nursing Education, 46*(5), 211–216.

Vacek, J. E. (2009). Using a conceptual approach with concept mapping to promote critical thinking. *Journal of Nursing Education, 48*(1), 45–48.

Wagner, W. (1994). *Teaching/learning process*. Presented at the Teaching Skills for Health Professions Educators, St. Simon's Island, GA.

CHAPTER 28

The Preceptored Clinical Experience

Brian M. French and Miriam Greenspan

The preceptored clinical experience provides an opportunity for students, new graduate clinicians, experienced clinicians new to a work setting or practice area, or others to work with an experienced staff member in order to begin socialization and role transition, as well as gain exposure to the healthcare arena. This experiential teaching and learning methodology provides clear benefits to the learner, preceptor, school, and healthcare setting.

DEFINITION AND PURPOSES

In 15th-century England, the word preceptor was first used to identify a tutor or instructor. The term first appeared in the nursing literature in the mid-1970s (Peirce, 1991). The more recent use of the term preceptorship denotes an experience lasting a designated period of time, during which an experienced clinician or preceptor enters into a one-on-one relationship with a novice clinician learner (the student, preceptee, or orientee) to assist the novice in the transition from learner to practitioner (Baggot, Hensinger, Parry, Valdes, & Zaim, 2005; Benner, Tanner, & Chesla, 1996; Marcum & West, 2004; O'Malley, Cunliffe, Hunter, & Breeze, 2000). The preceptorship is a process during which the preceptor, through role modeling, information sharing, coaching, and direction, teaches the preceptee the art of professional practice. The precepted clinical experience is a planned and organized instructional program with specific objectives and goals. It can be useful in supporting the learning process of students at all levels during a clinical, management, education, or research practicum. Other uses include orienting new graduate clinicians or experienced clinicians transferring between clinical areas. Visitors to the clinical area, such as clinicians from another country seeking exposure to the US healthcare system and roles, can also benefit from being precepted.

Student precepted experiences typically take place within a capstone clinical course during the latter part of the curriculum. Such a course might be designed to promote synthesis of theoretical knowledge, allow for more in-depth study of a specific patient population, and apply evidenced-based research to the clinical practice area. In addition, preceptors can assist students to demonstrate leadership and collaborative skills and provide experiences to enhance understanding of organizational behavior as well as ethical, legal, economic, and political issues.

Preceptorship is often used as a way of facilitating the role transition of novice clinicians. Preceptorship can also be used as a methodology for orienting experienced clinicians who are new to a particular patient population or institutional setting. This offers the clinician learner the opportunity to apply previously acquired knowledge in an experiential manner while safely accumulating new knowledge and experiences for future reference (Benner et al., 1996). During the preceptorship, a partnership is formed between the preceptor and the preceptee in which both contribute to the outcome (Godinez, Schweiger, Gruver, & Ryan, 1999; O'Malley et al., 2000). The partnership becomes an ongoing mutual exchange between the preceptor and the learner, in a mutually trusting, supportive environment. The preceptor offers information, direction, and feedback and the preceptee offers insight about personal goals, learning needs, and learning styles. During the preceptorship both the student and the graduate clinician learn the rules, language, and behaviors of the work environment (Godinez et al., 1999; Horsburgh, 1989; O'Malley et al., 2000; Tradewell, 1996).

The preceptored experience differs from spend-the-day shadowing experiences or informal pairing relationships that are typically geared toward providing a broad exposure to the healthcare environment or to promote individual career awareness or understanding of the clinician role. It also differs from the mentor–mentee experience, which is generally a more long-term relationship designed to promote career growth and development and may be mutually supportive and collaborative in nature (Alspach, 2000).

The preceptorship is the opportune time for the novice to be socialized into the new work setting. In the case of students, it may be the first exposure to the roles, responsibilities, and accountabilities of the clinician role. For the graduate clinician, the preceptorship serves as a period of transition from the role of student to that of professional. The experienced clinician moving into a new work setting also requires assistance with socialization, and must adjust previous experiences to fit into the current work setting with new rules, new languages, and new patient populations.

THEORETICAL FOUNDATIONS

Socialization has been defined as the passing of a role from one person to the next, the process by which a person acquires and internalizes new knowledge and skills (Horsburgh, 1989; Santucci, 2004; Tradewell, 1996). Socialization enables the transition from previous roles to new roles, and from familiar to unfamiliar work environments. Tradewell also states that socialization occurs through observing the preceptor role model behaviors and language as well as by exposure to incumbent staff as they reflect on their practice through stories of their own work experiences. Santucci states that the socialization period involves the learning of work systems, staff roles, and employer expectations for students and new employees alike. The preceptor informs, guides, and supports the clinician in navigating the social mores of the workplace and applying knowledge gained from past clinical and classroom experiences to the technological and physiological aspects of patient care in the new setting.

During this period, preceptees may experience a loss of confidence in their abilities to perform skills and think critically. For experienced clinicians entering a new practice arena, the loss of their self confidence is particularly difficult. In their previous work setting, they have been capable, experienced practitioners, relying on past experiences and intuition to function effectively. They were comfortable in their practice, and felt knowledgeable about the expectations of the work environment, resources, and sources of support. In the new work environment, their self image has changed as they find themselves unsure of how to behave or practice and lacking in knowledge regarding resources and support systems. This unfamiliarity engenders a self image or vision that is difficult to accept, even if the period is transient.

During the transition, the preceptee begins to leave behind previously learned beliefs and behaviors and integrates new standards and expectations into their practice. Kramer (1974) described this difficult process as reality shock, a period in which the learner begins to recognize differences and inconsistencies in the new environment, in comparison to the old environment. Students transitioning to the professional role are exposed to the realities and contradictions of the real world, as compared to the known and ordered world of academia. The preceptee may question the value of what was learned as well as the ethics of what is observed in the workplace. Finding a balance and learning to mesh the academic and work environments in a way that is acceptable for the learner may be difficult and emotionally stressful as familiar support and social systems are left behind. The work of learning, performing in a new role, balancing new and old roles, and making meaning of new work is an exhausting process that requires high-energy consumption by the learner and significant support from the preceptor.

Communication and feedback are the backbone of the preceptor–preceptee relationship. Open, honest, compassionate, and timely feedback is valued by the preceptee. Such communication requires mutual trust and respect. While it takes time to develop this trust, the reality of the preceptorship experience is that it is of the moment, existing only within a limited time frame. It is critical that an initial meeting between the learner and preceptor include a discussion of their past experiences, expectations, and goals for the relationship, and personal, work, learning, teaching, and communication styles. This conversation sets the stage for a successful, sharing relationship.

The preceptor is called on to be teacher, counselor, and clinician, to guide the preceptee through this complex transition (O'Malley et al., 2000). A safe, supportive, and informative environment is vital during this period (Goh & Watt, 2003). While the key relationships are between preceptor and preceptee, supportive faculty and unit staff is critical. Faculty, managers, and clinical specialists must meet with preceptors to describe the course or orientation program objectives and enlist the assistance of other staff as necessary to assist in designing the preceptorship. In this way, there is an investment and support for the program from the beginning. Consideration should be given to the kind of support that will be given to the preceptors throughout the experience. Support can be in the form of public acknowledgement of their work, scheduled meetings with the preceptor to ascertain whether assistance is needed, or with the preceptor and preceptee to discuss progress, support for the types of assignments the preceptor selects, and possible schedule adjustments for the preceptor to enhance the learning experience.

TYPES OF LEARNERS

Whether the individual involved in the precepted experience is a student, new graduate, experienced clinician, or a temporary visitor, all are adult learners who actively participate on some level in the identification of their individual learning needs and designing or choosing learning experiences intended to meet those needs. The precepted experience takes place in a complex and dynamic clinical environment with the preceptor facilitating the learning. The experience is enhanced by learners who exhibit well-developed adult learning characteristics. This includes an independent self concept, willingness to freely share their life experiences with others, active engagement in the process in order to meet learning goals, an openness to learning opportunities regardless of when they occur in the experience, and a problem-centered approach to learning.

CONDITIONS FOR LEARNING

The two most commonly named goals for the preceptored learning experience reported in the literature include the facilitation of socialization into the work setting and role transition from student to graduate clinician or from newly hired orientee to staff member (Gaberson & Oermann, 1999; Guhde, 2005; Smith &

Chalker 2005). Gaberson and Oermann also reported benefits for students in terms of the ability to integrate classroom theoretical knowledge with actual clinical practice within a healthcare organization. In addition, the preceptor has the ability to provide individualized attention and guidance to the learner, and improve the learner's clinical competence and confidence. The schools also benefit from preceptored experiences because students have less dependence on faculty because preceptors serve in the educator role. In this way, a faculty member can more effectively manage a group of students through collaborative relationships with preceptors.

From the organizational perspective, student-preceptored clinical rotations may assist in meeting mission statement goals, such as a commitment to educating future clinicians. In addition, preceptorships may facilitate recruitment of employees because the learner has a relationship within the organization and is exposed to the workplace and staff. The supportive relationship between an orientee and preceptor may also impact new employee recruitment, job satisfaction, and retention rates (Casey, Fink, Krugman, & Propst, 2004; Gaberson & Oermann, 1999).

RESOURCES

Although the preceptored experience may take place in any organization that delivers health care, it is important to ensure that the clinical environment matches the goals of the experience from either the course and student or program and orientee perspective. The length of the experience is dependent on the goals to be achieved. In short, the experience can be of any length but must be long enough to provide the varied clinical exposure and experiences to ensure achievement of course or orientation objectives.

Whether it is a student or orientee experience, the preceptor and learner will benefit from contact and guidance from a faculty member or organization-based educator, clinical specialist, or manager. Preceptors should have access to a student's goals and objectives or an orientee's competency checklist in order to facilitate planning, track achievements, and evaluate performance.

Organizations that provide clinical placements to student clinicians require qualified staff to precept. In addition, they require qualified staff to precept new or transferring employees. Depending on the staff mix in a given clinical area, there may not be an adequate supply of interested, committed, and educationally prepared staff to serve in the preceptor role, and this could be a limiting factor for the numbers of students or new hires a unit or department is able to absorb. This is particularly true if the unit or department also welcomes groups of students with clinical instructor at the same time, thus creating competition for patient assignments. Staff may view the role of preceptor and the teaching and evaluation responsibilities as added work and this may also limit the number of students or orientees for a given clinical area. All of these scenarios require commitment on the part of the unit or department manager, clinical specialists, educators, and faculty to creating a learning environment that supports staff throughout the process so that they are prepared to serve and feel valued in their role as preceptor.

Recognition for clinicians who are preceptors can take many forms. Schools may appoint preceptors to adjunct faculty status, provide access to continuing education programs, provide certificates of appreciation or recognition receptions, and, in some cases, vouchers for free or reduced tuition for selected courses. Although these recognition and reward efforts may have a budgetary impact on the academic institution, benefits may also be realized through recruitment of preceptors to enroll in academic programs. Healthcare organizations may or may not provide similar incentives for staff who are preceptors including certificates of appreciation, preceptor awards, luncheons, less off-shift or weekend scheduling, lighter than usual patient assignments, or pay differentials. Again, these methods of recognizing staff for their role as preceptor may have a budget impact but may also encourage staff to participate in this key role and contribute to job satisfaction and retention through recognition of their hard work. Speers, Strzyzewski, and Ziolkowski (2004) report that nonmaterial benefits had greater relative importance for staff in their decision to serve in the preceptor role.

USING THE METHOD

Under the guidance of an experienced clinician preceptor, the student or novice clinician begins to apply the knowledge and theory learned in the classroom to the reality of patient care and begins to transition from learner to professional. It is equally important that the environment is one in which the novice feels safe enough to ask questions and take risks. Having clear expectations for the precepting experience for both the preceptor and the novice further contributes to a successful experience. Faculty should review the goals prior to the experience if the novice is a student. If the novice is a new graduate clinician or an experienced clinician new to a particular work setting, he or she should come with expectations for the precepting experience and be prepared to discuss them with the preceptor. The preceptor, working with unit-based leadership, should also develop a set of goals and expectations for the precepting experience. During the initial meeting between the preceptor and the preceptee, goals and expectations for the experience should be shared and reworked into a mutually agreed upon plan with time frames for achievement.

The preceptor is the key to the success of this experience. When designing the precepting experience, time and attention should be paid to the selection, preparation, and ongoing support of the preceptor. Attention should also be given to the roles and responsibilities of the learner, the clinical faculty, and the unit leadership in this learning experience.

The Preceptor

Precepting requires an individual who is committed to nurturing and teaching the next generation of professionals, someone who is both caring and clinically competent. On occasion, preceptors are selected based on their availability, convenience, and clinical abilities but an outstanding clinician does not always translate into a skillful preceptor. There are four criteria for selecting a qualified preceptor. The first criterion in selecting a preceptor should be the clinician's interest in and willingness to assume the role in addition to their patient care responsibilities.

The second criterion is ensuring a positive relationship between the preceptor and the preceptee. The relationship must include trust and understanding if learning is to take place. Factors that can facilitate this trusting relationship include ensuring that the preceptor reviews written goals and objectives for the experience to facilitate upfront planning; reviewing preceptor and preceptee expectations for communication, behavior, and timelines for goal achievement; and providing time for meetings for discussion, reflection, and feedback throughout the experience. Other factors that may influence the relationship include involving the potential preceptor in the interview process for a new staff member and having a manager or clinical specialist choose a preceptor that matches their perceptions of the preceptee based on their knowledge of both individuals including such factors as communication, learning, and teaching styles.

Clinical knowledge, skill, and ability are the components of the third criterion for choosing an ideal preceptor. A practitioner with a depth of understanding of the patient population and a high level of technical skill is necessary when selecting a preceptor. Benner et al. (1996) state that the competent practitioner often provides the best guidance for the new clinician. The competent practitioner is adept at assessing and diagnosing patient needs in a step-by-step fashion. This attention to detail and use of a logical and orderly process is useful when teaching the student or novice practitioner. Proficient, expert clinicians have a breadth of knowledge and intuition not possessed by the competent practitioner but their skill often proves to be too abstract for the novice and therefore may not be the best choice to serve as a preceptor. As a task-focused learner, the novice is more comfortable with the more concrete precepts of the competent practitioner.

The ability to listen and communicate with respect describes the fourth criterion for the preceptor. During the transition from student or orientee to practitioner, the amount of new information, new experiences, and new responsibilities may be overwhelming. Students and orientees may experience a range of emotions from excitement and eagerness to anger and frustration during the transition period. The preceptor will need to be attuned to these reactions and adapt the learning experience accordingly. In order to manage this, the preceptor will need to be able to listen closely and assess the needs of the preceptee, much as they assess the needs of the patient.

The preceptor's role will be multifaceted. As teacher and guide, the preceptor will be introducing the novice to clinical practice (Godinez et al., 1999). In the first meeting between the preceptor and preceptee, the preceptor will discuss the goals for the precepting experience. The preceptor will also determine the preceptee's learning needs and learning style. This can be done by simply asking how the preceptee learns best (e.g., visual, auditory, audiovisual, verbal, or kinesthetic) or through a more formal assessment process using any of a number of standardized tools such as Kolb's learning style inventory (Kolb, 2005; Kolb & Kolb, 2005).

Role modeling patient care skills from interpersonal interactions to assessment and diagnosis, and finally to intervention and evaluation, will be the initial primary method of teaching. Ongoing explanations for each action will inform the learner of the reasons for the choices the preceptor makes. In addition to modeling practice at the bedside, the preceptor will model skills in communication with the interdisciplinary team involved in patient care, as well as with the patient and family.

In the early phase of the precepted experience, the novice will observe and listen to the preceptor role model. As the experience progresses, the role of the preceptor will move to teacher, as the preceptor instructs the learner in providing direct patient care, using technology, interacting with the multidisciplinary team, and accessing the resources available within the work environment.

The preceptor will spend time coaching the preceptee by role-playing interactions before they occur. For instance, the preceptor may have the preceptee practice reviewing the plan for participating in patient care rounds before they occur or giving clinician-to-clinician report before the shift ends. The skill of the preceptor will be called into action, knowing when to hover close by the preceptee as he or she provides direct care, and knowing when to allow the learner to practice more independently. As the patient dynamic changes, so will the choices the preceptor makes relative to the autonomy of the novice. When the patient's condition is acute, or changes unexpectedly, the preceptor will work closely with the learner as he or she provides care, makes assessments, and plans with other members of the healthcare team. When the patient is well known to the preceptor and learner, with a stable or improved condition, the preceptor may choose to review the care plan with the learner and then observe and evaluate the learner's ability to implement the plan.

Along with the responsibility for teaching at the bedside, the preceptor must introduce and socialize the preceptee to the work environment in order to assist in the transition from student or orientee to professional clinician. It is incumbent upon the preceptor to introduce the preceptee to the culture of the unit, the values of the staff, the formal and informal roles occupied by members of the staff, and the formal and informal rules by which the unit functions. Preceptors will need to explain basics such as how the schedule works and how to manage the hospital's communication system, as well as how to cope with the realities of the healthcare environment. The preceptor becomes a guide to the learner who has left behind familiar environments and support systems and must form a new and stable base on which to grow as a clinician.

When working with new clinicians, the preceptor, with support from unit leadership, should attempt to carve out some time for reflection. While this is challenging in today's fast paced clinical environment, it does serve several important purposes. Time away from the clamor of the unit allows the preceptor and learner to review the patient experience and to discuss in greater depth how and why specific patient care decisions were made. Perhaps most importantly, this time provides a safe space for the learner to reflect on his or her own thoughts and feelings about what has occurred with the patient and how he or she has performed. Through these discussions, the relationship between the preceptor and preceptee is built, trust is developed, and communication is enhanced. This is vital for later discussions as they evaluate the success of the practicum or process of orientation and each person's behavior in the process. Most likely, students will be familiar with this time for reflection as this is common practice in an instructor-led clinical practicum.

The Preceptee

The preceptee is an active participant in the precepting experience and must assume a leadership role in ensuring the success of the experience. In addition to the initial sharing of goals for the experience, the learner is responsible for informing the preceptor when the goals are not being met, when new lessons are not clear, or when he or she is uncomfortable performing a new skill. Feedback from the learner helps the preceptor adapt and adjust the experience in a meaningful way that leads to a successful outcome. Without feedback, the preceptor will only be making assumptions, which may not always be correct. The learner is also accountable for following through on the suggestions and recommendations made by the preceptor.

This may include practicing a skill, researching an unfamiliar aspect of clinical care, or reading a suggested article or chapter about a particular patient condition.

The Faculty and Unit Leadership

A strong collaborative partnership between academic faculty and service providers, including both unit leadership and staff, is a critical factor in ensuring a successful experience for students (Corlett, Palfreyman, Staines, & Marr, 2003). The role played by faculty and unit leadership will vary depending on the level of experience of both the preceptor and preceptee. If the preceptor is new to the role, then the faculty or unit leadership will play a mentoring role in the process and may need to provide more guidance to ensure success. As the preceptor gains experience in the role, faculty and unit leadership may only need to meet with the preceptor and preceptee occasionally to monitor the process or consult on more complex issues that the preceptor is unable to solve independently. Regardless of the experience level of the preceptor, faculty or unit leadership must maintain open communication and monitor the experience on some level to ensure objectives are met and intervene if there are issues that arise in the preceptor–preceptee relationship. Such support can be offered in direct discussions that occur periodically throughout the preceptorship or by phone or email when specific questions or concerns arise.

Evaluating the Preceptored Clinical Experience

Ideally, evaluation should be a formative and ongoing process, part of the daily communication between preceptor and preceptee. Discussion and feedback about skill performance, assessment and diagnosis, and bedside interactions should be part of the regular communication of each day. By incorporating this process into the routine of the day, it becomes a respectful, helpful activity, and one that moves the precepting experience continuously forward. Competency-based tools, timelines, or lists of objectives can serve as valuable guidelines for such discussions. If goals have been set at the beginning of the precepting experience, discussion can be based on how closely the experience has come to meeting those goals. Asking simple questions such as, "How do you think you performed today?," "Is there anything you would do differently?," and "How close are we to reaching each goal?" provide a basis for self-reflection and allow the preceptor to evaluate the learner's understanding of his or her performance. The preceptor can then compare their assessment of the preceptee's performance with the learner's self-assessment and provide constructive feedback to support or improve the preceptee's performance. If only summative evaluation is used to evaluate the precepting experience, the learner will not benefit from the preceptor's suggestions and recommendations since it has not been provided in a time-sensitive or event-sensitive manner. As the orientation is nearing the end of its prescribed timeline, the burden of evaluating the orientee becomes more acute. Many schools and clinical units have created evaluation tools that consider the preceptor's actions, the preceptee's actions, or both. In addition, both the American Association for Critical-Care Nurses (AACN) and The Center for Nurse Executives have used survey data and focus groups to determine lists of core competencies (Berkow, Virksis, Stewart, & Conway, 2009; Hickey, 2009). Important generic competencies identified in these documents include basic knowledge application, assessment, technical skill attainment, time management, critical thinking, and communication. For the new clinician, such tools most often follow a competency-based format that cover the various aspects of caring for a particular patient population, including skill acquisition, problem solving, and decision making. For the student, tools generally focus on goal attainment and the overall clinical experience, including the effectiveness of the preceptor. Preceptors may use a self evaluation model focusing on the various aspects of the preceptor role or they may receive feedback from the preceptee, faculty, or unit leadership using a more inclusive method. Faculty or unit leadership should participate in the evaluation process periodically during the precepting experience. They can offer objective insight into the progress being made and recommendations gleaned from their expertise in patient care and teaching. They can also serve as a role model and support the preceptor in handling more complex feedback issues that might occur during the precepting experience. Preceptors take their role very seriously, and may feel they are solely responsible for the outcome of the experience. Indicators for lack of readiness for independent practice have been identified through focus groups and individual interviews. Preceptors have listed a lack of basic knowledge, followed by the inability to perform frequently taught and demonstrated skills as most concerning general indicators of a preceptee's lack of readiness for practice; specific behaviors that raise red flags include an inability to develop organizational skills, an apparent lack of interest in engaging with patients, and an unwillingness to participate in self reflection or critical self assessment (Luhanga, Yonge, & Myrick, 2008; Modic & Harris, 2008). Active and timely faculty or unit leadership involvement will help the preceptor manage some of the perceived burden of the preceptor's sense of responsibility for the outcome of the experience.

POTENTIAL PROBLEMS

In order for a successful partnership to develop, consistent, interested, capable preceptors are necessary (Boychuck-Duchsher, 2001; Boyle, Popkess-Vawter, & Taunton, 1996; Casey et al., 2004; Oermann & Moffitt-Wolfe, 1997). On the other side of the equation, there must be an engaged, participative preceptee (O'Malley et al., 2000).

The challenges described by students and new graduates during this transition include being able to set priorities and organize patient care needs, acquiring time management skills, fearing communication with physicians, lacking confidence in their performance, and struggling with dependence and independence in the preceptor–preceptee relationship (Casey et al., 2004; Oermann & Moffitt-Wolfe, 1997). The issue of independent practice is a dilemma for preceptors as well as preceptees. Knowing when to allow the preceptee to practice more independently or when to step in and actively guide and participate in the patient care is subjective and varies from moment to moment. An event that can be handled by a preceptee in one instance may require the direct involvement of the preceptor in another case because of the impact of individual patient characteristics. This seeming inconsistency in preceptor behavior may contribute to the preceptee's issues of confidence and highlights the need for open, honest communication between preceptor and preceptee.

Potential problems can arise in the preceptorial experience because of factors related to the preceptor, the learner, or the process. The importance of formal training in preparing a staff member to function effectively as a preceptor is well documented in the literature (Alspach, 2000; Neumann et al., 2004; Speers et al., 2004). Although clinicians chosen to be preceptors are typically well prepared to care for their patients, in order to be effective as staff preceptors they must also be knowledgeable regarding the principles of adult education and adult learning, learning styles, planning and implementing learning experiences, reality shock, and the principles of evaluation and providing constructive feedback. Faculty, managers, clinical specialists, and staff educators must provide opportunities for advanced education in these areas in order to adequately prepare clinicians to serve in their assigned role and to maximize the potential success of the preceptor–preceptee relationship and achieve a positive outcome. In addition, staff preceptors should have periodic contact with faculty and their managers, clinical specialists, and educators throughout the preceptorship in order to enhance communication, problem solve, and continue their development as preceptors through evaluative feedback of their performance. For preceptors, the sense of responsibility they feel for the experience extends beyond the clinical teaching that occurs. They often feel responsible for diagnosing and resolving all problems that occur, even those that are beyond their scope to manage. Frequent involvement of faculty or unit leadership helps to establish a relationship in which the preceptor feels comfortable sharing concerns and seeking an expert's advice.

The learner must receive clear, up front communication regarding their responsibility for the learning process, achievement of outcomes, preceptor expectations, and what they can expect of their preceptor as well as practical issues such as adhering to assigned schedules and completion of assignments. This helps avoid misunderstandings about their role as learner and the goals of the experience. It also removes the primary responsibility for the success of the experience from the preceptor and ensures that the preceptee is aware of his or her accountability for successful outcomes.

Beyond preparation of both preceptor and learner, other issues internal to the individual must also be considered as affecting the relationship. There are many potential causes for perceived or real personality conflicts between a preceptor and preceptee but many can arise when there is a clash of values and beliefs that can occur between different age groups. The need to manage generational issues in the workplace is well documented in the literature (Gerke, 2001; Weston, 2001). Differing world views, personal motivating factors, preferred work environments, perceptions of work–life balance, and individual strengths and differences can create conflicts between a preceptor of one generation and a preceptee of another. Awareness and understanding of these different generational values, behaviors, and expectations is the first step in working toward a successful preceptor–preceptee relationship. Integration of this information into preceptor preparation programs is key to assisting with the teaching and learning challenges created by a multigenerational workforce.

Preparation of preceptors and preceptees requires a structure to support expected outcomes. Educational preparation of preceptors to serve in their role, orientation of learners as to what to expect in the clinical setting, written course or orientation program objectives, competency or skill checklists, articulated time frames for outcome achievement, appropriate matching of preceptor and learner, and appropriate scheduling and identification of resources to assist in the process are all aspects of a well-planned and organized preceptorship. Effective planning and creation of tools to support the process allow the preceptor and learner to focus on the learning process within the context of the busy clinical environment.

The acuity and pace of the current clinical environment provides unique challenges for the preceptor and student or orientee. The preceptor is no longer serving in one role, that of caregiver and coordinator of care, but also as a teacher of caregiving and care coordination (Alspach, 2000). The challenge of teaching while providing high-quality care requires the preceptor to balance these roles. Most often, the student or new orientee has less clinical knowledge and skill than the more experienced preceptor. The preceptor must consider the rights of the patients and adhere to the ethical standard of beneficence, the duty to help, to produce beneficial outcomes, or at least to do no harm within the context of the teaching and learning process (Gaberson & Oermann, 1999). Patients must be aware that a learner is involved in their care as part of informed consent and preceptors should ensure that the learner has demonstrated the knowledge and skill to provide care safely prior to doing so independently. The challenge for the preceptor is to achieve not only the desired patient clinical outcomes but also the desired educational outcomes for the student or orientee. The preceptor's judgment must be used exquisitely to determine when a learner can provide care safely and learn safely to achieve both goals.

CONCLUSION

The preceptored clinical experience is a valuable teaching and learning methodology with clear benefits for academic institutions and healthcare organizations alike. Students and orientees who are in the preceptee role benefit from the real-world experience of seasoned clinical staff preceptors. Preceptors benefit by adding this credential to their experience and learning new and valuable teaching, communication, and evaluation skills. Planning and communication are the keys to ensuring a successful period of socialization and role transition for the preceptee.

NEW GRADUATE CRITICAL CARE PROGRAM

The New Graduate Critical Care Program (Mylott & Ciesielski, 2003; Mylott & Greenspan, 2005) is a 6-month orientation and continuing education program designed to develop and support baccalaureate prepared new graduate registered nurses (RNs) in the acquisition of experiential nursing knowledge and the application of theory and research in the care of critically ill patients. Using Benner's (1984) and Benner et al.'s (1996) concepts explicating the development of novice nursing practice, the program combines participative and reflective didactic sessions with a preceptored clinical practicum in the intensive care unit of hire. Preceptor development is facilitated through group workshops and individual consultation as requested. Eight intensive care units participate in the program including medical, surgical/trauma, cardiac surgery, neurological, pediatric, burn, postanesthesia, and coronary care. A team of central and unit-based critical care nurse directors, clinical nurse specialists, educators, and human resources staff meet regularly to provide program oversight and development.

The program is 6 months in length and the majority of participants complete it within the allotted time. Formal didactic instruction is completed within 5 months and the last month is class free to allow for immersion in practice. This approach serves as a transition period to full professional responsibility. This time frame is consistent with the literature on similar programs, and the nursing leadership believes that a 6-month orientation is needed for the new graduate to acquire the experiential knowledge and clinical skills to practice safely and independently. Preceptors and leadership believe that much of the variation in readiness to practice occurs in the last 2 months, when the work is largely about becoming an independent clinician.

PARTICIPANT CHARACTERISTICS

Through experience, the leadership group has identified several attributes that are associated with success. These attributes include experience working as a nursing assistant in critical care, passing the NCLEX RN licensing exam on the first attempt, and a committed desire to practice in critical care.

The average age of the program's new graduate nurse participants is 24.5 years as compared with an average age of over 46.8 years for the general nursing population in the United States (US Department of Health and Human Services [HHS], 2004). Implications for a growing proportion of younger nurses in the practice environment are described within the literature (Nursing Executive Center, 2002). In response, the program planners implemented a workshop on generational differences as an intervention to facilitate communication and the development of positive relationships

between preceptors and new graduates that is delivered as needed (Tyrrell, 2005). Program evaluations of this workshop are positive to date.

To evaluate the professional development of the new graduate participants, email surveys with questions targeted toward their achievements were sent to participants in the first four classes (n = 24) who are currently employed at the institution. An 88% response rate (n = 21) was achieved and collated responses indicate that respondents have accomplished much professionally and are highly involved in professional development activities. In addition to the items cited in the Table 28-1, five respondents have served as preceptors to subsequent new graduate program participants.

CURRICULUM

The curriculum addresses the learning needs of both the new graduate preceptees and the experienced nurse preceptors. For the preceptees, a variety of learning options and supports are offered throughout the 6-month experience. The style of teaching is case-based, including simulation, narrative, and discussion sessions. Topic areas cover pathophysiology encountered in critically ill children and adults and interventions for each illness discussed. Content focuses on managing the patient requiring mechanical ventilation as well as patients requiring close cardiac monitoring, invasive hemodynamic monitoring, and neurological monitoring. Simulation sessions include respiratory

Table 28-1 Professional Development Survey Responses

Professional Development Indicators	Affirmative Response (%)	Number
Enrolled in graduate school	37	8
CVVH competent	94	20
Serves as unit resource nurse	59	12
Have passed CCRN exam or completed review course with intent to take exam	37	8
Clinical Advancement Program participation	10	2
Project Hope humanitarian effort participation	6	1

CCRN, critical care registered nurse; CVVH, continuous veno-venous hemofiltration;

distress and failure, shock, dysrhythmias with hemodynamic consequences, and cardiopulmonary arrests. These sessions require participants to work as a team to assess the patient, identify actual and potential problems, communicate and collaborate with various members of the healthcare team to identify and initiate interventions, and evaluate outcomes.

The preceptors are offered a workshop prior to participating in the program. The content includes new graduate behavior as described by Benner et al. (1996), teaching strategies, learning styles, communication and feedback skills, and interventions for precepting challenges. Techniques include simulation, case-based discussions, reflection, and role modeling. There is a panel discussion with experienced preceptors. Throughout the course of the 6-month program, preceptors are offered the opportunity to meet and discuss challenges with their peers.

The program's effectiveness is evaluated using a variety of measures. A focus group of preceptors and orientees is held in the fifth month to review the effectiveness from the participant's perspective. An evaluation tool is given to both preceptors and orientees to determine program effectiveness and areas in need of change. The tool's elements require both preceptors and orientees to evaluate the orientees' readiness to practice independently. In addition, both preceptors and orientees complete self evaluations of how they fulfilled their program roles, as well as evaluating their partner's effectiveness in fulfilling program roles. Finally a postprogram review of each orientees' capabilities is done using standards agreed to by the intensive care unit leadership. The standards include participants' ability to:

- Manage patients requiring invasive, closely monitored treatments such as continuous venous to venous hemodialysis.
- Serve as a resource nurse responsible for managing the flow of patients and staff during a work shift.
- Function as a program preceptor within 2 years of program completion.

NEW GRADUATE IN CRITICAL CARE PRECEPTOR NARRATIVE

The following is an adaptation of a narrative written by an experienced staff nurse preceptor (Albert, 2004). It describes the events of a typical day spent orienting a new graduate nurse participating in the hospital's New Graduate Critical Care Program. The narrative was submitted as part of a portfolio in support of the preceptor's nomination as the first Norman Knight Preceptor of Distinction Award. Nominees are asked to submit a narrative that illustrates their abilities as a preceptor. The author of the narrative, Jennifer Albert, RN, BSN, a staff nurse in the surgical/trauma intensive care unit received the award. Awardees receive funds to attend a graduate course of their choice or protected paid time to complete a course of study with a clinical nurse specialist in their area of interest. An annual ceremony is held to announce the award and is followed by a reception for the hospital community and invited guests. A plaque that describes the award's purpose and lists the names of awardees is prominently displayed on the first floor of the hospital. The names of the patient and preceptee used in the narrative have been changed to ensure anonymity.

> I am a staff nurse in the Surgical Intensive Care Unit where I have practiced for the past 7 years. My nursing career began in 1989, 6 months before graduating from nursing school. As part of my senior practicum, I spent 20 hours per week working one-on-one with an experienced nurse on the surgical/trauma floor. I was blessed with a preceptor who was warm and welcoming, patient and professional, and who, above all, had the desire to share her knowledge and expertise with me, the neophyte nurse. I credit this positive experience with my willingness to take the challenge of reciprocating two years later when I was approached

about precepting a student nurse from my alma mater. I was a bit apprehensive, as I had no previous teaching experience. What I did have, however, was the desire to share my newly acquired knowledge and to make this a fulfilling experience for this student, just as had been done for me 2 years previously.

Since my first experience in 1991, I have had the opportunity and privilege to serve as a preceptor for over a dozen nurses, all with varied levels of experience. My intent here is not to sound boastful, but rather, grateful. For, it is I who has truly been enriched both professionally and personally by each of these individuals whom I've had the opportunity to precept over the years.

Presently, I am nearing the halfway mark in a 6-month orientation process with my preceptee, Sue, a new graduate nurse enrolled in the critical care program. The narrative that follows is a glimpse into one of our days together.

Andy is a 39-year-old with a history of psoriases who had presented to an outside hospital with diffuse erythema extending from his thigh to his ankle, fever, and worsening renal failure and mental status, despite having received a dose of IV antibiotics in this hospital the previous night. His symptoms were most likely the result of either renal failure or profound sepsis. He was transferred to our hospital for further evaluation and his admitting diagnosis was necrotizing fasciitis. Andy would most likely be the most challenging and complex patient Sue had cared for thus far. Yet, as a preceptor, I knew the circumstances couldn't be more ideal because Sue had already had some exposure to this patient, as she had had the opportunity to observe his surgery, as well as participate in admitting him to our unit.

We assemble outside of Andy's room at 7:00 AM with the flow sheet to get report from the night nurse. I make the calculated, but hopefully inconspicuous decision to move my seat, so that I am sitting next to Sue so that she is sandwiched between the night nurse and me. A few years ago, it never would have occurred to me that where I sat during report had any relevance. Yet, one of my former orientees commented to me one day, "Have you ever noticed that during report they (the nurses giving report) tend to always address you?" Frankly, I had never made this observation, but as I watched over the next few months, it became apparent that this was indeed true. My colleagues had the tendency to talk directly to me, almost turning their backs toward my orientee at times. To prevent this, I began to position myself directly next to my orientee, so that there was no confusion and we were both being addressed during report.

We were told that Andy was started on drotrecogin alfa. Other critical pieces of data we receive during report are that his platelet level has fallen to 40,000, his hematocrit is trending down, and his leg dressing, which had not been bloody during the night, was now saturated with blood, only 1 hour after the surgeons had changed it.

We enter the room together and Sue begins the morning routine of zeroing and leveling transducers, setting alarms, checking drug doses, and infusion rates. I note, but choose not to yet verbalize my own observation, that there is heparin in all of the transducer bags. I quietly wonder if Sue has made the same observation and, if she has, will she make the connection that even this small amount of heparin could be contributing to Andy's thrombocytopenia and therefore needs to be removed from the transducers. Sue begins a thorough physical assessment. Andy's neurological status is difficult to assess since he is heavily sedated. Recalling that with previous patients we had shut off the propofol drip in order to get a more thorough exam, Sue questions whether we should do this with Andy. Sue's ability to incorporate previous experiences is becoming evident and I support her plan, but cautiously remind her about what had been relayed to us in report—that Andy becomes dyssynchronous with the ventilator and tends to drop his oxygen saturation when awake or undersedated. My role as preceptor is to help Sue anticipate this potential instability and I do so by questioning her about how she plans to react and what interventions she plans to employ should Andy become unstable. With an action plan in place, Sue moves ahead.

Having completed her physical exam, Sue discusses her findings and observations. She is particularly concerned and focused on the continued bleeding from Andy's leg. His dressing is now saturated with blood. At this point in her orientation, Sue has no previous experience to draw on that would allow her to differentiate normal from excessive bleeding. I attempt to coax from her what she might expect to see in a patient who had lost significant blood volume by asking "How might the patient's hemodynamic profile change?," "What lab values would be of particular concern?," and "What medications might be contributing to this ongoing bleeding?" Together we explore the answers, examining the most recent vital signs, interpreting the reading from the Swan Ganz catheter, and discussing the signs of hypovolemia. Lastly I prompt Sue about the medication that may be contributing to the patient's condition. She reviews Andy's medication list, but is unable to identify the two drugs that I find concerning. I suggested that she take a close look at the transducer bags. I immediately see the smile go across her face as she identifies her earlier oversight, even before actually looking at the bags. Sue removes the heparin from the transducers and I recommend that she take a 10-minute break to read about drotrecogin alfa, knowing that once she does, she will be able to identify my second concern—that this medication increases the risk of bleeding and is contraindicated with acute bleeding.

Sue is far enough along in her orientation that she has begun to take a more active and participatory role in rounds. Today I will take a backseat role and allow her the primary role of interacting with the physicians during rounds. In preparation for this, I assist her in generating a list of questions in regards to the bleeding that she might want to have answered or addressed. Rounds begin and I step back into the patient's room, far enough away so that I can hear the discussion, yet not directly involved in it. This will allow Sue the opportunity to independently interact with the physicians, while providing her with the security of knowing I am close by should she need my assistance. Following rounds, I have Sue reiterate the plan for the day, which she may think is redundant, but I need to know she has extrapolated the correct information from rounds and that she is clear on how we are to proceed.

UNBUNDLING THE NARRATIVE

Ms. Albert's narrative provides an insightful view into the thinking and practice of an expert preceptor. She chose to become a preceptor based on her own positive experience working with a caring and skilled preceptor, her wish to continue that experience for others, and finally her realization of the rewards of precepting through her own personal and professional sense of enrichment. Ms. Albert's passion for the role comes through clearly in the course of the narrative.

The expertise of precepting is apparent from the way Ms. Albert introduces the patient she selected for the shift. She was thoughtful and goal directed in the choice of patient assignment and gave specific reasons for her selection. She also displayed her awareness of the level of acuity this patient presented and the challenge this would be for Sue, her preceptee. Ms. Albert's clinical expertise is woven throughout the narrative, as she is able to guide her preceptee while anticipating potential patient problems and possible interventions.

Ms. Albert describes the importance of having a sharing, respectful relationship with a preceptee. When a preceptee she had worked with previously presented her with a critical observation regarding staff behavior toward preceptees during report, Ms. Albert felt compelled to followed up to confirm. This resulted in a decisive change in her personal placement during report, underscoring her openness as a preceptor. She mirrors this behavior later in the narrative when she describes her placement in the background during rounds with the physician staff. Ms. Albert never leaves Sue completely alone, but choreographs her presence such that it will not prevent other healthcare team members from treating the preceptee as the patient's nurse.

Ms. Albert's awareness of the new graduate's need for routine is clear as she describes the daily regimen Sue must follow when starting the shift. She is constantly aware of the patient and his needs and is thinking many steps ahead of the preceptee, but allows the preceptee time to think through and problem solve for herself. Rather than specifically telling Sue directly what to look for, she coaches, provides clues, and asks thoughtful questions to guide her. In so doing, Ms. Albert teaches and informs the preceptee while preparing her to begin her own critical thinking process. Ms. Albert uses this process several times during the shift to help Sue identify actual and potential clinical issues and also to help her devise a plan for intervention. The tactic is also utilized to prepare Sue to participate in rounds with the healthcare team. Prepping the preceptee is another example of how an expert preceptor teaches and helps build the new graduate's self confidence and self esteem.

Finally, Ms. Albert is tuned into her preceptee's own needs. When she provides time for Sue to review drotrecogin alfa, she is aware of her preceptee's informational needs, but also her need to step back and consider all that had occurred to that point in the day. The same holds true when Ms. Albert reviews the discussion from rounds that creates an opportunity for Sue to not only review the care plan, but also to ask questions or clarify the points discussed. Finally, Ms. Albert is aware of how Sue may feel about this process and is prepared to explain her reasons for engaging in such a manner.

Ms. Albert's narrative exemplifies the characteristics of an expert preceptor, starting with her commitment to precepting, extending through her own clinical expertise, and concluding with her ability to teach, coach, and guide her preceptee in a compassionate, respectful, yet structured manner.

REFERENCES

Albert, J. (2004). Preceptor narrative. *Caring Headlines. 1*, 4–5.

Alspach, J. G. (2000). *From staff nurse to preceptor: A preceptor development program. Instructor's Manual* (2nd ed., pp. 11–13). Aliso Viejo, CA: American Association of Critical Care Nurses.

Baggot, D., Hensinger, B., Parry, J., Valdes, M. S., & Zaim, S. (2005). The new hire/preceptor experience: Cost-benefit analysis of one retention strategy. *Journal of Nursing Administration. 35*(3), 138–145.

Benner, P. (1984). *From novice to expert: Excellence and power in clinical nursing practice.* Upper Saddle River, NJ: Prentice Hall.

Benner, P., Tanner, C., & Chesla, C. (1996). Entering the field: Advanced beginner practice. In P. Benner, C. Tanner, & C. Chesla (Eds.), *Expertise in nursing practice: Caring, clinical judgment, and ethics* (pp. 48–77). New York: Springer.

Berkow, S., Virkstis, K, Stewart, J., & Conway, L. (2009). Assessing new graduate nurse performance. *Nurse Educator, 34*(1), 17–22.

Boychuck-Duchsher, J. (2001). Out in the real world: Newly graduated nurses in acute-care speak out. *Journal of Nursing Administration, 31*(9), 426–439.

Boyle, D. K., Popkess-Vawter, S., & Taunton, R. L. (1996). Socialization of new graduate nurses in critical care. *Heart and Lung, 25*(2), 141–154.

Casey, K., Fink, R., Krugman, M., & Propst, J. (2004). The graduate nurse experience. *Journal of Nursing Administration*, 34(6), 303–311.

Corlett, J., Palfreyman, J. W., Staines, H. J., & Marr, H. (2003). Factors influencing theoretical knowledge and practice skill acquisition in student nurses: An empirical experiment. *Nurse Education Today, 23*(3), 183–190.

Gaberson, K., & Oermann, M. H. (1999). *Clinical teaching strategies in nursing*. New York: Springer.

Gerke, M. L. (2001). Understanding and leading the quad matrix: Four generations in the workplace: The traditional generation, boomers, gen x, nexters. *Seminars for Nurse Managers, 9*(3), 173–181.

Godinez, G., Schweiger, J., Gruver, J., & Ryan, P. (1999). Role transition from graduate to staff nurse: A qualitative analysis. *Journal for Nurses in Staff Development, 15*(3), 97–110.

Goh, K., & Watt, E. (2003). From 'dependent on' to 'depended on': The experience of transition from student to registered nurse in a private hospital graduate program. *Australian Journal of Advanced Nursing, 21*(1), 14–20.

Guhde, J. (2005). When orientation ends . . . Supporting the new nurse who is struggling to succeed. *Journal for Nurses in Staff Development, 21*(4), 145–149.

Hickey, M. (2009) Preceptor perceptions of new graduate nurse readiness for practice. *Journal for Nurses in Staff Development,* 25(1), 35–41.

Horsburgh, M. (1989). Graduate nurses' adjustment to initial employment: Natural field work. *Journal of Advanced Nursing, 14*(8), 610–617.

Kolb, A. Y., & Kolb, D. A. (2005). *The Kolb learning style inventory-version 3.1: 2005 technical specifications*. Boston: Hay Resources Direct.

Kolb, D. A. (2005). *The Kolb learning style inventory-version 3.1: Self scoring and interpretation booklet*. Boston: Hay Resources Direct.

Luhanga, F., Yonge, O., & Myrick, F. (2008) Hallmarks of unsafe practice. *Journal for Nurses in Staff Development, 24*(6), 257–264

Kramer, M. (1974). *Reality shock: Why nurses leave nursing*. St. Louis, MO: C V Mosby.

Marcum, E. H., & West, R. D. (2004). Structured orientation for new graduates: A retention strategy. *Journal for Nurses in Staff Development, 20*(3), 118–124.

Modic, M. B., & Harris, R. (2007). Masterful precepting: Using the BECOME method to enhance clinical teaching. *Journal for Nurses in Staff Development, 23*(1), 1–8.

Mylott, L., & Ciesielski, S. (2003). It takes a village: New graduate nurses enter critical care at Massachusetts General Hospital. *Advance for Nurses,* 29–30, 32.

Mylott, L., & Greenspan, M. (2005). *MGH-IHP new graduate in critical care program annual report*. Executive summary presented to the Vice President for Patient Care and Chief Nurse, Massachusetts General Hospital and the Director, Graduate Program in Nursing, MGH Institute for Health Professions, Boston, MA.

Neumann, J. A., Brady-Schluttner, K. A., McKay, A. K., Roslien, J. J., Twedell, D. M., & James, K. M. G. (2004). Centralizing a registered nurse preceptor program at the institutional level. *Journal for Nurses in Staff Development, 20*(1), 17–24.

Nursing Executive Center. (2002). *Nursing's next generation: Best practices for attracting, training, and retraining new graduates*. Washington, DC: The Advisory Board Company.

Oermann, M. H., & Moffitt-Wolfe, A. (1997). New graduates' perceptions of clinical practice. *The Journal of Continuing Education in Nursing, 28*(1), 20–25.

O'Malley, C., Cunliffe, E., Hunter, S., & Breeze, J. (2000). Preceptorship in practice. *Nursing Standard, 14*(28), 45–49.

Peirce, A. G. (1991). Preceptorial students' view of their clinical experience. *Journal of Nursing Education, 30*(6), 244–249.

Santucci, J. (2004). Facilitating the transition into nursing practice: Concepts and strategies for mentoring new graduates. *Journal for Nurses in Staff Development, 20*(6), 274–284.

Smith, A., & Chalker, N. (2005). Preceptor continuity in a nurse internship program: The nurse intern's perception. *Journal for Nurses in Staff Development, 21*(2), 47–52.

Speers, A. T., Strzyzewski, N., & Ziolkowski, L. D. (2004). Preceptor preparation: An investment in the future. *Journal for Nurses in Staff Development, 20*(3), 127–133.

Tradewell, G. (1996). Rites of passage: Adaptation of nursing graduates to a hospital setting. *Journal of Nursing Staff Development, 12*(4), 183–189.

Tyrrell, R. (2005). *Understanding and leading a multigenerational workforce.* Boston: Massachusetts General Hospital.

US Department of Health and Human Services. (2004). The registered nurse population: Findings from the March 2004 national sample survey of registered nurses. Retrieved May 8, 2009 from http://bhpr.hrsa.gov/healthworkforce/rnsurvey04/

Weston, M. (2001). Coaching generations in the workplace. *Nursing Administration Quarterly, 25*(2), 11–21.

ADDITIONAL RESOURCES

Baltimore, J. (2004). The hospital clinical preceptor: Essential preparation for success. *Journal of Continuing Education in Nursing, 35*(3), 133–140.

Flynn, J. P., & Stack, M. C. (Eds.) (2006). *The role of the preceptor: A guide for nurse educators, clinicians, and managers* (2nd ed.). New York: Springer.

Johnson, S. A., & Romanello, M. L. (2005). Generational diversity: Teaching and learning approaches. *Nurse Educator, (30)*5, 212–216.

Yonge, O., & Myrick, F. (2004). Preceptorship and the preparatory process for undergraduate nursing students and their preceptors. *Journal for Nurses in Staff Development, 20*(6), 294–297.

CHAPTER 29

Student Learning in a Faculty–Student Practice Clinic

Jennifer E. Mackey, Marjorie Nicholas, and Lesley Maxwell

INTRODUCTION

If we are to pursue excellence in any field, we must go beyond knowledge and skills in our education of graduate students. We need to identify the qualities of mind that underlie excellence and leadership potential in our disciplines and we need to build those qualities into the foundations of our educational programs.

What does it mean to have a critical spirit? Experts in the field of critical thinking use this metaphorical phrase to mean, "a probing inquisitiveness, a keenness of mind, a zealous dedication to reason, and a hunger or eagerness for reliable information" (Facione, 2009). The faculty of the graduate program in communication sciences and disorders at the MGH Institute of Health Professions asked itself this question: What are the foundational qualities of mind that excellence and leadership in the field are built upon and how can they be identified and nurtured in our graduate students? The result has been the development of an enhanced clinical curriculum that emphasizes excellence and systematically develops critical thinking, innovation, collaboration, social perception, risk taking, and self knowledge and reflection in our students.

Professional licensure and program accreditation standards form the basis of the academic and clinical curriculum of clinical education programs. The American Speech-Language-Hearing Association (ASHA) requires that the education of graduate students who are seeking to become speech-language pathologists includes the acquisition of both *knowledge* and *skills* in a variety of content and disorder areas (ASHA, 2005). The breadth and depth of knowledge and skill that is required for recent healthcare graduates to practice effectively in current times is immense. Programs of all types are struggling to develop the sophisticated knowledge and skills in their graduates needed to meet an ever-expanding scope of practice. So why expand the demands on students and faculty by developing an extra set of requirements related to the esoteric ideas of excellence or leadership?

The reason is simple. In a world where knowledge is exploding and skill sets must keep pace, the most valuable education is one that teaches you to think critically, to be innovative, to collaborate effectively, to take the perspectives of others and modify your behavior accordingly, to understand the value of taking thoughtful risks, and to practice in a manner that is self reflective. Education should teach students how to unlock their personal potential to spend a lifetime pursuing excellence and becoming leaders in their chosen field.

As in most healthcare programs, ensuring that students gain the requisite knowledge base required by the accrediting body is accomplished primarily via academic coursework. And, like education models in many healthcare professions, most programs in speech-language pathology in the United States utilize a series of clinical externships in which students work in different healthcare and educational settings to acquire the clinical skills they will need to become professional practicing clinicians. Most also have onsite clinics in which students learn the preliminary clinical skills they need before venturing out to their externships. In this chapter, we describe the MGH Institute of Health Professions' faculty–student practice clinic, known as the Speech, Language and Literacy Center. The center operates as both an entry level and an advanced practice clinic. While the examples we provide will necessarily be related to speech-language pathology, we believe the lessons learned from this clinical educational model are pertinent to a broad range of healthcare professionals.

The model of clinical education we will describe in this chapter is known as the *teacher-practitioner model* (Meyer, McCarthy, Klodd, & Gaseor, 1995; Montgomery, Enzbrenner, & Lerner, 1991; Peach & Meyer, 1996). One of the important features that we will highlight of our implementation of this model is the integration of academic (knowledge based) with clinical (practical and excellence skills based) education. We describe both our entry level and advanced practice clinics and then discuss the positive outcomes and challenges of using this model.

DEFINITION AND PURPOSE OF THE TEACHER-PRACTITIONER MODEL

The essential principle of the teacher-practitioner model is that students learn best from individuals who have dual roles as teachers and practicing clinicians. In this model, the supervising faculty member teaches the student in the classroom and also directs the clinical interaction with clients in the clinic through modeling and guided practice. In one of the most well-known models of supervision in speech-language pathology (Anderson, 1981; McCrea & Brasseur, 2003), a continuum of skill development is emphasized for both the student and the supervisor. Interaction between the two parties is also a key feature of the continuum model. This interaction and the continuum of skill development are also fundamental features of the teacher-practitioner model. This model is used by many academic institutions and seeks to create a strong link between scholarly and professional roles of the supervisor. Students have opportunities to see firsthand how theory relates to their clinical work with individuals with communication disorders. This model is the foundation for our faculty–student practice clinic, which serves two primary purposes: (1) it operates as a site for the education of students and (2) it provides communication therapy services to the community.

In its main role as a setting focused on student learning, the clinic provides an atmosphere for the integration of academic knowledge and research-based practice in a clinical environment. As a place where supervisors mentor beginning clinicians, an onsite clinic is an ideal environment for linking clinical practice with theory and academic coursework. This setting encourages the development of excellence skills as well as the development of students' self evaluation and self reflection skills and the establishment of personal goals for clinical and professional growth. Superficially, it might appear that the "best" learning atmosphere is a "real world" setting, such as a hospital, rehabilitation center, or specialty clinic. While these settings offer diverse, rich, and important experiences, the pressures of productivity, insurance issues, and medically complex patients make these environments exceptionally challenging for beginning clinicians (ASHA, n.d.). Like many healthcare professionals, speech-language pathologists face personnel shortages and increased requirements for documentation. External supervisors, or preceptors, often struggle with the demands of high caseloads and not enough time to teach and support students with limited knowledge and experience. Therefore, these settings are often best suited to advanced students who have already developed a solid basis for the understanding of intervention planning, diagnosis, and professional interaction.

The design of the teacher-practitioner model at the MGH Institute is uncommon across graduate programs in speech-language pathology nationally. Because of institutional requirements related to tenure and financial pressures at many colleges, academic faculty rarely participate in clinical work and clinicians involved in supervising students within graduate school clinics are often not faculty and are frequently unfamiliar with the academic curriculum. Thus, the split between researcher/academic and clinician begins immediately in the educational process itself. Beginning students need clear paths drawn from the classroom to clinical application if they are to learn to think critically while developing a scholarly approach to practice based on evidence from research. A teacher-practitioner setting provides this bridge from the classroom to the clinic. It is a bridge that is crossed in both directions, because research in applied fields should be guided by questions that arise in the real world of practice.

A secondary purpose of the faculty–student practice clinic is to provide diagnostic and therapeutic services to community members with communication disorders. Since the faculty–student practice clinic is an integral part of the educational program, the hosting educational institution financially supports the clinic as a place for student learning. Therefore, the clinic is not dependent on outside sources such as state or governmental funding or payments from insurance or private pay individuals. Clients are requested to pay a nominal "user fee" to support purchase of materials used in the clinic such as books, diagnostic tests, treatment materials, and software. This fee can be waived or reduced depending on individual circumstances. No client is ever denied services because of the inability to pay this fee. Having a "free" clinic is possible because of the nature of the integration of academic and clinical resources, including teachers and supervisors. Furthermore, because the clinic is not dependent on outside funding, it is able to provide services to underserved and underprivileged populations.

USE OF THE TEACHER-PRACTITIONER MODEL

The Entry Level Clinic

The Speech, Language and Literacy Center was designed as a space for beginning graduate students to work with children and adults with various speech and language disorders, as well as for experienced graduate students to work in a simulated outpatient setting with adults who have acquired language disabilities. The physical layout of the center includes 14 individual treatment rooms and one large group/conference room. A digital observation system allows parents, caregivers, students, and supervisors to observe and record sessions. All treatment rooms have video cameras that project to a third observation room equipped with television monitors. Supervisors can observe sessions in this room and also have the ability to operate the camera remotely from the computer on their office desk. This gives student clinicians independence in the therapy room while they are carefully observed by a supervisor.

Students are supervised by licensed speech-language pathology faculty members with advanced expertise in their field. These supervisors, often called instructors, mentors, or preceptors, are faculty members in the communication sciences and disorders department. The majority of the supervisors also teach academic and clinical courses. This integration of academic and clinical information and experience allows for a unique learning atmosphere for the students, and a rich collegial environment for faculty. This model of blending academic with clinical instruction is the basis of the teacher-practitioner model, and allows students to more fully assimilate information from classes into direct therapy with clients.

Students in their first year of the graduate program will have two semesters of clinical experience in the center. During one of these semesters, students work with children with spoken language disorders such as toddlers, preschoolers, or early school-aged children who demonstrate difficulties in the areas of expressive or receptive language, articulation or phonology, or social communication. These children might also present with a specific diagnosis such as autism, cerebral palsy, or Down syndrome, but most often do not have a specific diagnosis. Students also spend one semester with school-aged children and adults with reading and writing disorders. Some of these clients may have a diagnosis of dyslexia.

These two semesters of clinical experience occur during the first and second semesters of the students' graduate program. In the first semester (fall), the entire class is divided in half and students are assigned randomly to one section: either spoken language or written language. Students move to the alternate section during the second semester (spring) in order to give them experience with another population. Within each section, each student is paired with another student as a dyad partner. Dyad partners share two clients who are each seen twice a week for individual sessions. Each partner is responsible for the creation of weekly lesson plans as well as participating in diagnostic and therapeutic activities. This experience of working with a partner was designed to explicitly facilitate the development of professional collaboration skills.

Beginning clinical work is often highly stressful for novice clinicians. Some students may have experienced some type of clinical environment during their undergraduate education, but many see the clinical world as foreign and daunting. Pairing students with another beginning graduate student fosters a feeling of companionship and collegiality. Since speech-language pathologists rarely work independently in the healthcare and educational fields, learning how to function on a collaborative team is a crucial skill. In addition, working in a partnership provides students with direct experiences with more than one client. This diversity of clients leads students to a greater understanding of a variety of disorders and fosters clinical growth in a manner that working independently with only one client would not allow.

In addition to the dyad partnership, students also participate in a weekly case discussion (CD) group. Students are provided written documentation of CD group expectations and responsibilities. These include examples of behaviors demonstrating the core clinical excellence skills as well as process requirements for case presentation. For example, students are expected to actively participate in group discussions by asking questions that demonstrate critical thinking, giving examples of innovative approaches that they have developed, taking the risk to discuss and analyze errors, reflecting on and assessing their performance, thinking from the perspective of their client, and communicating in a professional manner. Each week, students spend 2 hours with a small group of students in a discussion format, facilitated by a faculty member. Therapy sessions are videotaped so that students can then select a digital segment to present to the group. For example, students might select a clip of a therapy activity that yielded unexpected results, a positive outcome, or perhaps led them toward a question about the client and the therapeutic process. Each student is given time to discuss issues pertaining to his or her client, and is also required to participate in discussions regarding other clients. This forum engages each student in a learning process that expands his or her knowledge base beyond a single client. Since multiple clients are represented, students learn about therapy techniques and treatment planning for a variety of disorders. This type of "peer group supervision" allows students to expand their perspectives to include different viewpoints and to learn from their peers as well as their supervisor (Williams, 1995).

A clinical discussion group syllabus guides the faculty member in facilitating the group. The syllabus includes the core excellence skills to be targeted that week and the knowledge and skill objectives and activities for the week. A questioning hierarchy based on Bloom's Taxonomy of Educational Objectives (Anderson & Krathwohl, 2001; Bloom & Krathwohl, 1956) is used by faculty to facilitate growth in critical thinking. Students are provided with the hierarchy and Bloom's Taxonomy, which are also used to guide written feedback in planning documentation. Students are given explicit information about how to advance through the hierarchy of critical thinking toward advanced skills and self supervision (Anderson, 1988) and how that progress is facilitated by supervisory scaffolding and the use of facilitative questions (Facione, 2009).

Encouraging active engagement in the learning process as a group facilitates critical thinking and self evaluation in all members. The goal of supervision should be to assist students in their own development of self analysis and evaluation as well as problem-solving skills in order for the student to become independent (Anderson, 1988). Active engagement in one's own learning encourages students to maintain an inquisitive nature and nurtures the development of critical thinking (Facione, 2009). These critical thinking concepts and self evaluation measures are outlined for students in a tool that we developed (Table 29-1) that states the expectations for participation in case discussions as well as guidelines to help students consider their own development of communication skills and application of theory to practice within the group setting. The tool was based on the descriptive work of Peter A. Facione (2009) in the area of critical thinking.

This self evaluation tool uses a directional arrow to illustrate a continuum of development of skills. One would expect a beginning student to be toward the left-hand side of the continuum (or the beginning) with such critical thinking skills as analysis or inference. Similarly, one might also expect to see a beginning student at a less developed level in his or her ability to self reflect or demonstrate innovation and creativity. This continuum allows students to see their own growth as clinicians as a developmental process. Few, if any, students in their first term in graduate school would be at a well-developed level for all of these skills.

Table 29-1 Student Self Assessment Form of Clinical Excellence and Critical Thinking Skills

Clinical Excellence Skills		
Skill	**Ranking of Performance**	
	Not Yet Present	**Well Developed**
Facilitates discussions Comes prepared, summarizes information, poses questions, analyzes strengths and weaknesses of session	├──────────	──────────►
Uses professional communication style Uses appropriate vocabulary, grammar, voice, speech rate, and articulation	├──────────	──────────►
Demonstrates self reflection		
• Fair-minded in appraising reasoning	├──────────	──────────►
• Honest in facing one's own biases, prejudices, stereotypes, or egocentric tendencies	├──────────	──────────►
• Prudent in suspending, making, or altering judgments	├──────────	──────────►
• Willing to reconsider and revise views where honest reflection suggests that change is warranted	├──────────	──────────►
• Accurate in identifying strengths and weaknesses	├──────────	──────────►
• Able to self correct	├──────────	──────────►
Demonstrates innovation and creativity	├──────────	──────────►
Collaborates effectively	├──────────	──────────►

(continues)

Table 29-1 Student Self Assessment Form of Clinical Excellence and Critical Thinking Skills *(continued)*

Critical Thinking		
Skill	**Ranking of Performance**	
	Not Yet Present	**Well Developed**
Analysis Identifies the intended and actual inferential relationships between concepts, facts, questions, descriptions, judgments, experiences, reasons, information, or opinions	├──────────────►	
Inference Identifies and secures elements needed to draw reasonable conclusions; forms conjectures and hypotheses; considers relevant information and induces consequences	├──────────────►	
Explanation States the results of one's reasoning; justifies that reasoning in terms of the evidential, conceptual, methodological, and contextual considerations; presents one's reasoning in the form of cogent arguments	├──────────────►	
Evaluation Assesses the credibility of statements or other representations; assesses the logical strength of the actual or intended inferential relationships among statements, descriptions, or questions	├──────────────►	

The concept of a continuum utilizes a mastery approach to clinical learning and gives the students a feeling of acceptance of current skills, with appropriate vision for areas of needed growth. Students are asked to self evaluate and identify strengths and areas of growth in the beginning of the first term. Students then return to this form to reevaluate their own progress periodically throughout the first and second terms of clinic. Supervisors also look at the student's self assessment of skills and progress and use this information as a point of discussion during midterm and final evaluations. It is common, for example, for students to either overestimate or underestimate their skill level in a particular area. Discussions between supervisors and students about perceived skills allow for the self evaluation process to become a part of the supervision process. Supervisors can then guide students in determining appropriate goals and objectives for growth. Students are encouraged to take this self assessment tool into external practicum experiences and share it with supervisors in these environments in order to continue the learning process with new populations and professional communication situations.

Communication skills are of great importance to anyone practicing in the health professions, yet they do not always come naturally to beginning clinicians. Supervisors seek to encourage students to use both higher level vocabulary and clear definitions when defining diagnostic terms as well as when discussing specific therapeutic strategies and techniques. Within the case discussion group, students have weekly opportunities to orally present information to their peers and supervisor. This develops oral skills of summarization of information, use of clear terminology, and improved professional interaction with colleagues, clients, and caregivers.

Application of theory to practice is not only part of the beginning student's self assessment process, but a journey for everyone throughout his or her career. Application involves taking information learned from an academic class, a journal article, or a professional presentation and applying it to clinical practice in a meaningful way. This is a skill that all professionals should strive for and is a major component of both the clinical and academic experiences in our program. We believe that the teaching of this skill begins with the individuals who are instructing our students.

Faculty members are often engaged in both the teaching process and the supervision of students in our clinic. Most faculty continue to practice within their field of expertise, which allows individuals to keep in close contact with their populations of interest. Some examples include serving as a consultant in early intervention agencies or schools and working in area hospitals or clinics. This also allows a faculty member to remain clinically active, which in turn provides an immediate experience to share with students who are beginning to understand the clinical process. All too often, clinical skills are taught by individuals who have not had an opportunity to practice clinically for many years. The teacher-practitioner model, in contrast, allows students to benefit not only from an instructor's past experience, but also from recent interactions in the clinical field.

Our model encourages faculty to perform in dual roles as clinical supervisors and academic teachers. First of all, new clinical supervisors attend weekly clinical seminars and courses on the theory of speech and language development along with beginning students. This allows new supervisors to understand the perspective and philosophy of the program and to also experience firsthand the coursework required of students. The supervisor can then refer students to readings from class, specifics of class lectures, or comments made by the course professor. Often, the professor of the class will engage the new supervisor in a discussion within the class. Perhaps a particular therapeutic approach is the class topic and the professor might have the supervisor discuss a personal experience or clinical opinion on the use of such an approach. If questions about a particular theory or clinical application arise in a subsequent clinical supervisory session, the professor of the related course can be consulted.

This integration of academic and clinical practice is beneficial to all involved. Students gain a deeper appreciation for course material when it can be applied to clinical experiences. They view the link between information taught in a course and planning for a therapy session as an integration of ideas. Academic information fuels intervention planning and vice versa. Clinical supervisors gain an understanding of the students' academic experience and its relation to current clinical issues. Academic professors find opportunities to link what is taught in the classroom with what happens in the clinical world. This regular interaction among faculty fosters a rich learning environment for students, as well as a rewarding intellectual atmosphere for everyone. The idea that all professionals should continue to explore and grow is an important lesson for students to learn.

The participation of supervisors in academic courses is extended into direct teaching experiences. For example, supervisors might teach a class on a particular topic within a course, or they could teach an entire course in their field of expertise. When clinical faculty teach in academic courses, students benefit from the overt integration of academic information to its practical application to the clinic.

Another way our program uses the teacher-practitioner model is to have primarily academic faculty supervise in the clinic. Professors teaching academic courses also offer professional opinions regarding challenging cases in the clinic. Thus, the program purposely chooses not to draw a clear distinction between faculty who are primarily academic instructors and those who are primarily clinical supervisors.

The Advanced Practice Clinic

The Advanced Practice Clinic specializes in providing diagnostic and treatment services to adults with acquired neurogenic speech and language disorders such as aphasia, dysarthria, alexia, agraphia, and other cognitive-linguistic disorders resulting from brain damage. The clinic was started to provide a site for a subset of the second year graduate students to gain clinical experience working with adults.

It is modeled on a "typical" outpatient rehabilitation clinic that provides speech-language pathology services to people who have had strokes and other adults with acquired communication disorders. The advanced practice clinic operates simultaneously with the entry level clinic, so that both first and second year students are seeing clients in the clinic at the same time. Many other speech-pathology graduate programs throughout the country operate on a similar model.

The clinical excellence curriculum and the teacher-practitioner model provide the base for clinical education across terms. In keeping with the philosophy of the entry level clinic, clinical supervision is provided in the advanced practice clinic by faculty members who also teach the acquired communication disorders courses. This allows for a meaningful integration of the academic knowledge students gain in their courses with the mentored clinical experiences they have with actual clients. As stated previously, we believe that this aspect of the clinical education model is perhaps the most important and novel feature of the program. Students in the advanced practice clinic are expected to develop their clinical excellence and critical thinking skills identified in the curriculum (Table 29-1) to a more advanced level than is expected for the students in the entry level clinic. In addition, because they have already taken the academic coursework relevant to their clientele, they are expected to be more independent in developing evidence-based treatment plans for their clients.

In addition to providing a clinical practicum experience, the advanced practice clinic also allows the students to learn several important realities of the larger healthcare arena. With the high costs of health care in the United States and the limited availability of funds to pay for services, many adults with communication disorders no longer qualify for services. The reasons for this are varied but generally arise from severe limitations in funds for chronic conditions such as aphasia. While a variety of therapies are generally covered by insurance plans in the first few months poststroke or injury, many insurance plans will no longer cover treatments for communication disorders in the chronic phase. As they enter the postacute period, many people with brain injuries from stroke or head trauma are denied further treatment. This is particularly true for individuals with limited means or those without family members to advocate for extended coverage beyond the acute period.

Settings such as the advanced practice clinics in universities and other healthcare education institutions can serve as bridges across this gap in service. Patients can receive the treatments they require and students gain valuable insights into both the nature of chronic impairments and how variably people respond to their chronic conditions.

Individuals in need of services are referred to the advanced practice clinic usually by speech-language pathologists at local hospitals and rehabilitation centers. In addition, many clients are self-referred. Like the entry level clinic, clients are requested to pay the nominal clinic user fee. In the advanced practice clinic, because the majority of clients are middle-aged or elderly adults who were forced to retire from working because of their strokes or other injuries, most have requested waivers of the fee.

The clinical supervisors in the advanced practice clinic manage all new referrals and discharges of clients. Clients may continue to receive services in the clinic for as long as they are benefiting from the intervention provided. Both impairment-based and life participation–based treatments are incorporated into the clinical practice model. Impairment-based therapies are those that would be considered standard treatments to improve a specific speech or language deficit that is interfering with communication to some extent. For example, direct treatment targeting impairments in syntax (the rules for combining words in language) would be a type of impairment-based therapy that could be provided. Life participation–based treatment approaches are attempts to take a step further to address the effects the communication impairment has on an individual's quality of life.

In their academic coursework covering acquired adult language disorders, students learn about the life participation approach to aphasia (LPAA; Chapey et al., 2001). A group of practitioners adhering to the LPAA has published a set of core values that stress that services should be provided to people with aphasia as long as they are needed, that the explicit goal of intervention should be the enhancement of life participation, and that both personal and environmental factors should be the targets of intervention. Similarly, the National Aphasia Association has recently published its Aphasia Bill of Rights, which stresses similar values (National Aphasia Association, n.d.). Students learn about this approach and other recent advances in their academic coursework, but experiencing them firsthand in the advanced practice clinic makes them come alive for the students.

Students have experiences providing both impairment-based therapies in individual treatment sessions and focusing on life participation enhancements with each client. For example, there is a cafe adjacent to the clinic where many clients meet to have lunch prior to the weekly aphasia support group meeting. Within the model of the LPAA, an appropriate intervention target would be to work with the staff at the cafe to educate them about aphasia and to teach them strategies to maximize communication interactions with people who may have communication impairments. Another target might be to work with the cafe to encourage them to have "aphasia-friendly" menus and signs that had pictures in addition to words. These actions would result in an improved quality of life for our clients, even though the clients themselves did not receive the interventions directly.

Each semester, in addition to developing and carrying out individualized treatment plans, the students are also required to assist with the aphasia support group and help plan group outings into the community. These outings have included events such as lunch at a nearby restaurant, seeing an IMAX movie at the local science museum, and attending a major league baseball game. Making the arrangements for these events has forced the students to think about how their clients must cope with physical, cognitive, and language disabilities in everyday life situations. As a result of their participation in these events, every student in the advanced practice clinic has commented on how inspired they have been by these experiences.

Students may also gain research experience in either the entry level or advanced practice clinic. They have an option to complete a master's thesis during their 2-year program, and many have completed projects either fully or partially within the onsite clinic. Individual case studies, small-group assessment studies, and short-term treatment studies are possible types of projects that can be conducted within the clinic. In planning and conducting their research, students become familiar with the process necessary to complete a research project, from the initial step of getting approval from an institutional review board (IRB) to the final stages of data analysis and interpretation. While students are not required to do their research projects in the clinic, the availability of subjects of all ages with a variety of communication disorders onsite makes the process easier to accomplish for many students.

Students who elect not to do a master's thesis have been able to gain research experience by participating in various faculty members' projects. For example, one of the clinical supervisors had an ongoing project investigating the efficacy of an alternative communication treatment software program. Students assisted in the project by delivering the treatments according to the research protocol and conducting the periodic assessment sessions.

Having the advanced practice clinic onsite at the Institute operating year-round also provides opportunities for first year students to observe second year students, as well as opportunities for students from other programs (e.g., nursing, physical therapy) to watch sessions. In addition, students are assigned projects in their academic coursework that require them to observe a treatment session and carefully document what they observed, and to determine what they think the treatment goals were in that session. Individual clients with aphasia and other neurogenic communication disorders have also been invited to be guest speakers in the class on aphasia. While students have many opportunities to watch videotaped examples of people with aphasia, they find that live interactions with people are even more valuable.

Finally, the mix of clients in our waiting areas, who are attending either the entry level or the advanced practice clinic, has resulted in some interesting learning experiences pertaining to living with disabilities among our students, faculty, clients, and their families. For example, we observed children attending the clinic reading books with an adult with aphasia in the waiting room. Young children have direct observation of individuals with disabilities and adult clients have opportunities to interact with young people in a social communication situation that might not otherwise be available to them. Similarly, students, faculty, and staff members benefit from the environment. For example, students in the entry level clinic have the opportunity to interact with adults who have aphasia in the social environment of the waiting room before they have the course on aphasia. This gives the students initial exposure to a population that they will learn about later in their education.

TYPES OF LEARNERS

A faculty–student practice clinic can support a wide range of student learning styles and needs, including students who have little experience with clinical application as well as those who are moving toward independence. Using the teacher-practitioner model, supervisors can often be matched to students with specific needs. For example, an instructor who is an expert writer might supervise a student who needs assistance with the development of clinical writing skills. This model also facilitates the learning styles of students who lack confidence, as well as those who may be considered overconfident.

It is common for students facing their first clinical encounter to feel unprepared, anxious, and frightened. Although many of these students find they are able to move beyond this fear and quickly become acclimated to the clinical environment, some students continue to lack confidence in their clinical and interpersonal skills. The teacher-practitioner model allows the instructor to approach this type of student in a positive, supportive manner. Supervisors might spend time in the therapy room with the student clinician in order to model techniques and strategies before moving outside of the room to observe via camera. Students are encouraged to use self evaluation and peer discussion as a means of improving self confidence and awareness of areas of strength.

Likewise, students who have exaggerated perceptions of their knowledge and clinical skills (Brasseur, McCrea, & Mendel, 2005; Dowling, 2001) can also be supported in a faculty–student practice clinic. It is for these students that the development of self evaluation skills is most critical prior to sending a student into an external placement. Analysis of a video after the session can be useful in order for the student to have a more objective view of what occurred in the session. For example, a supervisor might assist a student in analyzing a video clip of a session where a client's desired behavioral objective was not met. The supervisor can then help the student identify clinical and personal skills that need to be further developed.

CONCLUSION

Many positive outcomes have emerged as a result of this clinical training model. First, the teacher-practitioner model has allowed our students to be highly prepared when entering external practicum experiences. In fact, many external supervisors report that students are good critical thinkers and adopt professional roles easily. As a result, our students receive multiple job offers upon graduation and have become highly successful professionals in the field. The emphasis on excellence throughout the program allows students to become lifelong learners who see their professional growth as a continuum of development. Many alumni currently volunteer to precept our students in their clinical setting and several former students have returned to our program to teach courses and supervise students in our onsite clinic.

The onsite clinic is a student learning environment that enhances the integration of academic and clinical experiences and provides a rich atmosphere for the sharing of knowledge and expertise among faculty and students. The use of peers as dyads during the students' first year fosters personal growth in a collegial, supportive environment. Students learn to work as team members and to interact with a variety of clients as they learn to apply academic knowledge to clinical practice.

Some challenges of this model are common to many clinical education settings. These include logistical matters such as coordinating academic and clinical schedules with students, faculty, and clients; space management; parking; and maintenance of clinical materials. Another challenge is ensuring the right mix of clients each semester for our student clinicians. Clients with complex communication disorders who require expert therapeutic intervention may not be appropriate for a clinic geared toward the education of beginning clinicians. Similarly, clients with mild disorders are often challenging for novice clinicians because mild disorders are sometimes difficult to perceive. Therefore, finding clients that will benefit from working with graduate students is an important consideration when planning a faculty–student practice clinic.

It is crucial that faculty have time built into their schedules to meet and discuss student issues, academic planning, and coordination of course topics with clinical needs. For example, conducting a class about how to use diagnostic materials is especially helpful if this class comes before a student needs to test a client in the clinic. This is one example of how the teacher-practitioner model can function at its highest level.

This model in a faculty–student practice clinic allows for the integration of academic knowledge, the development of clinical skills, and the beginning preparation for a lifetime of excellence. The onsite practice clinic is a well-traveled bridge between the classroom and the clinic.

Leadership and the pursuit of excellence are not something that universities "train into" students. Students sit before us with the potential for a lifetime of excellence in service; it is our job to facilitate the unfolding of that potential.

REFERENCES

American Speech-Language-Hearing Association. (2005). *2005 Standards and implementation procedures for the certificate of clinical competence*. Retrieved September 1, 2009, from http://www.asha.org/certification/slp_standards.htm.

American Speech-Language-Hearing Association. (n.d.). *Responding to the changing needs of speech-language pathology and audiology students in the 21st century*. Retrieved September 1, 2009, from http://www.asha.org/academic/reports/changing.

Anderson, J. (1981). Training of supervisors in speech-language pathology and audiology. *ASHA, 23,* 77–82.

Anderson, J. L. (1988). *The supervisory process in speech-language pathology and audiology*. Boston: College-Hill Press.

Anderson, L., & Krathwohl, D. (2001). *A taxonomy for learning, teaching and assessing: A revision of Bloom's Taxonomy of Educational Objectives*. New York: Longman.

Bloom, B. S., & Krathwohl, D. (1956). *Taxonomy of educational objectives: The classification of educational goals, by a committee of college and university examiners. Handbook I: Cognitive Domain*. New York: Longmans, Green.

Brasseur, J. A., McCrea, E. S., & Mendel, L. L. (2005). Remediating poorly performing students in clinical programs. *Perspectives on Issues in Higher Education, 9*(2), 20–26.

Chapey, R., Duchan, J. F., Elman, R. J., Garcia, L. J., Kagan, A., Lyon, J.G., et al. (2001). Life participation approach to aphasia: A statement of values for the future. In R. Chapey (Ed.), *Language intervention strategies in aphasia and related neurogenic communication disorders*. Philadelphia: Lippincott Williams & Wilkins.

Dowling, S. (2001). *Supervision: Strategies for successful outcomes and productivity*. Boston: Allyn & Bacon.

Facione, P. A. (2009). *Critical thinking: What it is and why it counts*. California Academic Press, Insight Assessment. Retrieved September 1, 2009, from http://www.insightassessment.com/pdf_files/what&why2004.pdf.

McCrea, E. S., & Brasseur, J. A. (2003). *The supervisory process in speech-language pathology and audiology*. Boston: Allyn & Bacon.

Meyer, D. H., McCarthy, P. A., Klodd, D. A., & Gaseor, C. L. (1995). The teacher-practitioner model at Rush-Presbyterian-St. Luke's Medical Center. *American Journal of Audiology, 4,* 32–35.

Montgomery, L., Enzbrenner, L., & Lerner, W. (1991). The practitioner-teacher model revisited. *Journal of Health Administration Education, 9,* 9–24.

National Aphasia Association. (n.d.). *Aphasia Bill of Rights*. Retrieved September 1, 2009, from http://www.aphasia.org.

Peach, R. K., & Meyer, D. H. (1996, April). The teacher-practitioner model at Rush University. *Administration and Supervision Newsletter*, 9–13.

Williams, A. L. (1995). Modified teaching clinic: Peer group supervision in clinical training and professional development. *American Journal of Speech-Language Pathology, 4,* 29–38.

CHAPTER 30

Service Learning

Hendrika Maltby

Students in clinical placements are expected to acquire skills, problem solve, and prepare for future employment in professional fields. Many courses also require students to reflect on their practice: what went well, what did not, and how could practice be improved for the future. Experiential learning and reflection are two of the components of service learning. The involvement of the agency as a true partner in the meeting of agency needs and student learning adds the third component. The focus needs to be on both the students and the recipients of care in partnership (Bailey, Carpenter, & Harrington, 2002). That is, meeting community needs, students' learning objectives, and formal reflection of the experience are the components of service learning. This chapter describes the use of service learning in the health professions.

DEFINITION AND PURPOSE

The Community-Campus Partnerships for Health (CCPH) organization has defined service learning as:

> A structured learning experience that combines community service with preparation and reflection. Students engaged in service-learning provide community service in response to community-identified concerns and learn about the context in which service is provided, the connection between their service and their academic coursework, and their roles as citizens. (CCPH, 2009)

Using this definition, healthcare professionals have discovered that there are many opportunities to work with communities in enhancing health, as well as working with each other. "Service-learning not only connects theory with application and practice but also creates an environment where both the provider of service and the recipient learn from each other" (Norbeck, Connolly,

& Koerner, 1998, p. 2). This ties in with the philosophy of a liberal education, common in North American universities:

> [Liberal education] has always been concerned with cultivating intellectual and ethical judgment, helping students comprehend and negotiate their relationships with the larger world, and preparing them for lives of civic responsibility and leadership. It helps students, both in their general-education courses and in their major fields of study, analyze important contemporary issues like the social, cultural, and ethical dimensions of the AIDS crisis or meeting the needs of an aging population. (Schneider & Humphreys, 2005, p. B20)

Service learning operationalizes liberal education. Its purpose is to involve students in the community to provide a service that is determined by the community and connected to learning objectives in a course. Students begin to "understand that the people of a community are the true experts in knowledge of their community, because both the problems and the assets belong to them" (Mayne & Glascoff, 2002, p. 194).

THEORETICAL FOUNDATIONS

Service as a concept in the community has been implemented since ancient times when people provided support and care to families (Cohen, Johnson, Nelson, & Peterson, 1998). Dewey was one of the first champions of service learning in the early 1900s when service and educational goals were connected (Bailey et al., 2002). Over the years, various American presidents have established a variety of organizations that provided service to communities such as the Peace Corps, VISTA volunteers, the Foster Grandparents program, and the Office of National Service.

Increasingly, community partnerships and interdisciplinary education are coming to the forefront of health professional education. In the Pew Health Commission's 1998 final report, a number of recommendations were made and a set of 21 competencies for the 21st-century health professional were outlined that transcend disciplinary differences (Bellack & O'Neil, 2000). A main recommendation of this report was the requirement that all health professionals have interdisciplinary competence. This incorporates the competencies of partnering with communities to make healthcare decisions, and working in interdisciplinary teams. More recently, the Institute of Medicine (IOM) has made recommendations for education of public health professionals for the 21st century citing that "effective interventions to improve the health of communities will increasingly require community understanding, involvement, and collaboration" (IOM, 2003, p. 15). Service learning is part of this education.

CCPH is a nonprofit organization founded in 1996 that assists in fostering health promoting partnerships between communities and health professional schools (CCPH, 2009; Seifer & Vaughn, 2002). It is a "network of over 1000 communities and campuses throughout the United States and increasingly the world that are collaborating to promote health through service-learning . . . partnerships . . . for improving health professional education, civic engagement and the overall health of communities" (CCPH, 2009). Seifer (1998) also clarifies the differences between service learning, traditional clinical education, and volunteerism. In service learning there is a balance between service and learning objectives, and an emphasis on reciprocal learning, developing citizenship skills and achieving social change, reflective practice, addressing community-identified needs, and the integral involvement of community partners. Seifer emphasizes that service learning is not required volunteerism which lacks reciprocity and reflection and may not be connected to course objectives.

Using service learning in nursing and other health professions enables the development of perceptions and insight as described in cognitive learning theories in the opening chapter (Bradshaw, 2007). Developing a variety of teaching strategies to complement student learning styles is necessary to enhance this development. Students in health professions are usually practice oriented and want to "do something" which relates to the adult learning principles of Knowles (1975) of recognizing the meaning or usefulness of the information learned. Service learning allows the student to implement classroom learning objectives while providing a wanted service to a community.

TYPES OF LEARNERS

Service learning is suitable for any level of student in any program. Diversity and cultural understanding can be key elements. The Corporation for National and Community Service (2006) released a strategic plan for 2006 to 2010 with four focus areas. Focus three describes the elements for engaging students in their communities with the following goals: "engage 5 million college students in service, up from 3.27 million in 2005; and ensure at least 50 percent of America's K-12 schools incorporate service-learning into their curricula" (p. 21). Chapdelaine, Ruiz, Warchal, and Wells (2005) found that approximately 500 college and university presidents have signed the Declaration on the Civic Responsibility of Higher Education which challenges higher education to become engaged with the community so that the knowledge gained by the students can benefit society. Service learning has been added to courses and programs outside of health care as well such as geography, political science, education, and mathematics (C. Williams, personal communication, University of Vermont, Community University Partnership and Service-Learning office, January 14, 2006).

Examples in health care include a variety of professions in multiple settings. Cashman, Hale, Candib, Nimiroski, and Brookings (2004) had medical and nurse practitioner students provide depression screening at a community clinic through the application of service learning providing a mutually beneficial opportunity. Chabot and Holben (2003) integrated service learning into dietetics and nutrition education. Graduate rehabilitation students worked with inner city seniors to provide primary prevention through service learning and also learned about interdisciplinary roles and advocacy for those in need (Hamel, 2001). Occupational and physical therapy students provided service at a childcare facility (Hoppes, Bender, & DeGrace, 2005). The nursing profession uses service learning in partnership with many community agencies including a Sheriff's Department (Fuller, Alexander, & Hardeman, 2006), a tuberculosis screening clinic (Schoener & Hopkins, 2004), women's health (Callister & Hobbins-Garbett, 2000; Mayne & Glascoff, 2002), a Community Health Improvement Center (Carter & Dunn, 2002), and a variety of community health agencies (Mallette, Loury, Engelke, & Andrews, 2005; Redman & Clark, 2002; Simoni & McKinney, 1998). Service learning has also been used as a tool for developing cultural awareness with prenursing students in a first-year experience course (Worrell-Carlisle, 2005).

All of the examples cited here use service learning; students provided a necessary service that was tied into the coursework they were undertaking. Reflection on the service and the process was a key element. Students were able to examine issues such as homelessness in the elderly (Hamel, 2001), disabled children (Hoppes et al., 2005), social justice (Redman & Clark, 2002), underserved rural populations (Simoni & McKinney, 1998), financially disadvantaged (Scott, Harrison, Baker, & Wills, 2005), and culture (Worrell-Carlisle, 2005). Additionally, students had their worldview challenged and often changed their view in the process.

CONDITIONS FOR LEARNING

Service learning courses can be placed anywhere in the curriculum and students can be partnered in groups or as individuals working with homeless people, those with diabetes, residential living centers, health departments—in fact, almost anyone and anywhere. The learning environment becomes very broad and not bound by classroom walls. The first step is to build partnerships with community agencies that match course goals and objectives.

Prerequisites include teaching students what service learning is and the difference with volunteerism. Outlining reflection requirements and how to incorporate this component is essential because reflection helps students to connect the service to course objectives and to understand why service is important. Reflection can be done in a variety of ways such as in-class writing assignments, final papers, or journals.

RESOURCES

Resources can be as much or as little as needed depending on partnerships. Many placements will be able to provide necessary supplies for projects while others may rely on students providing the materials they need. For example, the agency may be able to fund clinics (screening for tuberculosis, cholesterol, etc.); other funding may be found through other sources such as Area Health Education Centers (AHEC) or the university. AHECs were begun by the US government in the late 1970s "to address health staffing distribution and the quality of primary care through community-based initiatives . . . designed to encourage universities and educators to look beyond institutions to partnerships that promote solutions which meet community health needs" (University of Vermont, College of Medicine, 2006). Research grants can also be applied for to incorporate service learning into the curriculum and to evaluate partnerships.

One of the major requirements is time, particularly when developing partnerships. Partners can be found anywhere. This may be through a partnership-type office at the educational institution that keeps a list of partners and their needs (e.g., a town planning office looking for geography students). The faculty member may have contacts via other courses, clinical experiences, service, or research in which they are involved.

Students also need time to provide the service. For example, a 3–credit hour course takes about 9 hours of preparation time for students outside of class; therefore, the service can be a part of the 9 hours. Time can range from 10 to 15 hours over a semester to a concentrated 90 to 135 hours. The revision of assignments for the course can also incorporate the service learning projects. Suggested Web sites that may serve as a resource for faculty are listed at the end of this chapter

USING THE METHOD

Health seldom takes place in a vacuum. It requires the efforts of the individual, family, group, university, and community working in partnership. Service learning works to address the needs identified by a partner. Therefore, one of the first essential steps is to identify a partner. This can be done over a summer, the semester prior to the service learning, or at the beginning of the course. Maurana,

Beck, and Newton (1998) have outlined some principles of good partnerships including common goals, mutual trust and respect, building on strengths, clear communication, and continuous feedback. They list three key themes in building successful partnerships: "1. Always remember that community members are experts in their community, 2. Promise less and deliver more, and 3. Be committed for the long haul" (p. 51). Once the partner has been identified, the contract can be as informal as a verbal agreement ("students will help . . .") or can be a formal written agreement outlining the roles and responsibilities of faculty, students, and partners. Web sites listed at the end of the chapter provide examples of different types of contracts. Partnerships can become one of the strengths of the course and can be utilized each time the course is offered.

The course syllabus needs to incorporate service as part of the course and not as a "mere sidebar" (Heffernan, 2001, p. 1). Heffernan goes on to describe six models of service learning (Table 30-1). The model of service learning chosen for the course will depend on the goals and objectives that students need to meet.

Decisions on the partners and model of service learning lead to the other required components that should be included in the syllabus. How are the students going to engage with the partner? Will students work individually or in groups? Will the partner be a guest speaker in the class? Will students meet partners on their own or will the faculty arrange formal meetings? Will projects be outlined in the syllabus or will the partner and student(s) decide on this together? Will the projects be presented?

The reflection on service in conjunction with course objectives needs to be clear. How are these going to be done (in-class writing assignments that are announced or unannounced, final paper, etc.)? How will they be graded? Are there specific criteria to be used? Will students have a grading rubric? Ash and Clayton (2004) provide an articulated learning structure for reflection through four questions: What did I learn? How did I learn it? Why does this learning matter? In what

Table 30-1 Models of Service Learning

1. Pure service learning where the service is the course content.
2. Discipline-based service learning that makes the link between content and experience explicit.
3. Problem-based service learning in which students may act as consultants.
4. Capstone courses usually offered to students in their final year.
5. Service internships, intense experiences with regular and ongoing reflection.
6. Community-based action research (or community-based participatory research) using research to act as an advocate for the community.

Source: Heffernan, K. (2001). *Fundamentals of service-learning course construction*. Providence RI: Campus Compact.

ways will I use this learning? Similarly, Kuiper (2005) suggests prompts for reflection such as: The problems I encountered . . . I think I solved them by . . . When I had difficulty I . . . Using prompts guides students to critically reflect on the experience and how it affects both the partner and themselves. Table 30-2 provides two examples of grading rubrics.

Table 30-2 Grading Rubric

Health Promotion Across the Life Span: In-Class Reflections
There will be **FOUR** in-class writing assignments based on the readings and your work to date. A question will be posed during the class. You will need to tie in your reading and other work in the response. These will be assessed by how well you link the readings to your work and your thoughts about the two. They will be short and unannounced ahead of time (five marks each).

Community/Public Health Nursing

Journal
Students will complete a journal every 2 weeks (for a total of 6) throughout the semester. The journal will be submitted electronically to the clinical faculty with whom you are working.

Due dates: Journal entries are due Monday mornings.

You will need to address the following items:

1. Summary and reflection of practice: This is a general overview of activities over the past 2 weeks including your thoughts, feelings, judgments, and an evaluation of your experience to this point. It should consist of no more than one to two pages (typed).
2. Describe how you used previous knowledge and experience during the past 2 weeks. Link experiences to specific course objectives. For example, if you are teaching children about asthma, you would incorporate child development, teaching, and learning strategies, coping skills, respiratory diseases, chronic illness, environmental issues, etc. By the end of the semester you need to have addressed all course objectives. Be sure to include the ethical standards.
3. What research and/or practice questions can you generate based on your 2-weeks experience? What additional knowledge do you require for your practice in the next 2 weeks? How will answering these questions improve your practice?
4. Discuss one research-, practice-, or theory-based article that relates to each question in number 3 and reflects evidenced-based practice. How does what you learned from the article relate to your practice?
5. Describe the value of activities to your individual learning and meeting personal objectives.
6. Discuss the impact on your personal beliefs about nursing, health care, the nurse in community and public health, and community partnerships.

(continues)

Table 30-2 Grading Rubric *(continued)*

Topic (Possible Marks)	Your Mark
Summary (5)	
Previous knowledge/course objectives (5)	
Question/additional knowledge improvement for practice (10)	
Article and relation to practice (10)	
Value of activities (5)	
Impact on personal beliefs (5)	
Total (40)	

Finally, how will reciprocity be accomplished? Usually, evaluations by and of all partners (the community, the students, the faculty) are necessary. These can be formal or informal. Shinnamon, Gelmon, and Holland (1999) have developed evaluation of service-learning tools for students, faculty, and community partners and asked questions about attitude, experiences, and influence on future work using a Likert scale. Evaluations help to create better relationships and a stronger experience. Showcasing service-learning projects during class presentations or a campus-wide poster presentation contributes to reciprocity by recognizing the work of the students and the partners.

INTERNATIONAL SERVICE LEARNING

Another option for service learning is study abroad—immersion experiences of living and learning in another culture. This has several advantages: increased student awareness of their own beliefs, values, practices, and behaviors and how that affects care; ability to learn from clients and provide culturally appropriate care; and ability to cope with factors affecting health and living conditions (Lipson & DeSantis, 2007). A number of authors described study abroad experiences. This included preparation of students and faculty (Doyle, 2004; Robinson, Sportsman,

Eschiti, Bradshaw, & Bol, 2006); descriptions of the study abroad opportunities (Anders, 2001; Bentley & Ellison, 2007; Harrison & Malone, 2004; Johanson, 2006; Tabi & Mukherjee, 2003); as well as learning cultural competence through these types of experiences (Caffrey, Neander, Markle, & Stewart, 2005; Koskinen & Tossavainen, 2004; Walsh & DeJoseph, 2003; Warner, 2002). Readers are encouraged to explore the literature concerning these experiences.

Service learning during study abroad experiences requires a long-term commitment (at least 5 years) for both learning and service with a partner outside of the country. Jacoby and associates (2003) outline three principles for international partnerships: trust, mutuality of benefit, and open communication. Trust entails being clear about goals, budgets, and limitations and includes being sure promises made can be kept. There must be a benefit for both partners (inherent in service learning). Open and complete communication is essential, ranging from the formal evaluation plans to the more informal "check-ins." Adaptability is indispensible in the process. All principals of service learning still hold for international experiences: linking community needs, students' learning objectives, and formal reflection of the experience.

Faculty interested in this type of experience for their students are encouraged to contact their Office of International Education (or equivalent) as they will provide logistical support. Many times it is the faculty themselves who have contacts in another country that is further developed for study abroad opportunities. As Bosworth et al. state, "it began with one professor of nursing . . ." (2006, p. 34). An example of international service learning in Bangladesh is provided at the end of the chapter.

POTENTIAL PROBLEMS

Teaching in, and the facilitation of, a service-learning course takes time, so a major potential problem is lack of time. Time is required to form partnerships, prepare students, and involve partners in the design and implementation of the course. Another potential problem is the lack of preparation of the students (partnerships, reflection). The information needs to be in the course syllabus and class time needs to be devoted to describing service learning, explaining reflection, and the process of partnership. It is recommended that faculty teach only one service learning course at a time.

Lack of involvement of community partners in the design and implementation of the service-learning projects can be a potential problem. As one of the components of service-learning is reciprocity, involvement of community partners is mandatory. This can be remedied by clear and open communication. Regular contact with faculty is necessary so that issues can be dealt with early.

Another potential issue that has arisen is presenting service-learning work for promotion and tenure. CCPH has developed a resource kit (available on their Web site) to provide health professional faculty with a set of tools to carefully plan and document their community-engaged scholarship and produce strong portfolios for promotion and tenure (CCPH, 2009).

CONCLUSION

Service learning provides students the opportunity to develop transferable skills such as "the ability to synthesize information, creative problem solving, constructive teamwork, effective communication, well-reasoned decision making, and negotiation and compromise . . . and an increased sense of social responsibility" (Jacoby, 1996, p. 21). Service learning fits well with health professional education. Students need to get out of the classroom and more involved in the community and with each other in order to make knowledge alive. This strategy can provide students with insight into community conditions; community collaboration is lived, not just talked about in class.

APPLIED EXAMPLES

1. **Health Promotion Across the Life Span**

   The Health Promotion class is a junior nursing class and is now service learning based. The semester-long service-learning project produces 30-second public service announcements (PSAs) to meet the course objectives of family education strategies, learning to give concise messages, and realizing that health education could be more than handing out pamphlets. Our community partner is the regional educational television network (RETN), the local producer and provider of media for learning and a public service organization. The production coordinator came to the class to teach the basics of developing and producing the PSAs. Groups of four to six students (78 students altogether, 14 groups) chose a health promotion issue for a particular age group and drafted a script and storyboard. This is approved by faculty and RETN. Although this sounded simple, it actually took more time than we anticipated. Having both faculty and RETN approve the scripts enabled students to incorporate their advice without stifling creativity. For example, one group who developed their PSA on toddler poisoning had the child carry the mock poison bottle rather than be seen drinking from the bottle. Once the scripts were approved, groups videotaped their PSAs with equipment borrowed from the university. It takes about an hour of video tape to edit down to a 30-second message. Editing was done by RETN. The outcome was 14 health messages that are being shown throughout the state over the next several months. Reflection on the process is done through in-class writing assignments (unannounced) and outcomes indicated that the students learned about communication, the value (and difficulty!) of providing short messages, and found this a very enjoyable experience in which to learn about health education.

2. **Community/Public Health Nursing: Bangladesh**

At the University of Vermont, two faculty members (nursing and medical laboratory sciences) in the College of Nursing and Health Sciences and four faculty members (three infectious disease and one international health specialists) in the College of Medicine received a 2-year grant to explore and increase global health opportunities for students in both Colleges. Two of the physicians had worked in Bangladesh, so two team members (Maltby and Khan) travelled to Bangladesh for a week to investigate the possibilities for students. Both nursing and medical students were able to be accommodated but only nursing will be discussed here.

The majority of the Bangladeshi population is rural, and more than half live in poverty. It is the eighth most populated country in the world and third poorest. Between 1991 and 2003, the infant mortality rate dropped from 87 to 53 per 1,000 live births (in the US, the rate is 7 per 1000); the under-five mortality rate is 76 per 1,000 live births in 2002 (US, 8 per 1000); and the maternal mortality ratio declined from 470 in 1991 to 380 per 100,000 live births in 2002 (US, 14 per 100,000 in 2000) (World Health Organization, 2007). Although the rates have declined, infant and maternal mortality are still high.

Following this preliminary visit, a 3-week public health nursing immersion experience for senior undergraduate nursing students in a baccalaureate program was organized in partnership with the Independent University, Bangladesh (IUB). Permission was granted by the Department of Nursing and the proposal was submitted to the Office of International Education (OIE). OIE assisted with budget preparation, student applications, visas, flights, and risk-management details. IUB provided the on-the-ground logistics as well as two faculty members to collaborate in planning and facilitating the course and five students who were interpreters and cultural brokers for the nursing students. Nursing students met about twice per month during the fall semester prior to departure to complete necessary paperwork, learn about Bangladesh, and begin to come together as a team.

The first group of nursing students arrived in Dhaka (the capital of Bangladesh) in January 2008. The immersion experience began at the airport: Small children dressed only in a pair of shorts came begging for food and money. Just in front of them was a fence lined with people at least 10 deep also holding out their hands. The noise and the smells of Dhaka poured over them. After piling luggage and themselves onto the bus, the trip, while only a few miles, took almost an hour due to traffic that was crowded with buses, trucks, cars, rickshaws, tempos (a very small pickup truck-style motorized vehicle), and people. The next few days were spent travelling to an arsenic affected village, different historical sites in the city, and then out to the village where we stayed for the next 12 days. The students interviewed families and learned about health care in Bangladesh. Classes were held in the evening and discussed the events and sights of the day, connecting with the history, sociology, and health of Bangladesh with our partner IUB professor. Students kept reflective journals throughout the experience and had some profound insights related to cultural competency: "We went to Bangladesh with the intention of learning about the community/public health in a developing country. We discovered the common need for quality nursing care and access to resources and education. Visiting Bangladesh opened our eyes to the similarities of human health needs in that we all have common goals for our health. Our future nursing practice will be forever impacted by this experience."

During the first trip, the girls' high school in the rural village invited the nursing students to provide health education for their classes. This began with learning about schooling in Bangladesh,

especially for girls. The following year, a photovoice project was completed to discover what nutrition and hygiene habits were already practiced by the families. Photovoice, a community-based participatory research method, is a photographic technique that enables people to record and reflect their community's strengths and issues leading to discussion and policy considerations (Wang & Redwood-Jones, 2001, p. 560). Following permission from the headmistress, five high school girls were given a digital camera to photograph their families' nutrition and hygiene habits. After training and discussion about the project, the girls returned with at least 50 photographs each. Using a portable photo printer and an interpreter, each girl told her story. Preliminary data analysis is providing indigenous beliefs, practices, and knowledge of food preparation and habits of these families. These stories will be the basis of a future nutrition program at the high school to be taught by the nursing students and IUB student–interpreters.

NOTES

One major resource is the CCPH Web site (http://depts.washington.edu/ccph/index.html). It contains a plethora of information, including sample syllabi that include service learning to provide assistance to faculty who want to use this methodology.

There is also a National Service-Learning Clearinghouse (NSLC) Web site (NSLC, 2009). This has a range of information for elementary, high school, and tertiary education settings. It includes information on national and international conferences and an invitation to join a listserv forum for "discussion on such issues as, curriculum requests, class assignments and the institutionalization of service-learning as they pertain to the Higher Education service-learning community" (NSLC, 2006). This site has a link to the Corporation for National and Community Service (2006) which lists opportunities in a variety of organizations. Access for the strategic plan is through this Web site for further information on service learning from kindergarten to graduate school.

Service learning is being used for international projects such as faculty-led study abroad courses. International Service Learning (ISL) is incorporated as a nonprofit organization in Costa Rica and operates under Good Samaritan Missions, a 501c3 nonprofit organization, in the United States. As an international educational agency, ISL provides medical and educational teams of volunteers to provide services for the underserved populations of Central and South America, Mexico, and Africa. The International Partnership for Service Learning and Leadership (IPSL) is another organization that links academic programs and volunteer service, giving students a fully integrated study abroad experience. "The service enlivens the formal learning, and the learning informs the service. Both students and the host communities benefit from the substantial service each student gives. By studying at a local university and serving 15–20 hours per week in a school, orphanage, health clinic, or other agency addressing human needs, students find their knowledge of the host culture—and of themselves—take on greater depth and meaning" (IPSL, 2009). Faculty who want to incorporate service learning into study abroad options will need to consult with their own institution's international offices.

REFERENCES

Anders, R. L. (2001). A nursing study abroad opportunity. *Nursing and Health Care Perspectives, 22*(3), 118–121.

Ash, S. L., & Clayton, P. H. (2004). The articulated learning: An approach to guided reflection and assessment. *Innovative Higher Education, 29*(2), 137–154.

Bailey, P. A., Carpenter, D. R., & Harrington, P. (2002). Theoretical foundations of service-learning in nursing education. *Journal of Nursing Education, 41*(10), 433–452.

Bellack, J. P., & O'Neil, E. H. (2000). Recreating nursing practice for a new century: recommendations of the Pew Health Professions Commission's final report. *Nursing and Health Care Perspectives, 21*(1), 14–21.

Bentley, R., & Ellison, K. J. (2007). Increasing cultural competence in nursing though international service-learning experiences. *Nurse Educator, 32*(5), 207–211.

Bosworth, T., Haloburdo, E., Hetrick, C., Patchett, K., Thompson, M. A. & Welch, M. (2006). International partnerships to promote quality care: Faculty groundwork, student projects, and outcomes. *The Journal of Continuing Education in Nursing, 37*(1), 32–38.

Bradshaw, M. J. (2007). Effective learning: What teachers need to know. In M. J. Bradshaw & A. J. Lowenstein (Eds.), *Innovative teaching strategies in nursing and related health professions* (4th ed.). Sudbury, MA: Jones and Bartlett.

Caffrey, R. A., Neander, W., Markle, D. & Stewart, B. (2005). Improving the cultural competence of nursing students: Results of integrating cultural content in the curriculum and an international immersion experience. *Journal of Nursing Education, 44*(5), 234–240.

Callister, L. C., & Hobbins-Garbett, D. (2000). "Enter to learn, go forth to serve": Service learning in nursing education. *Journal of Professional Nursing, 16*(3), 177–183.

Carter, J., & Dunn, B. (2002). A service-learning partnership for enhanced diabetes management. *Journal of Nursing Education, 41*(10), 450–452.

Cashman, S. B., Hale, J. F., Candib, L. M., Nimiroski, T. A., & Brookings, D. R. (2004). Applying service-learning through a community-academic partnership: Depression screening at a federally funded community health center. *Education for Health, 17*(3), 313–322.

Chabot, J. M., & Holben, D. H. (2003). Integrating service-learning into dietetics and nutrition education. *Topics in Clinical Nutrition, 18*(3), 177–184.

Chapdelaine, A., Ruiz, A., Warchal, J., & Wells, C. (2005). *Service-learning code of ethics*. Bolton, MA: Anker.

Cohen, E., Johnson, S., Nelson, L., & Peterson, C. (1998). Service-learning as a pedagogy in nursing. In J. S. Norbeck, C. Connolly, & J. Koerner (Eds.), *Caring and community: Concepts and models for service-learning in nursing* (pp. 53–63). San Francisco: American Association for Higher Education.

Community-Campus Partnerships for Health. (2009). Home page. Retrieved December 6, 2009, from http://depts.washington.edu/ccph/index.html

Corporation for National and Community Service. (2006). Strategic plan 2006–2010. Retrieved December 6, 2009, from http://www.nationalservice.gov/pdf/strategic_plan_web.pdf

Doyle, R. M. (2004). Applying new science leadership theory in planning an international nursing student practice experience in Nepal. *Journal of Nursing Education, 43*(9), 426–429.

Fuller, S. G., Alexander, J. W., & Hardeman, S. M. (2006). Sheriff's deputies and nursing students: Service-learning partnership. *Nurse Educator, 31*(1), 31–35.

Hamel, P. C. (2001). Interdisciplinary perspectives, service learning, and advocacy: A nontraditional approach to geriatric rehabilitation. *Topics in Geriatric Rehabilitation, 17*(1), 53–70.

Harrison, L., & Malone, K. (2004).A study abroad experience in Guatemala: Learning first-hand about health, education, and social welfare in a low-resource country. *International Journal of Nursing Education Scholarship 1*, (1), Article 16.

Heffernan, K. (2001). *Fundamentals of service-learning course construction*. Providence RI: Campus Compact.

Hoppes, S., Bender, D., & DeGrace, B. W. (2005). Service learning is a perfect fit for occupational and physical therapy education. *Journal of Allied Health, 34*, 47–50.

Institute of Medicine. (2003). *Who will keep the public healthy? Educating public health professionals for the 21st century*. Washington, DC: Author.

International Partnership for Service-Learning and Leadership. (2009). International service-learning programs. Retrieved December 6, 2009, from http://www.ipsl.org/defaultIPSL.aspx

Jacoby, B. (1996). *Service-learning in higher education: Concepts and practices*. San Francisco: Jossey-Bass.

Jacoby, B. and Associates. (2003). *Building partnerships for service-learning*. San Francisco, CA: Jossey-Bass.

Johanson, L. (2006). The implementation of a study abroad course for nursing. *Nurse Educator, 31*(3), 129–131.

Knowles, M. (1975). *Self-directed learning: A guide for learners and teachers*. New York: Cambridge.

Koskinen, L., & Tossavainen, K. (2004). Study abroad as a process of learning intercultural competence in nursing. *International Journal of Nursing Practice, 10*(3), 111–120.

Kuiper, R. A. (2005). Self-regulated learning during a clinical preceptorship. *Nursing Education Perspectives, 26*(6), 351–356.

Lipson, J. G., & DeSantis, L. A. (2007). Current approaches to integrating elements of cultural competence in nursing education. *Journal of Transcultural Nursing* (Supplement), *18*(1), 10S–20S.

Mallette, S., Loury, S., Engelke, M. K., & Andrews, A. (2005). *The integrative clinical preceptor model: a new method for teaching undergraduate community health nursing. Nurse Educator, 30*(1), 21–6.

Maurana, C. A., Beck, B., & Newton, G. L. (1998). How principles of partnership are applied to the development of a community-campus partnership. *Partnership Perspectives, 1*(1), 47–53.

Mayne, L., & Glascoff, M. (2002). Service learning: Preparing a healthcare workforce for the next century. *Nurse Educator, 27*(4), 191–194.

National Service-Learning Clearinghouse. (2006). *The national site for service-learning information*. Retrieved December 6, 2009, from http://temp.servicelearning.org/hehome/index.php

National Service-Learning Clearinghouse. (2009). Retrieved December 6, 2009, from http://www.servicelearning.org/.

Norbeck, J. S., Connolly, C., & Koerner, J. (1998). *Caring and community: Concepts and models for service-learning in nursing*. San Francisco: American Association for Higher Education.

Redman, R. W., & Clark, L. (2002). Service-learning as a model for integrating social justice in the nursing curriculum. *Journal of Nursing Education, 41*(10), 446–449.

Robinson, K., Sportsman, S., Eschiti, V. S., Bradshaw, P., & Bol, T. (2006). Preparing faculty and students for an international nursing education experience. *The Journal of Continuing Education in Nursing, 37*(1), 21–29.

Schoener, L., & Hopkins, M. L. (2004). Service learning: A tuberculosis screening clinic in an adult residential care facility. *Nurse Educator, 29*(6), 242–245.

Schneider, C. G., & Humphreys, D. (2005). Putting liberal education on the radar screen. *The Chronicle of Higher Education*. Retrieved December 6, 2009, from http://chronicle.com/article/Putting-Liberal-Education-on/26781

Scott, S. B., Harrison, A. D., Baker, T., & Wills, J. D. (2005). Interdisciplinary community partnership for health professional students: A service-learning approach. *Journal of Allied Health, 34*(1), 31–35.

Seifer, S. D. (1998). Service-learning: Community-campus partnerships for health professions education. *Academic Medicine, 73*(3), 273–277.

Seifer, S. D., & Vaughn, R. L. (2002). Partners in caring and community: Service-learning in nursing education. *Journal of Nursing Education, 41*(10), 437–439.

Shinnamon, A., Gelmon, S. B., & Holland, B. A. (1999). *Methods and strategies for assessing service-learning in the health professions*. San Francisco, CA: CCPH.

Simoni, R. S., & McKinney, J. A. (1998). Evaluation of service learning in a school of nursing: Primary care in a community setting. *Journal of Nursing Education, 37*(3), 122–128.

Tabi, M. M., & Mukherjee, S. (2003). Nursing in a global community: A study abroad program. *Journal of Transcultural Nursing, 14*(2), 134–138.

University of Vermont, College of Medicine. (2006). *What is an AHEC?* Retreived December 6, 2009, from http://www.med.uvm.edu/ahec/TB8+BL+I.asp?SiteAreaID=91

Walsh, L. V., & DeJoseph, J. (2003). "I saw it in a different light": International learning experiences in baccalaureate nursing education. *Journal of Nursing Education, 42*(6), 266–272.

Wang, C. C., & Redwood-Jones, Y. A. (2001). Photovoice ethics: Perspectives from Flint photovoice. *Health Education & Behavior, 28*(5), 560–572.

Warner, J. R. (2002). Cultural competence immersion experiences. Public health among the Navajo, *Nurse Educator, 27*(4), 187–190.

World Health Organization. (2007). *Bangladesh country profile*. Retrieved December 6, 2009, from http://www.searo.who.int/EN/Section313/Section1515_6121.htm

Worrell-Carlisle, P. (2005). Service-learning: A tool for developing cultural awareness. *Nurse Educator, 30*(5), 197–202.

CHAPTER 31

Study Abroad as a Strategy for Nursing Education: A Case Study

Carol Holtz and Richard L. Sowell

INTRODUCTION

The United States is experiencing the largest sustained immigration wave in its history with an estimated 44.3 million documented and undocumented immigrants arriving each year from all parts of the world. At present, 15% of the US population is comprised of individuals who have immigrated both legally and illegally from Latin America. It is estimated that by 2050, the Latino population could be 102.6 million, or 24% of the US population (US Census Bureau, 2007). However, immigrants to the United States represent diverse populations from Africa, Asia, Europe, and the Pacific Islands ("African immigration to the United States," 2009; Min, 2006). The United States accepts more legal immigrants as permanent residents than any other country in the world ("Immigration to the United States," 2006). The number of immigrants naturalized in the United States reached 1,046,539 (Lee & Rytina, 2008). Yet, it is estimated that there may be significant numbers of immigrants to the United States who have illegally entered the United States ("US Populations Hits 300 million," 2006). Often these individuals are poor, do not speak English, and are leaving adversity in their own country. This increase in global immigration to the United States in recent years has resulted in dramatic changes in the cultural tapestry of American society. It has challenged our public and private institutions to respond to individuals and groups that are of different religions, cultural beliefs, and traditions. Among US institutions, the healthcare system has been disproportionately impacted by immigration. Language, unfamiliar health beliefs and practices, and inability to pay for care are all challenges for healthcare institutions and healthcare providers. For many immigrants who come to the United States to work, their immigration is the result of seeking a better life and escaping poverty in their home country. They arrive in the United States with poor nutrition and are potentially at risk for a number of conditions, such as diabetes or tuberculosis (TB), which will require ongoing health care. The Centers for Disease Control and Prevention (CDC) has indicated that TB cases among foreign-born persons are nearly nine times the rate of US-born individuals (CDC, 2005). While there is an ongoing debate as to the ethics and cost of providing care to immigrants, especially those who have entered the United States illegally, there is no debate that immigration has changed the healthcare system. The US healthcare system has historically been focused on providing health care for individuals of European decent and African Americans. Increasingly, the healthcare system is responding to a global population, which is placing new demands on the system. It has become critical that healthcare providers gain a broader perspective of health and treatment in order to adequately perform their roles. This challenge to gain a more multicultural perspective of health and traditions of health care is particularly essential among nurses who represent the largest group of healthcare providers in the United States.

As described by Bennett and Holtz (2008), nursing as a profession is constantly striving to improve the delivery of health care to clients of all races, nationalities, and socioeconomic statuses. Clients from cultures other than that of the nurse often do not benefit from nursing care because of miscommunications, misunderstandings, and/or conflicts of values, beliefs, norms, and attitudes between themselves and the nurse. Because of the recent influx of international patients in the United States, comprehensive knowledge of the culture of the client is imperative in order to adequately assess, plan, implement, and evaluate nursing care. In addition, understanding the client's culture is likely to increase the patient's satisfaction with their nursing care. Cultural competence is an ongoing process of seeking cultural awareness, cultural knowledge, cultural skill, and cultural encounters (Campinha-Bacote, 1994; Leininger, 1978; Purnell & Paulanka, 2003; Spector, 2004).

Hall, Stevens, and Meleis (1994) have shown that the future of successful transcultural nurse–patient communication depends on the nurse's abilities to meet the needs of an ever-growing diverse population. Madeline Leininger, the author of transcultural nursing theory stated, "Our American nursing care practices tend to rely upon unicultural values which are largely derived from our Anglo-American caring values and expectations" (p. 11). Maintaining an open attitude in examining one's own prejudices, attitudes, and stereotyped perceptions is essential before one can learn about people of other cultures. It is not the client's responsibility to be understood, but the nurse's responsibility to understand and meet the client's needs (Leininger, 1978). In our pluralistic society nurses must develop an understanding about culture and its relevance to competent care. To provide this care nurses must understand specific factors that influence individual health and illness behaviors.

OVERVIEW OF THE GROWTH OF STUDY ABROAD PROGRAMS

It is the responsibility of universities to provide an education for students that will allow them to compete in the global market and it will be important for all students' education to help them become global citizens. For educators in the health disciplines, facilitating students in gaining a more global perspective, including cultural understanding of individuals from different health traditions, is an evolving component of their role as educators. Cultural competence is relative term that suggests a level of understanding of another's culture expectations related to that culture. There are a variety of educational strategies that are used to introduce students to other cultures. However, the strategy of using study abroad experiences to introduce students to other cultures, traditions, and beliefs is one that is gaining popularity. Study abroad programs can be effective in exposing students, as well as faculty members to individuals from other backgrounds than their own, providing a new level of understanding of these individuals' experiences, beliefs, and cultural traditions. The goal of such study abroad experiences is to expand the student's perspectives of world, promote a new sensitivity to beliefs and traditions different from their own, and promote a sense of intellectual openness that supports ongoing learning that extends beyond the student's formal education (Bennett & Holtz, 2008).

Study abroad programs for university faculty members and students vary from short tourist-like visits, which can often give a quick and sometimes superficial glimpse of a country (with its language, culture, and various special attractions), compared to a long-term, more intense experience (an immersion experience) in which the participants live, work, and study within local populations. As described by Leininger and McFarland (2002), an "etic" experience involves only the view and belief of an observer which may or may not be an accurate reflection of the genuine culture of a given people.

IMPORTANCE OF STUDY ABROAD PROGRAMS FOR STUDENTS' EDUCATION

Study abroad education provides students with a distinct advantage upon graduation. In today's global economy, study abroad experiences are an enormous asset to a student's resume and academic experiences. An increasing number of healthcare corporations are looking for candidates who have the ability to communicate and work with people from various cultural backgrounds. This is especially true in the healthcare professions where more and more healthcare industries are legally and competitively challenged to provide safe and culturally appropriate patient care. In addition, having a broader world perspective provides for greater depth of understanding of global health challenges, which gives nursing students greater opportunities to become better local citizens within their communities.

COMMON GOALS OF STUDY ABROAD PROGRAMS

Personal Growth

Students and faculty who return from a study abroad program often see it as an experience that matured them personally and intellectually. They praise being exposed to new ways of thinking and living, which encourages growth and independence. For many, going abroad to study is the first time they have really been away from home, from familiar surroundings of the United States, as well as from friends and family. This is seldom an easy experience, but it is worthwhile, often even life-transforming. After immersing themselves in a new culture, mastering the challenges of learning in a new and different academic environment, and having the experience of being a foreigner, they often return home with increased self confidence and pride in what they have achieved.

A Broad Perspective of the World

Study abroad can broaden intellectual horizons and deepen knowledge and understanding of international, political, social, and economic issues. By having this experience a person will learn how others view the United States and its world role. When living in a country where English is not the native language, or is spoken only by some, a person will learn the practical importance of learning another language and using it.

Career Enhancement

Study abroad also can enhance employment prospects, especially in the fields of business, international affairs, health care, and government service. Employers increasingly seek graduates who have studied abroad. They know that students who have successfully completed a study abroad program are likely to possess international knowledge and often second language skills. Such students are also likely to have other competencies that graduate and professional schools and employer's value highly such as cross-cultural communication skills, analytical skills, an understanding of and familiarity with local customs and cultural contexts, flexibility, resilience, and the ability to adapt to new circumstances and deal constructively with differences.

STUDY ABROAD IN HEALTH PROFESSIONS VERSUS MISSION TRIPS

Study abroad in health professions within a university setting, such as a nursing elective course, provides a student with specific goals and objectives to achieve within an academic setting. The emphasis is intellectual, professional, and objective. Students must conduct themselves professionally, complete all necessary goals with activities within a certain time frame, and their professional performance and personal conduct is evaluated. Funding sources for the trip may differ. The entire course is evaluated by faculty teaching the course, by others within the university system, and by outside accrediting agencies. Mission trips may have similar goals, but may also have a religious, political, or economic focus with other evaluation criteria.

CASE STUDY: AN IMMERSION STUDY ABROAD PROGRAM

The state of Georgia has experienced one of the highest rates of Mexican immigrants of all of the United States. In particular, the Latino population of metropolitan Atlanta increased by 400% over the last decade (US Census Bureau, 2007). The recent immigration of Spanish-speaking Latinos from a variety of cultural backgrounds has challenged the local healthcare system to provide culturally competent health care to the new Hispanic immigrants. As described by Bennett and Holtz (2008), the Wellstar School of Nursing at Kennesaw State University (KSU) has developed an immersion experience in Oaxaca (*Wa-ha-ka*), Mexico, for nursing students to respond to the need for nurses to gain greater understanding of this growing immigrant population. By learning about the people of Oaxaca, their language, customs, values, and beliefs, the student nurses and faculty can become more experienced in their knowledge of Hispanic culture (specifically Oaxacan) and Spanish language skills. These experiences will be invaluable to students when they communicate with their Hispanic patients in the US healthcare setting. In addition, alternative learning settings for nurses facilitates caring, cultural sensitivity, interdisciplinary relationships, and helps nursing students to form new ways of thinking about health care.

The mission of KSU, as well as the Wellstar College of Health and Human Services, is to increase intercultural contacts and global awareness for faculty, staff, and students. In order to carry out this mission, the university established the Global Institute on the campus. Additionally, the Wellstar College has established the Global Center for Social Change. One of the programs that support these initiatives among future nurses is a 2-week intensive nursing elective program in capital city of the state of Oaxaca, Mexico. The study abroad program has been implemented for the past 14 years and represents a proven strategy for introducing nursing students to a population and culture that they will frequently encounter in their clinical practice. The development, content, and evaluation of this program will be described within this chapter. The Oaxaca Study Abroad Program can serve as a model for the development of similar educational programs. The principles used to implement the program and the lessons learned from 14 years of offering the program have application beyond nursing and can be adapted for the development of programs in countries and communities worldwide.

The Nursing Practicum in Oaxaca Program Objectives

The intent of the nursing practicum in Oaxaca is to give the visiting faculty members and students the "emic" or lived experience, seeing a culture more through the eyes of the native people. Students in the KSU program experience hands-on activities by speaking the local language, as well as studying the Spanish language at the local university. In addition, students and faculty visit cultural sights to further understand the local culture.

The objectives of the nursing practicum program reflect the mission of the university and the community needs for college graduates, which is to possess global awareness and cultural sensitivity. More specifically, the objectives reflect the needs of nurses who will be working with Hispanic patients in the community. The course syllabus objectives include the following:

1. Explore one's personal attitudes and beliefs about patients in Oaxaca, Mexico.
2. Examine the structure and function of healthcare delivery to patients in the Oaxacan community.
3. Explore the main health issues of Oaxaca as identified by the local residents.
4. Actively participate in the healthcare delivery to patients in Oaxaca.
5. Improve Spanish language skills and communicate with patients, staff, and others in the Oaxacan community.
6. Explore the health beliefs and local cultural customs and practices of the Oaxacan community.

Description of the Kennesaw State University Program

The nursing practicum in Oaxaca is a 2-week intensive 3–credit hour nursing elective course, which is available every May, during the university's break after spring semester and prior to summer semester. This time period is known as "Maymester." The program was designed and implemented by a nursing faculty member who has continuously taught this course for the past 14 years. Students enroll in the course and pay for a package that includes course tuition and round trip airfare from Atlanta, Georgia, to Oaxaca, Mexico. Also included are 15 days of food and housing with a local middle-class family, daily Spanish lessons at the University of Oaxaca's language center (Centro de Idiomas), weekend excursions to the Monte Alban pyramids, a visit to Doña Rosa's famous black pottery center in nearby San Bartolo Coyotapec, a visit to Arrozola where the very unique animal carvings (alebrijes) are made, and another trip to the village of Teotitlan del Valle where the famous weavers are located. Medical supply donations and health insurance for the 15 days in Mexico are also included in this package. Several scholarships are available to students based on grade point average and need, which further assists students in payment for the course package. The group consists of 8 to 16 students with one or two nursing faculty members.

Setting

The capital city of the state of Oaxaca is also called Oaxaca. It has approximately 200,000 inhabitants, is located in the southwestern region of Mexico, and is 5,000 feet above sea level in the Sierra Madre Mountains. In Oaxaca, Spanish is the official language; however, there are more than 15 non-Hispanic ethnic groups, each with their own indigenous dialect and customs, yet most of the people are descendants of the ancient Zapotec and Mixtec groups (Ewing, 1996).

The State of Oaxaca is one of the most ethnically diverse states in Mexico, with a population of over 4 million inhabitants of a variety of indigenous ethnic groups, speaking primarily Spanish but also an estimated 30 other indigenous dialects (Ewing, 1996). Oaxaca is one of the poorest states in Mexico, having an extremely high infant mortality rate in some isolated rural areas.

The city of Oaxaca (currently the capital of the state of Oaxaca) was founded in 1529 by Hernan Cortez (Ewing, 1996). Economic factors have resulted in the immigration (both legal and illegal) of young people from Oaxaca to the United States for work. These workers often come to the metropolitan Atlanta region to seek employment and live in large communities with other recent Hispanic immigrants. They seek health care in local hospitals, from private physicians, and nurse-managed clinics.

Local Health and Healthcare Issues

Students often hold the assumption that health care is available to all, but find in Oaxaca that poor and rural populations are increasingly unable to compete for scarce health resources. In Oaxaca, the maternal mortality rate is twice that of the national Mexican average. Health problems include the inability to access fresh, clean water; childhood malnutrition; and exposure to communicable diseases, which all contribute to common causes of morbidity and mortality. Mexico ranks second in Latin America in incidence of HIV/AIDS and 11th in the world. Air pollution is a major problem throughout the country resulting in chronic bronchitis, emphysema, asthma, lung cancer, and eye infections. Cholera and other gastrointestinal disorders resulting from poor sanitation and unclean water are particularly devastating to infants and children (Barry, 1992). Many employed workers carry private health insurance, but the majority of people receive their health care from the government's Pronasol program. Lustig (1992) states that the Mexican Institute of Social Security (IMSS), one of the national health insurance programs, has been strained because of the inflationary economy. Infant and preschool mortality and morbidity have increased because of avitaminosis and other nutritional deficiencies (Lustig, 1992).

Several universities, schools of nursing and medicine, and language schools make Oaxaca a city with a large population of students. While KSU students are reminded to maintain measures to protect personal security, Oaxaca remains a comparatively safe city for students. The healthcare infrastructure is welcoming to students and provides a rich diversity of primary, secondary, and tertiary care experiences with very diverse populations. KSU faculty members decided that these characteristics made Oaxaca an ideal site for a clinically based nursing study abroad course (Bennett & Holtz, 2008).

Setting up the Program

The initial process in developing the nursing practicum in Oaxaca began by visiting the area to determine the feasibility of establishing a 2-week intensive study abroad nursing course. Contact with the leaders of health care in the community was essential. The KSU professor contacted the Secretary of Health for the State of Oaxaca. A discussion with the Secretary and key healthcare community leaders in Oaxaca produced a dialogue regarding goals and expectations of the experience for students, the facilities and experiences available to students, the type of nursing faculty supervision expected for students working in Oaxaca healthcare facilities, and potential benefits to the local healthcare system. When setting up a program such as this one, it is essential to establish a network of local people who will agree to coordinate student housing, Spanish language courses at the University of Oaxaca, student work experiences in local hospitals or public health department clinics, and transportation for local cultural excursions.

A housing coordinator, who already had experience in working with students from other study abroad university programs (nonnursing) from other US universities was next located. The housing coordinator was essential in giving the students opportunities for home stays with local families who could provide a private bedroom in their home located in a safe neighborhood, and also provide three nutritious, well-prepared meals per day. The network of families knew what foods would be appealing and safe for American students to eat. A coordinator for local excursions was also found. This person would assist with all transportation and agenda arrangements for weekend cultural outings to nearby villages to see the pyramids and local crafts. Contact and establishment of a relationship with the director of the Language Center at the University of Oaxaca was also needed in order to set up the daily Spanish conversation classes for students and faculty.

Student Prerequisites and Preparation

Prerequisites for all student nurses was having completed at least the basic nursing course with a clinical component, giving them skills in vital signs, bed and baths, etc. Most students were more advanced, with greater experiences in psychiatric, obstetric, and pediatric experiences and skills, and also had experience with more complex medical–surgical patients. Students were also required to have completed at least one Spanish language class prior to coming on the trip. KSU student nurses were all required to attend a very extensive orientation on campus prior to departure. During this orientation, students were encouraged to invite parents, spouses, or other interested parties to ask pertinent questions and feel reassurance about the student's participation in the Oaxaca experiences. In addition, reading material assignments were given along with the student course syllabus so that students could prepare for their experiences ahead of time. All students were told that included in their payment for the course was health insurance coverage during their stay in Oaxaca. Insurance also included emergency air evacuation to the United States if needed. A list of CDC-required vaccines for the Oaxaca region of Mexico was given. Students could obtain needed immunizations from the university's health clinic or another healthcare agency.

Recruitment of Students

Faculty conducted recruitment sessions about 7 months prior to departure. Colorful and detailed flyers depicted photos of Oaxaca and a few very brief excerpts about the nursing elective course. Several recruitment parties with free pizza and soda were given, and students were encouraged to learn about the special course and ask questions. Explanations regarding the costs, many available scholarships, and course elements were given. Some students signed up immediately with a down payment while others took a few months to think it over and carefully plan their finances. Parents, particularly single parents, needed to creatively find ways to cover their childcare needs. Students were able to make several partial payments that eventually covered all the costs. Some students were very creative in finding payments with a combination of scholarships, gifts from parents or other relatives, church donations, or finding extra overtime work in the hospitals. Others used partial credit card payments to fulfill their obligations. All in all, most students who really wanted to go found a way to achieve their wishes.

Orientation

The mandatory 3-hour student orientation with snacks was held about 5 weeks before departure. Students and other interested members (parents and spouses) attended this session. During this orientation, students were given a written handout and a group discussion addressed personal safety needs, documents, money, packing needs, special health challenges, housing, transportation, working in the clinics or hospitals, culture shock and adjustments, Spanish tutoring sessions, cultural excursions, and, perhaps most important of all, cultural sensitivity and appropriate dress and behavior. Many were very concerned about food, health, safety, and local customs, while others were more concerned about direct patient care in the clinical settings. Students were expected to be dressed professionally in white uniforms, nursing shoes, and name tags.

Donations of Supplies and Equipment

Faculty members noted that the Oaxaca Health Department did not have sufficient medical supplies and equipment both in the hospitals and outpatient satellite clinics. To thank the Oaxacan Health Department hosts, yearly donations of medical supplies and equipment were made and given directly to the Secretary of Health for the State of Oaxaca. These materials were assembled from a variety of sources. Some came from direct donations from physicians' private practices and some from local health departments within the greater Atlanta area. Others were purchased from a fee that was included from each student package price for the course itself. All donations were assembled, counted, and packed by faculty and students. A formal list, with types of supplies and quantities, was translated into Spanish for the Oaxaca customs office. This was sent ahead of the arrival to make the entrance into the country with the supplies an easier experience. Each student checked one box of supplies with their luggage, so that there were no additional fees for bringing the supplies into Mexico. This experience taught the students in the beginning about sharing goods and thanking the health department ahead of time for hosting their medical experiences. The Health Department of Oaxaca responded with a small reception for the students and thanked them for their donations.

Experiences in Oaxaca

Students lived separately with local middle-class families within the community. They were encouraged to participate in family activities to learn more about local culture and lifestyles. A local Oaxacan housing coordinator was responsible for making sure that all families were approved for hosting students from the program, were familiar with the needs and routines of the students, and were willing to provide a private bedroom and meals within their home. Living independently with local families provided an extra experience of local culture and language (families only spoke Spanish) that helped students obtain an insiders' prospective rather than a tourist prospective of their experiences.

Students participated in daily 1-hour Spanish conversation classes at the University of Oaxaca's Language Center, every evening during the week from 5 to 6 PM. These classes were for self improvement only, with no grade given. Students evaluated themselves and stated whether they would like to be in a beginning or intermediate Spanish class. Occasionally there were fluent Spanish speakers who could optionally not take the classes and visit museums during the time. Most fluent students opted to participate in the intermediate classes because they claimed that they gained special valuable knowledge of Spanish vocabulary used in the clinical areas. The KSU faculty also participated in Spanish lessons to improve their conversation skills.

Each student worked 6 hours per day for 5 days a week at an assigned clinical site for a total of 2 weeks. One to two students were assigned to each site and each had a Oaxacan nurse as a mentor during the entire experience. Faculty made continuous visits to each site to see the students, talk to them about their ongoing experiences, troubleshoot if problems existed, and observe student–staff and student–patient behaviors. They also talked with staff and patients daily to continue the relationship with the student mentors.

The KSU student nurses worked primarily in the public acute care hospital within the city of Oaxaca and also the major pediatric hospital located in a nearby village. At other times, students worked in satellite health department clinics. These facilities serve local indigent Oaxacan residents as well as others who come from distant isolated regions of the state of Oaxaca. The majority of the patients are indigenous Indians from various subcultures of Oaxaca. Students completed various levels of the nursing program and performed at the level in which they were most comfortable. They assisted the local registered nurses with patient care, but did not administer any medications because of the potential of errors with possible language barriers.

Transportation to and from the clinical sites was either by walking, local buses, or very inexpensive taxi service. Their nursing assignments in the clinics or hospital sites included patient physical assessment exams, health teaching, and basic care including vital signs. Students who worked in the health clinics also made visits to schools and homes to administer health care. Among the most frequently taught subjects were daily basic hygiene, purification of the local water, treatment of cholera and dehydration, birth control measures, and prevention and treatment of tuberculosis and other lung infections. Within the pediatric hospital students learned that malnutrition during pregnancy caused many of the preterm, low birth weight babies, and also much of the congenital anomalies, such as spina bifida, cleft lip, and cleft palate.

Students found the Oaxacan healthcare system workers to be welcoming and enthusiastic in providing them with interesting clinical experiences. Students bonded with Oaxacan nurses, nursing students, physicians, and medical students. The exchange of cultural information and language lessons in English and Spanish make the bonds even stronger. Students are placed throughout the hospital with nurse mentors on each clinical unit and faculty members circulate throughout the hospital, translating if necessary and facilitating the experience.

Course Grade Requirements

The course grading criteria included mandatory student participation in all clinical work as well as Spanish conversation classes and cultural activities unless they were ill. The clinical participation was graded on a pass/fail basis. To promote reflection of their experiences, each student was asked to keep a daily journal. Their feelings, thoughts, responses, observations, and activities were recorded. Journal recordings addressed the housing and living with a local family, clinical experiences, Spanish classes, cultural excursions, as well as new sounds, smells, and tastes. Students were encouraged to write about their prior thoughts about Oaxaca before they began the trip, and compare and contrast them to their actual experiences that they encountered. They wrote a journal summary paper according to specific criteria and were given a grade that counted as 25% of their final course grade. Also they were given an assignment to write a scholarly paper or participate in a group project (specific criteria were given) that addressed a health issue in Oaxaca, in Mexico, or within the Mexican American US population. This paper or project represented the remaining 75% of their grade. Both the journal summary paper and the scholarly course project/paper were due at the end of the following semester, giving them ample time to collect information in Oaxaca (if they chose to do so) and complete the assignments well after they returned home. This way, students would not be pressured to complete course assignments during their 2-week cultural experience.

Examples of Some Student Perceptions of the Study Abroad Experience

The experiences of living with an Oaxacan family were a vivid contrast to the everyday life experiences for the students at home in the United States. Most students were in their late 20s to mid-30s, married, and already parents. They paid for their own college tuition, living expenses, held a part-time job, studied, and were full-time parents and spouses, running a household. In contrast, while living with a family in Oaxaca they often became dependent children/adults. One student made the following comment:

> This family has show nothing but genuine love and caring behaviors for me. When I woke up in the morning they all were assembled at the table for breakfast. There was music in the house, and plenty of wonderful foods such as fresh mangoes, papayas, tortillas, beans, and Oaxacan cheese. The locally grown coffee is exceptional in smell and taste. The family mother walked me to the taxi, holding my hand, and repeated the directions I just gave to the cab driver, just to make sure I didn't get lost. I got a kiss and hug from my Oaxacan Mom as I hopped into the cab to go to the clinic. Later in the afternoon around 2 PM the whole family reassembled for the main meal, "la comida." My Oaxacan father returned from his job, the children returned from school (they attend the local college), and I came back from the clinic. Again we are all greeted with love, affection, hugs, and kisses.

Another student revealed the family dynamics during the main noon meal, which serves not only for feeding the family, but an important time for communication, which appears to facilitate the closely knit family structure. She stated the following:

> At lunch we discussed all that has transpired during the day. I was asked how I was feeling, what I had done at the clinic, and what was my response to my experiences in the clinic. I also attentively listened to the high school aged children talk about school, their friends, and their sports activities. La comida consisted of roasted chicken or beef, homemade vegetable soup, rice, tortillas, homemade lemonade, and a dessert of flan or fruit. The high school children planned an evening at a local disco with their dates and wanted me to attend with them. I'm a good 15 years older, a wife and mother myself, and yet they wished for me to hang out with them!

The siesta, or afternoon nap, is a family ritual that is very much part of the whole local culture of Oaxaca. All shops, businesses, and schools in the city close down around 1:30 PM and reopen at 4:00 PM. Another student described her experiences with the siesta time in the following comments:

> After the main midday meal everyone retreated to their own bedroom for a nap. This pattern makes so much more sense for the body. Eating the largest meal in the middle, rather than the end of the day, gives the body more opportunity for digestion and exercise before going to sleep at night. The heat of the day is during the siesta period and after a large meal it is immensely relaxing to take a little nap. At first this behavior seemed quite odd to me. Since I was a small child I haven't rested midday. I started by reading a novel I brought with me, and also making some journal entries. Later I actually became drowsy and fell asleep for about 45 minutes. After the siesta everyone arose and went back to school, work, or family related duties. Again, the family returned around 7 PM for a light snack of a sandwich and juice.

Evenings and weekend days with the family were also quite different from typical experiences that students experienced with their US families. One student stated the following:

> In the evenings they attended Mass at church about twice a week. On Saturday, early in the evening, they went to Mass and then later at night had friends come to their home for dinner, or they went to their friends' houses. Sunday was family day. All the children and grandchildren came to the home for a large family dinner and a family get-together for the afternoon. Midweek evenings were spent talking in the living room, watching television (they had cable TV and a VCR), or reading.

Some students thought that they would be "roughing it" in primitive housing with little or no running water and were shocked to see the homes in which they stayed. One student described the following:

> The houses were very lovely and some were old, and others were very new and modern. None had air conditioning, or screens. Most had large thick walls around them. The yards were small with very beautiful patios with gardens in them. Tropical flowers, and fruit trees decorated the courtyard. No one owned a washer or dryer, or even a dishwasher. Everyone had at least one household servant who lived with them, cooked, shopped for food in the markets, and cared for the yard. The servants cleaned the houses, washed the clothes by hand and hung them on the line to dry. All food was purchased daily in the market, and cooked during the day. A tiny refrigerator held a few fruit juices and some milk. There was no freezer compartment. No canned goods were ever used for any meals. All food was fresh. Clean drinking water was delivered to the house once a week and was in a large urn in the kitchen. Due to a water shortage everyone was careful not to use too much water at once, especially while taking a shower.

The Mexican families also appreciated the transcultural experiences. Families appeared to be interested in discovering more about what the students' lives were like in the United States. One student described the following:

> The family members had a great interest in learning about me and my family. They wanted to know what daily life like in the United States was. They wanted an explicit description of my home in Atlanta, my present family, birth family, job, and my friends. They inquired about our religious customs, festivals, and family experiences. They devoured the few family photos that I brought with me. I was careful to talk about my life, but not to compare and contrast my lifestyle with theirs. I tried to stress the wonderful things I experienced about Oaxacan culture that was superior to our life in the US. The slower pace of living, the strong family units' emphasis on enjoying the moment rather than always worrying about long-term goals were emphasized. The customs of eating less junk food, more fresh foods, eating in the middle of the day with a siesta were discussed. The clean fresh air, less traffic, and less internal pressures were evaluated. Yes, the US had a more technologically sophisticated environment, but what about daily quality of life? What about more frequent encounters with the extended family? We diplomatically came to the conclusion that each of our cultures had good and less favorable aspects, but it was most interesting to learn about each other.

Student Outcomes

The outcomes that the students have achieved in this study abroad practicum have been diverse, rewarding, and have affected practice patterns on return to the United States. Students have gained knowledge in a variety of healthcare issues affecting Latino immigrants, improved their Spanish language skills, developed an appreciation of the similarities and differences of cultures, and improved in their abilities to provide culturally competent care.

A review of the topics chosen by students for their analysis and synthesis papers reveals the wide range of learning that has occurred. Some examples of paper or project topics include: The Incidence of Neural Tube Defects Among Hispanics and Its Implication for Nursing Care; Some Major Health Issues in the Oaxacan Community; The Provision of Health Care in Mexico; A Comparison of the Mexican and US Healthcare Systems; Embracing Transcultural Nursing Theory Experientially; The Problem of Dehydration of Patients in Mexico; How the Government and Economy Affect the Quality and Availability of Healthcare in Mexico; The Practice of Transcultural Nursing Theory in Community Care for the Oaxacan Client; and Giger and Davidhizar's Transcultural Nursing Theory Applied to Mexican Culture. Several students have presented to their *Sigma Theta Tau* (nursing honor society) chapters or the Transcultural Nursing Society. Other students presented their experiences in other nursing classes, while a few have had their papers published in refereed nursing journals. Some students have been invited to present their work at statewide study abroad meetings sponsored by the Georgia Board of Regents.

Student Course Evaluations

Perhaps most revealing of the impact of the course on student participants are course evaluations. When asked, "What did you learn from your nursing practice in this setting?" the following responses are representative of the majority of evaluations. One student responded, "It gave me a better appreciation for the culture, the importance of family unity, and increased my language skills." Another stated, "I was impressed with what the nurses and doctors accomplished with so little supplies and materials. They were resourceful and careful. My experience in Oaxaca was very helpful to me with my nursing practice at home in Atlanta. I am better able to relate and care for my Hispanic patients." One student who is currently a labor and delivery nurse at a large urban hospital in Atlanta wrote, "This course was definitely a peak life experience for me. I have felt very drawn to Hispanic people since I have worked at my hospital. This experience, being immersed in the culture, working with nurses, mothers and children in Mexico, living with a Hispanic family, was an opportunity to see inside a world that is rarely opened to outsiders or tourists. I am very grateful to have had this course." Another student made the following comment, "I believe that I'm more knowledgeable about the Mexican culture, especially related to health care, as well as the language and medical care. With this knowledge I have been better equipped to plan and administer care that is individualized for the Mexican population I come in contact with every day in my practice here in Georgia. I consider this course to be the best I ever had. I learned so much besides nursing; I learned about politics, economics, the Spanish language, music and art, archeology, history, etc."

Lessons Learned

Many lessons have been learned from setting up this nursing elective program in Oaxaca, Mexico. First, it is imperative to have university support. The university must see the need for the program and be willing to invest time and money for faculty to go to the area and meet with local health officials, set up a housing program, review the clinical sites, and learn about the local culture, customs, and special cultural sites to visit. All faculty must be able to speak at least a functional level of Spanish and have a basic appreciation of what it is like to live, work, and study in a developing country with different customs, food, language, health issues, and cultural behaviors. Health insurance for local care for faculty and students is necessary as well as insurance for possible evacuation to the United States. Checking with the Mexican Embassy or Consulate is necessary beforehand when bringing in valuable supplies through customs into Mexico. Transportation, transferring planes, immigration, and customs issues with a group of students, some of whom may never have traveled before, are among the many issues that must be considered. Preparation for physical safety, potential loss of passport, money, plane tickets, and illness must be planned for well ahead of the trip with students. Even with the best of intentions of both Americans and Mexicans, problems will occur in language and cultural interpretation and each experience is a lesson learned. Finally, the willingness of the Mexican healthcare administrators to tolerate placement of students with varying levels of Spanish proficiency in their hospitals and clinics is a humbling and eye-opening experience. Extensive orientation to the hospital, careful pairing of students with compatible nurses, and, in some cases, placing a student with limited Spanish skills with a student with a higher level of proficiency increases the potential for successful placements. The nurses, physicians, medical students, and nursing students of Oaxaca are overwhelmingly welcoming, willing to teach, and eager to communicate. One has to ask if under similar circumstances would the American healthcare system would be as welcoming?

The process of developing and implementing the Oaxacan study abroad nursing program has been a challenge, especially since a new Secretary of Health for the State is appointed every 3 years. Each year, things have been slightly different and new challenges have been encountered under varying healthcare administrators in Oaxaca.

The nursing practicum in Oaxaca is a valuable and rich learning adventure for faculty as well as students. Much time in preparation is necessary in order for this to be a safe and beneficial learning experience. Every aspect must be thoroughly planned ahead, and all participants must reasonably expect the unplanned and unknown to still occur. In general, the student's cultural competence has been enhanced after the experience of attending the nursing practicum in Oaxaca, Mexico, and both students and faculty are better prepared to work with Latino/Hispanic clients in their own local community.

GUIDELINES FOR SETTING UP A STUDY ABROAD PROGRAM FOR A NURSING ELECTIVE COURSE FOR CREDIT FOR STUDENT NURSES

1. Create a proposal with the following:
   a. Goals and objectives of proposed program
   b. Location: distance, safety, costs, local interest and support for program, easy accessibility

   c. Experiences for students and faculty: clinical experiences, participation in cultural activities, local language lessons
   d. Safety plan: political safety and stability, environmental (climate, local disease threats), health insurance and local health care available for participants, emergency evacuation plan
   e. Student prerequisites: nursing skills, language background, grade point average, orientation, disciplinary rules
   f. Number of faculty needed
   g. Number of students expected (interest survey given to students may give a more precise idea)
   h. Transportation: round trip to destination, local transportation
   i. Estimated costs
2. Obtain support from university's president, provost, dean, department chairs, and whoever else who may need to approve of the endeavor. Obtain "seed money" to investigate the feasibility of the program, provide transportation, housing, and other costs needed to explore an area to make initial preparations for the proposed program. Gifts may also be required in some cultures to facilitate appointments for key people in the local proposed site of the community.
3. Preparation visit to proposed location
   a. Arrange all transportation and housing if possible as you would expect to visit with students. Stay in hotel or with a local family as you would expect students to experience in order to see how the experience would be for students. Ask permission, always, to take pictures to show the university administrators as well as prospective students.
   b. Keep a detailed record book of all costs encountered. This will help in designing a course with an accurate price to reflect real costs.
   c. Find a person who has experience and is willing to coordinate housing for students. This person will require a placement fee per student. Often the local university has such a person, or a secretary may be able to handle this. See if they already have someone who assists foreign students with housing. Visit several homes or hotels for proposed housing and get specifics with prices.
   d. Local language lessons: find a local university or language school that is willing to give lessons to students at a reasonable price for 1 hour per day. This will help students to enhance their language and cultural background while they are at the proposed location.
   e. Meet with the Minister of Health (or equivalent person of high ranking in the community) to discuss the students' participation in caring for local patients within a healthcare setting (hospitals or clinics). Discuss

exactly what are student roles, supervision by faculty, dress codes, hours of work, length of stay, etc. If culturally appropriate, get a written contract. Ask what types of supplies or equipment are needed for the purpose of donations in the future. After the meeting, send flowers and a thank you note to the person for giving time and attention. Note: Students working within a different culture and language should not be giving medications because of the safety issue which could be further threatened by a language barrier.

f. Meet with a tourist travel agency or find a specific person in the community who will agree to provide transportation and help with an agenda for visiting sites of interest. Take advantage of all local tourist attractions, emphasizing anything reflecting health care if available. (Example: Students and faculty in Oaxaca, Mexico visited a local curandera [village healer] and watched her treat patients.) Note all costs for entrance fees, meals, transportation, tips, etc.

4. Student recruitment
   a. Prior to recruitment make all decisions about transportation, tuition, housing, food, cultural sites, donations, health insurance, availability of scholarships, etc., and prepare a formal budget. Decide how much it will cost per student for the entire package.
   b. Create a brochure for the course/trip with detailed specifics of costs, inclusions, dates, course credits, prerequisites, etc., and print flyers for a recruitment session. Several different recruitment sessions may be necessary to contact all available students who may be interested in the program. Arrange a date, time, and location for the recruitments and order food. If possible, bring photos or show a PowerPoint of pictures of the area. Obtain a list of interested students with names and email contacts and provide a way for students to sign up for the course. If the university already has other study abroad programs in place, they may be extremely helpful in planning your program.
   c. Collect all fees prior to departure. Assemble supply or equipment donations. Pack donations and send boxes with students to avoid mailing costs and possible theft of items.
   d. Create a mandatory orientation program prior to departure. Make sure that all students have all needed passports and vaccinations. Supply food and invite all family or friends who are interested in the trip details. Review and give written handouts relating a typical day, dress and behavior codes, and health guidance including what to eat and what medications to bring. Include a list of what to pack, and weight and number limitations for luggage. State where to meet at the airport and at what time.

Emphasize the safety and health plan. Review rules and regulations. Pass out course syllabus and review pretrip readings available. A survey of student perceptions of the trip prior to leaving would make an interesting contrast when compared to impressions after having had the experience. Encourage students to bring a small gift for host family and/or nurse mentors at their location.

   e. Have students review and sign a code of behavior while studying in the location. Include the following:
      i. No alcohol or drug use is permitted.
      ii. Dress codes and expected behavior with family, faculty, all members of local community are to be written and enforced.
      iii. No leaving of city under any circumstances without permission of faculty is permitted.
      iv. All students will stay all night with host family, with no exceptions.
      v. Students will always follow the faculty's instructions and are subject to be sent home, incurring their own extra expenses if not behaving.
      vi. Students will fail course if not behaving as instructed by faculty.

5. Experience while at location
   a. Plan an orientation with local health administration for tours, work assignments, give donations of supplies, and offer to pay for snacks served. Bring a gift for key health administrator contacts.
   b. Keep a daily journal of visits, contacts, phone numbers and emails, costs, problems to be solved, and daily agenda.
   c. Make student assignments with local agency administrators. Give students preferences when possible according to their previous experiences and language abilities.
   d. Make local community contacts on own time. Meet the directors of all hospitals, clinics, housing, group excursions, and language centers. Bring small gifts or take them for coffee and pastries when meeting with them. Emphasize how much you appreciate the help that they are giving to you.
   e. Make friends in the local community with merchants, taxi drivers, restaurant owners, etc., and if relationships are successful, bring students to them. Often you will receive a group discount on tickets, transportation, food, etc., with these relationships.
   f. Participate in all student activities. Take local language classes with students and assist with supervision in hospitals, clinics, and on all cultural excursions. Find out about other interesting activities in the community that may interest students.

THINGS TO EMPHASIZE TO AVOID PROBLEMS

The following is from many experiences in which faculty have learned the hard way with no idea of what to expect, especially the first few years. It is never possible to know ahead of time what problems may occur. Faculty, as well as students, need to be flexible and adaptable to new challenges.

1. Always write a code of behavior, emphasize it at recruitment, orientation, and during the visit to the host country. Have students sign the behavior code.
2. Always have health insurance with evacuation coverage for all students and faculty. It is very reasonable. Do not rely on local healthcare facilities for serious accidents or illnesses. For minor problems they usually will be fine.
3. Make sure that all students stay in the local city at all times and spend the night with host families every night.
4. Review safety precautions for money (under-the-clothing money bags for traveling) and locking valuables such as passports, money, credit cards, and cameras with local family.
5. Constantly remind students about what and where is safe to eat and drink, and be sure that they are always aware.
6. Always watch luggage and carry-ons at airports. Things may disappear very quickly especially in developing countries if they are valuable and unattended.
7. Be prepared to deal with culture shock. Language, customs, and, in some locations, tremendous, never before seen poverty can overwhelm faculty and students. Many poor people including those begging in the streets can be overwhelming. Giving away prepared sandwiches and fruit or bread can be a group activity that can help some of the overwhelming feelings of frustration.
8. Have students always travel in groups and always carry information with them regarding their host family homes and contact information for reaching faculty 24/7.
9. Always be available to students 24/7. This is not like the responsibility of a classroom on campus.

Acknowledgment

The authors, Carol Holtz and Richard Sowell, wish to acknowledge the contributions of Drs. David Bennett, June Laval, Janice Long, and Astrid Wilson for their support, creativity, and challenging work with students enrolled in the nursing practicum course in Oaxaca, Mexico.

REFERENCES

African immigration to the United States. (2009). Retrieved June 7, 2009, from http://en.wikipedia.org/wiki/African_immigration_to_the_United _States

Barry, T. (1992). *Mexico: A country guide*. Albuquerque, NM: The Inter-Hemisphere Resource Center.

Bennett, D., & Holtz, C. (2008). Building cultural competence: A nursing program in Oaxaca, Mexico. In C. Holtz (Ed.), *Global health care*. Sudbury, MA: Jones and Bartlett.

Camphina-Bacote, J. (1994). *The process of cultural competence in health care: A culturally competent model of care* (2nd ed.). Wyoming, Ohio: Perfect Printing Press.

Centers for Disease Control and Prevention. (2005). Tuberculosis in the United States, 2004–2005. Retrieved June 8, 2009, from http://www.cdc.gov/od/oc/media/pressrel/fs050317.htm

Ewing, R. (1996). *Six faces of Mexico: History, people, geography, government, economy, literature, and art*. Tucson, AZ: The Arizona Board of Regents.

Hall, J. M., Stevens, P. E., & Meleis, A. I. (1994). Marginalization: A guiding concept for evaluating diversity in nursing knowledge development. *Advances in Nursing Science, 16*(4), 2–41.

Immigration to the United States. (2006). Retrieved June 7, 2008, from http://en.wikipedia.org/wiki/Immigration to the United_States 2006

Lee, J., & Rytina, N. (2008). *Naturalizations in the United States: 2008*. Retrieved June 7, 2009, from http://www.dhs.gov/xlibrary/assets/statistics/publications/natz_fr_2008.pdf

Leininger, M. (1978). *Transcultural nursing: Concepts, theories, and practices*. New York: John Wiley & Sons.

Leininger, M., & McFarland, M. (2002). *Transcultural nursing: Concepts, theories, research, and practices* (3rd ed.). New York: McGraw Hill.

Lustig, L. (1992). *Mexico: The making of an economy*. Washington, DC: Brookings Institution.

Min, P. G. (2006). Asian immigration: History and contemporary trends. In P. G. Min (Ed.), *Asian Americans: Contemporary trends and issues* (2nd ed., pp 7–31). Thousand Oaks, CA: Pine Forge Press/Sage.

Purnell, L., & Paulanka, B. J. (2003). *Transcultural health care: A culturally competent approach*. Philadelphia: F.A. Davis

Spector, R. (2004). *Cultural diversity in health and illness* (6th ed.). Norwalk, CT: Appleton & Lange.

US Census Bureau. (2007). *Hispanic population of the United States*. Retrieved August 11, 2007, from http://www.census.gov/population/www/socdemo/hispanic.html

US Population Hits 300 Million. (2006). Retrieved June 7, 2009, from http://www.msnbc.msn.com/id/15298443/

SECTION VI

EVALUATION

The final section of this text presents a brief glimpse at a key aspect of any educational program: evaluation. Whereas the importance of evaluation is often overlooked, it is an essential part of the teaching–learning process. Educators predominately think of evaluation either in the form of testing and grading, or in clinical evaluation. Chapters in this section describe innovative approaches to evaluation that include student evaluation of teachers and evaluation of the strategies and resources that educators use. Feedback from students as consumers provides useful, practical information. This information then feeds into total program evaluation and provides data on the curriculum, teaching effectiveness, and the use of learning activities. A thorough evaluation provides information for quality attainment.

CHAPTER 32

Programmatic Evaluation

Jill M. Hayes

INTRODUCTION

Educational programs in healthcare-related fields strive to provide competent practitioners for a variety of healthcare delivery settings, which is based on a sound empirical body of knowledge (DeSilets & Dickerson, 2008). These programs are dependent on consumers enrolling in their programs, the resources needed to support and sustain the programs, and the external environment that provides educational experiences and settings in which program graduates may pursue their careers in health care. Programmatic evaluation is one method of validating the accomplishment of this mission, both to consumers of education and the various stakeholders or recipients of services. All educational institutions providing professional programs have a focus on teaching and student outcomes and the role of faculty involves a complex set of expectations that vary within the context of the individual program, and institutional, mission. The teaching role of the faculty includes all aspects of facilitating student learning, including the evaluation of that learning, which in turn contributes to the overall programmatic evaluation.

There is a growing demand from consumers and stakeholders of education that colleges and universities be more accountable for the product they are graduating. In addition, mandates from accrediting associations and education commissions state that effectiveness of educational programs must be addressed, placing an emphasis on measuring student learning and documenting student learning outcomes. Historically, the quality of educational programs has been measured in terms of resources, program offerings, faculty qualifications, and student services. However, these definitions of quality are being challenged, and educators are being charged with the task of documenting program effectiveness in terms of student learning. Therefore programmatic evaluation is essential to the success of professional healthcare-related academic programs.

PURPOSE

According to Bell, Pestka, and Forsyth (2007), the purpose of programmatic evaluation is the determination of the program's worth. This includes collecting and analyzing data for use in judging the educational program and the product of the program, its graduates. Programmatic evaluation is an expectation of numerous stakeholders in the healthcare environment (DeSilets & Dickerson, 2008). Consumers of education look to a program's status/reputation to assist them in their decision to enroll. The professional student of today considers many aspects of a program when choosing to enroll. In addition to location, cost, scheduling of classes, and accessibility of resources, these students consider the success rate of graduates in licensure requirements as significant to their decision. A second significant characteristic of a professional education program is their accreditation status. Although not mandated (Grumet, 2002), accreditation status of a program potentially affects the availability of external funding and other resources, clinical educational opportunities, and students' advanced educational opportunities upon graduation from the program. Programmatic evaluation is a method to accurately reflect and validate a program's success in accomplishing stated outcomes—principally the graduation of competent practitioners capable of successful completion of licensure requirements and the pursuit of their professional healthcare career (DeSilets & Dickerson, 2008). The attainment of national accreditation requires thorough programmatic evaluation using valid measurable outcomes with accurate data to support the achievement of these outcomes. Benefits of a rigorous programmatic evaluation include the ability to attract a diverse student population and qualified faculty. Additionally, the attainment of national accreditation status and the ability to obtain internal and external funding and educational resources to support and sustain the program mission are contingent on the results of overall programmatic evaluation. The education of competent healthcare practitioners is critical to meet the needs of, and to enhance, the current healthcare environment.

DEFINITION

Effective programmatic evaluation is defined as the "application of evaluative approaches, techniques, and analysis to systematically assess and improve the planning, implementation and effectiveness of the program" (Chen, 2005). Fink (2005) defines programmatic evaluation as "the diligent investigation of a program's characteristics and merits" and examines the effectiveness of programs or activities performed to optimize outcomes, efficiency, and quality of healthcare delivery. Davidson (2005) further elaborates, stating the purpose of evaluation is to "determine the overall quality or value of something and to find areas of improvement." According to Worral (2008), the process of evaluation is the collection, summation, interpretation, and utilization of data to identify the extent to which an action was successful; in the case of professional healthcare-related education programs, the education of competent practitioners able to successfully complete professional licensure requirements.

EVALUATIVE STRATEGIES

Although the evaluation of programmatic outcomes (summative evaluation) is valuable to determine the effectiveness of the program, it is insufficient to ensure the program's success. Worral (2008) proposes that the use of both formative and summative evaluation are essential to effective programmatic evaluation. Summative or process evaluation helps programs to determine the effectiveness of the program in question through the analysis of data reflective of the extent to which the learners' needs and terminal program outcomes were met. Formative evaluation enables the program to examine whether the program and the learners are proceeding as planned and desired and to make adjustments in educational activities as needed to enhance the successful accomplishment of programmatic outcomes.

THEORETICAL FOUNDATION

Programmatic evaluation is intrinsic to programs of professional healthcare education, and the entire academic arena (Gard, Flannigan, & Cluskey, 2004). To be effective, the evaluation should be based on established standards, which for professional healthcare education are most often set by external accrediting agencies. Inherent in the evaluative process is decision making relative to program outcomes, based on the evaluative findings. Reliability and validity of the findings are strengthened through the application of a systematic approach to the evaluation, guided by established guidelines and implemented by a formalized group of faculty and/or administrators with expertise in the process of evaluation.

Because the process of decision making is inherent in evaluation, valid and reliable data must be collected. Validity and reliability can be obtained only through a systematic approach to evaluation. A systematic approach can be ensured when an evaluation design is used to guide the process. An evaluation design is defined as a plan that identifies what decisions will be made, when and from whom data will be gathered, as well as what instruments will be used to obtain the data. General considerations include what evaluation model will be used, what type of data needs to be collected, how the data will be analyzed and by whom, and how the evaluation results will be disseminated. Deliberate decisions about the evaluation design ensure that the evaluation plan is valid, reliable, timely, pervasive, and credible.

The use of a theoretical framework is essential to systematic program evaluation. Once measurable outcome criteria are selected, theoretical foundations assist in the identification of data to be collected, the timing of data collection, and how this data then directs and contributes to the evaluation of program outcomes. A valuable theoretical framework for programmatic evaluation is the widely known systems theory (Chen, 2005).

Systems theory includes the identification/analysis of five elements, applicable to programmatic evaluation. These elements are input, throughput, output, environment, and feedback. Each of these elements impacts all other elements and the analysis of each provides valuable data for effective overall programmatic evaluation (Figure 32-1).

According to the Chen (2005), the terms identified within systems theory provide a means to clarify the nature and characteristics of any given program. To be successful, any program must accomplish two functions. Internally, "inputs" must be transformed into desirable "outputs"; externally, the program must continuously and successfully interact with its environment to procure resources to support and sustain itself and meet the environmental need—in this case, the needs of the healthcare environment. Because of this essential element of environmental interaction, successful programs must exist as "open systems," open to the

Figure 32-1 Systems theory.

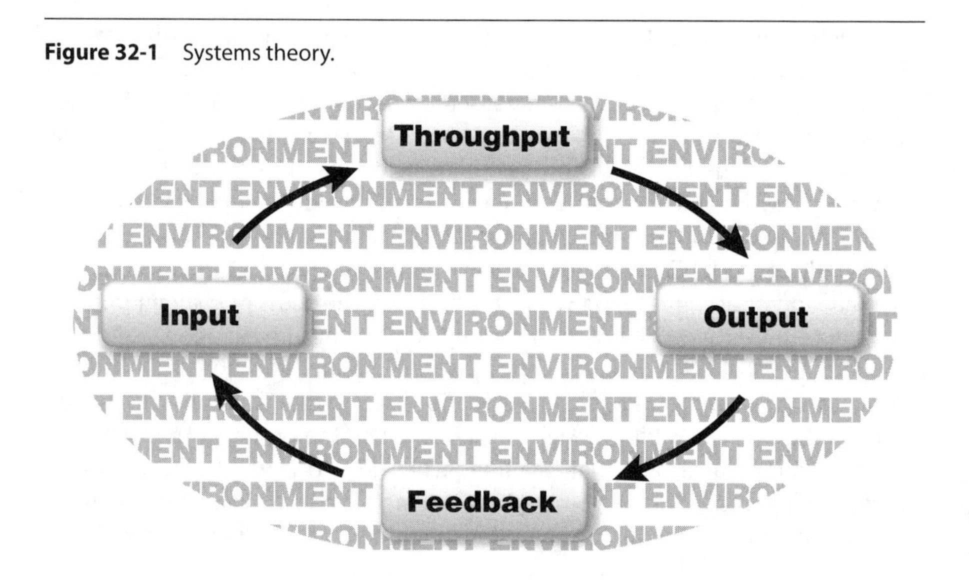

influence of their environments. This theoretical framework readily guides programmatic evaluation, both formative and summative, and in this manner requires professional healthcare programs to clearly demonstrate the role of each program component in the evaluative process.

Application to the Evaluative Process

Applying systems theory to the process of programmatic evaluation in professional education, *inputs* may be identified as students enrolling in the program, educational resources provided both from the educational environment and the external environment, faculty teaching in the program, and the curriculum. The *throughput* or *transformation* element of the program is viewed as including the implementation of the curriculum by the faculty, the use of classroom/teaching resources, and/or clinical practice settings available to the students. In addition, the administration of the program which involves the hiring/evaluating of faculty, ensuring that teaching resources are available to the students, and determining the conceptual framework/teaching philosophy that guides the teaching/learning is considered to be "throughput" within the context of the program. *Outputs* are the actual graduates of the program, measures of their knowledge acquisition in all settings where teaching/learning occurs, and their success in meeting licensure requirements and providing competent practice within a variety of healthcare environments. In addition, outputs may be viewed as the productivity of the faculty outside of the classroom, such as research and scholarly activities as well as service to the community.

Environment is identified as the community(ies) within which the program is located and provides services. This may include the academic environment where the program is established, and the political environment that influences the availability/accessibility of healthcare settings for student learning experiences, resources for such services, and availability of and support for graduates in professional nursing. In addition, the type of stakeholders associated with the educational and practice institutions and their philosophical view of education are considered to be environmental influences on program effectiveness. Finally, the direct consumer of this education, the students, significantly influence both the academic environment and the external environment, dependent on their learning needs and expectations of the program.

The fifth element, *feedback*, is essential to the creation of an effective educational program and valid programmatic evaluation. This informational loop provides data relative to characteristics inherent to its inputs, throughputs, and outputs (both formative and summative) and is used to make adjustments to all aspects of the program. Data is gathered from student evaluations both while enrolled in the program (formative) and following graduation (summative); the environmental response to program throughputs and outputs; healthcare organization evaluations of program graduates; measures of healthcare quality as provided by these graduates. Utilizing this theoretical framework clearly provides a means to perform valid and accurate programmatic evaluation, valuable to both program administrators, national accreditation agencies/program stakeholders as well as a means to demonstrate how all elements of the program contribute to the evaluative process.

Process of Evaluation

Utilizing this theoretical framework, it is clear how each component of an educational program is essential to overall programmatic evaluation. Faculty frequently do not consider elements of their role in the development of teaching/learning activities and their course materials as significantly impacting programmatic evaluation. However, to be effective, an educational program's mission statement, philosophy, and conceptual framework must be reflected in all elements of the program—course descriptions, course objectives, teaching/learning activities, etc., which are developed by individual faculty. For example, if the mission statement addresses the need for graduates to serve a diverse client population, then the course objectives in each course must reflect teaching/learning that allows the students to care for a diverse client population within the context of course content. If cultural sensitivity is viewed as a program outcome for its graduates, then cultural sensitivity education must be a part of all courses within the curriculum. If successful completion of licensure requirements is stated as a program outcome, then assessment in all courses must reflect activities to ensure students meet testing criteria and mastery of content requisite for meeting the licensure standards.

As stated previously, all elements of an educational program must be clearly guided by programmatic evaluation and contribute data to support that evaluative process. Feedback from the environment—healthcare environment needs and expectations—help to determine admission requirements for applicants to the program and faculty expertise for teaching in the program. Relative to the throughputs aspect of the program, classroom/educational environments and clinical experiences are selected to meet the learning needs of the students to ensure environmental needs are met and students successfully meet the licensure agency requirements. In addition, faculty research and service activities will be guided by community needs, student learning needs, and demands of the university environment for faculty effectiveness. Feedback from both the outputs (graduates) and the external environment provides data to support adjustments to curriculum and teaching/learning to better meet the community and learner needs. The use of a theoretical framework also assists in the determination of outcome criteria selected by the evaluator. Program outcomes, when reflected throughout the curriculum and all program elements, assist in the setting of admission criteria (i.e., cultural diversity of students) and also the selection of faculty to teach in the program. Faculty are selected based on their area of expertise to assist in meeting the needs of the current healthcare environment. In turn, curriculum development is guided by the needs of the current healthcare environment, the needs of the learners, and the research and service focus of faculty. Teaching and learning activities are guided by the availability and diversity of practice environments, and also guide the selection of specific learning activities incorporated into the curriculum. In addition, community alliances enhance the diversity of the learning experiences offered to students and faculty, as well as provide resources to support and sustain the program.

ELEMENTS OF PROGRAM EVALUATION

Clearly, there are a wide variety of criteria that may be selected as program outcomes within the context of programmatic evaluation. Simpler is often better when selecting evaluative criteria, so long as the essential elements of the program are analyzed. In professional healthcare education, learning must be viewed as essential as a program outcome, since clinical practice is dependent on a sound knowledge base for that practice (DeSilets & Dickerson, 2008). Outcome evaluation measures changes in clinical practice following a learning experience. Evaluation of learning incorporates not only the objectives of the learning experience but also the characteristics of the learner. Evaluation of learning enables faculty members to determine the progression of students toward meeting the educational objectives. Specifically, the goal is to discover to what degree learners have attained the knowledge, attitudes, or skills emphasized in a learning experience. As a result of the dearth of available instruments to measure the student's brain to determine if learning has occurred, simulated or designed situations are developed to measure learning. Therefore, evaluation of learning is a value judgment based on the data obtained from the various designed measurements taken in the classroom and clinical settings. In addition, the evaluation methods should match the nature of the course and the outcomes. For example, if students are enrolled in a course that contains 45 clock hours of didactic and 150 clock hours of clinical, it would be important that most of the measurements used to evaluate this course would measure learning in the clinical area.

The process for evaluating learning is similar to the process for program evaluation, in that it is based on a planned design, and in turn contributes significantly to the overall programmatic evaluation. Deliberate planning and thought are needed to decide what evaluation methods should be used in a course of study. First, faculty members need to identify what is to be evaluated. What are the outcomes of learning? Inherent in this process is the specification of the domain of learning. In the health professions, learning occurs not only in the cognitive or knowledge domain, but also in the affective or value domain and in the psychomotor or competency domain. Each domain of learning requires different evaluation measures. For example, a multiple choice exam measures a student's cognitive understanding of a concept but does not measure the student's ability to perform a clinical skill.

In addition, in measuring the domain of a learner, the faculty must determine the complexity of the learning. Complexity of learning is determined when one considers the characteristics of the learner (i.e., level of learning, prerequisite courses, past clinical experiences). Integrated into this determination is the identification of the content or concepts associated with the learning experience. All of these factors clearly describe the behavior to be measured that indicates that learning has occurred. One should construct a matrix that identifies all of the factors to ensure that all concepts are integrated and the best measurement is chosen.

If licensure success rate is selected as a program outcome, data from curriculum, teaching/learning activities, and practice environments may be collected to support this criterion. Data relative to retention/attrition of students as well as student progression through the program may be used to evaluate admission requirements and make adjustments as needed. Cost-effectiveness of the program may be reflected through practice and learning environments as well as community partnerships utilized to enhance available resources. Data related to time from admission to graduation also includes curriculum, faculty expertise, assessment techniques, and teaching/learning activities.

Classroom Assessment

Formative evaluation provides valuable data when evaluating student learning and the teaching strategies being used. Classroom assessment is a type of formative evaluation that involves ongoing assessment of student learning and assists faculty in selecting teaching strategies (Melland & Volden, 1998). This technique involves both students and instructors in the continuous monitoring of student learning. The purpose of classroom assessment parallels the purpose of formative evaluation. The purpose is to collect data during the learning experience to make adjustments so that students can benefit from the modifications before the final measurement of learning occurs. This approach is learner centered, teacher directed, mutually beneficial, formative, context specific, ongoing, and firmly rooted in good practice (Angelo & Cross, 1993).

Classroom assessment differs from other measurements of learning in that it is usually anonymous and is never graded. It is context specific, meaning that the technique used to evaluate one class or a content-related learning experience will not necessarily work in another experience.

The use of classroom assessment provides feedback about learning not only to the faculty but to the student as well. Assessment techniques (e.g., asking student to identify the muddiest point discussed or a one-sentence summary of the discussion) are simple to use, take little time, and yet are fun for the student. An example of a popular assessment technique is muddiest point. Close to the end of the learning session, the student is asked to write, "What was the muddiest point in this lecture?" (or whatever teaching strategy was used). The faculty then reviews the responses to determine if a concept is mentioned frequently or if a pattern emerges indicating that a concept or content was misunderstood. Based on the results, the faculty may choose to address the "muddiest point" in the next class. Answering the question also causes students to reflect on the session and identify concepts needing further study.

Clinical Evaluation

Health professions are practice disciplines, and therefore student learning involves more than acquiring cognitive knowledge. Learning includes the practice dimension where the student demonstrates the ability to apply theory in caring for patients. Clinical evaluation addresses three dimensions of student learning—cognitive, affective, and psychomotor—and is the most challenging of the evaluative processes. Inherent in this process is the need to demonstrate progressive acquisition of increasingly complex competencies. Evaluating student learning and student competency in clinical is challenging. The faculty must make professional judgments concerning the student's competencies in practice, as well as the higher-level cognitive learning associated with application. Yet, the clinical environment changes from one learning experience to another, making absolute comparisons among students even in the same clinical setting impossible. In addition, role expectations of the learners and evaluators are perceived differently. The evaluations of a student's performance frequently are influenced by one's own professional orientation and expectations. Evaluation in the clinical setting is the process of collecting data in order to make a judgment concerning the students' competencies in practice based on standards or criteria. Judgments influence the data collected; therefore, it is not an objective process. Deciding on the quality of performance and drawing inferences and conclusions from the data also involves judgment by the faculty. It is a subjective process that is influenced by the bias of the faculty and student and by the variables present in the clinical environment. These factors and others make evaluating the clinical experience a complex process.

In clinical evaluation, the faculty members observe performance and collect data associated with higher-order cognitive thinking, the influence of values (affective learning), and psychomotor skill acquisition. (This process is addressed in more depth in Chapter 25.) The judgment of a student's performance in the clinical area can either be based on norm- or criterion-referenced evaluation. With norm-referenced evaluation, the student's clinical performance is compared with the performance of other students in the course, whereas criterion-referenced evaluation is the comparison of the student's performance with a set of criteria. Regardless of the type of evaluation used, providing a fair and valid evaluation is challenging. Although the use of criterion-referenced tools reduces the subjectivity inherent to this process, using multiple and varied sources of data (i.e., observation, evaluation of written work, student comments, staff comments) increases the possibility that a valid evaluation occurs. Also, making observations throughout the designated experience in an effort to obtain a sampling of behaviors that reflect quality of care provided and the extent of student learning helps to validate the evaluation.

It has been established that, even with the best-developed evaluation criteria, clinical evaluation is subjective and therefore efforts must be made to ensure that the process is fair. Oermann and Gaberson (1998) addressed the following dimensions associated with fairness in clinical evaluation:

- Identifying the faculty's own values, attitudes, beliefs, and biases that may influence the evaluation process
- Basing clinical evaluation on predetermined objectives or competencies
- Developing a supportive clinical environment
- Basing judgments on the expected competency according to curriculum and standards of practice
- Comparing the student's present behavior performance with past performance, other students' performances, or to the level of a norm reference group

The process of evaluating a student's performance in a clinical setting poses several challenges to evaluation theory. Extensive documentation exists in the nursing literature addressing clinical evaluation and providing examples of evaluation tools. Students are demonstrating their ability to apply knowledge in caring for patients in an uncontrolled environment, and therefore it is difficult for them to hide their lack of understanding or inability to "put it all together." However, although this setting is ideal for learning, the variables that exist in the setting make each learning experience different. Faculty members also struggle with the concept of when the time for learning ends and the time for evaluation begins. Again, the literature provides guidelines addressing this issue.

A solution to the challenges of clinical evaluation may exist within the context of clearly defining the parameters of formative and summative evaluation. Although not without its flaws, this solution worked as long as the clinical experiences existed in the hospital setting and were defined by discrete units of time; however, educating students in a managed care environment has changed the settings and the focus of the clinical experience. Faculty members no longer have the security of the familiar hospital setting and the discrete time units. Patients receive health care in a variety of settings such as day surgery, outpatient clinics, community settings, and in the home. Patients admitted to the hospital stay shorter periods, require more extensive care, and present with more complex situations. Thus, many past strategies that were successful in clinical evaluation are no longer applicable.

Clinical Concept Mapping

Clinical concept mapping was developed by an educational researcher as an instructional and assessment tool for use in science education (Novak, 1990). In general, the technique is a hierarchical graphic organizer developed individually by students. It demonstrates their understanding of relationships among concepts. Key concepts are placed centrally, and subconcepts and clusters of data are placed peripherally. All concepts are linked by arrows, lines, or broken lines to demonstrate the association between and among the concepts and the data (Baugh & Mellot, 1998).

Clinical concept mapping is applicable in evaluating students in the clinical setting because it facilitates the linking of previously learned concepts to actual patient scenarios. The diagramming of the concepts allows faculty members to evaluate the student's interpretation of collected data and how it applies to the student's patient and to management of patient care. It also provides data for faculty members to evaluate the student's ability to apply class content and concepts to implementing care. Faculty members are also able to evaluate the student's ability to solve problems and to think critically. Clinical concept mapping can be applied to a variety of clinical settings (Bentley & Nugent, 1998) and to a variety of learning experiences (see Chapter 26).

Portfolio Assessment

Portfolio analysis can serve as an important component of the process of assessing student learning outcomes and the achievement of overall program outcomes. When used appropriately, portfolio assessment provides valid data for clinical evaluation of students and may be used to clearly demonstrate a correlation between competencies gained and curricular or program outcomes. A portfolio is a compilation of documents demonstrating learning, competencies, and achievements, usually over a period of time. Used extensively in business to demonstrate one's accomplishments, the portfolio is often used in education to track academic achievement of outcomes (Ryan & Carlton, 1990). Although portfolios are discussed here in relation to clinical evaluation, they also can be used in different aspects of program evaluation. Portfolios are valid measures in clinical evaluation in that students provide evidence in their portfolios to confirm their clinical competence and to document their learning. They may be used in either formative or summative evaluation. Portfolio assessments are a positive asset in clinical settings in which students are not directly supervised by faculty.

Nitko (1996) describes the use of portfolios in terms of best work and growth and learning portfolios. Best work portfolios provide evidence that students have mastered outcomes and have attained the desired level of competence (summative evaluation), thus contributing to the accreditation process. Growth and learning portfolios are designed to monitor students' progress (formative evaluation). Both types of portfolios reflect the philosophy of clinical evaluation.

Portfolios are constructed to match the purpose and objectives of the clinical experience. Faculty members need to clearly delineate the purpose and outcomes and to identify examples of work to be included. Likewise, the criteria by which the contents of the portfolio will be evaluated must be provided for the students. Students need to understand that portfolios are a reflection of their learning and an evaluation of their performance. The portfolio can be used in conjunction with the clinical pathway (Chapter 35 for evaluation).

Although still in the exploratory stage, portfolios are evolving as effective measurements in outcome evaluation. If portfolios are used in clinical evaluation, then faculty members benefit from data that demonstrate the clinical progression of students through the curriculum toward the program outcomes. Although portfolio development has been shown to increase student responsibility for learning, increase faculty/student interaction, and facilitate the identification of need for curricular revision, they are time consuming to compile and present challenges related to document storage. In addition, faculty struggle with the lack of research-based evidence to establish validity and reliability of grading measures related to program outcome evaluation.

Clinical Journals

Teaching/learning in the clinical setting is broad and diverse, including much more than can be identified superficially. Journaling is a technique that has been successfully used to bring together those elusive bits of information and experience associated with the clinical experience (Kobert, 1995). Clinical journals provide an opportunity for students to not only document their clinical experience but also to reflect on their performance and knowledge, and demonstrate a level of critical thinking. Journals provide an avenue for students to express their feelings of uncertainty and to engage in dialogue with the faculty concerning the experience. Journaling also can be structured to include nursing care, problem solving, and identification of learning needs. Whereas journals provide valuable evaluation data, the challenge is to obtain from the students the quality of journal entries needed.

Hodges (1996) addressed this issue in a proposed model in which four levels of journal writing were identified. These levels of journal writing progressed from summarizing, describing, and reacting to clinical experience, then to analyzing and critiquing positions, issues, and views of others. Examples of journal entries that parallel this progression are moving from writing objectives or a summary to writing a critique or a focused argument. The key to this progression lies in providing a clear purpose for the journal entry. To think critically, students need to know what they are thinking about (Brown & Sorrell, 1993). Once faculty members have identified the desired outcome of the clinical journal, they can assist the students in attaining these outcomes by providing clear guidelines.

Although keeping a journal requires a substantial commitment of time by both faculty and students, it is a valuable evaluation tool for both groups. Controversy exists concerning whether journals should be used for evaluation of students' learning or to be graded (Holmes, 1997). Some educators maintain that grading journals negates the students' ability to be reflective and truthful concerning clinical experiences; however, as students document their evolution of clinical experiences, their journal entries are laden with expressions of self evaluation (Kobert, 1995). If journals are to be graded, then clear and concise criteria must exist that not only identify how they are graded but also what is to be included in the journal. Regardless of the decision to grade or not to grade them, clinical journals provide important evaluation data concerning the student's performance in the clinical setting and can be used effectively to monitor the student's development in terms of program outcomes.

In summary, evaluation of learning is an important component of the faculty teaching role and contributes significantly to overall programmatic evaluation. Because the purpose of evaluation is to provide valid data concerning learning in all domains, a variety of measurements is needed. The key to successful evaluation is to match the evaluation tool with the learning in order to provide reliable and valid data on which to make judgments.

In addition to making a judgment concerning a student's performance in clinical, it is important to remember that the other purpose of clinical evaluation is to provide feedback to the student regarding his or her performance and to provide the student with an opportunity to improve in the needed areas. Clinical evaluation should be a consistent and frequent means of communicating the student's progress. Using an adopted clinical evaluation tool ensures that all students are counseled using the same criteria. The evaluation process needs to be constructed so that active student participation is included. Feedback should be stated in the specific terms of the measurement tool and the outcomes of the course. Comments should be based on data and should not contain general global clichés such as "will make a good nurse." Strengths, as well as areas needing improvement, should be documented. If a student needs to improve to pass the clinical experience, then the student should be given, in writing, those areas needing improvement with specific guidelines on what behavior is required to pass. Again, all comments should be stated in terms of the criteria on the evaluation tool.

CONCLUSION

This chapter has addressed some aspects of the role of evaluation in program development and student success. Clearly, evaluation is an important part of the faculty role, and contributes significantly to the overall success of professional academic programs. An understanding of evaluation and how it impacts the teaching/learning environment is critical. Proper use of evaluation techniques requires an awareness of both their limitations and their strengths and requires matching the appropriate measurement with the purpose or role of evaluation. In addition, the role of evaluation in the success of professional healthcare education programs and their ongoing existence to meet the needs of the health environment must not be under emphasized. As faculty and program administrators are increasingly held accountable to external stakeholders, program evaluation becomes increasingly significant to a program's success and continued existence. All elements of a professional education as mentioned previously, contribute valuable data to the process of rigorous programmatic evaluation, and assist in the ongoing enhancement of the program offerings. Professional practice in healthcare environments is entering a new era with increased use of, and dependence on, technology and advancements in knowledge and skills acquisition. This new era will significantly alter the traditional roles of faculty and students. Inherent in this new era of teaching is the mandate to evaluate teaching and learning using less traditional methods to demonstrate success in meeting program outcomes and meeting the needs of the healthcare community.

REFERENCES

Angelo, T., & Cross, K. P. (1993). *Classroom Assessment techniques: A handbook for college teachers* (2nd ed.). San Francisco: Jossey-Bass.

Baugh, N., & Mellott, K. (1998). Clinical concept mapping as preparation for student nurses' clinical experiences. *Journal of Nursing Education, 37*(6), 253–256.

Bell, D. F., Pestka, E., & Forsyth, D. (2007). Outcome evaluation: Does continuing education make a difference? *The Journal of Continuing Education in Nursing, 38*(4), 186–190.

Bentley, G., & Nugent, K. (1998). A creative student presentation on the nursing management of a complex family. *Nurse Educator, 23*(3), 8–9.

Brown, H., & Sorrell, J. (1993). Use of clinical journals to enhance critical thinking. *Nurse Educator, 18*(5), 16–18.

Chen, H. (2005). *Practical program evaluation: Assessing and improving planning, implementation, and effectiveness*. London: Sage Publications.

Davidson, E. J. (2005). *Evaluation Methodology Basics: The Nuts and Bolts of Sound Evaluation*. Thousand Oaks, CA: Sage.

DeSilets, L. D., & Dickerson, P. S. (2008). Assessing competency: A new accreditation resource. *The Journal of Continuing Education in Nursing, 39*(6), 244–245.

Fink, A. (2005). *Evaluation fundamentals: Insights into the outcomes, effectiveness, and quality of health programs*. London: Sage Publications.

Gard, C. L., Flannigan, P. N., & Cluskey, M. (2004). Program evaluation: An ongoing systematic process. *Nursing Education Perspectives, 25*(4), 176–179.

Grumet, B. R. (2002). Quick reads: Demystifying accreditation. *Nursing Education Perspectives, 23*(3), 114–117.

Hodges, H. (1996). Journal writing as a mode of thinking for RN-BSN students: A leveled approach to learning to listen to self and others. *Journal of Nursing Education, 35*, 137–141.

Holmes, V. (1997). Grading journals in clinical practice. *Journal of Nursing Education, 36*(10), 89–92.

Kobert, L. (1995). In our own voice: Journaling as a teaching/learning technique for nurses. *Journal of Nursing Education, 34*(3), 140–142.

Melland, H., & Volden, C. (1998). Classroom assessment: Linking teaching and learning. *Journal of Nursing Education, 37*(6), 275–277.

Nitko, A. (1990). *Educational assessment of students* (2nd ed.). Englewood Cliffs, NJ: Prentice Hall.

Novak, J. (1990). Concept mapping: A useful tool for science education. *Journal of Research in Science Teaching, 27*(10), 937–949.

Oermann, K., & Gaberson, M. (1998). Evaluation of problem-solving, decision-making, and critical thinking: Context-dependent item sets and other evaluation strategies. In M. Oermann and K. Gaberson (Eds.), *Evaluation and testing in nursing education*. New York: Springer Publishing.

Ryan, M., & Carlton, K. (1990). Portfolio applications in a school of nursing. *Nurse Educator, 22*(1), 35–39.

Worral, P. S. (2008). Evaluation in healthcare education. In S. B. Bastable (Ed.), *Nurse as educator: Principles of teaching and learning for nursing practice* (3rd ed.). Sudbury, MA: Jones & Bartlett.

CHAPTER 33

Assessment of Learning and Evaluation Strategies

Eric Oestmann and Joanna Oestmann

INTRODUCTION

This chapter will examine the current literature involved in the assessment of learning and various evaluation strategies; discuss the relevant educational issues and teaching techniques with examples of each provided; identify common problem areas; and offer solutions to these problems accordingly.

LEARNING ASSESSMENT AND EVALUATION TOPICS

The assessment of learning and corresponding evaluation strategies and methods is a complex process. Learning styles/types must be considered first.

Learning Styles/Types

There are three primary modalities for learning: visual, auditory, and kinesthetic (Fig. 33-1). Each student may be dominant in one area, but all areas must be considered in the assessment of learning and evaluation of learning therein.

To assess learning style dominance, the following exercise may be used:

Learning Style Exercise 1

To better understand how you prefer to learn and process information, place a check in the appropriate space after each statement, then use the scoring key that follows to evaluate your responses. Use what you learn from your scores to better develop learning strategies that are best suited to your particular learning style. Respond to each statement as honestly as you can.

	Often	Sometimes	Seldom
1. I can remember best about a subject by listening to a lecture that includes information, explanations, and discussion.			
2. I prefer to see information written on a chalkboard and supplemented by visual aids and assigned readings.			
3. I like to write things down or to take notes for visual review.			
4. I prefer to use posters, models, or actual practice and other activities in class.			
5. I require explanations of diagrams, graphs, or visual directions.			
6. I enjoy working with my hands or making things.			
7. I am skillful with and enjoy developing and making graphs and charts.			
8. I can tell if sounds match when presented with pairs of sounds.			
9. I can remember best by writing things down several times.			
10. I can easily understand and follow directions on a map.			
11. I do best in academic subjects by listening to lectures and tapes.			
12. I play with coins or keys in my pocket.			
13. I learn to spell better by repeating words out loud than by writing the words on paper.			
14. I can understand a news article better by reading about it in the newspaper than by listening to a report about it on the radio.			
15. I chew gum, smoke, or snack while studying.			
16. I think the best way to remember something is to picture it in your head.			

17. I learn the spelling of words by "finger spelling" them.			
18. I would rather listen to a good lecture or speech than read about the same material in a textbook.			
19. I am good at working and solving jigsaw puzzles and mazes.			
20. I grip objects in my hands during learning periods.			
21. I prefer listening to the news on the radio rather than reading about it in the newspaper.			
22. I prefer obtaining information about an interesting subject by reading about it.			
23. I feel very comfortable touching others, hugging, handshaking, etc.			
24. I follow oral directions better than written ones.			

Figure 33-1 Learning styles 1.

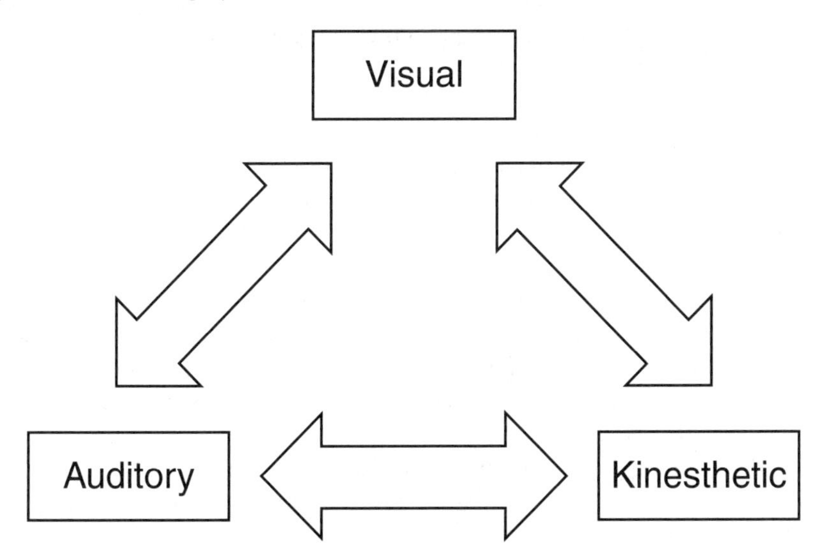

Learning Style Exercise 1 Scoring Key

Place the point value on the line next to the corresponding item. Add the points in each column to obtain the preference score under each heading: Often, 5 points; Sometimes, 3 points; Seldom, 1 point. VPS is visual preference score, APS is auditory preference score, and KPS is kinesthetic preference score.

Visual	**Auditory**	**Kinesthetic**
No. Points	No. Points	No. Points
2 ____	1 ____	4 ____
3 ____	5 ____	6 ____
7 ____	8 ____	9 ____
10 ____	11 ____	12 ____
14 ____	13 ____	15 ____
16 ____	18 ____	17 ____
19 ____	21 ____	20 ____
22 ____	24 ____	23 ____
VPS = ____	APS = ____	KPS = ____

If you are a visual learner, by all means be sure that you look at all study materials. Use charts, maps, filmstrips, notes, videos, and flash cards. Practice visualizing or picturing words and concepts in your head. Write out everything for frequent and quick visual review.

If you are an auditory learner, you may wish to use tapes. Tape lectures to help fill in gaps in your notes. But do listen and take notes—and review your notes frequently. Sit in the lecture hall or classroom where you can hear well. After you have read something, summarize it and recite it aloud. Talk to other students about class material.

If you are a kinesthetic learner, trace words as you are saying them. Facts that must be learned should be written several times. Keep a supply of scratch paper on hand for this purpose. Taking and keeping lecture notes is very important. Make study sheets. Associate class material with real world things or occurrences. When appropriate, practice role playing.

Another learning classification system is based on the following categories: concrete experience (CE), reflective observation (RO), abstract conceptualization (AC), or active experimentation (AE) (Fig. 33-2). Again, each person may be

Figure 33-2 Learning styles 2.

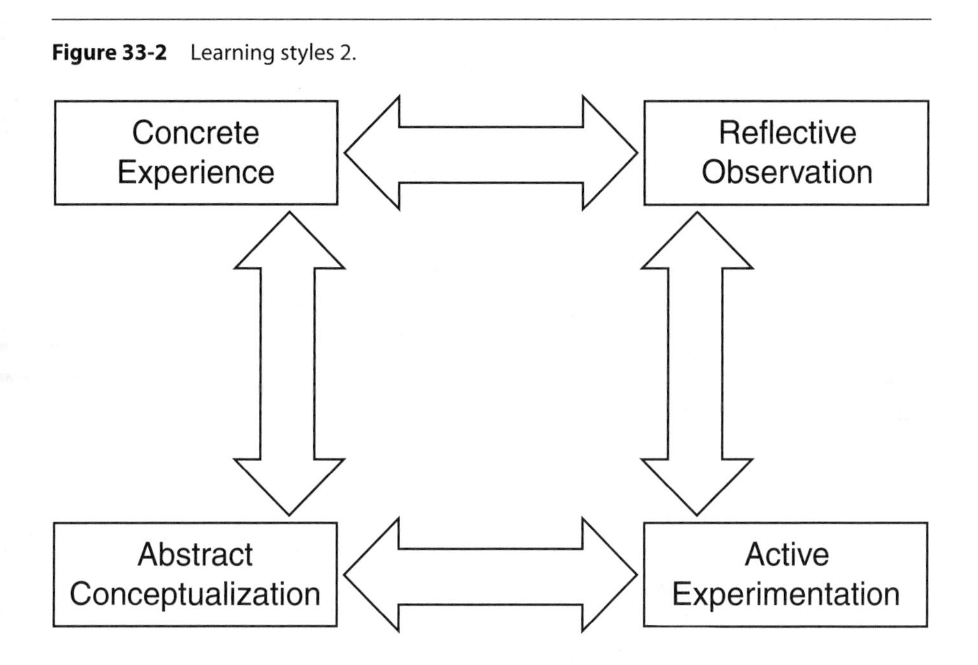

dominant in one area, but all must be considered in the assessment of learning and evaluation of learning therein.

To assess learning style dominance per CE, RO, AC, or AE, the following exercise may be used.

Learning Style Exercise 2

In the following assessment instrument, you are asked to complete 12 sentences that describe learning. Each has four endings. To respond to these sentences, consider some of the recent learning situations you have just written about. Then rank the endings for each sentence according to how well you think the ending describes the way you learned. Write a *4* next to the sentence ending that describes how you learn *best,* and so on down to *1* for the sentence ending that seems *least* like the way you learned. Be sure to rank all the endings for each sentence unit.

1. When I learn:
   a. _____ I like to deal with my feelings.
   b. _____ I like to think about ideas.
   c. _____ I like to be doing things.
   d. _____ I like to watch and listen.

2. I learn best when:
   a. ______ I listen and watch carefully.
   b. ______ I rely on logical thinking.
   c. ______ I trust my hunches and feelings.
   d. ______ I work hard to get things done.
3. When I am learning:
   a. ______ I tend to reason things out.
   b. ______ I am responsible about things.
   c. ______ I am quiet and reserved.
   d. ______ I have strong feelings and reactions.
4. I learn by:
   a. ______ Feeling
   b. ______ Doing
   c. ______ Watching
   d. ______ Thinking
5. When I learn:
   a. ______ I am open to new experiences.
   b. ______ I look at all sides of the issues.
   c. ______ I like to analyze things, break them down into their parts.
   d. ______ I like to try things out.
6. When I am learning:
   a. ______ I am an observing person.
   b. ______ I am an active person.
   c. ______ I am an intuitive person.
   d. ______ I am a logical person.
7. I learn best from:
   a. ______ Observation
   b. ______ Personal relationships
   c. ______ Rational theories
   d. ______ A chance to try out and practice
8. When I learn:
   a. ______ I like to see results from my work.
   b. ______ I like ideas and theories.
   c. ______ I take my time before acting.
   d. ______ I feel personally involved in things.
9. I learn best when:
   a. ______ I rely on my observations.
   b. ______ I rely on my feelings.
   c. ______ I can try things out for myself.
   d. ______ I rely on my ideas.

10. When I am learning:
    a. _____ I am a reserved person.
    b. _____ I am an accepting person.
    c. _____ I am a responsible person.
    d. _____ I am a rational person.
11. When I learn:
    a. _____ I get involved.
    b. _____ I like to observe.
    c. _____ I evaluate things.
    d. _____ I like to be active.
12. I learn best when:
    a. _____ I analyze ideas.
    b. _____ I am receptive and open minded.
    c. _____ I am careful.
    d. _____ I am practical.

Learning Style Exercise 2 Scoring Key

To compute your learning profile based on the four dimensions of the learning style inventory, add your scores for each of the items listed here.

LEARNING STYLE DIMENSION **ITEMS**

1	2	3	4	5	6	7	8	9	10	11	12
Concrete Experience											
a	c	d	a	a	c	b	d	b	b	a	b
										Total CE	
Reflective Observation											
d	a	c	c	b	a	a	c	a	a	b	c
										Total RO	
Abstract Conceptualization											
b	b	a	d	c	d	c	b	d	d	c	a
										Total AC	
Active Experimentation											
c	d	b	b	d	b	d	a	c	c	d	d
										Total AE	

The style with the most points indicates your primary learning style, next highest is your second style, and so on.

ANDRAGOGICAL VERSUS PEDAGOGICAL CONSIDERATIONS

Once information is known about the primary modes in which learning takes place, considerations for the teaching and evaluation of that learning revolves around a central argument of andragogical versus pedagogical techniques (Conner, 2003).

Andragogy, popularized by Malcolm Knowles (1973), is based on student-centered learning, also referred to as Socratic or learner-centered styles, that embrace experiential learning and social interaction from which to improve cognitive development. The andragogical teacher plays an interactive role, coaching the students, guiding them to epiphanies and applications, and keeping them on track. The facilitator's experience and background cannot be emphasized enough. Active and open participation by teachers and students drive the andragogical learning process based largely on Vygotsky's socio-cultural cognitive theory.

Lev Vygotsky's social-cultural cognitive theory (1987) is related to education effectiveness that states basically that the more social interaction, the better the learning outcomes. Therefore, "team" based intervention/groups would be theoretically more effective than those that are not. In application of Vygotsky's theory, educational institutions have focused the majority of content delivery systems using various learning applications to create an atmosphere where students have maximal interaction with other students and instructors in order to optimize learning outcomes and cognitive development.

Oestmann and Oestmann (2006) completed a research study based on Vygotsky's social-cultural cognitive theory related to online class size and learning outcomes. Discussion interactivity (i.e., the number of substantive discussion posts) and final course grade percentages between large online classes (> 20 students) and small online classes (< 10 students) were evaluated for significant differences and correlations. A retrospective comparison between five large and small online master's level healthcare management courses delivered between 2004 and 2005 was evaluated. The results indicated significantly different substantive discussion posts in the large class cohort at 76.3 as compared with the small class cohort at 49.9. Similarly, the average final grade percentage in the large class cohort was 91.1% and significantly higher than the average final grade percentage in the small class cohort of 84.9%. The correlation between average number of substantive discussion posts and final grade percentages in the large class cohort was qualified as "strong" at 0.864 and significantly different from the small class cohort value qualified as "moderate" at 0.670. Consequently, more learning occurred in the larger online classes as compared with the smaller online classes.

Anecdotally, traditional brick-and-mortar educational institutions have generally found smaller class sizes result in the most interaction between students and faculty, according to Parbudyal and William (2004). Achilles, Finn, and Bain (1998) reported in a traditional higher education classroom setting that small classes (13 to 17 students), compared with regular class sizes (23 to 26 students), provided higher student learning outcomes as determined by final grades, also citing anecdotal evidence of more student discussion interactivity in the smaller classes. Lou, Abrami, and Spence (1996) also reported increased student achievement in traditional higher education classroom settings favored small group learning sizes. In Abrami, Lou, Chambers, Poulsen, and Spence's (2000) latest study involving class size and learning outcomes in traditional higher education classroom settings, the results confirmed previous research findings related to smaller class sizes and higher student learning outcomes. However, the authors stated that this is most likely because smaller class sizes allow for more social interaction among the instructor and student peers, which is not as prevalent in larger class sizes.

In regard to online versus face-to-face learning environments, several research studies have concluded there are no significant differences in learning outcomes. Sims, Dobbs, and Hand (2002) reported that studies have demonstrated both positive and negative impacts in terms of effectiveness and achievement of outcomes between online and traditional higher education delivery modalities. This may directly reflect the fundamental differences in learning styles between the traditional face-to-face and virtual (online) classroom being structural: speaking and listening in the traditional classroom versus typing and reading in the online classroom. Moreover, studies by Parbudyal and William (2004); Driver (2002); and Dutton, Dutton, and Perry (2001) all reported that once courses are effectively managed by instructors, online education can be the same quality as, or even better than, the regular in-class method due in part to fostering an increase in participation by students.

Glahn and Gen (2002) summarized the "no significant difference" phenomena by stating, "Online teaching is not better than face-to-face teaching, nor is it worse. It is simply different" (p. 777). Both online and traditional methods of higher education delivery are unique and have their own advantages and disadvantages. However, the goal in both traditional and online educational delivery systems is to maximize the best features of teaching in order to promote optimal, active student-centered learning that is directly related to student learning.

Although the large versus small class size argument may never be unanimously agreed upon in regard to optimizing learning, according to Knowles

(1973), five characteristics of adult learners maximize learning within the andragogical approach.

1. Self concept: As adults mature, they move from dependence to self direction.
2. Experience: As a person matures, he or she develops experience, which becomes a resource for learning.
3. Readiness to learn: Adults' readiness to learn is related to a task- or problem-centered approach. They are motivated to learn what is useful to them.
4. Orientation to learning: Adults desire immediacy of application and prefer experiential learning.
5. Motivation: Adults have an internal motivation to learn (Smith, 2001).

Conversely, pedagogy is based on teacher-centered and teacher-directed learning in which teachers select the applicable topics and determine the structure of the learning process. The student is the vessel for receiving knowledge imparted by the teacher. Most often, this model of teaching/learning involves a lecture-based process (Conner, 2003). Despite the longstanding history of pedagogical teaching/learning, critics state the passivity of the student learning is the primary weakness of this approach.

COURSEROOM ASSESSMENT TECHNIQUES

Setting the stage for effective learning and assessment of that learning is therefore a complex process that involves, at a minimum, considerations for learning style; andragogical versus pedagogical teaching style; class size; class venue (online versus traditional face-to-face); and student age, experience, and other demographic characteristics before assessment of learning and the corresponding evaluation strategies can be implemented. Two primary resources were used for this section.

1. Angelo and Cross' book entitled *Classroom Assessment Techniques* (1993) has been the gold standard by which educators have based learning assessments and evaluation for nearly two decades.
2. Diamond's book entitled *Designing and Assessing Courses and Curricula* (1998).

The assessment of learning has become a focal point for accreditation bodies of higher education for obvious reasons. Not only is knowledge and application of educational materials important to validate and justify the educational curriculum and process, but in the cases of educational trades (e.g., health care, vocational jobs, etc.) learning outcomes are required to ensure competence of service provision, safety, and reduction of malpractice/litigation. Consequently, the teaching goals are a primary consideration and answers to the following questions are required:

1. What should the students learn?
2. How should the materials best be presented to achieve the learning?
3. How can we objectively measure the learning outcomes of students?

While course knowledge is traditionally measured by examination (multiple choice, true/false, short answer, essay), Bloom (1956) is credited with historical research that suggests the action verbs associated with six cognitive levels (e.g., knowledge, comprehension, application, analysis, synthesis, evaluation) for particular assignments are related with various progressive levels of knowledge. Moving from simple rote memory to evaluation and synthesis of the information demonstrates higher levels of thinking and course-related knowledge. Again, this is important for the teacher to understand because rote memorization can yield outstanding results on standardized testing and yet fail to demonstrate application of the course knowledge in the real world.

1. *Bloom's Level 1 Knowledge*. At the knowledge level, the instructor's questions require students to recognize or recall information and to remember facts, observations, and definitions that have been learned previously. Although there is substantial criticism among educators of factual or knowledge level questions, this level of question does have its place in the instructional spectrum. The overuse or abuse of this level of questioning is the main reason for criticism. It is important for instructors to realize that the learner must function at the knowledge level before being expected to perform at higher levels. Memorization of information is also required in order to perform a variety of tasks. The meaning of words, correct spelling, multiplication facts, and rules of the road are examples of important information that must be committed to memory. (Examples: remembering, memorizing, recognizing, recalling identification, recalling information, who, what, when, where, how?, describing.)
2. *Bloom's Level 2 Comprehension*. Questions at the comprehension level require students to interpret and translate information that is presented on charts, graphs, tables, as well as specific facts. It is important to realize that the student must have certain factual information in order to gain the understanding necessary to organize and arrange the material mentally. For questions of this type, the student must demonstrate a level of understanding by rephrasing, describing, or making comparisons. (Examples: interpreting, translating from one medium to another, describing in one's own words, retelling, organization and selection of facts and ideas.)
3. *Bloom's Level 3 Application*. Questions at the application level require a student to apply previously learned information to solve a specific problem. At this level, it is not sufficient for the student to relate or even to paraphrase and interpret previously memorized information. Instead,

students must use the information to answer questions or solve problems. For example, a student who has learned the definitions of latitude and longitude may be asked to locate a given point on a map. (Examples: problem solving applying information to produce some result; use of facts, rules and principles how is _______ an example of _______? how is _______ related to _______? why is _______ significant?)

4. *Bloom's Level 4 Analysis.* Questions at this level of cognition require students to look for hidden meaning or inferences of acquired information. As information is analyzed, one must reach sound conclusions or draw generalizations based on available information. Analysis questions ask students to identify motives, reasons, and/or causes of specific occurrences or events; reach certain conclusions, draw inferences, or generalizations based on given information; or identify evidence needed to support or refute conclusions, inferences, or generalizations. In many instances, there are no absolute answers to the analysis question, as several answers are plausible. Furthermore, because it takes time to analyze these questions, they cannot be answered quickly or without careful thought. (Examples: subdividing something to show how it is put together; finding the underlying structure of a communication; identifying motives; separation of a whole into component parts; what are the parts or features of _______?; classify _______ according to _______ outline/diagram; how does _______ compare/contrast with _______?; what evidence can you list for _______?)
5. *Bloom's Level 5 Synthesis.* Synthesis questions require higher order thinking processes. Students must make predictions, use creativity in developing original approaches, or solve problems that do not have single answers. Instructors can use synthesis questions to help develop and reinforce students' creative abilities. These questions demand a substantial amount of information and a thorough understanding of many factors as students consider possible responses. (Examples: creating a unique, original product that may be in verbal form or may be a physical object; combination of ideas to form a new whole; what would you predict/infer from _______? what ideas can you add to _______? how would you create/design a new _______? what might happen if you combined _______? what solutions would you suggest for _______?)
6. *Bloom's Level 6 Evaluation.* Evaluation questions require students to judge the meaning of an idea or to assess the plausibility of a solution. These actions require that a student possess substantial information and be able to establish criteria for making a judgment. (Examples: making value decisions about issues; resolving controversies or differences of opinion; development of opinions, judgments or decisions; do you agree that _______? what do you think about _______? what is the most important _______? place the following in order of priority; how would you decide about _______? what criteria would you use to assess _______?)

According to Cross and Cross (1993) and Diamond (1998), there are over 50 courseroom assessment techniques (CATs) that may be implemented to measure student learning. While there is no singular and universal CAT that can be applied for all classes and all situations, generally two or three CATs are both effective and efficient based on teaching goals and other variables previously identified.

Obviously both knowledge and skills (application) are important in many higher education classrooms. However, the CATs to achieve these results are again specifically designed for each course based on the individual goals. Common CATs related to this level of learning include background knowledge probe; focused listing; misconception/preconception check; empty outlines; memory matrix; minute paper; muddiest point.

How do we measure skill in analysis and critical and creative thinking? Moving to the higher levels of Bloom's taxonomy, evaluation, analysis, and synthesis become important components of CATs implemented. As indicated previously, this is important for the teacher to understand as rote memorization can yield outstanding results on standardized testing and yet fail to demonstrate application of the courseroom knowledge in the real world. For example, a student can recite verbatim theory, theorists, indications, contraindications, and goals, but if they cannot apply the theory, or specific details of a particular case, the knowledge application is ineffective and inefficient. This has particular consequences in health care as ineffective and inefficient treatment provision may result in legal ramifications and productivity/cost inefficiencies. In addition, healthcare careers are unique in the fact that they deal with the complexity of the human condition. It is rare that two patients in any profession present to a treating professional with exactly the same symptoms and conditions. Therefore, the ability to critically think, analyze, and act in a safe, effective, and efficient manner are imperative in the application of CATs, which commonly include categorizing grid, defining features matrix, pro and con grid, content, form and function outlines, analytic memos, one sentence summary, word journal, approximate analogies, concept maps, invented dialogues, and annotated portfolios.

How do we measure skill in problem solving? Perhaps one of the most important educationally related goals for educators is to impart the skill of problem solving for students. Regardless of the profession or educational category, problem solving is a universal skill required for almost every college educated person working in government or private industry. Problem solving CATs commonly include: problem recognition tasks, what's the principle, documented problem solutions, audio and videotaped protocols, directed paraphrasing, applications cards, student-centered test questions, human tableau or class modeling; and paper or project prospectus.

How do we assess learner attitudes, values, and self awareness? As teachers and clinicians, it is easy to assume that we know best for our students. However, as times change and multiple generational cohorts represent our students, teachers need to periodically evaluate learner attitudes, values, and self awareness. The CATs commonly associated with the evaluation of learner attitudes, values, and self awareness include classroom opinion polls, double-entry journals, profiles of admirable individuals, everyday ethical dilemmas, course-related self confidence surveys, focused autobiographical sketches, interest/knowledge/skills checklists, goal ranking and matching, and self assessment of ways of learning.

How do we assess student learning and study skills? Again, what sounds good in theory may not provide the best student learning and study skills given a particular area of education. However, the assessment by educators is another important component of effective and efficient teaching and learning. Common CATs related to assessing student learning and study skills include productive study time logs, punctuated lectures, process analysis, and diagnostic learning logs.

How do we assess learner reactions to educational instruction? In almost every higher education venue, educators are evaluated by their students. This is an accreditation requirement and common practice among higher education schools of all types. While often criticized as a forum for students to voice complaints about a particular instructor or instructional technique, this feedback is imperative to improving the effectiveness and efficiency of education. In that, it is imperative for the educators and administrators to decipher what is legitimate in terms of complaints and what is not. Obviously, the theory behind this practice is simple. Students learn more when the teaching method/educational instruction is highly regarded. In addition to student satisfaction, many educators advocate cross comparison of these reports with student learning outcomes (e.g., final grades primarily). While other measures of student learning can be used, the premise of this practice is based on the following examples. If student satisfaction reports are high and final grades are high, two conclusions can be drawn. First, teaching and learning is both effective and efficient. Second, teaching is pleasant but learning is ineffective as grades are artificially inflated. This second conclusion requires verification of teaching/learning ineffectiveness as indicated on standardized national exams. The additional outcomes (student satisfaction reports low; final grades low) and any combination can also yield various conclusions as to teaching and learning efficacy. Per Angelo and Cross (1993), assessing learner reactions to educational instruction involves more than just simple satisfaction surveys. The following CATs related to assessing learner reactions to educational instruction include chain notes, email feedback, teacher-designed feedback forms, group instructional feedback technique, and classroom assessment quality circles.

How do we assess learner reactions to class activities, assignments, and materials? Each classroom assessment method needs to be chosen for a specific purpose and then evaluated for its success, or lack thereof. This is referred to as the classroom assessment project cycle which is similar in nature to continuous quality improvement (CQI) programs. Class activities often consist of individual or group projects. Sometimes personality differences may confound the learner reactions to group activities, whereas the logistics of crossing several time zones in online group projects may represent a legitimate reason to decrease or even eliminate group assignments, despite Vygotsky's social learning theory tenets. Materials used in each course should be pertinent and timely in nature, which is the reason for course content revision as part of most educational programming. For example, if learner reactions to class activities, assignments, and materials are negative and learning outcomes are negative (e.g., poor final grades, poor final performance on clinical applications or national standardized testing), it would represent an immediate change in curriculum and activity/assignment for that particular course. In addition, the grading rubrics used in a particular course are also involved in the assessment of learner reactions to class activities, assignments, and materials. Perhaps there is an unequal distribution of grading weight for a particular assignment to the time required to complete the assignment. If, on the other hand, grading rubrics are too subjective (e.g., not quantitative and specific), poor learner reactions to class activities and assignments may also result with resulting grades being overly inflated or overly strict without substantial objective justification. CATs related to assessing learner reactions to class activities, assignments, and materials include recall, summarize, question, comment, connect (RSQC2); group work evaluations; reading rating sheets; assignment assessments; and exam evaluations.

Despite the plethora of CATs available to measure student learning, one must objectively quantitate in order to avoid grade inflation and subjective biases. In order to accomplish this task, grading rubrics become invaluable considerations.

EDUCATIONAL ISSUES: GRADING RUBRICS

As education has evolved over the years, fundamental flaws of subjective grading were replaced with more objective (quantitative) rubrics in the search for measuring learning outcomes of students. How often have you attempted to grade your students' work only to find that the assessment criteria were vague and the performance behavior was overly subjective? Would you be able to justify the assessment or grade if you had to defend it? The rubric is an authentic assessment tool that is particularly useful in assessing criteria that are complex and subjective (Miller & Miller, 1999).

The *advantages* of using rubrics in assessment are that they:

1. Allow assessment to be more objective and consistent.
2. Focus the teacher to clarify his or her criteria in specific terms.
3. Clearly show the student how their work will be evaluated and what is expected.

4. Promote student awareness of about the criteria to use in assessing peer performance.
5. Provide useful feedback regarding the effectiveness of the instruction.
6. Provide benchmarks against which to measure and document progress.

Rubrics can be created in a variety of forms and levels of complexity; however, they all contain common features that:

1. Focus on measuring a stated *objective* (i.e., performance, behavior, or quality)
2. Use a range to rate performance.
3. Contain specific performance characteristics arranged in levels indicating the degree to which a standard has been met.

A number of options for evaluating papers exist. Evaluating a paper need not involve correcting every surface error and writing voluminous comments at the end.

1. Give separate grades for form and content.
2. Use performance grading: If students do the assignment, they get credit (or points). You make no value judgments about the quality of the work, merely decide what is an acceptable amount of work.
3. Use impression marking: Scan the paper and mark it based on your general impression of the paper's effectiveness. Again, have a clear set of criteria in mind—or even written down—as you read.
4. Use portfolio evaluation: Rather than evaluating individual papers, evaluate a student's entire output at the end of the course.
5. Evaluate based strictly on clearly defined criteria, which may be set out in the form of: (1) contracts (you create a contract which spells out how much work and/or what sort must be done to receive a particular grade—the student chooses what grade to work for); or (2) checksheets (you list the criteria for an acceptable piece of work and evaluate based on how many criteria are met).
6. Scales: rank a student's work based on your criteria. Analytic and dichotomous are just two of a variety of scales; examples are included in Tables 33-1 and 33-2 (Miller & Miller, 1999).

Two grading rubrics that the authors have developed and modified over the year of teaching include a general grading rubric (i.e., 5-point grading rubric) and a formal paper grading form (Table 33-3).

Five-Point Grading Rubric Example

Grading Rubric 4, Exemplary competency. Regarding how well a student understands terms and concepts in context. Highest level of mastery (e.g.,

Table 33-1 Sample Analytical Scale

		Low				High
General merit	Ideas	2	4	6	8	10
	Organization	2	4	6	8	10
	Wording	1	2	3	4	5
Mechanics	Spelling and punctuation	1	2	3	4	5
	Grammar and usage	1	2	3	4	5
	Format	2	4	6	8	10
Comprehension	Understanding of terms	2	4	6	8	10
	Application of concepts	2	4	6	8	10
Total score:						

synonymous use of a concept, introduction to a new concept, identification of misunderstood concept). Includes American Psychological Association (APA) formatting and referencing compliance few to no errors.

A = Clearly stands out as an excellent performer. Has unusually sharp insight into material and initiates thoughtful questions. Sees many sides of an issue. Articulates well and writes logically and clearly. Integrates ideas previously learned from this and other disciplines; anticipates next steps in progression of ideas. **Example:** A work should be of such a nature that it could be put on reserve for all students to review and emulate. The A student is, in fact, an example for others to follow.

Grading Rubric 3, Accomplished competency. Regarding how well a student understands terms and concepts in context. Mastery of terms and concepts in context. Develops argument and cites prior material in support. Includes APA formatting and referencing compliance with a few errors (1–5 per page).

B = Grasps subject matter at a level considered to be good to very good. Participates actively in class discussion. Writes well and complies with the majority of APA formatting and referencing rules. Accomplishes more than the minimum requirements. Produces high-quality work. **Example:** B work indicates a high

Table 33-2 Sample Dichotomous Scale

	Yes	No	
Content	___	___	Ideas are insightful.
	___	___	Ideas are original.
	___	___	Ideas are logical.
	___	___	Ideas are clearly expressed.
Organization	___	___	There is a thesis.
	___	___	Thesis is adequately developed.
	___	___	Each paragraph is developed with concrete and relevant details.
Mechanics	___	___	Many misspellings.
	___	___	Awkward sentences.

quality of performance and is given in recognition for solid work; a B should be considered a high grade.

Grading Rubric 2, Developing competency. Regarding how well a student understands terms and concepts in context. Interpreting terms and concepts in context. Begins to develop argument beyond opinion. APA formatting and referencing is semicompliant with consistent errors noted throughout (6–10 errors per page).

C = Demonstrates a satisfactory comprehension of the subject matter. Accomplishes only the minimum requirements, and displays little or no initiative. Communicates in writing at an acceptable level for a college student. Has an acceptable understanding of all basic concepts. **Example:** C work represents average work. A student receiving a C has met the requirements, including deadlines, of the course.

Grading Rubric 1, Beginning to meet competency. Regarding how well a student understands terms and concepts in context. Distinguishing terms or concepts in context. APA formatting and referencing is awry throughout with consistent errors noted throughout (10+ per page).

D = Quality and quantity of work is below average and barely acceptable. **Example:** D work is passing by a slim margin.

Grading Rubric 0, Failure to meet competency. Regarding how well a student understands terms and concepts in context. Failure to meet competency. APA formatting and referencing is literally nonexistent.

F = Quality and quantity of work is unacceptable. Academic credit is not earned for an F. **Example:** F work does not qualify the student to progress to a more advanced level of coursework.

Table 33-3 Formal Paper Grading Example

Content and Organization (70%)	**Points Earned**	**Comments**
All key elements of the assignment are covered in a substantive way. • [Add assignment requirements as needed]		
The content is comprehensive, accurate, and/or persuasive.		
The paper develops a central theme or idea, directed toward the appropriate audience.		
The paper links theory to relevant examples of current experience and industry practice and uses the vocabulary of the theory correctly.		
Major points are stated clearly; are supported by specific details, examples, or analysis; and are organized logically. • [Add major points as needed]		
The introduction provides sufficient background on the topic and previews major points.		
The conclusion is logical, flows from the body of the paper, and reviews the major points.		
Paragraph transitions are present and logical and maintain the flow throughout the paper.		

(continues)

Table 33-3 Formal Paper Grading Example *(continued)*

Readability and Style (15%)	**Points Earned**	**Comments**
The tone is appropriate to the content and assignment.		
Sentences are complete, clear, and concise.		
Sentences are well constructed, with consistently strong, varied sentences.		
Sentence transitions are present and maintain the flow of thought.		
Mechanics (15%)	**Points Earned**	**Comments**
The paper, including the title page, reference page, tables, and appendices, follow APA guidelines for format.		
Citations of original works within the body of the paper follow APA guidelines.		
The paper is laid out with effective use of headings, font styles, and white space.		
Rules of grammar, usage, and punctuation are followed.		
Spelling is correct.		
Total (100%)	**Points Earned**	**Comments**

Grading Feedback

In addition to the use of grading rubrics as noted previously, two common types of grade feedback include (1) formative and (2) summative (Fig. 33-3). However, they are not mutually exclusive concepts (Weimer, 1987).

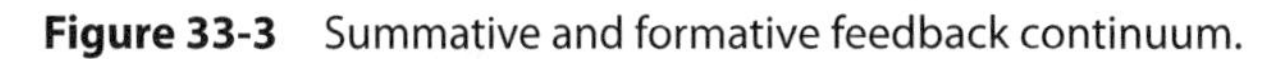

Figure 33-3 Summative and formative feedback continuum.

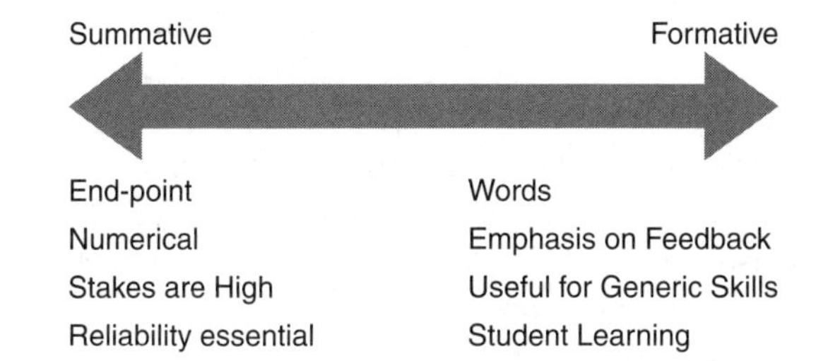

Source: Adapted from Weimer, M. G. (1987). Translating evaluation results into teaching improvements. *AAHE Bulletin* (1) 4, 8–11.

Assessment feedback used to sum up a person's achievement on a particular assessment is often called *summative*. Conversely, *formative* feedback is intended to inform students how to improve their learning. The emphasis in formative assessment is in encouraging more understanding in the students in relation to their strengths, weaknesses, and gaps in knowledge from which additional learning opportunities occur. In both instances, feedback should ascribe to the following parameters:

1. Always begin your comments by saying something positive about the writing. Writers need to know what parts are effective (clear, original, well worded, etc.) as well as what needs work.
2. Marking every error or covering a student's paper with comments will not only drive you crazy, it may also overwhelm your student. Research has shown that many student writers ignore or react negatively to a large amount of written feedback, even if many comments are positive!
3. Correcting students' errors or rewriting parts of their papers makes a lot of work for you, and does not necessarily help them. A better technique—easier for you and more thought-provoking for the writer—is indicating an error with a squiggly underline or putting a check in the margin next to the line in which the error occurs.
4. Criteria for evaluating essays may differ depending on whether or not the student has a chance to revise the writing. Some instructors expect less grammatical and mechanical accuracy on in-class essays.
5. It is reasonable to require even short answer in-class essays to be written in complete sentences rather than just lists of words or phrases; the act of putting ideas into sentences requires a higher level of thinking.

When responding to student writing to enhance learning, instructors should bear in mind two points: (1) comments should be brief enough to provide attainable goals for the students and (2) comments should emphasize how communication fails rather than labeling problems. Try to form your comments as questions, avoiding questions with simple yes and no responses. Begin the questions with why, how, or what to generate most substantive thought from the student. Avoid imperatives such as "proofread next time"; these point out problems but do not help the student learn how to solve them.

Avoid labeling problems unless you give students a way to solve the problem. For example, rather than writing "unclear," write, "Did you intend to say _____ or _______" or explain what is awkward and why. You can also highlight passages in which the writer successfully avoided the problem. Praise work that will lead to improvement. For example, explain why something is good or appeals to you. This kind of evaluation can be much more difficult than the identification of problems (we arere just not used to doing it), but it is extremely important to the young writer to know what works well and why. Avoid doing the student's work. Rewriting a passage or two for modeling purposes is fine, but only if you clarify the principle that you are modeling. You can place a check in the margin of the line in which the problem occurs and then ask the student to identify and correct it. This will work quite well if the student feels comfortable checking with you to determine what the check means. Write a careful endnote that (1) recognizes what you have legitimately liked about the paper, (2) identifies one or two problems and explains how and why they harm the quality of the paper, (3) sets a goal for the student to work toward in the next assignment, and (4) suggests specific strategies for reaching that goal.

Even when the feedback to students is not positive, it must always be constructive and respectful. We must be conscious of the manner in which feedback is presented, especially when pointing out the shortcomings of an assignment. As with all messages, it is the listener who dictates what is actually received, and facilitators need to thoughtfully consider their communication to students when addressing areas in need of improvement. Comments need to encourage performance improvement without discouraging students from trying. Lastly, grade feedback should exemplar the following characteristics:

1. *Timeliness*. Prompt feedback can serve as a valuable motivator for students at all levels of performance. It also serves to help students improve their performance on subsequent assignments. Faculty members must return student assignments in a timely manner (within 7 days of the assignment being submitted) with specific, objective feedback that will assist students in learning from the experience and improving future submissions.
2. *Clarity*. The evaluation is communicated in a form and style that can be understood easily by the student. Include your own narrative remarks on student papers that inform the student why his or her conclusions are sound and which statements need more substantiation. Add questions that prompt the student to further investigate the selected topic.

3. *Thoroughness.* The evaluation covers all the areas of student performances as requested by the faculty member. Assignments that earn an A need feedback as much as assignments that earn a C. Feedback means informing students of what they have done well in addition to that which they need to improve.
4. *Consistency.* Expectations and guidelines established by faculty in the beginning are not repudiated later on in the course.
5. *Equitability.* Faculty follow through on a commitment to make discriminatory judgments. It is not advisable to cater to student interests by putting everyone in only two categories, such as A and A-. Likewise, it is not necessary to designate a large percentage of the course grade to the instructor's subjective judgment, just for the sake of creating an artificial grade variance.
6. *Professionalism.* The facilitator is respectful in his or her communications with the student because the tone affects how students interpret and use that feedback. If facilitators use a supportive, encouraging tone when making suggestions for improvement, the feedback comes across as constructive rather than critical.

TEACHING TECHNIQUES/EXAMPLES

CATs and the teaching particulars based on the aforementioned considerations for effective and efficient assessment of learning are now posited by the authors. A *baker's dozen* of learning assessment best practices that should be considered in addition to the standard techniques of written essays and examinations are based on the applicable teaching goals.

Assessing Skills in Problem Solving

1. *Problem recognition.* Giving the students examples of problems and looking at the depth, breadth, and clarity of their responses can give the instructor a lot of information about how well they are integrating the information. Group discussions of their responses also will help them discover other ways of thinking, and help them understand other perspectives. Give the students a case study and have them work in small groups to identify the important issues. I find that this is a quick, effective technique to identify the patient issue and apply it to the learned information.

2. *Documented problem solutions*. How can we get our students to adapt the problem-solving skills to real life situations? How do they synthesize the information being presented and apply it to real life?
3. *Audio and videotaped protocols*. Instructors could look at the video with the students and see if the student recognizes strengths and weakness, and then they can talk about ways to improve handing or interactions. This is very time consuming.

Assessing Skill in Applications and Performance

1. *Directed paraphrasing*. This is a very useful CAT. It is important to know how the student understands the information they are learning, and if they can put it in their own words. Additionally, it allows you to find out if the student can put the diagnosis/theory into words their patients, family members, physicians, and coworkers can understand. In a clinical setting, I would ask my students to paraphrase the theoretical perspective and approach they were using prior to going into a session. This provides the instructor with a quick feedback to the student's knowledge base. Very useful and effective in the education of practitioner students.
2. *Application cards*. These are one of the easiest CATs to give. Students are just asked to write down one application for what they have just learned. For example: In a kinesiology class, students could be asked how shortening a lever arm could be used to make an exercise easier or harder. Or, after discussing a treatment technique, students could be asked to describe how they might apply it in an outpatient setting.
3. *Student generated test questions*. Students are asked to generate the midterm or final exam. Their task would be to create 50 multiple-choice questions (4+ responses: a, b, c, d) highlighting the correct answer with the page number in the text in which the material and answer was found. This lets us know what is important to the student and that they actually read the text and spent time critically thinking through the material and processed the information. The responsibility is on them to create the work from what they studied.
4. *Human tableau or class modeling*. The instructor has to be very skilled in teaching the subject matter to make it work well. The students create "living" scenes of patient/management situations. Great for assessing application.
5. *The categorizing grid*. Provides the faculty with a picture of the students sorting ability. This technique is most useful in introductory courses. It

helps students reorganize their learning to make new associations and contextual meaning and it (1) assesses students' basic analytic and organizing skill; (2) reinforces effective organization of material/recall; and (3) moves from broad concept to specific subcategories with mastery.

6. *Analytic memos*. This is a simulation exercise that allows the students to organize their thoughts and present them in a concise manner, connecting all the concepts together with practice application.
7. *One sentence summary*. This tool assesses the student's ability to summarize quickly. This is a powerful technique for helping students grasp the complex techniques and explain to others in nontechnical language.
8. *Word journal*. Summarizing a text or lesson in a single word and writing two paragraphs explaining why the student chose that word. This forces the students to critically and analytically read and assesses the student's skill at defending or explaining. This skill will help students learn to write abstracts skillfully. This allows for active learning through reading. By choosing a word the faculty member gains insight to the student's personal connections with the subject.
9. *Concept maps*. Drawings of diagrams showing mental connections that students make between major concepts presented in class. This technique allows the faculty member to see the web of relationships that students bring to the task at hand and then can easily identify gaps.
10. *Invented dialogues*. Students synthesize their knowledge of issues, personalities, and historical perspectives. Students might create dialogues using a series of primary quotes of get into the character and summarize how the conversation might have gone with the characters in real time. This technique forces the students to internalize and process course material in profound ways.

PROBLEM AREAS AND SOLUTIONS

Common problem areas in the assessment of learning can be illuminated through the process of self reflection. According to Nater and Gallimore (2006), the following questions should therefore be answered by each instructor as part of an ongoing process to improve the learning opportunities and minimize problem areas:

1. What are my best practices in teaching? What are the strengths I can build on? How will I do that?
2. How will my teaching practice change (or will it?) as the result of my self reflection?
3. How comfortable do I feel in creating and delivering online courses? How comfortable do I feel in mentoring or conducting directed studies? What do I need to do to increase my level of comfort with these activities?

4. How comfortable do I feel with my ability to give learners constructive feedback on their work and in the courseroom? What do I need to do to increase my level of comfort with these activities?
5. What questions remain unanswered for me, and how will I get the information I need (i.e., find resources on the topic or topics, take a class, shadow another instructor, etc.)?

According to Cloud (2006), one of the central problems in the assessment of learning is based on the lack of student generational cohort considerations by faculty, which leads to ineffective instructor questioning. It is desirable to enhance the quality of student thinking through the questioning process. A questioning strategy leads the student from one level of thinking to higher levels by a careful series of questions. *Probing questions* should follow students' responses and attempt to stimulate thinking about their answers. This type of questioning may be used to prompt students to think more effectively at the higher levels of analysis, synthesis, and evaluation. *Leading questions* guide the discussion to focus or refocus the discussion to where you want it to go. In addition to questions, instructors must also be prepared to react to student-initiated comments and questions. Relevant student questions indicate a need for clarification or a desire to know more about the subject. Relevant comments suggest that students are actively thinking about the subject matter and relating it to past experiences. (This, too, is a great way to lead to good threaded discussions.) These questions and comments present unique opportunities that demand attention. Instructors should welcome such questions and comments and, when possible, should respond positively.

Another central problem in the assessment of learning, according to Palmer (1998), is based on faulty assumptions regarding the teaching process of critical thinking. One of the biggest challenges facing a faculty member is how to encourage students who are not using their critical thinking skills to reach their fullest potential. The reason for this lack of use could be cognitive, affective, or a mix of both areas. Noncritical thinkers are missing many great learning opportunities in their lives because of placing their focus on following, rather than generating, new ideas and possibilities. We all would probably agree that critical thinking is hard work, but the rewards are worth the effort.

Closely related to the concept of noncritical thinkers is the concept of weak sense critical thinkers (Peterson, 2001). Weak sense critical thinkers are more motivated to defend their beliefs or egocentricity. Egocentric thinking puts the person into a defensive mode. These students react to probing questions/challenges with a defensive, "me against you" attitude. We can typically break down thinkers into three types.

1. *Fair-minded thinkers*. These individuals try to understand ideas and situations and attempt to be honest, empathetic, and fair. They are willing to put forth the effort necessary to think critically.

2. *Naïve thinkers*. These individuals usually do not know or do not care about the concepts of critical thinking. They tend to not think things through, and to go along with the decisions of others.
3. *Selfish thinkers*. These individuals are good at thinking, but not fair to others. They tend to be manipulative and are not always intellectually honest.

There are a variety of methods for dealing with noncritical thinkers. In addressing both naïve and selfish thinkers, one should encourage them to do the following:

1. Be clear; ask them to state what they mean, explaining in different ways and giving examples.
2. Be accurate; ask them to justify or explain how they know their claims are true or how they might find out.
3. Be relevant; ask them to explain how their ideas are related to the topic at hand.
4. Be logical; ask them to explain how the ideas fit together and why they make sense. Also ask how they came to their conclusions.
5. Be fair; ask them to consider how their ideas/behaviors will make others feel or think.
6. Practice intellectual integrity.
7. Treat oneself and others with respect.

When asking noncritical thinkers to address problems (or assignments), Brookfield (1987) encourages faculty to do the following:

1. Consider the purpose/goal.
2. Restate the question in numerous ways.
3. Gather information.
4. Be aware of inferences.
5. Be aware of assumptions.
6. Clarify the ideas you use to understand the problem.
7. Understand their point of view.
8. Think through the implications/possibilities.

Lastly, learning is an individual and continuous process with a variety of motivating factors that also need to be considered by teachers (Nater & Gallimore, 2006). At least six factors serve as sources of motivation for adult learning:

1. *Social relationships*: to make new friends, to meet a need for associations and friendships.
2. *External expectations*: to comply with instructions from someone else; to fulfill the expectations or recommendations of someone with formal authority.

3. *Social welfare*: to improve ability to serve humankind, prepare for service to the community, and improve ability to participate in community work.
4. *Personal advancement*: to achieve higher status in a job, secure professional advancement, and stay abreast of competitors.
5. *Escape/stimulation*: to relieve boredom, provide a break in the routine of home or work, and provide a contrast to other exacting details of life.
6. *Cognitive interest*: to learn for the sake of learning, seek knowledge for its own sake, and to satisfy an inquiring mind.

According to Nater and Gallimore (2006), the best way to motivate adult learners is simply to *enhance* their reasons for enrolling and *decrease* the barriers. Instructors must learn why their students are enrolled (the motivators); they have to discover what is keeping them from learning. Then the instructors must plan their motivating strategies. Instructors can motivate students via several means.

1. Set a feeling or tone for the lesson. Instructors should try to establish a friendly, open atmosphere that shows the participants the instructor will help them learn.
2. Set an appropriate level of concern. The level of tension must be adjusted to meet the level of importance of the objective. If the material has a high level of importance, a higher level of tension/stress should be established in the class. However, people learn best under low to moderate stress; if the stress is too high, it becomes a barrier to learning.
3. Set an appropriate level of difficulty. The degree of difficulty should be set high enough to challenge participants but not so high that they become frustrated by information overload. The instruction should predict and reward participation, culminating in success.

In addition, students need specific knowledge of their learning results (feedback). Feedback must be specific, not general. Participants must also see a reward for learning. The reward does not necessarily have to be monetary; it can be simply a demonstration of benefits to be realized from learning the material. Finally, the participant must be interested in the subject. Interest is directly related to reward. Adults must see the benefit of learning in order to motivate themselves to learn the subject.

Reinforcement is a very necessary part of the teaching/learning process; through it, instructors encourage correct modes of behavior and performance.

1. Positive reinforcement is normally used by instructors who are teaching participants new skills. As the name implies, positive reinforcement is good and reinforces good (or positive) behavior.
2. Negative reinforcement is normally used by instructors teaching a new skill or new information. It is useful in trying to change modes of behav-

ior. The result of negative reinforcement is extinction; that is, the instructor uses negative reinforcement until the bad behavior disappears, or it becomes extinct.

Students must also retain information from classes in order to benefit from the learning. The instructors' jobs are not finished until they have assisted the learner in retaining the information. In order for participants to retain the information taught, they must see a meaning or purpose for that information. They must also understand and be able to interpret and apply the information. This understanding includes their ability to assign the correct degree of importance to the material. The amount of retention will be directly affected by the degree of original learning. Simply stated, if the participants did not learn the material well initially, they will not retain it well either.

Transfer of learning (*transference*) is the result of training. It is the ability to use the information taught in the course but in a new setting. As with reinforcement, there are two types of transfer: positive and negative.

1. Positive transference, like positive reinforcement, occurs when the participants use the behavior taught in the course.
2. Negative transference, again like negative reinforcement, occurs when the participants do not do what they are told not to do. This results in a positive (desired) outcome.

Transference is most likely to occur in the following situations:

1. Association: participants can associate the new information with something that they already know.
2. Similarity: the information is similar to material that participants already know; that is, it revisits a logical framework or pattern.
3. Degree of original learning: participants' degree of original learning was high.
4. Critical attribute element: the information learned contains elements that are extremely beneficial (critical) on the job.

CONCLUSION

The following checklist is a useful tool for faculty to consider in the assessment of learning and evaluation strategies:

1. What are the primary teaching goals/objectives?
2. How do these teaching goals/objectives fit within the appropriate Bloom's taxonomy (knowledge, comprehension, application, analysis, synthesis, evaluation)?

3. What are the student's predominant learning style(s): visual, auditory, and kinesthetic or concrete experience (CE), reflective observation (RO), abstract conceptualization (AC), or active experimentation (AE)?
4. What type of educational setting is involved (face-to-face, online, hybrid)?
5. What teaching philosophy is applicable given the student demographic characteristics (pedagogical, andragogical)?
6. What is the predominant teaching theory applicable with consideration of class size (group-based learning, Vygotsky, individual-based learning)?
7. What are the potential CATs available to assess learning based on numbers 1 to 6 considerations?
8. What type of grading rubric(s) need to be used/developed or modified in order to match the CAT used?
9. What type of feedback is most appropriate to maximize learning (formative, summative)?
10. What kind of problems may be involved with the chosen CAT and how will you best minimize these based on the techniques shared in this chapter?

Answer these questions, and you are well on your way to successful teaching and learning assessments!

REFERENCES

Abrami, P. C., Lou, Y., Chambers, B., Poulsen, C., & Spence, J. C. (2000). Why should we group students within-class for learning? *Educational Research and Evaluation, 2*, 158–179.

Achilles, C. M., Finn, J. D., & Bain, H. P. (1998). Using class size to reduce the equity gap. *Educational Leadership, 55*, 40–43.

Bloom, B. S. (1956). *Taxonomy of educational objectives, Handbook I: The cognitive domain*. New York: David McKay.

Brookfield, S. (1987). *Developing critical thinkers*. San Francisco: Jossey-Bass.

Cloud, H. (2006). *Integrity: The courage to meet the demands of reality*. New York: Harper Collins.

Conner, M. L. (2003). Andragogy and pedagogy. Retrieved December 20, 2008, from http://ageless-learner.com/intros/andragogy.html

Cross, T. A., & Cross, K. P. (1993). *Classroom assessment techniques: A handbook for college teachers* (2nd ed.). San Francisco: Jossey-Bass.

Diamond, R. M. (1998). *Designing and assessing courses and curricula: A practical guide*. San Francisco: Jossey-Bass.

Driver, M. (2002). Investigating the benefits of Web-centric instruction for student learning: An exploratory study of an MBA course. *Journal of Education for Business, 77*(4), 236–245.

Dutton, J., Dutton, M., & Perry, J. (2001). Do online students perform as well as lecture students? *Journal of Engineering Education, 90*(1), 131–141.

Glahn, R., & Gen, R. (2002). Progenies in education: The evolution of internet teaching. *Community College Journal of Research and Practice, 26*, 777–785.

Knowles, M. (1973). *The adult learner: A neglected species.* Houston: Gulf Publishing.

Lou, Y., Abrami, P. C., & Spence, J. C. (1996). Within-class grouping. *Review of Educational Research, 66,* 423–458.

Miller, W. R., & Miller, M. F. (1999). *Handbook for college teaching.* Atlanta: PineCrest Publications.

Nater, S., & Gallimore, R. (2006). *They haven't taught until they have learned.* Morgantown, WV: Fitness Information Technology.

Oestmann, E., & Oestmann, J. (2006). Significant difference in learning outcomes and online class size. *Journal of Online Educators, 2*(1), 1–8.

Palmer, P. J. (1998). *The courage to teach.* San Francisco: Jossey-Bass.

Parbudyal, S., & William, P. (2004). Online education: Lessons for administrators and instructors. *College Student Journal, 38*(2), 302–308.

Peterson, D. (2001). *Critical thinking in the strong sense in the weak sense non-critical thinking.* Retrieved on December 29, 2007, from http://www.santarosa.edu/~dpeterso/permanenthtml/Phil.CT.lessonsP5.html

Sims, R., Dobbs, G., & Hand T. (2002). Enhancing quality in online learning: Scaffolding planning and design through proactive evaluation. *Distance Education, 23*(2), 135–148.

Smith, M. K. (2001). *Andragogy: The history and current use of the term plus an annotated bibliography.* Retrieved December 20, 2008, from http://www.infed.org/lifelonglearning/b-andra.htm

Vygotsky, L. S. (1987). *Thinking and speech: The collected works of L.S. Vygotsky.* New York: Plenum.

Weimer, M. G. (1987). Translating evaluation results into teaching improvements. *AAHE Bulletin, (1)*4, 8–11.

CHAPTER 34

Student Evaluation of Teaching

Jill M. Hayes

INTRODUCTION

The shortage of professionals in the healthcare industry continues, contributed to by increased career options for women, advances in science and technology, and changes in the role of professional staff, particularly that of the registered nurse (Poorman, Mastorovich, & Webb, 2008). A consequence of this phenomenon is increased pressure on the academic environment to expand their enrollments in professional programs.

Innovative efforts are underway to recruit the most eligible students into professional educational programs and to design programs to meet the unique needs of the current student population. Curricula are planned to include flexible scheduling to accommodate the nontraditional student and students may enroll in part- or full-time study. Many professional educational programs are accountable to external agencies for funding and/or for approval of the program through formalized accreditation standards. Although accreditation is voluntary (Gard, Flannigan, & Cluskey, 2004; Grumet, 2002), most professional programs seek accreditation in response to the public sector's demands for demonstrated accountability, requirement of federal funding agencies, and to provide their graduates with opportunities for educational mobility into higher degree programs.

Program evaluation, discussed in depth in Chapter 32, requires comprehensive assessment of every aspect of the program. A significant component of this assessment is the evaluation of teaching effectiveness from the direct consumer of teaching: the professional student.

Student evaluation of teaching effectiveness has long been recognized as valid and reliable (Miller, 1988; Raingruber & Bowles, 2000) and considered a significant input into the quality of faculty performance and overall program quality. Education in the health professions is inherently multidimensional, and thus feedback on the effectiveness of teaching/learning strategies must be sought from all arenas where educational experiences occur: the classroom, the simulation laboratory, supervised clinical settings, and precepted experiences (Raingruber & Bowles, 2000).

BACKGROUND

Historically, research in education has focused on teaching strategies to enhance student and faculty success in their respective roles. In addition, numerous attempts have been made to evaluate teaching effectiveness to promote the development of expert faculty, meet the accountability requirements for funding sources, and to satisfy consumer demands for quality educational experiences.

Prior to further discussion of evaluation, definitions of terms commonly employed in such a discussion will be helpful. Evaluation is viewed as "a means of appraising data or placing a value on data gathered through one or more measurements" (Bourke & Ihrke, 2005). Evaluation also is utilized to render a judgment relative to a process or product, identifying the strengths and weaknesses of the features or dimensions of the product. Formative evaluation takes place during the activity, focusing on the progress being made toward achieving the stated objectives or outcomes of the activity. Summative evaluation refers to data collected following completion of the activity and focuses on the extent to which the objectives or outcomes have been met.

According to Miller (1988), efforts to evaluate faculty effectiveness have been primarily summative in nature, directed toward satisfying funding agency requirements and facilitating faculty attainment of tenure and promotion. Formative evaluation, when it occurs, is intended to assist the faculty to grow and develop in their roles. Outcomes measured through student evaluation to meet these goals strive to identify the amount of learning that occurs, the resultant ability of students to integrate and apply knowledge gained, and a cost benefit analysis of the program. Student ratings are considered highly reliable, highly correlated with other types of observational evaluation, and positively correlated with student achievement.

Hoyt and Pallet (1999) consider faculty evaluation as providing data on two aspects of faculty performance: direct and indirect contributions. Indirect contributions are described as activities that contribute to the learning environment such as collegiality, curriculum development, and sharing of effective teaching strategies with colleagues. Direct contribution activities are described as those contributing to the achievement of program outcomes. The area of direct contribution is where student evaluation and/or feedback is considered an important element.

THEORETICAL FRAMEWORK

As stated previously, research in evaluation began with a focus on identification of behavioral learning objectives, the development of tools to measure learning outcomes, and then the evaluation of students to determine if the objectives had been met (summative evaluation). As the process of evaluation has evolved, more emphasis has been placed on formative evaluation and the compilation of both formative and summative data to enhance educational program effectiveness. Perhaps because nursing historically sought to identify sound frameworks by which to collect and interpret data to build on the body of professional knowledge, theoretical frameworks or models have been integrated into evaluative research activities. Although several models are useful guides to the evaluative process, the concepts of the context, input, process, and product model (CIPP) (Stufflebeam & Webster, 2005) are easily applicable when attempting to collect data useful in decision making relative to the evaluation of professional programs.

This model addresses the need to evaluate context, input, process, and product (see Table 34-1). Within this model, ***context*** refers to the target population of any teaching/learning activities; in the case of nursing education and student evaluation,

Table 34-1 CIPP Model of Evaluation

Evaluative Element	Examples
Context	Target/student population Unique needs of students
Input	Programmatic strategies Implementation of educational strategies Program design Curriculum design Teaching/learning strategies
Process	Implementation of curriculum Course design and presentation Course sequencing Clinical site selection
Product	Student outcomes Certification/licensure examination pass rate

this refers to the student population currently enrolling in these programs and the assessment of their unique needs. ***Input*** evaluates the target system's capabilities including program strategies and mechanisms to implement those strategies. In the case of student evaluation of teaching effectiveness, the overall educational program design, curricular arrangement of courses, and teaching/learning strategies are examined. ***Process*** evaluation involves the assessment of the curricular implementation: how courses are designed and implemented; course sequencing; clinical site selection, etc. ***Product*** evaluation assesses the end product: the graduates' success relative to program outcomes and pass rates on licensure examinations.

Using this model, a discussion of student evaluation demonstrates the ease of use of this model, and how it facilitates decision making relative to student feedback on programmatic quality and teaching effectiveness. Evaluation of teaching in professional education must consider the current target population (context) and assess their unique needs within the arena where the teaching/learning occurs. This includes consideration given to the type of setting and the level of student within the program structure—such aspects as acute care settings versus outpatient settings; high-acuity patients versus ambulatory; novice student versus advanced beginner. Decisions then must be made relative to what teaching/learning strategies are appropriate to the particular setting, content being presented, and the expected student learning activities (input). Process evaluation examines the teaching/learning strategies selected and the effectiveness in transmitting required knowledge. Product evaluation would examine expected educational outcomes of the learning experience, and correlate these with student success in meeting expected outcomes, course design (input), and teaching/learning strategies employed (process). Student evaluation is pertinent to all aspects of this decision making model and elements of the model are identifiable in the two instruments to be discussed later in this chapter.

IMPLEMENTATION

As stated previously, education in the health professions is viewed as multidimensional and is strongly influenced by the particular setting in which it occurs. Raingruber and Bowles (2000) proposed that student evaluation feedback must be sought in all four major areas in which the educational experiences occur: supervised clinical settings, simulation laboratory settings, preceptor-led experiences, and didactic/classroom settings. The evaluation of faculty should be guided by a need for feedback on faculty performance, opportunities for student input into the curriculum, information for personnel decisions, and a focus on educational research. In addition, evaluation is considered to be significant for its impact on faculty and student satisfaction, faculty promotion and tenure decisions, and the overall quality of instruction provided. These authors also acknowledge the significant reliability and validity of student evaluative data.

In an effort to enhance the evaluative process, and its meaningfulness in terms of program quality and faculty and student success, recent educational research has focused on identifying the characteristics of effective teachers and the perceptions of students related to what constitutes effective teaching. According to Raingruber and Bowles (2000), adequate measures of faculty performance must address the following: clinical competency, continuing education activities, national certifications, participation in curriculum development, research/scholarship activities, community service, and self and peer evaluation. Most research supports the need for student evaluation as a valuable supplement to evaluation of overall faculty performance and as essential to program success. To this end, the authors advocate for the development of evaluative instruments that address the diverse settings in which teaching occurs, and attempt to capture or match the essential skills required for effective instruction in the four major settings in which professional education occurs. Individual factors identified as important to assess are: method of instruction, course design, course objectives, mode of delivery, feedback mechanisms, and clinical competencies. Through their research, characteristics of effective teaching were identified (see Table 34-2). Overwhelmingly, in all settings, the significance of faculty attitude toward students is essential to student learning. Within the context of attitude, faculty enthusiasm, the ability to establish strong positive interpersonal relationships with students, staff, and patients; and the ability to create an atmosphere of mutual respect were viewed as characteristic of effective teaching.

Tang, Chou, and Chiang (2005) recognized the contribution to student success of faculty attitude toward students. Teachers receiving low scores on interpersonal relationships and personal characteristics received significantly lower scores on teaching effectiveness, in spite of relatively positive scores on professional competency. A need for a feeling of mutual respect and concern for students' unique needs contributes significantly to student success. Bietz and Wieland (2005) support this premise, advocating for behavior supportive of student learning needs as essential to student perceptions of teaching effectiveness.

More recently, Clark (2008) discusses the impact of "uncivil" behavior on student success. According to this author, civility is "treating others with dignity and respect and involves time, presence, and an intention to seek common ground. Academic incivility is defined as rude, discourteous speech or behavior that disrupts the teaching-learning environment" (p. 458). This author proposes that academic civility is possible during lively debates within the teaching/learning environment, while maintaining an atmosphere of mutual respect and safety. Students experiencing uncivil behavior from faculty report feeling traumatized, powerless, helpless, and angry, which in turn resulted in less than favorable learning experiences and diminished learning. Poorman et al. (2008) report on a study examining how

Table 34-2 Characteristics of Effective Teaching

Raingruber & Bowles, 2000	Faculty attitude toward students Faculty enthusiasm Interpersonal skills Ability to demonstrate mutual respect
Tang, Chou, & Chiang, 2005	Faculty attitude Interpersonal skills Concern for students Demonstration of mutual respect
Bietz & Wieland, 2005	Supportive of student learning needs
Poorman, Mastorovich, & Webb, 2008	Ability to "attend" to students Attempt to understand students' unique needs Instill "hopeful attitude" in student Provide clear expectations for student outcomes
Clark, 2008	Demonstrate civil behavior in teaching/learning settings Promote civil behavior in teaching/learning settings

faculty most commonly assist or hinder students at risk. This phenomenological study identified "attending" as a common mechanism utilized by faculty who were seen as assisting students at risk and therefore effective teachers. This behavior was conceptualized as faculty being present to students, spending time with them, paying attention to them, and listening to them to gain an understanding of how they were struggling and which strategies would be helpful to enhance their learning experience. These behaviors created a hopeful attitude for the student whereby they would be more inclined to ask for assistance, which resulted in a "turning point" for the student and enhanced success. Faculty demonstrating presence with the student also conveyed their expectations to students more clearly, contributing to enhanced success.

Within the process of programmatic assessment, an important element is the teaching/learning environment created by the faculty and administration. This includes physical facilities, instructional resources, faculty, and the teaching/learning environment. Schaefer and Zygmont (2003) analyzed types of learning environments created in nursing education and categorized them as either student centered or teacher centered. Results of quantitative analysis of the findings demonstrated a predominance of teacher-centered environments, which in turn impacts students' perceptions of teacher effectiveness. However, qualitative data analysis indicated a desire on the part of faculty to create student-centered learning environments but an inability to achieve this, arising most often from a tendency on the part of faculty "to teach the way they were taught." Student-centered environments are viewed as promoting critical and reflective thinking, creativity, and a foundation of trust, as well as higher student and faculty satisfaction and more active engagement of the student. The authors advocate a move to student-centered environments by supporting faculty in this endeavor to better meet the needs of the current student population. Student-centered environments have been shown to be better suited to the student of today and the demands of the current healthcare environment for graduates with the ability to think critically and creatively within their work environment.

Nelson (2007) studied the use of distance education/online learning within a nursing education program, but the findings are applicable to most professional programs. This author posits that support services for both students and faculty are essential to the successful learning within this teaching/learning format. Absence of, or inadequate, support services lead to diminished learning, reduced satisfaction, and increased attrition. Student-centered environments where all support services available to on-campus students are also provided to the distant students promote greater recruitment of students, more program satisfaction among both faculty and students, higher rates of program completion, and more actively engaged alumnae.

According to Tanner (2005), nursing education and practice would greatly benefit from students who anticipate positive clinical learning experiences, practice for the "love of it" for knowledge sake, and not out of fear of the consequences for not preparing, and for learning experiences that are positive and beneficial. Characteristics of effective teaching are described as the ability to strengthen links between theory and practice, provide information on a continuum of simple to complex, present information as an inductive process, and creating trusting relationships inclusive of appropriate constructive feedback in a timely and caring approach.

Poorman et al., (2008), when discussing the concept of "attending," posit that this behavior is essential to creating a supportive environment for student learning and ensuring positive learning experiences. Faculty express this behavior in teaching/learning encounters through paying attention (attending) to student needs and with efforts to listen, observe, and understand the students' experiences. Research revealed two themes associated with the concept of attending. Attending as understanding and attending as expecting. Attending as understanding is expressed when faculty listen and observe students' behavior to identify why and attempt to understand how they are struggling in a particular learning encounter. Attending as expecting is conceptualized as faculty behavior that ensures that expectations are clearly conveyed in two ways—faculty to student and student to faculty. To exhibit this behavior, faculty should clearly state their expectations for student behavior and also ask students their expectations of the faculty. Both of these attending behaviors lead to a greater understanding of student learning needs and learning experiences on the part of the faculty. In turn, faculty are better able to craft teaching/learning encounters to enhance student learning and exhibit behavior viewed as supportive by the student.

Although student evaluation of teaching effectiveness is viewed as highly reliable and the most common mechanism used, there remains a recognized need to enhance the process of faculty evaluation with meaningful measures (Raingruber & Bowles, 2000). In the academic environment, faculty performance is increasingly being evaluated for reasons other than the measure of student satisfaction. These measures are being used, as discussed previously, to respond to funding agency requirements, consumer demand, and faculty reward systems. As the use of these data increases, additional measures that are objective and provide accurate information must be developed and employed. In addition, supplemental measures such as self evaluation, peer evaluation, and administrative evaluation are being explored.

Bietz and Wieland (2005) present two clinical evaluation instruments with established validity and reliability, and advocate their use in obtaining feedback on students' perceptions of teaching effectiveness in clinical settings. The Nursing Clinical Teaching Effectiveness Inventory (NCTEI) is a 48-item Likert-scale instrument that is used to determine students' perceptions of effective clinical teaching behaviors (Knox & Mogan, 1985; Mogan & Warbinek, 1994). The five specific areas of clinical teaching addressed in the instrument are teaching ability, interpersonal relationships, personality traits, nursing competency, and evaluation. Higher scores on the instrument are indicative of a higher level of teaching ability. Applying the CIPP model to this instrument, it is easy to see that teaching ability corresponds to process as do interpersonal relationships and personality traits, nursing competency corresponds to input, and evaluation corresponds to product. A second tool discussed by Bietz and Wieland (2005) as useful in assessing teaching effectiveness in nursing education is the effective clinical teaching behaviors (ECTB) tool (Zimmerman & Westfall, 1988). This instrument is a 43-item Likert-scale tool with established reliability and validity. Similar behaviors are identified in this instrument as in the NCTEI and higher scores are indicative of more frequently observed effective teaching behaviors.

Other tools exist for use in the evaluation of faculty performance in all settings, many of which are developed by professional programs in response to the demand of accrediting agencies for outcome data and/or the need to meet individual institutional requirements for faculty evaluation. These tools often are developed as required, and efforts to establish validity and reliability are time consuming and the result tenuous at best. Research in health profession education should emphasize the development of accurate, valid, and reliable tools to collect data on teacher effectiveness to meet accrediting requirements, consumer demand for a quality product, and the demand of healthcare agencies for competent providers.

CHALLENGES

Challenges to valid and reliable evaluation of teaching effectiveness exist within the instrument in use, the student population enrolling in health profession educational programs, and the analysis of data collected. Overall challenges to effective evaluation are identified as lack of training for effective self, peer, and administrative evaluation; demand for a time commitment for both peer and administrative evaluation; a need for multiple observational experiences for adequate evaluative feedback; and validity and reliability of tools specific to teaching activities in all major arenas where educational experiences occur (Raingruber & Bowles, 2000).

As stated, valid and reliable instruments are time consuming to develop and often characterized as setting specific—clinical teaching, classroom teaching, seminar teaching. Poorly constructed and nonstandardized evaluative tools, associated with an inability to account for extraneous factors such as class size, all lead to inadequate reliability and validity of the instruments currently in use. Research focused on instrument development, although incorporated into advanced degree programs for educators, is lacking but clearly needed to provide for accurate meaningful faculty evaluation.

Current professional education literature is rife with discussions related to the characteristics of the student of today, and their impact on healthcare related education. The nursing students encountered today differ significantly from the nursing students of the late 20th century. According to the American Association of Colleges of Nursing (AACN), (2003), the average student enrolling in nursing education today possesses prior degrees, is more mature and older chronologically, has more pressure from personal responsibilities and accountabilities, is embarking on a second career, and is more assertive. The same may be found to be true today. Bietz and Wieland (2005) posit the idea that, considering the characteristics of the current student, educators are compelled to develop new strategies and approaches to the presentation of content to meet these students' unique learning needs. In addition, the settings and/or modes of delivery of content, such as through distance learning technology, require that supportive services be provided in all educational settings (Nelson, 2007). Student characteristics also have significant implications for the *context* of nursing education (curriculum design, settings for educational experiences, *input* (course sequencing, instructional strategies, content presented), *process* (teaching/learning activities employed in particular settings, competencies of the faculty,interpersonal relationships), and *product* (student expected outcomes, learning behavioral outcomes).

It is clear how the aforementioned characteristics of students lead to the elements of teaching effectiveness identified in recent research literature. Raingruber and Bowles (2000) identified the importance of faculty attitude; interpersonal relationship building with students, staff, and patients; and an atmosphere of mutual trust to students' perceptions of teaching effectiveness. Multiple theories of learning abound in an attempt to develop an understanding of how learning occurs and what activities are best suited to facilitating learning in a group of individuals, and adult education models provide assistance to faculty in the planning of curricula and associated teaching/learning processes to present content. Within the context of adult education, Knowles (1980) too characterizes adult learners as individuals who perform best when required to use their life experiences when learning new material, have a desire to apply new knowledge to solve real-life problems, and are motivated to learn by pragmatism and a need to solve problems. Further assumptions relative to adult learners include that they are self directed, their life experiences serve as a resource for other learning, and their readiness to learn arises from the need to perform life tasks and solve problems. Additionally, Jackson and Caffarella (1994) characterize adult learners as having preferred styles of personal learning; prefer being actively involved in their learning; have a desire to be connected to, and be supportive of, each other in the learning process; and having responsibilities and life circumstances that provide a social context within which learning occurs. When students of today are characterized as adult learners—self directed, possessing life experience, more personal responsibilities, and a higher level of potential talent for future career choices—it is easy to see the applicability of the premise that faculty attitude and an environment of mutual trust are important.

Student characteristics impact the teaching/learning environment and faculty must be prepared and willing to adjust their approach to education to meet the unique needs of these students—most often best met through student-centered learning environments (Nelson, 2007). Failure to do so will result in poor student evaluations, reduced student and faculty satisfaction, and a lower level of student and faculty success. In addition, students are viewed as poorly qualified to evaluate subject matter presented, course and curriculum design, individual commitment of faculty to teaching, institutional support of faculty, evaluative methods for student work, and methods and materials used for content delivery (Hoyt & Pallet, 1999).

The connection between the perceptions of students in programs of postsecondary education in the health professions, such as nursing, as to what constitutes effective teaching, and the characteristics of adult learners is clear. If curricula are developed without considering the need for these students to be actively engaged in their learning, and their need to be connected and supported, then students will not perceive their needs are being addressed and evaluative feedback will be less than positive (Nelson, 2007). When content is developed, the teaching/learning strategies employed to present the content should reflect consideration of the need for students to apply this new knowledge immediately to solve problems, to be supported in the learning process, and to learn in an environment that is individualized and personalized for self directed mature students who desire to be actively engaged in the learning process. Attention to these unique student needs will potentially be reflected in more positive evaluative feedback, and enhanced student and faculty satisfaction.

Challenges also exist within the processes of data analysis, and interpretation, and the use of evaluative findings. The instruments currently in use have questionable reliability because of the difficulty in accounting for the impact of class size, course level, and whether the course is a requirement of the curriculum or an elective when data is interpreted. In addition, analysis must take into consideration the setting in which the teaching occurs, the mode of delivery of content, and the teaching strategies employed. Since teaching/learning in healthcare education often occurs within a social context, additional factors of space, access to educational experiences, privacy issues, agency policies governing and constraining student activities, and staffing plans must all be considered. Few, if any, instruments exist that account for these factors, all of which have the potential to significantly impact the quality of any educational experience.

CONCLUSION

Clearly, student evaluation of teaching is an essential element of successful faculty performance and professional development, student success, and programmatic success. Much effort has been expended to develop tools to capture the essence of teaching, but much still remains to be done. Although student evaluation of teaching effectiveness is viewed as highly reliable and the most common mechanism, there remains a recognized need to enhance the process of faculty evaluation with additional measures (Raingruber & Bowles, 2000). In the academic environment, faculty performance is increasingly being evaluated for reasons other than the measure of students' satisfaction. In addition, these measures are being utilized, as discussed previously, to respond to funding agency requirements, consumer demand, and faculty reward systems. As the use of these data increases, additional measures of faculty performance must be developed and employed. Supplemental measures such as self evaluation, peer evaluation, and administrative evaluation are being explored.

Considering the characteristics of the student of the 21st century, and their stated need for concerned and caring faculty (Nelson, 2007; Norman, Buerhaus, Donelan, McCloskey, & Dittus, 2005; Poorman et al., 2008), further investigation is needed to identify characteristics of effective teaching from the students' perspective, and then match those needs to the other demands placed on faculty in higher education.

REFERENCES

American Association of Colleges of Nursing. (2003). *Faculty shortages in Baccalaureate and Graduate Nursing Programs: Scope of the problem and strategies for expanding the supply*. Washington, DC: AACN.

Bietz, J. M., & Wieland, D. (2005). Analyzing the teaching effectiveness of clinical nursing faculty of full- and part-time generic BSN, LPN-BSN, and RN-BSN nursing students. *Journal of Professional Nursing, 21*(1), 32–45.

Bourke, M. P., & Ihrke, B. A. (2005). The evaluation process: An overview. In D. M. Billings, & J. A. Halstead (Eds.), *Teaching in nursing: A guide for faculty* (2nd ed., pp. 443–464). St. Louis, MO: Elsevier Saunders.

Clark, M. C. (2008). Faculty and student assessment of and experience with incivility in nursing education. *Journal of Nursing Education, 47*(10), 458–465.

Gard, C. L., Flannigan, P. N., & Cluskey, M. (2004). Program evaluation: An ongoing systematic process. *Nursing Education Perspectives, 25*(4), 176–179.

Grumet, B. R. (2002). Demystifying accreditation. *Nursing Educational Perspectives, 23*(3), 114–117.

Hoyt, D. P., & Pallett, W. H. (1999). Appraising teaching effectiveness: Beyond student ratings. *Idea Paper No. 36.* Manhattan, KS: Idea Center, Kansas State University.

Knox, J. E., & Mogan, J. (1985) Important clinical teaching behaviors as perceived by university nursing faculty, students, and graduates. *Journal of Advanced Nursing, 10*(1), 25–30.

Knowles, M. S. (1980). The modern practice of adult education. Chicago: Follett.

Jackson, L., & Caffarella, R. S. (1994). *Experiential learning: A new approach*. San Francisco: Jossey-Bass.

Miller, A. (1988). Student assessment of teaching in higher education. *Journal of Higher Education, 17,* 3–15.

Mogan, J., & Warbinek, E. (1994) Teaching behaviors of clinical instructors: An audit instrument. *Journal of Advanced Nursing, 20*(1), 160–166.

Nelson, R. (2007). Student support services for distance education students in nursing programs. *Annual Review of Nursing Education, 5,* 181–205.

Norman, L., Buerhaus, P. I., Donelan, K., McCloskey, B., & Dittus, R. (2005). Nursing students assess nursing education. *Journal of Professional Nursing, 21*(3), 150–158.

Poorman, S. G., Mastorovich, M. L., & Webb, C. A. (2008). Teachers' stories: How faculty help and hinder students at risk. *Nursing Educational Perspectives, 29*(5), 272–277.

Raingruber, B., & Bowles, K. (2000). Developing student evaluation instruments to measure instructor effectiveness. *Nurse Educator, 25*(2), 65–69.

Schaefer, K. M., & Zygmont, D. (2003). Analyzing the teaching style of nursing faculty: Does it promote a student-centered or teacher-centered learning environment? *Nursing Educational Perspectives, 24*(5), 238–245.

Tanner, C. A. (2005). The art and science of clinical teaching. *Journal of Nursing Education, 44*(4), 151–152.

Stufflebeam, D. L., & Webster, W. J. (2005).The evaluation process: An overview. In D. M. Billings, & J. A. Halstead (Eds.), Teaching in nursing: A guide for faculty (2nd ed., pp.449-450). St. Louis MO: Elsevier Saunders

Tang, F., Chou, S., & Chiang, H. (2005). Students' perceptions of effectiveness and ineffective clinical instructors. *Journal of Nursing Education, 44*(4), 187–192.

Zimmerman, L., & Westfall, J. (1988). The development and validation of a scale measuring effective clinical teaching behaviors "Effective Teaching Clinical Behaviors" (ETCB). *Journal of Nursing Education, 27*(6), 274–277.

CHAPTER 35

The Clinical Pathway: A Tool to Evaluate Clinical Learning

Martha J. Bradshaw

INTRODUCTION

The clinical pathway is a strategy that uses specific, essential evaluation criteria in unique clinical learning settings.

DEFINITION AND PURPOSE

The clinical pathway is an abbreviated form of clinical evaluation that provides a means for the instructor to evaluate student progress using specified criteria. Clinical pathways can be used to evaluate nursing practice and clinical learning that occur in time-limited, less traditional care settings. Learning activities are directed toward the same clinical outcomes as would be expected in traditionally structured patient care settings. The emphasis is on application of nursing principles in a new setting versus gaining experience via repeated opportunities in a familiar setting. As students apply principles, they recognize the development of individual nursing judgment and decision making, and they begin to visualize themselves as professional nurses. Faculty can determine how well the student uses guided thinking in unfamiliar settings and, at the same time, provides familiar nursing interventions.

THEORETICAL FOUNDATIONS

Clinical pathways, also called critical pathways, are being used by nurses and other members of the healthcare team as a directed approach to goal-based outcomes; they are especially beneficial in case management and quality improvement (Dickerson, Sackett, Jones, & Brewer, 2001). Most nursing literature describes pathways for use in complex patient care situations, but pathways are also used for orientation of new nursing staff, quality improvement, and for student-precepted experiences (Kersbergen & Hrbosky, 1996; Kinsman & James, 2001). One of the advantages of a pathway is that it is a cost-effective means, in both time and money, by which the individual is directed to the goal(s) and progress is measured (Renholm, Leino-Kilpi, & Suominen, 2002). Pathways also enable all individuals involved to know exactly what the goals are, thus clarifying expectations and making energy expenditure more efficient (Kersbergen & Hrbosky, 1996). Nursing faculty are able to collaborate on student evaluations by examining how well the student meets outcome criteria from more than one perspective. This principle is similar to how integrated care pathways are used in interdisciplinary clinical situations in that student progress and achievement of outcomes is the focus (Atwal & Caldwell, 2002).

CONDITIONS

In selected situations, student clinical learning activities are one-time experiences and may deviate from the more structured patient care experiences. In addition, many clinical experiences are short term because of decreases in hospitalization length and emphasis on wellness programs. Examples of these clinical experiences are community health fairs, outpatient surgery, and pediatric health screenings in daycare settings. Whereas these unique clinical opportunities provide expanded observations and open up new areas of practice, one-time experiences do not always lend themselves to achievement of established clinical learning outcomes. If the learning outcomes are not readily identified, then the clinical instructor cannot easily evaluate clinical progress based on the experience. Therefore, instructors traditionally create one-time experiences as observation only activities, or as task-focused activities that may not represent a professional nursing approach. In doing so, many valuable learning opportunities may be lost to the students. Instructors also lose the opportunity to determine the extent to which students are able to adapt to unique settings, apply principles, and enact new roles.

Use of a clinical pathway for student experiences enables continued learning by students and maximizes the benefits of the one-time clinical opportunities. Just as the critical pathway is an abbreviated version of a patient's plan of care, the student clinical pathway is an abbreviated version of the clinical evaluation tool. A major advantage of the pathway for both the student and course faculty is that it reduces the inconsistency or inadequacy of evaluation of one-time or isolated clinical learning opportunities. Variations in expectations and evaluation lead to variations in outcomes among students (Holaday & Buckley, 2008), and the pathway is a means to correct this problem.

At the time of the clinical experience, the student uses the pathway as a guide for fulfilling selected roles and completing specific responsibilities. Simultaneously, the student is aware of the criteria by which evaluation will take place. Therefore, use of clinical time and experience is maximized. The clinical pathway makes unique clinical experiences more purposeful, thus improving student clinical learning outcomes (Kinsman, 2004). Student clinical pathways are based on the same purposes as are patient- or staff-oriented pathways: They are goal directed, designed to be efficient, and effective in terms of time and energy. The components of the clinical pathway are derived directly from the clinical evaluation tool used by faculty in student evaluation.

TYPES OF LEARNERS

Whereas the clinical pathway could be used with learners of all levels, it is best used with undergraduate students. The clinical pathway offers specific learning outcomes and can include recommended or structured activities that enable the student to meet these outcomes. Students in undergraduate clinical settings generally have more faculty supervision, which creates opportunity for direct observation and evaluation. The clinical pathway is designed for intended learning, even though students often acquire additional personal growth during the clinical experience.

The pathway also is quite suitable for students of all levels in brief clinical learning settings with a preceptor, such as a one-day event. The preceptor should not be expected to conduct an in-depth evaluation of the student, but preceptor feedback is exceedingly helpful in compiling comprehensive information on a student. Therefore, a succinct and purposeful tool can be easily completed and provide needed information. Preceptors also feel more empowered in their ability to make decisions about students and promote accountability for care (Kersbergen & Hrbosky, 1996).

RESOURCES

The basis for a clinical pathway is the learning outcomes for the course. These outcomes are based on professional competencies (Oermann & Gaberson, 2006). Evaluation tools used by all clinical instructors are directed toward course outcomes and ultimately professional standards for practice. Instructors supervising students in selected experiences identify outcomes and expected behaviors from the evaluation tool. Based on anticipated clinical learning opportunities, the instructor develops a clinical pathway that guides the student in what will be accomplished during the experience and the activities or behaviors the instructor expects to observe in each learner.

USING THE METHOD

Implementation of an education-focused clinical pathway enables the faculty to develop student learning experiences that are directly related to the outcomes for the total clinical course. Two examples demonstrate how pathways are derived from the clinical evaluation tool and how components of the tool can be applied to more than one setting. Hearing and vision screening with school-aged children can be conducted with nursing students at any level in the educational program. Such screenings have a place in a fundamentals course, a course on nursing care of children, or in a community nursing course. A more sophisticated version of the screening (to include patient referral) can be developed for nurse practitioner students.

When students are assigned to a unique, one-time clinical experience, they may have some apprehension about being responsible for patient care in a new setting. Knowing that they have only one opportunity to demonstrate competence, students benefit from the direction that a pathway provides. In fact, many students like the opportunity to test themselves in the new setting. Time and opportunity do not permit the students to meet all criteria on the standard, comprehensive course evaluation tool. To maximize the learning experience, a sample pathway (see Table 35-1) was developed based on the following items from the course clinical evaluation tool.

- Demonstrates preparation for assignment
- Performs nursing skills correctly
- Maintains professionalism
- Demonstrates professional inquiry activities

As can be seen by the example in Table 35-1, other expectations are specified under the broad clinical outcomes. The pathway expectations are derived from the clinical evaluation tool and applied to the situation, such as communications with children or use of critical thinking. The expectations also indicate specific behaviors related to the clinical activity that must be demonstrated by the student, such as ability to complete vision screening.

Additional information that leaves no room for guesswork regarding preparation and professional behaviors is provided in the pathway for the student. Also, the standard for acceptable behavior (pass) is indicated as part of the directions, so that in the event a student demonstrates unacceptable behaviors, he or she has a clear understanding of how the final evaluation was determined (see Exhibit 35-1).

In developing the pathway, the focus is on outcomes (student learning), not process (tasks or activities). Therefore, the instructor may designate specified activities or behaviors that direct the student to the outcomes; not all behaviors must be seen in order to attain the goal. Furthermore, other, unanticipated activities

Table 35-1 Course Outcomes Applied to Clinical Pathways

Learning Outcomes of Clinical Pathways

1. Demonstrates professional behaviors and inquiry activities
2. Demonstrates preparation and use of principles in screening techniques
3. Assesses behaviors of patient and family/support in ambulatory surgery and provides appropriate nursing interventions
4. Provides nursing interventions for a patient in the ambulatory surgery/operative unit

Clinical Learning Outcomes of Course

1. Demonstrates professional behavior and accountability
2. Demonstrates preparedness for assignment
3. Provides a safe environment
4. Complies with the regulations of the school of nursing and clinical agency
5. Performs nursing skills or interventions appropriate to the patient's health
6. Demonstrates safe administration of medications
7. Establishes rapport and demonstrates good communication skills
8. Demonstrates collaboration with other care disciplines
9. Demonstrates patient and family teaching
10. Demonstrates appropriate documentation
11. Maintains confidentiality and respect for others
12. Completes assignments on time
13. Seeks assistance/guidance appropriately
14. Adapts to changing or stressful situations
15. Uses critical thinking skills
16. Demonstrates professional inquiry activities

related to the patient situation that enable the student to meet the outcomes may present themselves.

An evaluation sheet provides feedback to the student regarding the experience and serves as the evaluation measure and anecdotal record for the instructor. Information regarding clinical activities and evaluation is found in the clinical section of the course syllabus. In that section is the detailed information indicating that the one-time activity is a clinical day of equal importance to a day caring for a hospitalized patient. Clinical instructors use the information from the pathway when formulating a final clinical evaluation report on each student.

Exhibit 35-2 is a clinical pathway developed for use with nursing students in an ambulatory surgery unit. In addition to typical nursing activities related to an operative experience, an emphasis of this experience includes patient and caregiver interaction, alleviation of anxiety, provision of information about

EXHIBIT 35-1

Clinical Pathway: Hearing and Vision Screening

The clinical pathway identifies the specific nursing activities that will enable the student to meet the objectives for this one-time clinical experience. The student will be evaluated based on completion of items on this pathway. A student who fails this clinical pathway (i.e., fails to pass at least 7 of the 12 items on the clinical pathway) has failed the clinical day.

Objectives and Student Nursing Activities

1. Demonstrates preparation and use of principles in screening techniques:
   - Attends clinical experience promptly, appropriately attired, and with own supplies
   - Establishes a positive working relationship with patient(s)
   - Initiates and completes screening in timely manner
   - Correctly follows sequence of steps in screening assessment(s)
   - Shows familiarity with equipment, screening criteria, and documentation
   - Individualizes assessments as needed based on unique attributes of each patient
2. Demonstrates professional behaviors and inquiry activities:
   - Uses principles of therapeutic and professional communications when interacting with patient(s)
   - Shows appropriate level of independence and self direction
   - Demonstrates critical thinking and problem-solving skills regarding screenings or patient interactions
   - Documents or reports results of screening exam
   - Seeks guidance or advice from instructor as needed
   - Discusses screening results and/or patient responses with instructor and fellow students

Student Preparation

- Complete check-off on hearing and vision screening equipment in the skills lab. If needed, practice again before clinical experience.
- You are permitted to bring your H&V booklet or some guidelines written on a card. This does not take the place of preparation and familiarity with the procedure. If you make too many references to the guidelines, your instructor will consider you unprepared. Bring these pathway sheets to give to your instructor.

EXHIBIT 35-2

Clinical Pathway: Ambulatory Surgery Experience

For this one-time clinical experience, the clinical pathway identifies the specific nursing care activities on which the student will be evaluated. Items on this pathway will enable the student to meet the objectives for the ambulatory surgery experience for NUR (listed below). A student who fails the ambulatory surgery experience (i.e., receives a failing evaluation on two of the three sections of the clinical pathway) has failed a clinical day.

Objectives and Student Nursing Activities

1. Assesses behaviors of patient and family/support in ambulatory surgery and provides appropriate nursing interventions:
   - Introduces self to patient and family/support person; establishes a working relationship
   - Identifies behaviors related to hospitalization and surgery; discusses conclusions regarding behaviors with instructor, giving specific examples
   - Indicates how patient behaviors influence preoperative, surgical, and postoperative periods
   - Gives specific examples of family/support coping abilities
   - Makes conclusions and interventions that are correctly based on patient's developmental level
2. Provides nursing interventions for a patient in the ambulatory surgery/operative unit:
   - Demonstrates preparedness regarding knowledge of surgical procedure; discusses procedure and pertinent information with instructor
   - Reviews patient's health history, lab, and other data as available on unit
   - Teams with staff RN to provide care for patient
   - Conducts assessments, including vital signs, in a timely manner, using correct technique
   - Recognizes comfort and safety needs, specific for operative patients
   - Provides interventions promptly
   - Administers medications, based on the "five rights" and according to school of nursing guidelines
   - Practices professional therapeutic communication skills in the areas of teaching, reassurance, and collaboration
3. Demonstrates professional behaviors and inquiry activities:
   - Selects appropriate priorities for patient and family/support
   - Conducts self in dignified, professional manner, including conversation and general appearance
   - Shows organization and good use of time
   - Demonstrates initiative to be involved in patient care and to further own learning
   - Evaluates outcomes of patient's surgical experience; discusses patient responses and readiness for discharge/transfer with instructor

Ambulatory Surgery Experience Clinical Pathway: Evaluation

(Note: The student must receive a passing evaluation for at least two of the objectives in order to receive a passing grade for this clinical day.)

1. Assess behaviors of patient and family/support in ambulatory surgery and provide appropriate nursing interventions.

   Pass/Fail Comments:

2. Provide nursing interventions for a patient in the ambulatory surgery/operative unit.

   Pass/Fail Comments:

3. Demonstrate professional behaviors and inquiry activities.

   Pass/Fail Comments:

____________________________ __________
Instructor Date

the procedure, and presentation of postoperative teaching prior to discharge. The ambulatory surgery pathway also is constructed to indicate to the students what the expectations are for patient care. Prior to use of the pathway, students may be unsure of what they are permitted to do, and thus miss many learning opportunities.

Because the ambulatory surgery pathway is broader in scope, it uses both basic care items (same as in Table 35-1) and specific items.

- Provides a safe environment
- Establishes good rapport and maintains good communication
- Recognizes skill and knowledge limitations and seeks assistance appropriately
- Demonstrates safe administration of medications
- Uses critical thinking in decision making and applying various problem solving methods

For this clinical experience, the student may be evaluated either by a different instructor or by a staff preceptor. Evaluation information is shared with the clinical instructor, added to other evaluation data, and used as part of the final course evaluation. One benefit of using the pathway in total course evaluation is that it provides the instructor with a glimpse at behavior patterns in a student, regardless of setting. In the event that the pathway does not provide beneficial evaluative feedback, the faculty must determine if the clinical experience and learning opportunities cannot be measured the way the pathway was constructed, or if the course evaluation tool needs to be revised to better reflect student learning outcomes (Kinsman, 2004).

POTENTIAL PROBLEMS

Any difficulties encountered in using the clinical pathway are related to the nature of this evaluation measure. It is intended to evaluate the student in a one-time experience, based on selected criteria.

Potential problems with this method include:

- Inability of the instructor to observe and evaluate all behaviors. The type of clinical activity and spontaneous events govern the student's participation in care and types of care provided.
- The new environment may have a negative effect on the students' behavior. Some students adapt more quickly than others to working in new settings. This is especially true of more experienced students and field-independent students who are able to sort out and select relevant information about the clinical setting. Students who are less able to adapt are therefore hampered in their performance and may appear to be weak in clinical judgment or nursing skills.
- It is easy to rubber stamp evaluation remarks. For the instructor who has 40 or 50 students progressing through the one-time experience, the evaluation remarks become repetitive and tiresome. Instructors must endeavor to make individual comments that are an accurate description of the student. Remarks that reflect abilities in other clinical settings will validate the student's total clinical evaluation.
- To some instructors, the clinical pathway may be seen as too behavioral. In some cases, this is the intent of the pathway: to evaluate psychomotor skills. An immunization pathway is an example of psychomotor evaluation. The clinical pathway can be constructed in such a way to provide opportunities for the student to use critical thinking and problem-solving abilities in ways that the instructor can readily observe and evaluate. An example is priority setting and decision making related to immediate patient care needs. This is an advantage of the pathway in that it facilitates evaluation in spontaneous situations.

CONCLUSION

Clinical pathways are a means by which an instructor can objectively and effectively evaluate student learning and progress toward clinical outcomes. An advantage to use of pathways in one-time experiences is that the pathway serves as a criterion-based frame of reference for both the student and the instructor because the criteria are the same as for other clinical experiences in that course. The faculty member thus has an objective measure of student learning and performance, and the student always knows the measure on which he or she will be evaluated.

Clinical pathways are limited to brief experiences and are not designed to show professional growth and progress in learning over time. However, a pathway could be designed to appraise critical thinking and professional behaviors associated with spontaneous incidents, such as a problem patient. Nurse educators can use pathways as a creative means to address student performance in a variety of situations.

REFERENCES

Atwal, A., & Caldwell, K. (2002). Do multidisciplinary integrated care pathways improve interprofessional collaboration? *Scandinavian Journal of Caring Sciences, 16,* 360–367.

Dickerson, S. S., Sackett, K., Jones, J. M., & Brewer, C. (2001). Guidelines for evaluating tools for clinical decision making. *Nurse Educator, 26,* 215–220.

Holaday, S. D., & Buckley, K. M. (2008). A standardized clinical evaluation tool-kit: Improving nursing education and practice. *Annual Review of Nursing Education, 6,* 123–149.

Kersbergen, A. L., & Hrbosky, P. E. (1996). Use of clinical map guides in precepted clinical experiences. *Nurse Educator, 21*(6), 19–22.

Kinsman, L. (2004). Clinical pathway compliance and quality improvement. *Nursing Standard, 18,* 33–35.

Kinsman, L., & James, E. L. (2001). Evidence-based practice needs evidence-based implementation. *Lippincott's Case Management, 5,* 208–219.

Oermann, M. H., & Gaberson, K. (2006). *Evaluation and testing in nursing education* (2nd ed.). New York: Springer.

Renholm, M., Leino-Kilpi, H., & Suominen, T. (2002). Critical pathways: A systematic review. *The Journal of Nursing Administration, 32,* 196–202.

CHAPTER 36

Evaluation of Teaching Resources

Jill M. Hayes

INTRODUCTION

Professional education programs are confronted with the need to prepare graduates to meet the needs of diverse patient populations, while contending with an ever worsening availability of learning environments (Hedger, 2008). Within the context of current educational environments, geography and economics are presenting challenges to students seeking to pursue careers in health care, including the accessibility of professional programs, instructional methods to meet their learning needs, and resources to enable them to successfully complete their program of study. Professional programs are also challenged to find faculty with the expertise required to prepare healthcare practitioners of the future.

In addition, the shortage of professional staff in healthcare organizations in turn frequently leads to an inability of these organizations to accommodate students for clinical educational experiences, thus reducing enrollment capacity in the educational programs. According to Bogdanowicz (2006), the educator shortage in many professional programs is approaching crisis proportions and is resulting in concern for the quality of care provided. The process is cyclical and clearly healthcare arenas are being pressured to address this critical issue. Within the context of this crisis is a growing acknowledgment of the need for all parties involved to carefully evaluate resources utilized by professional programs.

BACKGROUND

The evolution of professional education has a clear and often articulated history. In the past, healthcare education occurred within healthcare settings and was directed by faculty with a dual role, that of providing patient care/service to the organization while concurrently educating new practitioners. The commitment of educational resources included some classroom space, simulation laboratory space, within the school and the patient care environment.

As professional programs strive to meet the needs of their current students and the critical shortages in the healthcare environment, faculty are compelled to learn and use innovative instructional resources in the classroom and simulation laboratory for the presentation of content (Finke, 2005; Landeen & Jeffries, 2008). In addition, faculty are actively engaged in the clinical practice component of the students' educational experiences and thus play a lesser role in the service aspect of the healthcare environment. Healthcare organizations are asked to provide sites for clinical experiences as an adjunct to the educational program.

More recent changes in higher education have contributed to a demand for new teaching/learning strategies to be incorporated into professional programs (Nelson, 2007). The student population continues to evolve as more people with a diversity of educational and work backgrounds seek educational opportunities at a later age. In addition, frequently education is no longer their only "job" (Poorman, Mastorovich, & Webb, 2008). This new student population and their associated learning needs are occuring concurrently with a need for faculty to constantly revise, adjust, and update the strategies used to present content in all four areas where professional education occurs: simulation laboratory settings, clinical settings, classroom settings, and preceptor led educational experiences (Raingruber & Bowles, 2000). Lecture is no longer the only acceptable format for the presentation of content. Faculty are increasingly required to incorporate technology into their course presentations to include sophisticated simulations and in many cases, online distance educational formats (Landeen & Jeffries, 2008; Nelson, 2007). These new modes of content delivery necessitate the development of support services for both students and faculty and ongoing evaluation of these services to ensure they meet the instructional needs of students and facilitate the role of faculty in the educational process (Nelson, 2007). In addition, faculty and administration are increasingly exploring innovative simulation activities that provide students with valuable learning experiences prior to their engagement in clinical practice environments, or as a replacement for these learning experiences. According to Rothgeb (2008), simulations are increasingly being used in professional education. The various modes of content delivery and use of technology have been presented in depth throughout this book.

As the learning needs of students change, the numbers of students entering into professional education increase, and faculty strive to ensure valuable educational experiences and positive learning outcomes in programs of higher education, new and varied teaching/learning strategies will be developed and introduced in the academic settings (Landeen & Jeffries, 2008). However, a balance must be sought between the need for a variety of educational resources to support these new innovative instructional strategies, the budgetary constraints currently being imposed on academic institutions, and clinical practice settings, along with the faculty training needed to effectively employ these strategies. In addition, the effective use of new strategies must be validated through empirical research to ensure positive program outcomes.

THEORETICAL FRAMEWORK

Jeffries (2005) proposes a framework to utilize when designing, implementing, and evaluating simulation activities in professional programs and this model is well suited to the evaluation of any instructional resource. Within the context of this model, antecedent factors that are to be considered when evaluating teaching/learning resources include instructor/teacher's use of the strategy relative to their areas of expertise, faculty members' historical or traditional teaching styles, and faculty familiarity with the teaching strategy. Additionally, students participating in the educational activity should also be considered relative to their program of study, level in the program, and their ages. The educational philosophy commonly held by the institution impacts the use of instructional strategies in the classroom, learning laboratory, and clinical setting by the faculty and requires evaluation in terms of factors such as what active learning strategies are used, the type of student/faculty interactive activities that occur, and the type and format of collaborative teaching activities that are employed. Antecedent and institutional factors must be considered prior to selecting and implementing an instructional intervention as all of these factors play a significant role in the planning of effective instructional interventions to present required content. In any academic setting, following the intervention, evaluation of the value of the resources/strategies used should focus on the planned outcomes of that intervention: knowledge gained, skill performance demonstrated, learner satisfaction with the intervention, level of critical thinking demonstrated, and overall confidence of the student in the performance of the acquired skills. This evaluative data is then used to enhance future instructional interventions. In addition, evaluation of the resource(s) relevant to their value to the educational experiences of the students, feasibility of the cost involved in their purchase, and the readiness of faculty to use them, all contribute to the activity's impact on program outcome—summative evaluation. Resource evaluation, in professional programs, should focus on skill performance and faculty/learner satisfaction following participation.

IMPLEMENTATION

Resource evaluation in the current academic environment must address how best to use teaching/learning resources in the presentation of required content. This evaluation must focus on which outcomes best "fit" with the use of which resources, and what is the best method to promote faculty and student development within the context of current budgetary restraints. Resource evaluation in professional education must involve all resources used to enhance students' learning experiences. This includes faculty resources, material resources, physical plant resources, and instructional resources, along with all support services in place for both students and faculty.

Faculty evaluation, a significant program resource and therefore an integral part of resource evaluation, is commonly formalized by the program administrator, and may include processes of peer evaluation, self evaluation, classroom and clinical observations, and student evaluation. According to Miller (1988), faculty evaluation typically is summative in format—as an annual performance review completed by the program administrator and focusing on the faculty member's performance within the tripartite mission of the university, to include teaching, service, and scholarship. Formalized student evaluations are incorporated into this evaluation process along with peer and self evaluation (see Chapter 34). Dependent on the primary mission of the university—scholarship or teaching—the three elements are weighted and the faculty counseled on identified areas of strengths and weaknesses. Raingruber and Bowles (2000) propose that student evaluations be solicited in all four areas in which most professional education occurs—classroom, clinical setting, laboratory, and precepted educational experiences—and address the clinical competency, scholarship, service, and knowledge base in area(s) of expertise. Multiple observational opportunities should be offered to ensure the accuracy of the data obtained.

Although student evaluations are recognized as highly reliable and valid (Raingruber & Bowles, 2000), using the aforementioned model, the evaluation of faculty should primarily focus on teacher factors such as knowledge base in area(s) of expertise, readiness to explore and use new instructional strategies, and support available to facilitate this innovative practice. According to Jeffries (2005), faculty are critical to the successful implementation of any instructional resource. Dependent on the philosophical perspective on teaching held by the institution, department, and/or the faculty member, the educator will employ student-centered or teacher-centered activities within the learning environment. Faculty steeped in the traditional pedagogical method of structured lectures (teacher centered) will use teaching/learning strategies that support that form of instruction such as overhead technology, handouts, and PowerPoint presentations. In addition, resistance to the adoption of new technology/simulation resources into instructional activities may well occur. This, in turn, will impact outcomes of student learning and learner satisfaction. Faculty whose teaching/learning philosophy is characterized by a readiness to engage in student/faculty interaction in the classroom, collaborative learning, and active participation in the learning process may use technology and simulation activities to facilitate their students' educational experiences and thus impact educational outcomes. Jeffries (2007) proposes that increasing use of simulation activities in the classroom and the learning laboratory will somewhat alleviate the impact of the current faculty shortage, along with improving learning outcomes. Creative use of technology to simulate "real clinical experiential learning" will reduce the dependency of professional educational programs on actual clinical experiences while continuing to provide valuable learning experiences for their students.

The current nursing faculty shortage is contributed to by the aging of faculty and diminishing enrollment in graduate professional education programs. Once faculty with the requisite academic credentials are hired, educational institutions must be willing to support additional resources to train the new educators in technology and innovative teaching/learning strategies appropriate to meet their students' needs (Blood-Siegfried et al., 2008; Nelson, 2007). The multifaceted role of educators necessitates training in the design of curriculum, programmatic evaluation, and skills in developing and implementing strategies to meet program outcomes and often accreditation requirements. Collaborative innovations between the service and academic environments will assist in the alleviation of the impact of current staff/faculty shortages. However, professional programs must also pursue creative and innovative methods of developing competent practitioners and use simulation activities to contribute meaningful learning experiences to the curriculum (Rothgeb, 2008). Feedback from the outcome evaluation must be recognized as valuable data to influence teacher/student factors and educational practices. Teacher evaluation should include this feedback data to assist in the development of faculty expertise and the "best educational practices" (Blood-Siegfried et al., 2008).

When evaluating faculty performance relative to resources used, it is imperative to remember that a faculty member's use of innovative teaching resources must be supported and facilitated by the institution (Childs & Sepples, 2006; Nelson, 2007). This support may range from the provision of financial resources to purchase needed equipment, to the provision of adequate facilities to house and use the resources, to providing faculty with the opportunity to develop new skills and tangible evidence of administrative support for the use of such resources.

Physical plant resources must be considered as critical elements of successful professional education—classroom space, simulation laboratory space, and clinical sites. In this time of budgetary constraints, classroom space is often inadequate. Large classrooms necessitate the use of varying teaching/learning strategies. For example, active engagement of students with group work is difficult when 50 students are crowded into a classroom designed to accommodate 30 to 40 students. In addition, the incorporation of technology as an instructional strategy requires the equipment be available and user-friendly for both faculty and students. This requires substantial financial commitment on the part of the institution to provide the needed and updated equipment, and support of the faculty in the design, setup, and use of the equipment. These factors, all considered as a part of educational best practices, must be considered when evaluating the use, and value of, instructional resources.

CHALLENGES

The procurement of adequate and valuable sites for clinical learning in professional education continues to be a critical factor (Jeffries, 2007). Questions center on: what competencies are needed for effective teaching in the clinical setting; how best to ensure faculty possess needed competencies; how to supplement faculty deficiencies in either numbers or clinical expertise to maximize student experiences to then meet the needs of the healthcare industry; how to ensure adequate numbers of qualified clinical faculty; and how to ensure adequate physical facilities for a diversity of clinical learning experiences. Once again, the theoretical model proposed by Jeffries (2005) may be used to evaluate clinical resources. The philosophy and mission of the program impacts the educational practices used to promote positive program outcomes. According to Jeffries (2005), sound educational practices, based on pedagogical principles, are crucial to good teaching, student learning, and learner satisfaction. Active learning, timely feedback, and collaborative learning are viewed as critical to successfully achieving positive student learning outcomes.

Rothgeb (2008) defines simulation as "the reproduction of essential features for the purpose of study or training; it is the imitation of something or an enactment of an experience" and "the process of illustrating an action" (Anderson, 2001, p. 489). As simulation activities along with appropriate teaching/learning resources are used more frequently to supplement or replace some clinical experiences, academic programs must evaluate their use to ensure the learning experiences of the students, that these activities not only meet their needs, but also the mandates of administration and the accreditation agencies. In nursing, for example, questions must be asked to determine what can and cannot be simulated, what aspects of simulation are important, when are live actors (standardized patients) appropriate, and how much actual patient experience can be replaced. With ever increasing enrollments in professional education, an ongoing shortage of staff in the healthcare arenas and faculty in academia, coupled with ongoing budgetary constraints, professional programs will continue to struggle with finding adequate clinical sites to provide meaningful education, and simulation will be increasingly viewed as an essential component of the educational experience.

Medley and Horne (2005) advocate for increased use of technological simulation activities in undergraduate professional education, citing improved skill acquisition, enhanced decision making and critical thinking, and team building. Challenges identified related to the implementation and use of technology that arise from faculty underestimation of their potential to enhance nursing education and their underuse by faculty. Clinical practice in nursing education programs, and other professional education programs, although viewed as critical to professional development, is associated with increasing challenges arising from inadequate faculty resources, increased numbers of students, decreased lengths of stay for patients in the hospital, high patient acuity in hospital settings, and the current shortage of practitioners in healthcare delivery settings. All these factors create a need for students who are highly competent in clinical practice and yet also contribute to increasing difficulties in the preparation of such a graduate. Complex, high-tech simulation learning resources are viewed as a highly valued supplement to the education of competent practitioners (Jeffries, 2007).

Relative to augmenting resources, Mathews (2003) proposes the establishment of creative collaborative relationships between academia and the service industry to enhance student learning experiences. Establishing partnerships that provide adjunct/joint faculty appointments enhance the availability of faculty and opportunities for the development of educators in the service sector. The faculty shortage is attributed, in part, to salary disparity between academia and the service industry, limited access to scholarships to fund advanced education for staff, inadequate access to information related to advanced degree programs, and the aging of the current faculty workforce. Joint appointments provide opportunities for creative job design for staff and an increase in the numbers of qualified educators to participate in student learning experiences. In addition, partnerships between academia and service promote careers in professional education, recognition of clinical expertise, and aid in the retention of educators in the service industry. As clinicians are encouraged to contribute their expertise to the students' educational experiences through these collaborative partnerships, evaluation data on learner satisfaction, critical thinking, knowledge and skill acquisition, and self confidence in their role will contribute significantly to the selection and utilization of innovative learning resources and academic institutions' willingness to provide and support these resources. Although the landscape of professional education has changed, faculty and program administration must continue to strive to maintain program integrity through ongoing evaluation of new instructional strategies, and identification of additional resources to support these strategies.

As technology becomes more evident in today's society, students in professional disciplines enter educational programs as computer savvy consumers. Feedback on the introduction of technology-based instructional strategies bring mixed results. According to Ndiwane (2005), instructional technology tools such as individual devices to store and communicate data enhance student learning and reduce student dependence on faculty presence in the clinical setting. Jang, Hwang, Park, Kim, and Kim (2005) advocate for the use of Web-based instruction to enhance the flexibility of educational programming; reduce faculty travel time and cost; and enhance student learning experiences through opportunities for self analysis, critical reflection, and sharing information with peers. However, Nelson (2007) advocates for strong support services for both faculty and students to ensure successful use of online learning formats, improved student and faculty satisfaction and enhanced learning. Although research on Web-based instruction and the use of other instructional technology produces mixed results, many efforts have demonstrated significant improvements in learner motivation, course satisfaction, and stimulation of learning. Blood-Siegfried et al. (2008) have developed a rubric to evaluate the quality of Web-based instruction and the need for faculty support to enhance the quality of instruction. Through the use of this rubric faculty may identify best practices in distance education and evaluate the delivery of online course content.

CONCLUSION

Students today are characterized as adult learners and virtual learners (Ostrow & DiMaria-Ghalili, 2005). Both types are described as adaptable, self directed, and possessing a strong desire for immediate application of knowledge. Based on principles of adult learning theory, these students require a learning environment that enables them to incorporate life experiences into their education, allows them to be actively engaged in the learning process, and immediately apply new knowledge to problem solving—be it in the clinical environment or any other environment which enhances their education (Knowles, 1980). To meet the needs of these students, technology-based instruction that is reliable, ensures complete and organized information, includes a detailed orientation to the instructional tools, and provides prompt feedback to the student results in positive learning outcomes (Ostrow & DiMaria-Ghalili, 2005). According to Hedger (2008), the faculty role vis a vis the technology is characterized by an ability to promote and develop a sense of community, encourage student engagement in the learning process, empower students to develop and maintain a learning community, and enlist student cooperation and active learning. However, this author has also identified challenges faculty face as they convert their traditional courses to an online format and/or develop new course offerings. These challenges include course design/redesign, student learning needs, and the availability of technical support for both students and faculty all viewed as crucial to successful implementation. The availability of these support services for both faculty and students are viewed as essential to ensure positive learning experiences, improved student and faculty satisfaction, and reduced attrition from professional programs (Nelson, 2007).

Educational practices conducive to positive learning outcomes are characterized as those that ensure a creative interactive learning environment, time devoted to the specific task, prompt feedback, active learning, and are viewed as contributing significantly to positive educational outcomes. Feedback data from formative and summative evaluation must be readily accessible and relevant to allow educators to make adjustments in instructional strategies and other services provided to students and faculty alike.

REFERENCES

Anderson, D. M. (2001). *Mosby's medical, nursing, & allied health dictionary* (6th ed.). St. Louis, MO: Mosby.

Blood-Siegfried, J. E., Short, N. M., Rapp, C. G., Hill, E., Talbert, S., Skinner, J., et al. (2008). A rubric for improving the quality of online courses. *International Journal of Nursing Education Scholarship, 5*(1), 1–13.

Bogdanowicz, H. (2006). Dental community faces shortage of educators as numbers steadily decline. Retrieved December 7, 2009, from http://www.aae.org/pressroom/releases/newseducators.htm

Childs, J. C., & Sepples, S. (2006). Clinical teaching by simulation: Lessons learning from a complex patient care scenario. *Nursing Education Perspectives, 27*, 154–158.

Finke, L. M. (2005). Teaching in nursing: The faculty role. In D. M. Billings, & J. A. Halstead (Eds.), *Teaching in nursing: A guide for faculty* (2nd ed., pp. 443–464). St. Louis, MO: Elsevier Saunders.

Hedger, A. (2008). Web-based education in graduate nursing programs. *Clinical Scholars Review, 1*(2), 121–124.

Jang, K. S., Hwang, S. Y., Park, S. J., Kim, Y. M., & Kim, M. J. (2005). Effects of a web-based teaching method on undergraduate nursing students' learning of electrocardiography. *Journal of Nursing Education, 44*(1), 35–39.

Jeffries, P. R. (2005). A framework for designing, implementing, and evaluating simulations used as teaching strategies in nursing. *Journal of Nursing Education Perspectives, 26*(2), 96–103.

Jeffries, P. R. (2007). Clinical simulations in nursing education: Valuing and adopting an experiential clinical model. *Create the future, 4*(7). Retrieved August 24, 2008, from http://www.nursingsociety.org/Publications/Newsletter/Documents/CTF_V4_7.pdf

Knowles, M. S. (1980). *The modern practice of adult education*. Chicago: Follett.

Landeen, J., & Jeffries, P. R. (2008). Simulation. *Journal of Nursing Education, 47*(11), 487–488.

Mathews, M. B. (2003). Resourcing nursing education through collaboration. *Journal of Continuing Education in Nursing, 34*(6), 251–257.

Medley, C. F., & Horne, C. (2005). Using simulation technology for undergraduate nursing education. *Journal of Nursing Education, 44*(1), 31–34.

Miller, A. (1988). Student assessment of teaching in higher education. *Journal of Higher Education, 17*, 3–15.

Nelson, R. (2007). Student support services for distance education students in nursing programs. *Annual Review of Nursing Education, 5*, 181–205.

Ndiwane, A. (2005). Teaching with the Nightingale Tracker Technology in community-based nursing education: A pilot study. *Journal of Nursing Education, 44*(1), 40–42.

Ostrow, L., & DiMaria-Ghalili, R. A. (2005). Distance education for graduate nursing: One state school's experience. *Journal of Nursing Education, 44*(1), 5–10.

Poorman, S. G., Mastorovich, M. L., & Webb, C. A. (2008). Teachers' Stories: How faculty help and hinder students at risk. *Nursing Educational Perspectives, 29*(5), 272–277.

Raingruber, B., & Bowles, K. (2000). Developing student evaluation instruments to measure instructor effectiveness. *Nurse Educator, 25*(2), 65–69.

Rothgeb, M. K. (2008). Creating a nursing simulation laboratory: A literature review. *Journal of Nursing Education, 47*(11), 489–494.

Index

Note: Page numbers followed by *t* or *f* indicate material in tables or figures, respectively.

I

P